Health, United States, 1999

With Health and Aging Chartbook

U.S. DEPARTMENT OF HEALTH AND HUMAN SERVICES
Centers for Disease Control and Prevention
National Center for Health Statistics
6525 Belcrest Road
Hyattsville, Maryland 20782-2003

September 1999
DHHS Publication number (PHS) 99-1232

U.S. Department of Health and Human Services (DHHS)

Donna E. Shalala
Secretary

Office of Public Health and Science, HHS

David Satcher, M.D., Ph.D.
Assistant Secretary for Health and Surgeon General

Centers for Disease Control and Prevention (CDC)

Jeffrey P. Koplan, M.D., M.P.H.
Director

National Center for Health Statistics, CDC

Edward J. Sondik, Ph.D.
Director

For sale by the U.S. Government Printing Office
Superintendent of Documents, Mail Stop: SSOP, Washington, DC 20402-9328
ISBN 0-16-050043-5

Health, United States, 1999 is the 23d report on the health status of the Nation submitted by the Secretary of the Department of Health and Human Services to the President and Congress of the United States in compliance with Section 308 of the Public Health Service Act. This report was compiled by the Centers for Disease Control and Prevention (CDC), National Center for Health Statistics (NCHS). The National Committee on Vital and Health Statistics served in a review capacity.

Health, United States presents national trends in health statistics. Major findings are presented in the highlights. The report includes a chartbook on health and aging and detailed tables on trends.

Health and Aging Chartbook

In each edition of *Health, United States*, a chartbook focuses on a major health topic. This year health and aging was selected as the subject of the chartbook because older people are major consumers of health care and their numbers are increasing. The United Nations' General Assembly proclaimed 1999 the "International Year of Older Persons." The health and aging chartbook consists of 34 figures and accompanying text.

Detailed Tables

The chartbook is followed by 146 detailed tables on trends organized around four major subject areas: health status and determinants, utilization of health resources, health care resources, and health care expenditures. A major criterion used in selecting the detailed tables is the availability of comparable national data over a period of several years. The detailed tables report data for selected years to highlight major trends in health statistics. Earlier editions of *Health, United States* may present data for additional years that are not included in the current printed report. Where possible, these additional data are available in Lotus 1–2–3 spreadsheet files as listed in Appendix III.

Racial and Ethnic Data

Several tables in *Health, United States* present data according to race and Hispanic origin consistent with Department-wide emphasis on expanding racial and ethnic detail in presenting health data. The presentation of data on race and ethnicity in the detailed tables is usually in the greatest detail possible, after taking into account the quality of data, the amount of missing data, and the number of observations. The large differences in health status by race and Hispanic origin that are documented in this report may be explained by several factors including socioeconomic status, health practices, psychosocial stress and resources, environmental exposures, discrimination, and access to health care.

Changes in This Edition

Similar tables appear in each volume of *Health, United States* to enhance the use of this publication as a standard reference source. However, some changes in the content of the tables are made each year to enhance their usefulness and to reflect emerging topics in public health. New to *Health, United States, 1999* are data on death rates for selected causes of death by educational attainment (table 35); additional notifiable diseases (table 53); the percent of children with untreated dental caries (table 72); the percent of adults with no usual source of care (table 81); student enrollment and number of schools of public health (table 107); and the percent of persons with private health insurance through health maintenance organizations (table 131).

Data for racial and ethnic groups have been expanded in tables showing the percent low-birthweight live births by State (tables 13 and 14), the percent of persons with fair or poor health (table 60), the percent of persons who currently smoke cigarettes (table 63), and the percent of children without a physician contact in the past year (table 79) and without a usual source of care (table 80). In addition new tables 72, 81, and 131 also present data for racial and ethnic groups.

Trends in overweight among adults, presented in table 70, have been revised to reflect current definitions and to include the proportion of persons with healthy weight and those with obesity. Data on procedures presented in tables 94 and 95 now include ambulatory procedures from the National Survey of Ambulatory Surgery and inpatient procedures from the National Hospital Discharge Survey. Some of the tables in the health care expenditures section (tables 116, 117, 120, and 127) were reformatted to simplify presentation of the data.

Appendixes

Appendix I describes each data source used in the report and the limitations of the data and provides references for further information about the sources. Appendix II is an alphabetical listing of terms used in the report. It also contains standard populations used for age adjustment and *International Classification of Diseases* codes for cause of death and diagnostic and procedure categories. Appendix III lists tables with additional years of trend data that are available electronically in Lotus 1–2–3 spreadsheet files on the NCHS homepage and CD-ROM.

Electronic Access

Health, United States can be accessed electronically in four formats. First, the entire *Health, United States, 1999* is available, along with other NCHS reports, on a CD-ROM entitled "Publications from the National Center for Health Statistics," featuring *Health, United States, 1999*, vol 1 no 4, 1999. These publications can be viewed, searched, printed, and saved using Adobe Acrobat software on the CD-ROM. The CD-ROM may be purchased from the Government Printing Office or the National Technical Information Service.

Second, the complete *Health, United States, 1999* is available as an Acrobat .pdf file on the Internet through the NCHS home page on the World Wide Web. The direct Uniform Resource Locator (URL) address is:

www.cdc.gov/nchswww/products/pubs/pubd/hus/hus.htm.

Third, the 146 detailed tables in *Health, United States, 1999* are available on the FTP server as Lotus 1–2–3 spreadsheet files and can be downloaded. The URL address for the FTP server is:

www.cdc.gov/nchswww/datawh/ftpserv/ftpserv.htm.

The detailed tables are also included as Lotus 1–2–3 spreadsheet files on the CD-ROM mentioned above.

Fourth, for users who do not have access to the Internet or to a CD-ROM reader, the 146 detailed tables can be made available on diskette as Lotus 1–2–3 spreadsheet files for use with IBM compatible personal computers. To obtain a copy of the diskette, contact the NCHS Data Dissemination Branch.

Questions

For answers to questions about this report, contact:
Data Dissemination Branch
National Center for Health Statistics
Centers for Disease Control and Prevention
6525 Belcrest Road, Room 1064
Hyattsville, Maryland 20782-2003
phone: 301-436-8500
E-mail: nchsquery@cdc.gov

Overall responsibility for planning and coordinating the content of this volume rested with the Office of Analysis, Epidemiology, and Health Promotion, National Center for Health Statistics (NCHS), under the general direction of Diane M. Makuc and Jennifer H. Madans.

Health, United States, 1999 highlights, detailed tables, and appendixes were prepared under the supervision of Kate Prager. Detailed tables were prepared by Alan J. Cohen, Margaret A. Cooke, Virginia M. Freid, Andrea P. MacKay, Michael E. Mussolino, Mitchell B. Pierre, Jr., Rebecca A. Placek, Anita L. Powell, and Kate Prager with assistance from La-Tonya Curl, Patricia A. Knapp, Mark F. Pioli, Sharon H. Saydah, and Catherine Duran of TRW, Information Services Division and Henry Xia of NOVA Research Company. The appendixes, index to detailed tables, and pocket edition were prepared by Anita L. Powell. Production planning and coordination were managed by Rebecca A. Placek with assistance from Carole J. Hunt and Camille Miller.

The **chartbook** was prepared by Ellen A. Kramarow, Harold R. Lentzner, Ronica N. Rooks, Julie D. Weeks, and Sharon H. Saydah. Data and analysis for specific charts were provided by Christine S. Cox, Mayur M. Desai, Thomas A. Hodgson, Nadine R. Sahyoun, and Clemencia M. Vargas.

The Office of the Demography of Aging, Behavioral and Social Research Program, National Institute on Aging, under the direction of Richard Suzman, provided support for the chartbook. Advice on the content of the chartbook was provided by Donna L. Hoyert, Raynard S. Kington, and Harry M. Rosenberg of NCHS; Suzanne M. Smith of the National Center for Chronic Disease Prevention and Health Promotion, CDC; and Robert Clark of the Office of Assistant Secretary for Planning and Evaluation, Department of Health and Human Services (DHHS).

Publications management and editorial review were provided by Thelma W. Sanders and Rolfe W. Larson. The designer was Sarah M. Hinkle. Graphics were supervised by Stephen L. Sloan. Production was done by Jacqueline M. Davis and Annette F. Holman.

Printing was managed by Patricia L. Wilson and Joan D. Burton.

Electronic access through the CD-ROM and NCHS internet site was provided by June R. Gable, Gail V. Johnson, Thelma W. Sanders, Julia A. Sothoron, and Tammy M. Stewart-Prather.

Data and technical assistance were provided by Charles A. Adams, Robert N. Anderson, Veronica Benson, Linda E. Biggar, Kate M. Brett, Ronette R. Briefel, Catharine W. Burt, Margaret D. Carroll, Robin A. Cohen, Achintya N. Dey, Thomas D. Dunn, Sylvia A. Ellison, Katherine M. Flegal, Nancy G. Gagne, Cordell Golden, Malcolm C. Graham, Edmund J. Graves, Barbara J. Haupt, Katherine E. Heck, Rosemarie Hirsch, Donna L. Hoyert, Deborah D. Ingram, Susan S. Jack, Elizabeth W. Jackson, Clifford L. Johnson, Kenneth D. Kochanek, Lola Jean Kozak, Robert J. Kuczmarski, Linda S. Lawrence, Karen L. Lipkind, Anne C. Looker, Marian F. MacDorman, Joyce A. Martin, Jeffrey D. Maurer, Linda F. McCaig, William D. Mosher, Sherry L. Murphy, Cheryl R. Nelson, Francis C. Notzon, Parivash Nourjah, Maria F. Owings, Elsie R. Pamuk, Gail A. Parr, Kimberly D. Peters, Linda S. Peterson, Linda J. Piccinino, Cheryl V. Rose, Harry M. Rosenberg, Colleen M. Ryan, Susan M. Schappert, J. Fred Seitz, Manju Sharma, Alvin J. Sirrocco, Betty L. Smith, Genevieve W. Strahan, Luong Tonthat, Clemencia M. Vargas, Stephanie J. Ventura, and David A. Woodwell of NCHS; Jeffrey Y. Liu of TRW, Information Services Division; Carolyn M. Sherman of Sherman and Holmes Associates; Tim Bush and Melinda L. Flock of the National Center for HIV, STD, and TB Prevention, CDC; Samuel L. Groseclose and Myra A. Montalbano of the Epidemiology Program Office, CDC; Lisa M. Koonin and Myra A. Montalbano of the National Center for Chronic Disease Prevention and Health Promotion, CDC; Monina Klevens and Edmond F. Maes of the National Immunization Program, CDC; Suzanne M. Kisner of the National Institute of Occupational Safety and Health, CDC; Evelyn Christian of the Health Resources and Services Administration; Mitchell Goldstein of the Office of the Secretary, DHHS;

Acknowledgments

Joseph Gfroerer, Janet Greenblatt, Andrea Kopstein, Patricia Royston, Michael Witkin, Richard Thoreson, and Deborah Trunzo of the Substance Abuse and Mental Health Services Administration; Ken Allison, Lynn A. G. Ries, and Arthur Hughes of the National Institutes of Health; Cathy A. Cowan, Janice D. Drexler, Leslie Greenwald, Paula Higger, Roger E. Keene, Helen C. Lazenby, Katharine R. Levit, Anna Long, Edward F. Mortimore, Anthony C. Parker, Madie W. Stewart, and Joanne Weller of the Health Care Financing Administration; Loretta Bass, Joseph Dalaker, and Terry Lugaila of the Census Bureau; James Barnhardt, Alan Blostin, Daniel Ginsburg, and Kay Ford of the Bureau of Labor Statistics; Elizabeth Ahuja of the Department of Veterans Affairs; Susan Tew of the Alan Guttmacher Institute; Wendy Katz of the Association of Schools of Public Health; Richard Hamer of InterStudy; and Patrick O'Malley of the University of Michigan.

Jacob J. Feldman, Ph.D.

This volume of *Health, United States* is dedicated to our colleague and friend, Dr. Jack Feldman, who served as Associate Director for Analysis, Epidemiology, and Health Promotion at the National Center for Health Statistics (NCHS) from the mid-1970's until he retired from Federal service in 1998. The development of *Health, United States* was one part of the analytic program that Jack oversaw during his tenure at NCHS.

Jack made innumerable contributions to *Health, United States* over a 23-year period, providing insightful direction and wise guidance on the content of the report. Jack's comprehensive knowledge of the public health literature as well as his strong grasp of emerging health issues have been key to ensuring that this report provides data on the most important health topics each year. Jack also brought a vast knowledge of and keen interest in survey methodology, data quality, and statistical analysis to his work on this report. He is equally knowledgeable about all of the wide range of topics and data sources that are included in this publication. More amazing is Jack's uncanny ability to absorb the large volume of statistics presented in the detailed trend tables of this report and to identify interesting and important trends that need to be brought to the attention of the health community. On the other hand, Jack's healthy skepticism of changes in trends and unusual patterns in the data has ensured that highlighted trends reflect true differences in health rather than changes in data collection methods or other data artifacts.

Although Jack is no longer in the office with us on a daily basis, the example he provided still serves to guide and inspire the work we do. We are challenged to continue the high standards that he set not only for this report but for all aspects of the collection, analysis, and dissemination of health data. A grateful staff acknowledges his unique contributions to this profile of the Nation's health and wishes Jack all the best in his new endeavors.

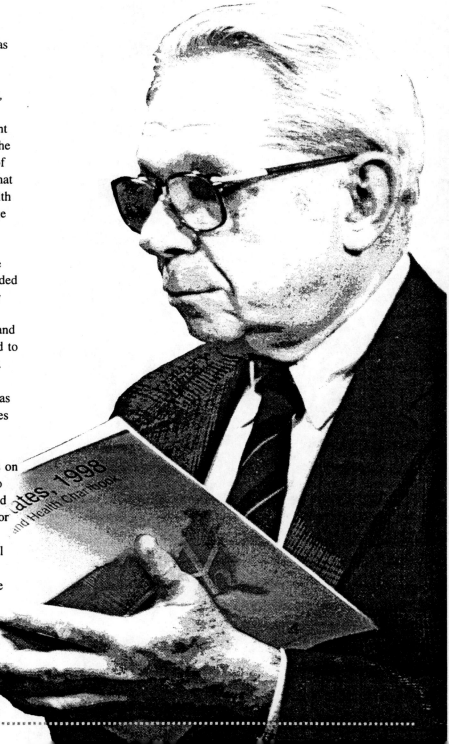

Contents

Contents ....

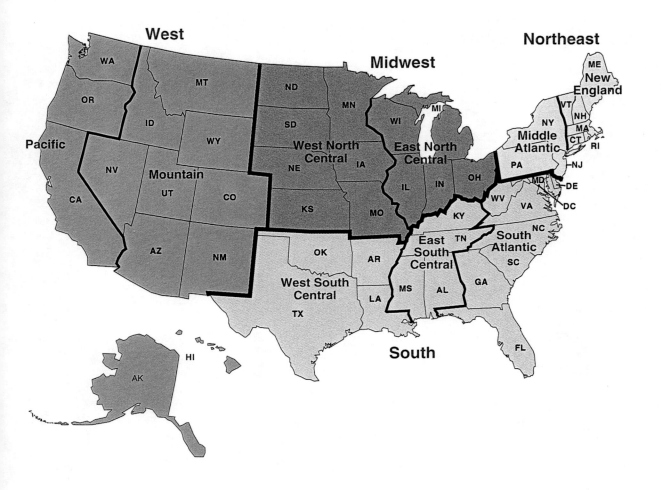

Health and Aging

Population

The older population of the United States is large and growing and will be more diverse in the twenty-first century. Women constitute the majority of the older population. Only a small proportion of older persons reside in institutions, and a significant proportion of community-dwelling elderly persons (particularly women) live alone.

■ In 1997, 13 percent of the U.S. **population** was 65 years of age and over. It is estimated that in 2030, 20 percent of Americans will be 65 years of age and over. In 1997 older persons made up a larger proportion of the non-Hispanic white population compared with other racial and ethnic groups. However, the older non-Hispanic white population is growing more slowly compared with other groups (figure 1).

■ The **living arrangements** of older persons vary greatly by age, sex, race, and marital status. While a majority of noninstitutionalized persons 65 years of age and over lived with family members in 1997, nearly one-third lived alone. Women in every age group were more likely than men to live alone (figure 2).

■ In 1997 approximately 4 percent of the older population lived in nursing homes. The rate of **nursing home residence** rises sharply with age. Approximately 1 percent of persons 65–74 years of age lived in nursing homes compared with almost 20 percent of persons 85 years of age and over. Women at all ages had higher rates of nursing home residence than men (figure 3).

■ Although **poverty** rates among the elderly have declined significantly since the 1960's, 1 out of 10 persons 65 years of age and over in 1997 was living in a family with income below the Federal poverty threshold. The poverty rate was higher among older black and Hispanic persons compared with older white persons (figure 4).

Health Status

Americans have longer lives than ever before. Persons who survive to age 65 today can expect to live on average nearly 18 more years. The health of the older population varies greatly. Rates of illness and disability increase sharply among the "oldest-old," persons 85 years of age and over, compared with younger persons. Nearly all measures reflect this variation by age.

■ **Life expectancy** at age 65 and age 85 increased over the past 50 years. Women have on average longer lives than men. In 1997 life expectancy at age 65 was higher for white persons than for black persons. However, at age 85 life expectancy for black persons was slightly higher than for white persons (figures 5 and 6).

■ Chronic diseases such as heart disease, cancer, stroke, and chronic obstructive pulmonary diseases are the **leading causes of death** among the older population, although pneumonia and influenza were responsible for approximately 7 percent of deaths among persons 85 years of age and over in 1997 (figure 9).

■ **Chronic conditions** are prevalent among older persons. In 1995 among noninstitutionalized persons 70 years of age and over, 79 percent reported at least one of seven chronic conditions common among the elderly. The majority of persons 70 years of age and over reported arthritis, and approximately one-third reported hypertension. Diabetes was reported by 11 percent (figure 11).

■ **Visual and hearing impairments** among older persons increase sharply with age. In 1995, 13 percent of persons 70–74 years of age were visually impaired compared with 31 percent of persons 85 years of age and over. For hearing impairments, the prevalence rose from 26 percent of persons 70–74 years of age to 49 percent of persons 85 years of age and over (figures 12 and 13).

Highlights

■ **Osteoporosis** is common among older persons and is a strong predictor of subsequent fractures. In 1988–94 just over one-half of noninstitutionalized persons 65 years of age and over had reduced hip bone density, either osteoporosis or osteopenia (a less severe form of bone loss than osteoporosis). The proportion of older persons with osteoporosis was higher among women than men and rose with age for both women and men (figure 14).

■ **Physical functioning and disability** rates among the older population vary by age and sex. Nearly 9 percent of noninstitutionalized persons 70 years of age and over were unable to perform one or more activities of daily living such as bathing, dressing, using the toilet, and getting in and out of bed or chairs. Women in every age group were more likely to be disabled than men, and the proportion disabled rose with age (figure 15).

■ **Oral health** indicators among the older population are improving over time. Yet, 30 percent of persons 65 years of age and over in 1993 were edentulous, that is, they had no natural teeth. Non-Hispanic white persons had lower levels of total tooth loss compared with non-Hispanic black persons and Hispanic persons (figure 20). In 1988–94 nearly one-third of persons 65 years of age and over with natural teeth had untreated dental caries in the crown or the root of their teeth (figure 19).

■ In 1995 nearly all noninstitutionalized persons 70 years of age and over participated in some **social activities** in a 2-week period. The most common activity was contact with family, either in person or by telephone. Persons who were disabled were less likely than nondisabled persons to participate in activities outside of their house (figure 21).

■ In 1995, 71 percent of nondisabled persons 65 years of age and over participated in some form of **exercise** at least once in a recent two-week period. Most older persons who exercise engage in light and moderate activities such as walking, gardening, and stretching. However, only about one-third of persons who exercised achieved recommended levels of 30 minutes each time on most days of the week (figure 22).

Health Care Access and Utilization

Changes in the health care system have affected the older population. Use of in-home contacts with medical providers has increased, and length of hospital stays has decreased. Approximately 12 percent of Medicare beneficiaries 65 years of age and over were enrolled in a managed care plan in 1997, although the percent varies widely by region. In general, persons 85 years of age and over use health care services more than those 65–84 years of age.

■ In 1995 approximately one-third of noninstitutionalized persons 70 years of age and over received help from a **caregiver** with daily activities such as dressing, bathing, shopping, housework, and managing money. The number of caregivers providing help to an older person increased with age (figure 23).

■ Thirty-nine percent of noninstitutionalized persons 70 years of age and over in 1995 used **assistive devices** such as hearing aids, diabetic and respiratory equipment, and canes and walkers during the previous 12 months. Rates of device use were twice as high among persons 85 years of age and over compared with persons 70–74 years of age (figure 25).

■ In 1994–96 the mean number of **ambulatory physician contacts** among persons 65 years of age and over was 11.4 per year. The number of contacts with physicians or with other personnel working under a physician's supervision increased with age. From 1990 to 1996 the proportion of contacts in the home increased by 63 percent (figure 26).

■ Older persons are major consumers of **inpatient health care.** Older men had higher rates of hospitalization than older women. Heart disease was the most common cause for hospitalization. The average length of hospital stay in 1996 was 6.5 days for persons 65 years of age and over, about two days less than in 1986 (figure 27).

■ **Influenza and pneumococcal vaccinations** are recommended for older adults. During 1993–95 an average of 55 percent of noninstitutionalized persons 65 years of age and over reported receiving a flu shot within the previous 12 months. Twenty-nine percent reported ever having received a pneumonia vaccination. Vaccination coverage for both influenza and pneumococcal disease was higher among non-Hispanic white persons than non-Hispanic black persons or Hispanic persons (figure 28).

■ On an average day in 1996, approximately 1.7 million persons 65 years of age and over, roughly 51 per 1,000 population, were **home health care** patients. In every age group women had higher rates of home health care usage than men, and the rate increased with age for both women and men (figures 29 and 30).

■ In 1994–96 persons 85 years of age and over were more likely to rely on Medicare alone or on Medicare combined with Medicaid for their **health insurance** coverage than persons under 85 years of age. Non-Hispanic black and Hispanic persons were less likely than non-Hispanic white persons to have private insurance to supplement their Medicare coverage (figure 31).

■ Participation in **Medicare health maintenance organizations (HMO's)** is increasing among the older population. In 1997 over 4 million persons 65 years of age and over who received Medicare were enrolled in a managed care plan, a four-fold increase since 1985. The highest levels of Medicare HMO participation are in the West. Several states had no Medicare managed care plans in 1997 (figure 32).

■ In 1995 the overall **cost of heart disease** among persons 65 years of age and over was estimated to be more than 58 billion dollars. Hospital care and nursing home care accounted for over three-fourths of the total personal health care expenditures for heart disease among the older population (figure 33).

■ In 1995 the **cost of diabetes** among persons 65 years of age and over was estimated to be 26 billion dollars. The largest personal health care expenditure attributed to diabetes, including chronic complications and comorbidities asssociated with diabetes, was for hospital care. Nursing home care accounted for one-fifth of expenditures (figure 34).

Highlights ....

Health Status and Determinants

Mortality

In 1997 life expectancy at birth increased to an all-time high and infant mortality fell to a record low. Life expectancy for black males increased for the fourth consecutive year.

■ In 1997 **life expectancy** at birth reached an all-time high of 76.5 years and **infant mortality** fell to a record low of 7.2 deaths per 1,000 live births (tables 22 and 28).

■ Between 1995 and 1997 **life expectancy** at birth for black males increased 2 years to a record high of 67.2 years, due in large part to declines in mortality from HIV infection and homicide. However, life expectancy was still 7.1 years shorter for black males than for white males in 1997 (table 28).

The death rate for HIV infection declined by almost one-half. Death rates for heart disease, cancer, unintentional injuries, and homicide also decreased. Although death rates for two leading causes of death, stroke and suicide, were lower in 1997 than in 1996, the longer-term trend shows little change.

■ Mortality from **heart disease**, the leading cause of death, declined 3 percent in 1997, continuing a long-term downward trend in mortality. The 1997 age-adjusted death rate for heart disease was almost one-half the rate in 1970 (tables 30 and 32).

■ Mortality from **cancer,** the second leading cause of death, decreased 2 percent in 1997, continuing the decline that began in 1990. Over the preceding 20-year period, 1970 to 1990, age-adjusted cancer death rates had steadily increased (tables 30 and 32).

■ Mortality from **HIV infection** declined 48 percent in 1997 following a 29-percent decline in 1996. This 2-year decline contrasts sharply with the period 1987–94, when HIV mortality increased at an average rate of 16 percent per year. In 1997 HIV infection fell from 8th to 14th in the ranking of leading causes of death (table 43).

■ Mortality from **unintentional injuries**, the fifth leading cause of death, declined 1 percent in 1997, continuing the generally downward trend in injury mortality since the 1980's (tables 30 and 32).

■ The age-adjusted **homicide** rate declined 6 percent in 1997. This decline continued a trend that began in the early 1990's (table 46).

■ Mortality from **stroke**, the third leading cause of death, was fairly stable between 1992 and 1997. Between 1980 and 1992 stroke mortality declined at an average rate of 3.6 percent per year (tables 30, 32, and 38).

■ The age-adjusted death rate for **suicide**, the eighth leading cause of death, fell 2 percent between 1996 and 1997, to 10.6 deaths per 100,000 population. Between 1980 and 1997 age-adjusted suicide rates ranged between 11 and 12 per 100,000 (tables 30, 32, and 47).

Despite overall declines in mortality, disparities among racial and ethnic groups in mortality for many causes of death are substantial. Disparities among persons of different education levels continue. Persons with less than a high school education have death rates at least double those with education beyond high school.

■ In 1996 **infant mortality** rates were highest among infants of non-Hispanic black and American Indian mothers (14.2 and 10.0 deaths per 1,000 live births). Infant mortality was lowest for infants of Chinese American mothers (3.2). Mortality rates for infants of Hispanic mothers and non-Hispanic white mothers were virtually the same (6.1 and 6.0) (table 19).

■ **Infant mortality** decreases as the mother's level of education increases. In 1996 mortality for infants of black, white, and Asian American mothers with less than 12 years of education was 42–60 percent higher than for infants whose mothers had 13 or more years of education. The disparity in infant mortality by mother's education was smaller for Hispanic mothers, ranging from 6 percent for Mexican American mothers to 32 percent for Puerto Rican mothers (table 20).

■ The **firearm-related death rate for young black males** 15–24 years of age declined 10 percent per year on average between 1993 and 1997. The rate for 1997

(119.9 deaths per 100,000) was still nearly 5 times the rate for young white males (table 48).

■ In 1997 the **homicide rate for young Hispanic males** 15–24 years of age was almost 7 times the rate for non-Hispanic white males. Among those 25–44 years of age the homicide rate for Hispanic males was more than 3 times as high, and the **HIV infection** death rate for Hispanic males was more than twice as high as for non-Hispanic white males (tables 43 and 46).

■ In 1997 among **American Indians** the age-adjusted death rates for **unintentional injuries** (58.5 deaths per 100,000 population) and **diabetes** (30.4) were at least double the rates for white persons and the death rate for **cirrhosis** (20.6) was nearly 3 times the rate for white persons. Death rates for the American Indian population are known to be underestimated (table 30).

■ In 1997 overall mortality was 55 percent higher for **black Americans** than for white Americans. In 1997 the age-adjusted death rates for the black population exceeded those for the white population by 77 percent for **stroke**, 47 percent for **heart disease**, 34 percent for **cancer**, and 655 percent for HIV infection (table 30).

■ In 1997 the overall age-adjusted death rate for **Asian-American** males was 39 percent lower than the rate for white males. However the **homicide** rate for Asian males was only 6 percent lower than for white males and the death rate for **stroke** was 10 percent higher for Asian males than for white males. Death rates for Asian Americans are known to be underestimated somewhat (tables 36, 38, and 46).

■ In 1997 the age-adjusted death rate for **chronic obstructive pulmonary diseases (COPD)**, the fourth leading cause of death, was 47 percent higher for **males than females**. Between 1990 and 1997 age-adjusted death rates for males were relatively stable while death rates for females increased at an average annual rate of nearly 3 percent (tables 32 and 42).

■ Death rates increase as **educational attainment** decreases. In 1997 the age-adjusted death rate for chronic diseases was more than twice as high among adults with fewer than 12 years of education as among those with more than 12 years of education. The death rate for injuries was 3 times as high for the least educated as for the most educated adults (table 35).

Natality

The overall fertility rate declined to a record low in 1997, continuing the decline that began in 1990. Birth rates for teens, especially younger teens, and birth rates for unmarried women also continued to decline in 1997. The proportion of babies born with low birthweight continued to edge upward.

■ In 1997 the **birth rate for teenagers** declined for the sixth consecutive year, to 52.3 births per 1,000 women aged 15–19 years. Between 1991 and 1997 the teen birth rate declined more for 15–17 year olds than for 18–19 year olds (17 percent compared with 11 percent) (table 3).

■ Between 1994 and 1997 the **birth rate for unmarried women** declined almost 11 percent for black mothers, to 73.4 births per 1,000 unmarried black women aged 15–44 years. The birth rate declined almost 10 percent for unmarried Hispanic mothers, to 91.4 per 1,000 (table 8).

■ **Low birthweight** is associated with elevated risk of death and disability in infants. In 1997 the rate of low birthweight (infants weighing less than 2,500 grams at birth) increased to 7.5 percent overall, up from 7.0 percent in 1990. Since 1990 the low birthweight rate increased for most racial and ethnic groups. However among black infants low birthweight declined slightly from 13.3 percent in 1990 to 13.0 percent in 1997 (table 11).

■ **Cigarette smoking during pregnancy** is a risk factor for poor birth outcomes such as low birthweight and infant death. In 1997 the proportion of mothers who smoked cigarettes during pregnancy declined to a record low of 13.2 percent, down from 19.5 percent in 1989. However the percent of teenage mothers who smoked increased between 1994 and 1997 (table 10).

Health Status

Morbidity

The two overall measures of morbidity presented in this report show little change over time. The percent of persons with activity limitation due to a chronic condition has remained stable from 1990 to 1996 as has the percent of persons who report fair or poor health status. As family income decreases the percent of persons reporting fair or poor health or reporting an activity limitation increases. Better summary measures of health for assessment of trends are needed and are under development. Trends in the incidence of specific diseases are additional measures of morbidity trends.

■ In 1996 the percent of persons reporting **fair or poor health** was four times as high for persons living below the poverty level as for those with family income at least twice the poverty level (22.2 percent and 5.5 percent, age adjusted) (table 60).

■ The number of **AIDS cases** newly reported in 1997 was 12 percent lower than in 1996. The number of newly reported AIDS cases decreased 14 percent for males and 5 percent for females in 1997. AIDS incidence continues to be more common among males than females. The incidence rate for males 13 years of age and over (38.5 cases per 100,000 population) was nearly 4 times the rate for females during July 1997–June 1998 (table 54).

■ Between 1995 and 1997 the number of hospital inpatient discharges with a diagnosis of **human immunodeficiency virus (HIV)** decreased 29 percent to 178,000 discharges, and average length of stay declined by 1.2 days to 8.1 days (table 91).

■ In 1997 **tuberculosis (TB)** incidence declined for the fifth consecutive year to 7.4 cases per 100,000 population. In 1997, 39 percent of TB cases occurred among foreign-born persons in the United States. This proportion has been increasing since the mid-1980's, in part attributable to changes in immigration patterns (table 53).

■ Between 1990 and 1997 the incidence of primary and secondary **syphilis** declined 84 percent to 3.2 cases

per 100,000. The incidence of **gonorrhea** declined 56 percent to 122.5 per 100,000 (table 53).

■ Overall **cancer incidence** has been declining in the 1990's, more so for males than for females. Between 1991 and 1995 overall cancer incidence rates declined 13 percent for white males, 6 percent for black males, 4 percent for black females, and 2 percent for white females (table 57).

■ **Prostate cancer and lung cancer** are the two most frequently diagnosed cancers among men. Between 1991 and 1995 the age-adjusted incidence rate for prostate cancer declined 23 percent for white males and 5 percent for black males. During this period lung cancer incidence declined by 9–11 percent for white and black males (table 57).

■ In 1995 **breast cancer** incidence was 12 percent lower for black females than for white females. However the 5-year relative survival rate for black females with breast cancer diagnosed in 1989–94 was 16 percentage points lower than for white females (71 and 87 percent). In 1997 breast cancer mortality was 41 percent higher for black women than white women (tables 41, 57, and 58).

■ Between 1990 and 1997 the **injuries with lost workdays** rate decreased 21 percent to 3.1 per 100 full-time equivalents (FTE's) in the private sector (table 74).

Health Risk Factors

Elevated blood pressure, high levels of serum cholesterol, and overweight are important risk factors for cardiovascular and other chronic diseases. Recent trends show improvements in the prevalence of hypertension and high cholesterol. However, the prevalence of overweight has increased. Overweight among children and adolescents has doubled since the early 1970's, raising concerns for long-term health effects.

■ Between 1976–80 and 1988–94 the age-adjusted prevalence of **hypertension** among adults 20–74 years of age declined sharply from 39 percent to 23 percent, after remaining relatively stable over the previous 20 years (table 68).

■ Between 1960–62 and 1988–94 the age-adjusted mean **serum total cholesterol** level for adults 20–74 years of age declined from 220 to 203 mg/dL. The age-adjusted percent of adults with cholesterol greater than or equal to 240 mg/dL declined from 32 percent to 19 percent (table 69).

■ Between 1960–62 and 1988–94, the prevalence of **overweight** (body mass index (BMI) greater than or equal to 25) among adults 20–74 years of age increased by one-quarter, from 44 to 55 percent. Almost one-half of overweight adults are obese (BMI greater than or equal to 30), and **obesity** increased by more than three-quarters from 13 to 23 percent during this time period (percents are age adjusted) (table 70).

■ Between 1971–74 and 1988–94 the prevalence of **overweight** among 6–11 year-old children increased from 6 to 14 percent. Among adolescents 12–17 years of age, overweight increased from 6 to 11 percent during the same period (percents are age adjusted) (table 71).

Cigarette smoking is the single leading preventable cause of death in the United States. It increases the risk of lung cancer, heart disease, emphysema, and other respiratory diseases. Cigarette smoking by adults has remained stable at about 25 percent since 1990. Heavy and chronic use of alcohol and use of illicit drugs increase the risk of disease and injuries.

■ **Cigarette smoking** is more prevalent among the American Indian population than among other groups. In 1993–95, 40 percent of American Indian males and 33 percent of American Indian females were current smokers compared with 27 percent of white males and 24 percent of white females (percents are age adjusted and are for persons 18 years of age and over) (table 63).

■ In 1998 **cigarette smoking** in the past month by high school seniors declined slightly, following 5 consecutive years of increase. In 1998 the proportion of white seniors who smoked cigarettes, 41 percent,

was nearly three times the proportion of black seniors who smoked, 15 percent (table 65).

■ In 1998, 23 percent of high school seniors reported using **marijuana** in the past month, nearly double the prevalence in 1992. Use among eighth graders nearly tripled to 10 percent during that time period (table 65).

■ Between 1993 and 1998 the proportion of high school seniors reporting **alcohol** use in the past month increased from 49 to 52 percent after declining from 72 percent in 1980 (table 65).

■ **Heavy alcohol use**, having five or more drinks on at least one occasion in the past month, is more common among young people 18–25 years of age than among younger or older persons. In 1997 among 18–25 year olds, heavy drinking was 1.5–2.5 times as likely for non-Hispanic white persons (33 percent) as for Hispanic and non-Hispanic black persons (22 and 13 percent) (table 64).

■ In 1996 there were more than 152,000 **cocaine-related emergency room visits**, almost twice as many as in 1990. The greatest increases occurred for persons 35 years and over, reflecting an aging population of drug abusers being treated in emergency departments. However, the proportion of adults age 35 years and over who reported using cocaine in the past month has remained stable during this period at less than 1 percent (tables 64 and 66).

Environmental factors are important determinants of health and disease. An environmental health objective for the year 2000 is that at least 85 percent of the U.S. population should be living in counties that meet the Environmental Protection Agency's National Ambient Air Quality Standards.

■ In 1996, 81 percent of Americans lived in counties that met standards for all pollutants. However, there were disparities among racial and ethnic groups. In 1996, 56–64 percent of the Hispanic and Asian American population lived in counties that met **air quality standards** for all pollutants compared with 81–83 percent of the white, black and American Indian populations (table 73).

Health Care Utilization and Resources

Ambulatory Care

Use of preventive health services has substantial positive effects on the long-term health status of those who receive the services. The use of several different types of preventive services has been increasing. However, disparities in use of preventive health care by family income and by race and ethnicity remain in evidence.

■ Between 1990 and 1997 the percent of mothers receiving **prenatal care** in the first trimester of pregnancy increased from 76 to 83 percent. The largest increases in receipt of early prenatal care have occurred for racial and ethnic groups with the lowest levels of use, thereby reducing disparities in use of early care. However in 1997 the percent of mothers with early prenatal care still varied substantially among racial and ethnic groups from 68 percent for American Indian mothers to 90 percent for Cuban mothers (table 6).

■ In 1997, 76 percent of children 19–35 months of age received the combined **vaccination** series of 4 doses of DTP (diphtheria-tetanus-pertussis) vaccine, 3 doses of polio vaccine, 1 dose of measles-containing vaccine, and 3 doses of Hib (Haemophilus influenzae type b) vaccine, up from 69 percent in 1994. Children living below the poverty threshold were less likely to have received the combined vaccination series than were children living at or above poverty (71 compared with 79 percent) (table 51).

■ In 1997 only 138 cases of **measles** were reported, down from 28,000 cases in 1990, providing evidence of the success of vaccination efforts to increase population immunity to measles (table 53).

■ Regular **mammography** screening for women aged 50 years and over has been shown to be effective in reducing deaths from breast cancer. In 1994, 61 percent of women aged 50 years and over reported mammography screening in the previous 2-year period, up from 27 percent in 1987. Women living below the poverty threshold were one-third less likely than their

nonpoor counterparts to report recent screening in 1994 (table 82).

Some indicators of children's access to health care services include having health insurance coverage, having a usual source of health care, having a recent physician contact, and treatment of health problems such as dental caries. Access to health care among children varies by family income, race, and ethnicity.

■ In 1997, 14 percent of children under 18 years of age had no **health insurance coverage**. More than one-quarter of children with family income just above the poverty level were without coverage compared with only 6 percent of those with income above twice the poverty level (table 129).

■ In 1995–96, 9.2 percent of children under 6 years of age did not have a **physician contact** within the previous 12-month period. Uninsured children were 2.5 times as likely as those with health insurance to be without a recent visit (18.5 percent compared with 7.3 percent) (table 79).

■ In 1995–96, 7.2 percent of children 6–17 years of age and 4.3 percent of children under age 6 had **no usual source of health care**. About one-quarter of older children without health insurance coverage had no usual source of health care (table 80).

■ In 1988–94, 23.1 percent of children 6–17 years of age had at least one untreated **dental cavity**, down from 55.0 percent in 1971–74. Although substantial declines in untreated dental cavities have occurred for children at all income levels, poor children were 2.5 times as likely as nonpoor children to have an untreated cavity in 1988–94 (36.3 percent compared with 14.5 percent) (table 72).

Inpatient Care

Major changes are occurring in the delivery of health care in the United States, driven in large part by the need to rein in rising costs. One important change has been a decline in use of inpatient services and an increase in outpatient services. About 60 percent of surgical operations in community hospitals were performed on an outpatient basis in 1997.

■ Between 1985 and 1996 the **inpatient discharge rate** declined by one-quarter from 138 discharges per 1,000 population to 102 per 1,000, while **average length of stay** declined by more than a full day, from 6.3 to 5.1 days (data are age adjusted) (table 90).

■ Use of **inpatient hospital care** increases as family income declines. In 1996 the age-adjusted hospital discharge rate for persons with low family income (less than $16,000) was almost 3 times the rate for those with high family income ($50,000 or more) and the average length of hospital stay was nearly 2 days longer (6.6 days and 4.8 days) (table 89).

■ In 1997, 61 percent of all **surgical operations** in community hospitals were performed on outpatients, up from 51 percent in 1990, 35 percent in 1985, and 16 percent in 1980 (table 96).

■ Between 1985 and 1997 the number of **community hospital beds** declined from 1 million to 853,000 and during the same period occupancy rates in community hospitals declined from 65 to 62 percent (table 110).

■ Between 1984 and 1994 the supply of beds in inpatient and residential **mental health organizations** declined 14 percent to 98 beds per 100,000 population. The decline was greatest for state and county mental hospitals with a reduction of 45 percent to 31 beds per 100,000 population (table 111).

■ In 1997 there were almost 1.5 million elderly **nursing home residents** 65 years of age and over. One-half of elderly nursing home residents were 85 years of age and over and three-quarters were women. (table 97)

■ In 1997 there were 1.7 million **nursing home beds** in facilities certified for use by medicare and medicaid beneficiaries. Nursing home bed occupancy in those facilities was estimated at 82 percent (table 114).

Health Care Expenditures

National Health Expenditures

After 25 years of double-digit annual growth in national health expenditures, the rate of growth has slowed during the 1990's. However the United States continues to spend more on health than any other industrialized country.

■ In 1997 **national health care expenditures** in the United States totaled almost $1.1 trillion, increasing less than 5 percent from the previous year and continuing the slowdown in growth of the 1990's. During the 1980's national health expenditures had grown at an average annual rate of 11 percent (table 116).

■ This slowdown in growth is also reflected in the **Consumer Price Index (CPI)**. The rate of increase in the medical care component of the CPI declined from 7.5 percent in 1985–90 to 3.0 percent in 1996–98 (table 117).

■ The combination of strong economic growth and the slowdown in the rate of increase in health spending over the last few years has stabilized **health expenditures as a percent of the gross domestic product** at 13.5–13.7 percent from 1993 to 1997, after increasing steadily from 8.9 percent in 1980 (table 116).

■ Despite the slowdown in the growth of health spending, the United States continues to spend a larger **share of gross domestic product (GDP)** on health than any other major industrialized country. The United States devoted 13.5 percent of GDP to health in 1997 compared with about 10 percent each in Germany, Switzerland, and France, the countries with the next highest shares. (table 115).

Highlights ....

Health Care Expenditures

Expenditures by Type of Care and Source of Funds

Expenditures for hospital care as a percent of national health expenditures continue to decline. The sources of funds for medical care differ substantially according to the type of medical care being provided.

■ **Expenditures for hospital care** continued to decline as a percent of national health expenditures from 42 percent in 1980 to 34 percent in 1997. Physician services accounted for 20 percent of the total in 1997 and nursing home care and drugs for 8 and 10 percent each (table 119).

■ Between 1993 and 1997 the average annual increase in **total expenses in community hospitals** was 3.5 percent, following a period of higher growth that averaged 9.3 percent per year from 1985 to 1993 (table 123).

■ In 1997, 35 percent of **personal health care expenditures** were paid by the Federal Government and 10 percent by State and local government; private health insurance paid 32 percent, and 19 percent was paid out-of-pocket. Between 1990 and 1997 the share paid by the Federal Government increased 6 percentage points, while the share paid out-of-pocket decreased 4 percentage points (table 120).

■ In 1997 the major **sources of funds** for hospital care were Medicare (33 percent) and private health insurance (31 percent). Physician services were also primarily funded by private health insurance (50 percent) and Medicare (21 percent). In contrast, nursing home care was financed primarily by Medicaid (48 percent) and out-of-pocket payments (31 percent) (table 120).

■ In 1995 **funding for health research and development** increased by 7 percent to $36 billion. Between 1990 and 1995 industry's share of funding for health research increased from 46 to 52 percent while the Federal Government's share decreased from 42 to 37 percent (table 127).

■ **The National Institutes of Health (NIH)** account for about 80 percent of Federal funding for research and development. In 1997 the National Cancer Institute

accounted for 20 percent of NIH's research and development budget, the National Heart, Lung and Blood Institute for 12 percent, and the National Institute of Allergy and Infectious Diseases for 10 percent (table 127).

■ In 1998 **Federal expenditures for HIV-related activities** increased 7 percent to $8.9 billion, a slowdown from an average annual increase of 11 percent between 1995 and 1997. Of the total Federal spending in 1998, 57 percent was for medical care, 21 percent for research, and 8 percent for education and prevention (table 128).

Publicly Funded Health Programs

The two major publicly-funded health programs are Medicare and Medicaid. Medicare is funded by the Federal government and reimburses the elderly for their health care. Medicaid is funded jointly by the Federal and State governments to provide health care for the poor. Medicaid benefits and eligibility vary by State. Medicare and Medicaid health care utilization and costs vary considerably by State.

■ In 1997 the **Medicare** program had 38.4 million enrollees and expenditures of $214 billion. The total number of enrollees increased less than 1 percent over the previous year while expenditures increased by 7 percent (table 134).

■ In 1997 **hospital insurance (HI)** accounted for 65 percent of Medicare expenditures. Expenditures for home health agency care increased to 14.4 percent of HI expenditures in 1997 up from 5.5 percent in 1990. Expenditures for skilled nursing facilities more than doubled to 9.0 percent of the HI expenditures over the same period (table 134).

■ In 1997 **supplementary medical insurance (SMI)** accounted for 35 percent of Medicare expenditures. Group practice prepayment increased from 6.4 percent of the SMI expenditures in 1990 to 14.8 percent in 1997 (table 134).

■ Of the 33.4 million elderly **Medicare** enrollees in 1996, 12 percent were 85 years of age and over and 11 percent were 65–66 years of age. Medicare payments increase with age from an average of $2,574

12

per Medicare enrollee for those aged 65–66 years to $6,666 for those 85 years and over (table 135).

■ In 1996 **Medicare payments per enrollee** averaged $5,048 in the United States, ranging from $3,500 in Nebraska, South Dakota, and Montana to more than $6,200 in Massachusetts, Louisiana, and the District of Columbia (table 143).

■ In 1997 **Medicaid** vendor payments totaled $124 billion, a 2-percent increase from the previous year. Recipients declined from 36.1 million in 1996 to 33.6 million in 1997, a 7-percent decrease (table 136).

■ In 1997 children under the age of 21 years comprised 46 percent of **Medicaid** recipients but accounted for only 13 percent of expenditures. The aged, blind, and disabled accounted for 30 percent of recipients and 74 percent of expenditures (table 136).

■ In 1997 one-quarter of **Medicaid** payments went to nursing facilities and 19 percent to general hospitals. Home health care accounted for 10 percent of Medicaid payments in 1997, up from 5 percent in 1990 (table 137).

■ In 1997 almost 6 percent of **Medicaid** recipients received home health care at a cost averaging $6,575 per recipient. Early and periodic screening, rural health clinics, and family planning services combined received less than 2 percent of Medicaid funds in 1997, with the cost per recipient averaging between $200 and $251 for each service (table 137).

■ In 1997, 48 percent of **Medicaid recipients were enrolled in managed care**, up from 40 percent the previous year. In 1997 the percent of Medicaid recipients enrolled in managed care varied substantially among the States from 0 in Alaska and Wyoming to 100 percent in Washington and Tennessee (table 144).

■ Between 1996 and 1997 spending on health care by the **Department of Veterans Affairs** increased by less than 5 percent to $17.1 billion. In 1997, 43 percent of the total was for inpatient hospital care, down from 58 percent in 1990, 37 percent for outpatient care, up from 25 percent in 1990, and 10 percent for nursing home care, unchanged since 1990 (table 138).

Privately Funded Health Care

About 70 percent of the population has private health insurance, most of which is obtained through the workplace. The share of employees' total compensation devoted to health insurance has declined in recent years. The health insurance market is changing rapidly as new types of managed care products are introduced. The use of traditional fee-for-service medical care continues to decline.

■ Between 1993 and 1997 the age-adjusted proportion of the population under 65 years of age with **private health insurance** has remained stable at 70–71 percent after declining from 76 percent in 1989. Some 92 percent of private coverage was obtained through the workplace (a current or former employer or union) in 1997 (table 129).

■ Nearly all persons 65 years of age and over are eligible for Medicare and most have additional health care coverage. However the percent with additional coverage has been declining. Between 1994 and 1997 the age-adjusted percent of the elderly with **private health insurance** declined from 78 to 70 percent while the percent with only Medicare coverage increased from 13 to 21 percent (table 130).

■ Between 1994 and 1998 **private employers' health insurance costs** per employee-hour worked declined from $1.14 to $1.00 per hour after increasing by 24 percent between 1991 and 1994. Among private employers the share of total compensation devoted to health insurance declined from 6.7 percent in 1994 to 5.4 percent in 1998 (table 122).

■ The average monthly contribution by full-time employees for family **medical care benefits** was more than 50 percent higher in small companies ($182 in 1996) than in medium and large companies ($118 in 1995) (table 133).

■ During the 1990's the use of **traditional fee-for-service** medical care benefits by full-time employees in private companies declined sharply. In 1996 in small companies, 36 percent of full-time employees who participated in medical care benefits were in fee-for-service plans, down from 74 percent in

1990. In 1995 in medium and large companies, 37 percent of participating full-time employees were in fee-for-service plans, down from 67 percent in 1991 (table 133).

■ In 1998, 29 percent of the U.S. population was enrolled in **health maintenance organizations (HMO's)**, ranging from 21–23 percent in the South and Midwest to 38–39 percent in the Northeast and West. HMO enrollment has been steadily increasing. Enrollment in 1998 was 77 million persons, double the enrollment in 1993 (table 132).

■ In 1997 non-Hispanic black and Hispanic persons were less likely to have private health insurance than non-Hispanic white persons. However among those with private health insurance coverage, non-Hispanic black and Hispanic persons were more likely than their non-Hispanic white counterparts to enroll in **HMO's**. The elderly were less likely to be enrolled in private HMO's than younger adults and children (table 131).

■ In 1998 the percent of the population enrolled in **HMO's** varied among the States from 0 in Alaska and Vermont to 54 percent in Massachusetts. Other States with more than 40 percent of the population enrolled in HMO's in 1998 include Connecticut, Delaware, Maryland, Oregon, and California (table 145).

■ In 1997 the proportion of the population without **health care coverage** (either public or private) was 16.1 percent, compared with 15.6 percent the previous year and 12.9 percent in 1987. In 1997 the proportion of the population without health care coverage varied from less than 10 percent in Hawaii, Wisconsin, Minnesota, and Vermont to more than 20 percent in Arkansas, Mississippi, Texas, New Mexico, Arizona, and California (table 146).

The older population in the United States is large and growing. The post-World War II baby boom generation is entering middle age, and in the early part of the twenty-first century, this group will swell the ranks of the older population both in the United States and in other Western industrialized countries.

The year 1999 has been proclaimed the International Year of Older Persons by the United Nations to draw attention to the aging of societies and to the contributions and needs of older persons. This chartbook on health and aging describes the health of older persons in the United States at the end of the twentieth century.

The health of older Americans affects everyone, either directly or indirectly. For older persons, quality of life in later years is directly influenced by their health and functional status. Persons who are disabled by chronic conditions or by injuries such as falls have difficulty living independently and managing their personal affairs. Young and middle-aged persons who care for aging parents, grandparents, relatives, and friends know first hand the challenges, both financial and emotional, of declining health in old age. For society as a whole, the financing of health care services for the elderly, particularly through Medicare, the Federal health insurance program for elderly and disabled persons, is a significant outlay of resources (1).

A long and healthy life is a universal goal. In the twentieth century great progress has been made toward increasing the years of life for most Americans. In the United States today, most persons can look forward to a significant number of years spent in old age. Whether these will be healthy years, with high levels of physical and cognitive functioning, the ability to live independently in the community, and access to affordable health care, is of concern to all.

Organization of the Chartbook

This chartbook focuses on the group that has traditionally been defined as elderly in the United States, persons 65 years of age and over. The definition of old age is social as well as biological. Certain roles (for example, being retired or being a grandparent) usually characterize old age, although these life events may occur at many different chronological ages. Within the population 65 years of age and over, there is much variation in health and levels of activity.

Age and sex differences are emphasized in this chartbook. Many of the health status and utilization measures are shown by three or four age groups to draw attention to the heterogeneity in health among the older population and to highlight the "oldest-old," persons 85 years of age and over, the fastest growing segment of the elderly population. Data for women are presented first, as they are the majority of the older population and represent 7 out of 10 persons 85 years of age and over. Race and ethnic variation in health among the older population, a topic of increasing interest among researchers, is discussed when the data sources allow for such analysis (2).

Characterizing the health of older persons requires not only measuring mortality and morbidity but also describing their living arrangements, their levels of activity, who assists them, and how they utilize the health care system.

This chartbook is divided into sections on population, health status, and health care access and utilization. The emphasis is on current measures of health and health care utilization among the older population. Important trends in health and health care are mentioned in the bullets accompanying the figures, and references are made to related tables in *Health, United States*. Highlights are presented first. The 34 figures and accompanying text are then followed by technical notes and data tables for each figure.

Here is a summary of each section:

Population

The first section of the chartbook describes some sociodemographic characteristics of older persons. The most notable characteristic is the increasing size of the older population (figure 1). Today, approximately 13 out of every 100 Americans are 65 years of age and over. It is estimated that in 2030, 20 out of 100 persons will be 65 years of age and over, and 2 out of 100 will be 85 years of age and over. There are more women than men at every age among the elderly population.

In 1997 approximately one-third of all noninstitutionalized older persons lived alone. Among women 85 years of age and over, 60 percent lived alone (figure 2). The proportion of all persons 85 years of age and over living alone rose from 39 percent in 1980 to 49 percent in 1997. Approximately 4 percent of persons 65 years of age and over were in nursing homes in 1997, and women had higher rates of nursing home residence than men (figure 3).

While poverty rates among the older population have declined since the 1960's, 1 out of 10 persons 65 years of age and over in 1997 lived in families with income below the poverty line (figure 4).

Health Status

The second section of the chartbook presents measures of health status. Figures on life expectancy (figures 5 and 6) show gains in years of life from 1950 to the present and differentials in life expectancy by race and sex. In 1997 life expectancy in the United States was 79.4 years for women and 73.6 years for men. Life expectancy at birth, as well as life expectancy at ages 65 and 85 years of age, has increased over time as death rates for many causes of death have declined.

The biggest decreases in mortality have been in death rates for heart disease and stroke. However, death rates for some causes of death among the elderly, for example pneumonia and influenza, have increased in the last two decades.

Many factors have contributed to mortality declines in the last 50 years: changes in health behaviors, for example, declines in smoking and improvements in nutrition, increases in the overall educational level of the older population, and innovations in medical technology.

Will life expectancy continue to increase? The above factors will likely also influence life expectancy in the future. For example, the percent of elderly persons who have completed high school will increase from almost 66 percent in 1997 to an estimated 83 percent in 2030. Nearly one-fourth of the elderly in

2030 will be college graduates (3). Government projections suggest that life expectancy in the United States will reach 84.3 years for women and 79.7 years for men by 2050 (4). Japan currently has the longest life expectancy in the world, 82.9 years for women and 76.4 years for men in 1995. At age 65 Japanese women have a life expectancy of 20.9 years. Considerable research is underway to determine what maximum life span is, how life expectancy may be enhanced, and what are the characteristics of long-lived families.

Next the chartbook presents measures of health and disability, including the prevalence of chronic conditions (figure 11), visual and hearing impairments (figures 12 and 13), osteoporosis (figure 14), physical functioning and disability (figure 15), conditions associated with disability (figure 16), overweight (figures 17 and 18), oral health (figures 19 and 20), and social activity and exercise (figures 21–22).

The wide differences by age in the health of the older population are clearly seen in nearly all measures. Rates of illness and disability increase sharply among persons 85 years of age and over compared with persons 65–74 years or 75–84 years of age. For example, 35 percent of white men 70–74 years of age in 1995 were hearing impaired compared with 56 percent of white men 85 years of age and over (figure 13). Nineteen percent of women 65–74 years of age had osteoporosis compared with 51 percent of women 85 years of age and over (figure 14). Five percent of women 70–74 years of age were unable to do one or more activities of daily living compared with 23 percent of women 85 years of age and over (figure 15). Increases in illness and disability are accompanied by decreases in social activity. Among women 70–74 years of age, 65 percent participated in at least five different social activities in a 2-week period compared with 39 percent of women 85 years of age and over (figure 21).

Health Care Access and Utilization

The last section of the chartbook focuses on health care access and utilization. These measures show that, in general, persons 85 years of age and over have higher rates of health care utilization than younger persons. Women 85 years of age and over were twice as likely to use assistive devices such as canes, walkers, and hearing aids as women 70–74 years of age (figure 25). Hospitalizations for fractures were 5 times as high among women 85 years of age and over as for women 65–74 years of age (figure 27). Rates of home health care use were over 4 times as high for the oldest women as for women 65–74 years of age (figure 29).

At the same time, persons 85 years of age and over were less likely than younger persons to be covered by private insurance in addition to Medicare. Less than one-half of non-Hispanic black persons and Hispanic persons 85 years of age and over had private insurance to supplement their Medicare coverage (figure 31). While the total costs of heart disease and diabetes were lower among the population 85 years of age and over compared with the population 75–84 years of age, per capita costs of health care for these illnesses were highest among the oldest members of the population (figures 33 and 34).

Data

The data presented in the charts are from nationally representative health surveys or vital statistics. One of the data sources (the Second Supplement on Aging to the 1994 National Health Interview Survey) is a survey of persons 70 years of age and over. Consequently, some figures present data for the population 70 years of age and over instead of the population 65 years of age and over. For data from the National Health Interview Survey (except for the Second Supplement on Aging and supplements on oral health in 1983 and 1993 and exercise in 1995), survey years are combined (1994–96 or 1993–95) to create a large enough sample for analysis.

Measures of health are based on the noninstitutionalized population that excludes residents of nursing homes, except where noted, for example rates of nursing home residence (figure 3), life expectancy and mortality (figures 5–9), or hospital discharge rates (figure 27). Consequently, the measures of health in the chartbook in general are biased slightly

upward; that is, the noninstitutionalized older population is healthier than the older population as a whole.

In national surveys that are not specifically designed to study the elderly, the number of observations may not be large enough to analyze differences among all age, sex, and race/ethnicity groups. For certain topics, data are presented for all races combined in the chart, and significant race differences (if they exist) are discussed in the accompanying text.

Data Gaps

Although the chartbook focuses on the elderly, the health of persons in old age is related to their health status and health behaviors throughout life. Those in their middle ages are of particular interest to researchers today in planning for the health care needs of the elderly of the twenty-first century. The large size of the baby boom cohorts ensures that their health, health care utilization, and financial status will have a large impact on society. The figures in this chartbook do not cover the population 50–64 years of age. However, many of the data sources used, for example the National Health Interview Survey, the National Health and Nutrition Examination Survey, the National Hospital Discharge Survey, and vital statistics, contain information on these age groups. In addition, many tables in *Health, United States* present data for middle aged persons.

This chartbook does not include measures of health by socioeconomic status. Although differences in health status and health care utilization by socioeconomic status exist, they are generally smaller for older persons compared with younger persons.

Most surveys have only income-based measures of socioeconomic status and do not capture the accumulated wealth and assets on which many older persons rely. In addition, many older survey respondents do not know their incomes or are not willing to share this information, resulting in large proportions of respondents with missing data. For example, in the Second Supplement on Aging, approximately one-fourth of the sample are missing data on the family income question.

Important work is in progress in this area to collect better information on the socioeconomic status of older adults. Two surveys conducted by the Institute for Social Research of the University of Michigan have collected wealth and asset information: the Health and Retirement Study that focuses on persons 51–61 years of age and a survey called Asset and Health Dynamics Among the Oldest Old, which studies persons 70 years of age and over (5).

Cognitive and emotional functioning are crucial to good health but are difficult to measure in surveys using traditional data collection tools. There is debate regarding the prevalence of Alzheimer's disease in the older population, and estimates of the number of older Americans suffering from the disease range from about 2 million to 4 million persons (6).

The prevalence of major depression among the noninstitutionalized elderly is estimated by some studies to be less than 3 percent, although the prevalence of depressive symptoms is higher. In addition, community-dwelling older persons have lower rates of depression than persons in nursing homes or care facilities (7). New approaches are being developed to provide better national, population-based estimates of cognitive functioning and mental health among the elderly.

Nutritional status is another area important to the health of older persons but difficult to measure in national surveys. What people eat and how well the food is absorbed, digested, and utilized are crucial in determining the health status of individuals.

Although the topic of nutrition is not presented directly in the chartbook, many of the risk factors that contribute singly or interactively to nutritional problems are covered here. For example, poverty and economic uncertainties are important contributors to malnutrition. Limited income decreases the variety and quantity of food purchased and consumed. Living alone and eating alone contribute to reduced food intake, while sadness and depression may exacerbate this situation and lead to social isolation with its potential for changes in appetite, energy level, weight and well-being.

The suppressing effect of certain medications on taste, smell, and appetite can also lead to reduced food intake. Physical disabilities such as difficulty walking, grocery shopping, and preparing food further restrict access to adequate amounts and types of food. Inability to carry heavy things during shopping can limit the selection of food products such as fresh fruits and vegetables, and, therefore, limit variety and complete nutrient intake. Similarly, missing, loose, or decayed teeth or ill-fitting dentures make it hard for elders to eat well.

In addition, altered mental status such as confusion and memory loss make it hard to remember what, when, and if one has eaten and limit the ability to modify diets in response to chronic diseases. To the extent that one has these risk factors, food insufficiency and/or malnutrition may be a problem.

The prevalence of food insufficiency in 1988–94 has been estimated from the Third National Health and Nutrition Examination Survey to be 1.7 percent among all persons 60 years of age and over and 5.9 percent among low-income persons in that age group (8). Forthcoming analyses from this survey will provide new data on the nutritional status of the older population.

Conclusion

The older population throughout the world is growing. The International Year of Older Persons proclaimed by the United Nations provides an opportunity to evaluate the health of older persons at the end of a century of remarkable advances in health and longevity.

Americans live longer than ever before. Persons who survive to age 65 in the United States today can expect to live on average nearly 18 more years.

This chartbook examines a variety of current measures of health and health care utilization from national data sources. The health of individuals in old age reflects the cumulative effect of health behaviors and health care over a lifetime as well as advances in medical technology and the biological process of aging. These factors cannot be disentangled by measuring health status at one point in time.

The health of the older population varies greatly. The largest differences are age related. Persons 85 years of age and over, the majority of whom (71 percent) are women, have noticeably higher rates of illness, disability, and utilization of health care services than older persons who are less than 85 years of age. Ensuring good health and quality of life in old age requires attention to differences in the population by race and ethnicity, sex, and age.

References

1. Waldo DR, Sonnefeld ST, McKusick DR, Arnett RH. Health expenditures by age group, 1977 and 1987. Health Care Financing Review 10(4):111–20. 1989.

2. Martin LG, Soldo BJ, eds. Racial and ethnic differences in the health of older Americans. Washington, DC: National Academy Press. 1997.

3. U.S. Bureau of the Census. Current population reports. Special studies, P23-190. 65+ in the United States. U.S. Government Printing Office, Washington. 1996.

4. Day JC. Population projections of the United States by age, sex, race, and Hispanic origin: 1995 to 2050. U.S. Bureau of the Census. Current population reports; P25–1130. Washington: U.S. Department of Commerce. 1996.

5. Soldo BJ, Hurd MD, Rodgers WL, Wallace RB. Asset and health dynamics among the oldest old: An overview of the AHEAD study. J Gerontol 52B(special issue): 1–20.1997.

6. U.S. General Accounting Office. Alzheimer's disease: Estimates of prevalence in the United States. GAO/HEHS-98–16. 1998.

7. Diagnosis and treatment of depression in late life. NIH Consens Statement Online 1991 Nov4–6. 9(3):1–27.<http://www.nih.gov>. November 1998.

8. Alaimo K, Briefel RR, Frongillo, Jr EA, Olson CM. Food insufficiency exists in the United States: Results from the Third National Health and Nutrition Examination Survey (NHANES III). AJPH 88(3):419–26. 1998.

Population

Demographic Characteristics

■   In 1997, 13 percent of the U.S. population was 65 years of age and over. Among these 34 million persons, nearly 4 million were 85 years of age and over. The population of the United States is aging; the elderly population is growing at a faster rate than the population as a whole. In addition, the proportion of the population 85 years of age and over is growing faster than the elderly population as a whole. Projections of the population indicate that 70 million persons will be 65 years of age and over in the year 2030, representing 20 percent of the total U.S. population. It is estimated that the population 85 years of age and over will more than double to approximately 8.5 million persons.

■   There are more women than men among the older population. Among persons 65 years of age and over in 1997, 59 percent were women. At the oldest ages, the sex ratio is even higher; 71 percent of persons 85 years of age and over were women.

■   In 1997 a larger proportion of the non-Hispanic white population was over the age of 65 compared with other racial and ethnic groups. Fifteen percent of the non-Hispanic white population was 65 years of age and over compared with 8 percent of the black population, 7 percent of the Asian or Pacific Islander population, and 7 percent of the American Indian or Alaska Native population. Among persons of Hispanic origin, 6 percent were 65 years of age and over. However, the older non-Hispanic white population is growing more slowly compared with other groups. From 1990 to 1997, the proportion of the population 65 years of age and over grew more than five times as fast among Hispanic persons as among non-Hispanic white persons.

Figure 1. Population 65 years of age and over: United States, 1950–2030

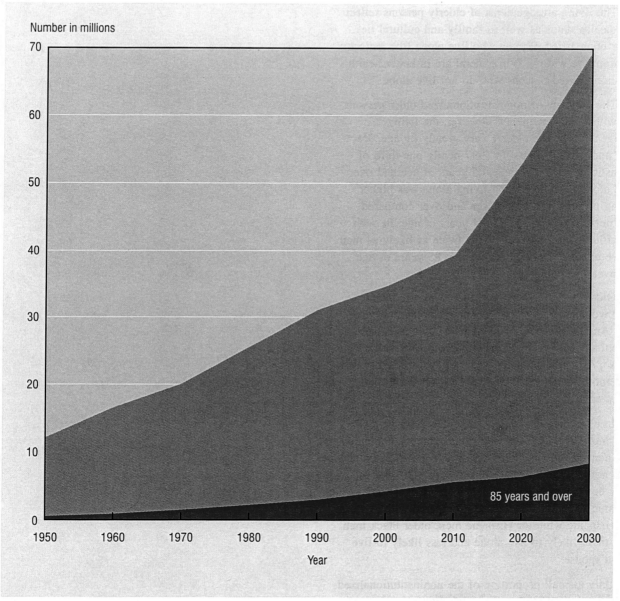

NOTES: Figures for 1950–90 are based on decennial censuses. Figures for 2000–30 are middle series population projections of the U.S. Bureau of the Census.

SOURCES: See *Health,United States, 1999*, table 1 for data years 1950–90. For data years 2000–30, see U.S. Bureau of the Census. Day JC. Population projections of the United States by age, sex, race, and Hispanic origin: 1995 to 2050. Current population reports; P25–1130. Washington: U.S. Department of Commerce. 1996.

Population

Living Arrangements

■   The living arrangements of elderly persons reflect their health status as well as family and cultural ties. Older nonmarried persons who live alone (the majority of whom are widowed) in general are in better health than nonmarried persons who do not live alone.

■   The majority of noninstitutionalized older persons live with family members; however, the living arrangements of the elderly vary greatly by age, sex, race, and marital status. In 1997 nearly one-third of noninstitutionalized persons 65 years of age and over lived alone. The proportion living alone was higher among persons 85 years of age and over compared with persons 65–74 and 75–84 years of age. In each age group, women were at least twice as likely as men to live alone. Six out of ten women 85 years of age and over lived alone.

■   Older men are more likely to be married than older women, in large part because women outlive men. Among persons 75–84 years of age, men were more than twice as likely as women to live with a spouse. Among persons 85 years of age and over, men were more than 4 times as likely as women to live with a spouse.

■   In every age group, black and Hispanic women were more likely to live with other relatives compared with non-Hispanic white women. At ages 75 years and over, non-Hispanic white women were 1.2 times as likely as black women and 1.7 times as likely as Hispanic women to live alone. Compared with non-Hispanic white or Hispanic men, older black men were more likely to live alone and less likely to live with a spouse.

■   Only a small proportion of the noninstitutionalized older population lived with nonrelatives. Among women 65 years of age and over, 2 percent lived with nonrelatives. Among men, the percent living with nonrelatives was 3 percent among persons 65–84 years of age and 7 percent among persons 85 years of age and over.

Figure 2. Living arrangements of persons 65 years of age and over by age and sex: United States, 1997

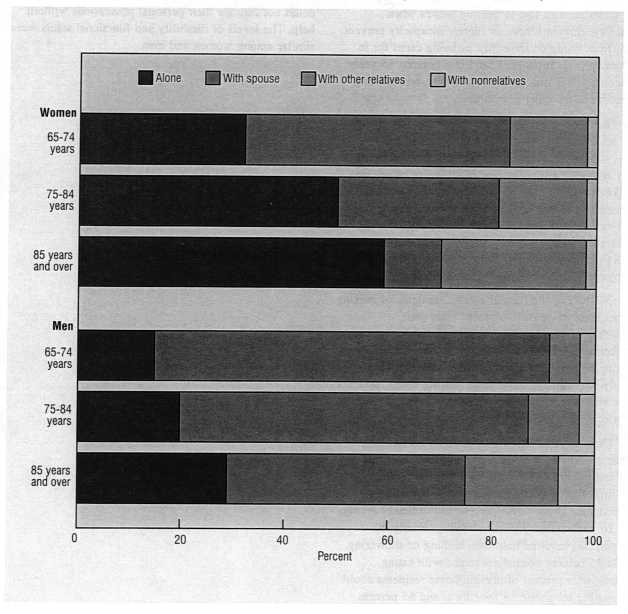

NOTES: Figures are based on the noninstitutionalized population. See Technical Notes for definitions of categories of living arrangements.

SOURCE: Lugaila TA. U.S. Bureau of the Census. Marital Status and Living Arrangements: March 1997 (Update), Series P20–506.

Nursing Home Residence

■ Older persons live in nursing homes when disability, chronic illness, or mental incapacity prevent them from living on their own or being cared for in the community. In 1997, 1.5 million persons 65 years of age and over were in nursing homes, representing 4 percent of the older population.

■ The rates of nursing home residence vary by age, sex, and race. In 1997, 11 in 1,000 persons 65–74 years of age were nursing home residents compared with 46 out of 1,000 persons 75–84 years of age and 192 out of 1,000 persons 85 years of age and over. Women had higher rates of nursing home residence than men, and the sex difference increased with age. Black persons 65–74 years of age and black men 75–84 years of age were more likely than their white counterparts to be nursing home residents.

■ One-half of the current elderly residents of nursing homes were 85 years of age and over, and three-fourths were women. Research has shown that unmarried elderly persons have a higher risk of nursing home admission than married persons (1). Nearly two-thirds of all current nursing home residents were widowed, with female residents twice as likely to be widowed as male residents.

■ There is variation in the health of nursing home residents. Among nursing home residents 65 years of age and over in 1997, 48 percent were receiving full-time skilled nursing care under a physician's supervision. Twenty-nine percent had difficulty seeing, and 26 percent had difficulty hearing. Nearly all (96 percent) required help with bathing or showering, while 45 percent needed assistance with eating. Seventy-nine percent of nursing home residents could not use the telephone on their own, and 65 percent

could not care for their personal possessions without help. The levels of disability and functional status were similar among women and men.

Reference

1. Freedman VA. Family structure and the risk of nursing home admission. J Gerontol (51B):S61–9. 1996.

Figure 3. Nursing home residents among persons 65 years of age and over by age, sex, and race: United States, 1997

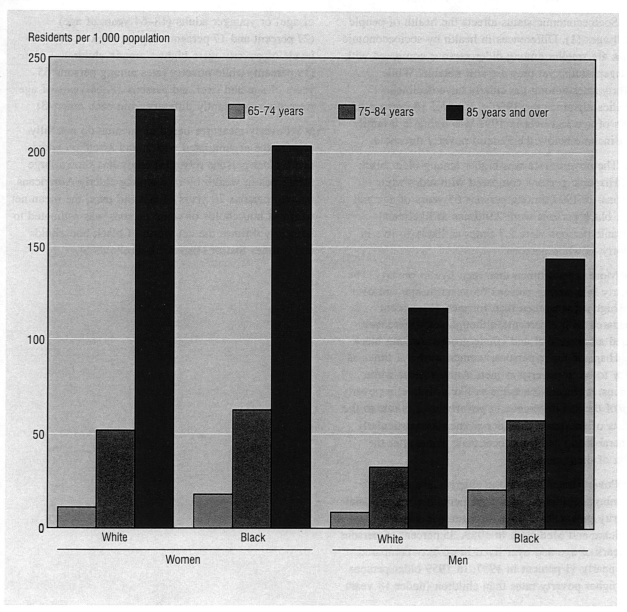

NOTES: Nursing home residents exclude residents in personal care or domiciliary care homes. Age refers to age at time of interview. Rates are based on the resident population as of July 1, 1997, adjusted for net underenumeration using the 1990 National Population Adjustment Matrix from the U.S. Bureau of the Census.

SOURCE: Centers for Disease Control and Prevention, National Center for Health Statistics, National Nursing Home Survey. See related *Health, United States, 1999*, tables 97 and 98.

Poverty

■ Socioeconomic status affects the health of people of all ages (1). Differences in health by socioeconomic status are smaller among older persons compared with younger adults, yet they are still notable. While poverty rates among the elderly have declined significantly since the 1960's, 1 out of 10 persons 65 years of age and over in 1997 was living in a family with income below the Federal poverty threshold.

■ The poverty rate was higher among older black and Hispanic persons compared with older white persons. In 1997 among persons 65 years of age and over, black persons were 2.9 times as likely and Hispanic persons were 2.7 times as likely to live in poverty as white persons.

■ More older women than men live in poverty. The poverty rate among persons 65 years of age and over was higher for women than for men (13 percent compared with 7 percent), although sex differences varied among racial and ethnic groups. Among black and Hispanic older persons, women were 1.3 times as likely to be in poverty as men. Among older white persons, women were twice as likely to live in poverty. Part of the sex difference in poverty rates is due to the effects of widowhood. Older women are particularly vulnerable to declines in economic status after the death of their spouse (2).

■ Poverty rates among the elderly have been declining as older persons have benefitted from Social Security payments and health insurance through Medicare and Medicaid. In 1959, 35 percent of persons 65 years of age and over lived in poverty compared with nearly 11 percent in 1997. In 1959 older persons had higher poverty rates than children (under 18 years

of age) or younger adults (18–64 years of age) (27 percent and 17 percent, respectively). In 1997 levels of poverty were highest among children (19 percent) while poverty rates among persons 65 years of age and over and persons 18–64 years of age were not significantly different from each other (3).

■ Poverty measures based on income do not fully capture the accumulated wealth and assets on which many older persons rely. One study has shown large disparities in wealth by race among elderly Americans. Among persons 70 years of age and over, the mean net worth of households of white persons was estimated to be nearly 4 times the net worth of black households and 3 times that of Hispanic households (4).

References

1. Pamuk E, Makuc D, Heck K, Reuben C, Lochner K. Socioeconomic status and health chartbook. Health, United States, 1998. Hyattsville, Maryland: National Center for Health Statistics. 1998.

2. Bound J, Duncan GJ, Laren DS, Oleinick L. Poverty dynamics in widowhood. J Gerontol (46): S115–124. 1991.

3. U.S. Census Bureau. "Historical Poverty Tables - People, (Table) 3. Poverty Status of People, by Age, Race, and Hispanic Origin: 1959–1997." Last revised September 24, 1998. <http://www.census.gov./hhes/poverty/histpov/hstpov3.html>.

4. Smith JP. Wealth inequality among older Americans. J Gerontol 52B (Special Issue): 74-81. 1997.

Figure 4. Percent in poverty among persons 65 years of age and over by sex, race, and Hispanic origin: United States, 1997

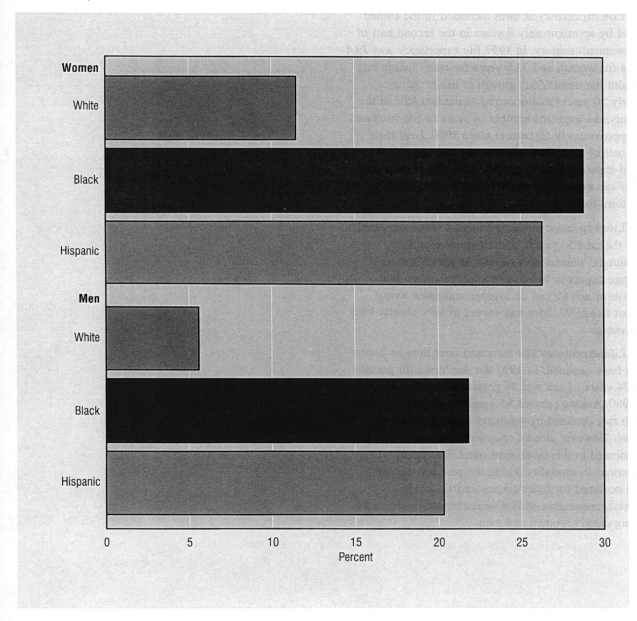

NOTES: Figures are based on the civilian noninstitutionalized population. The race groups white and black include persons of both Hispanic and non-Hispanic origin. Persons of Hispanic origin may be of any race. See Appendix II for poverty level definition.

SOURCE: Dalaker J, Naifeh M. U. S. Bureau of the Census. Poverty in the United States: 1997. Current population reports; Series P60–201. Washington: U.S. Government Printing Office. 1998.

Health Status

Life Expectancy

■   Life expectancy at birth increased in the United States by approximately 8 years in the second half of the twentieth century. In 1997 life expectancy was 79.4 years for women and 73.6 years for men. Taking into account the tremendous growth in life expectancy (nearly 20 years) that occurred in the first half of the century, the expected number of years of life increased by approximately 60 percent since 1900. Less than one-half of all children born at the turn of the century could expect to live to age 65. About 80 percent born today can expect to survive to age 65 and roughly one-third to age 85.

■   Life expectancy at ages 65 and 85 also increased over the past 50 years. Under current mortality conditions, women who survive to age 65 can on average expect to live to age 84, and women who survive to age 85 can on average anticipate living almost to age 92. Men can expect to have shorter lives on average.

■   Life expectancy has increased over time as death rates have declined. In 1997 the death rate for persons 65–74 years of age was 16 percent lower than the rate in 1980. Among persons 85 years of age and over, the death rate declined by 4 percent in the same time period. However, not all causes of death have contributed to this downward trend. The major reductions in mortality during the past two decades have occurred for heart disease and stroke. By contrast, pneumonia and influenza mortality increased among elderly women and men.

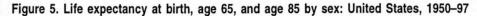
Figure 5. Life expectancy at birth, age 65, and age 85 by sex: United States, 1950–97

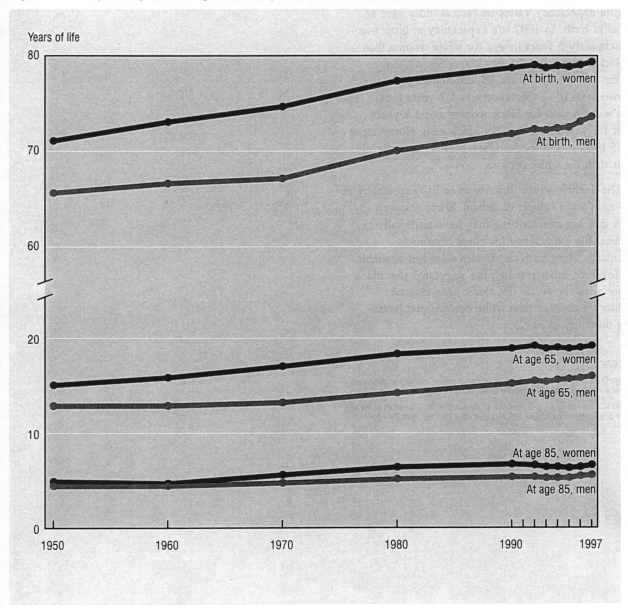

NOTE: See Technical Notes on life expectancy estimation.

SOURCE: Centers for Disease Control and Prevention, National Center for Health Statistics, National Vital Statistics System. See related *Health, United States, 1999*, table 28.

Life Expectancy by Race

■   Life expectancy varies by race at older ages as well as at birth. In 1997 life expectancy at birth was approximately 5 years longer for white women than for black women and 7 years longer for white men than for black men. At age 65, differences by race narrowed and life expectancy was 1.7 years longer for white women than for black women and 1.8 years longer for white men than for black men. However, at age 85 life expectancy for black persons was slightly higher than for white persons.

■   The declining race differences in life expectancy at older ages are a subject of debate. Some research shows that age misreporting may have artificially increased life expectancy for black persons, particularly when birth certificates were not available (1). However, other research has suggested that black persons who survive to the oldest ages may be healthier on average than white persons and have lower mortality rates (2).

References

1. Preston SH, Elo IT, Rosenwaike I, Hill M. African-American mortality at older ages: Results of a matching study. Demography 33(2): 193–209. 1996.

2. Manton KC, Stallard E, Wing S. Analyses of black and white differentials in the age trajectory of mortality in two closed cohort studies. Stat Med 10: 1043–59. 1991.

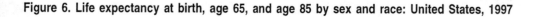

Figure 6. Life expectancy at birth, age 65, and age 85 by sex and race: United States, 1997

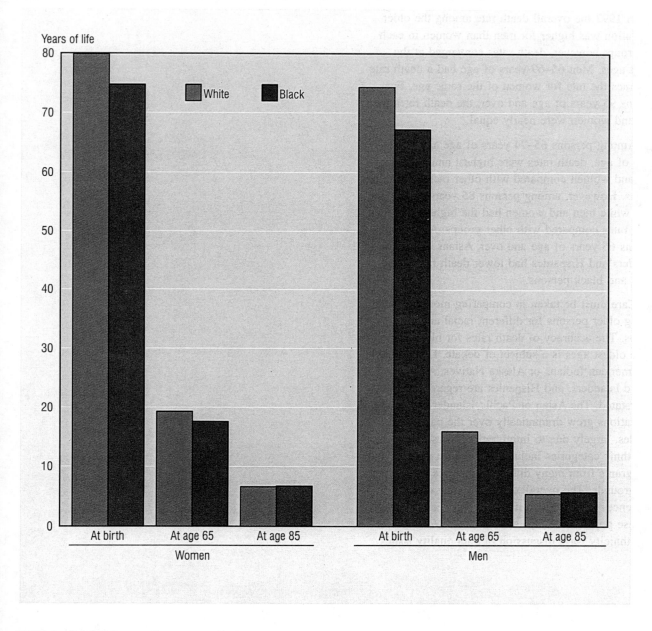

NOTE: See Technical Notes on life expectancy estimation.

SOURCE: Centers for Disease Control and Prevention, National Center for Health Statistics, National Vital Statistics System. See related *Health, United States, 1999*, table 28.

Health and Aging ....

Deaths From All Causes

■   In 1997 the overall death rate among the older population was higher for men than women in each age group; however, death rates converged at the oldest ages. Men 65–69 years of age had a death rate 1.7 times the rate for women of the same age. For persons 95 years of age and over, the death rates for men and women were nearly equal.

■   Among persons 65–74 years of age and 75–84 years of age, death rates were highest among black men and women compared with other racial and ethnic groups. However, among persons 85 years of age and over, white men and women had the highest recorded death rates compared with other groups. Among all persons 65 years of age and over, Asians or Pacific Islanders and Hispanics had lower death rates than white and black persons.

■   Care must be taken in comparing mortality levels among older persons for different racial and ethnic groups. The accuracy of death rates for black persons at the oldest ages is a subject of debate. Death rates for American Indians or Alaska Natives, Asians or Pacific Islanders, and Hispanics are regarded as understated. The Asian or Pacific Islander and Hispanic populations grew dramatically over the past two decades, largely due to immigration. These broad racial and ethnic categories include native-born persons and immigrants from many different countries and diverse backgrounds. The overall death rate may obscure differences in health and mortality between subgroups of these populations. See the Technical Notes on race and ethnicity for a discussion of data quality issues.

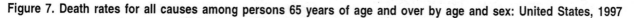

Figure 7. Death rates for all causes among persons 65 years of age and over by age and sex: United States, 1997

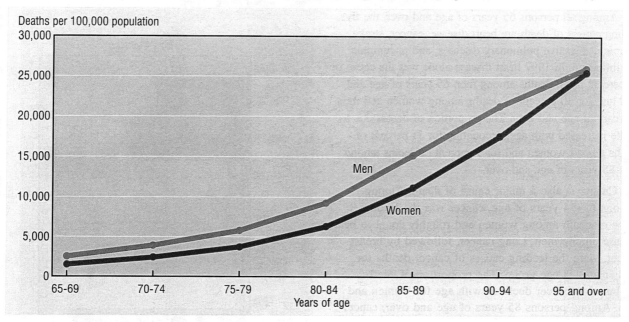

Figure 8. Death rates for all causes among persons 65 years of age and over by age, sex, race, and Hispanic origin: United States, 1997

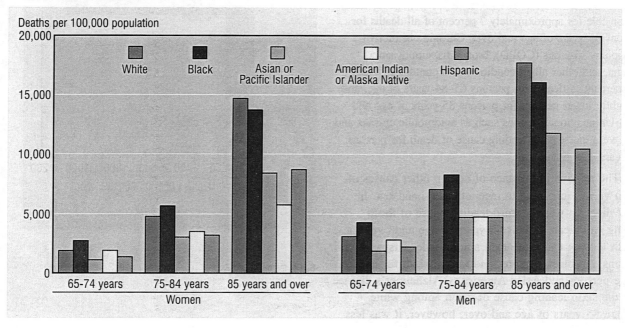

NOTE: Persons of Hispanic origin may be of any race.

SOURCE: Centers for Disease Control and Prevention, National Center for Health Statistics, National Vital Statistics System. See related *Health, United States, 1999*, table 36.

Health Status

Selected Leading Causes of Death

■ Among all persons 65 years of age and over, the five leading causes of death are heart disease, cancer, stroke, chronic obstructive pulmonary diseases, and pneumonia and influenza. In 1997 heart disease alone was the cause of 35 percent of all deaths among men 65 years of age and over and for 40 percent of deaths among women and men 85 years of age and over. The proportion of deaths due to stroke increased with age, accounting for 11 percent of deaths among women and for 9 percent of deaths among men 85 years of age and over.

■ Cancer is also a major cause of death. Among persons 65–74 years of age, cancer was the leading cause of death among women and roughly equal to heart disease among men. Lung cancer, followed by breast cancer, were the leading causes of cancer deaths for women in this age group. The proportion of deaths attributed to cancer declined with age for women and men. Among persons 85 years of age and over, cancer was responsible for 10 percent of deaths among women and for 16 percent of deaths among men.

■ Other major causes of death among the older population include pneumonia and influenza, which were responsible for approximately 7 percent of all deaths for persons 85 years of age and over. Chronic obstructive pulmonary diseases (COPD), bronchitis, emphysema, asthma, and other allied conditions, accounted for about 6–7 percent of deaths for persons 65–84 years of age, and a slightly lower percent for persons 85 years of age and over. Unintentional injuries such as automobile crashes and falls were the seventh leading cause of death for persons 65 years of age and over.

■ The relative importance of certain other causes of death varied according to race, ethnicity, and sex. In 1997 diabetes was the third leading cause of death among American Indians 65 years of age and over, the fourth leading cause of death among older Hispanic persons and black persons, and ranked sixth for older white persons and Asian Americans. Alzheimer's disease was the sixth leading cause of death among white women 85 years of age and over; however, it was less common among black women of the same age or men of either race.

Figure 9. Death rates for selected leading causes among persons 65 years of age and over by age and sex: United States, 1997

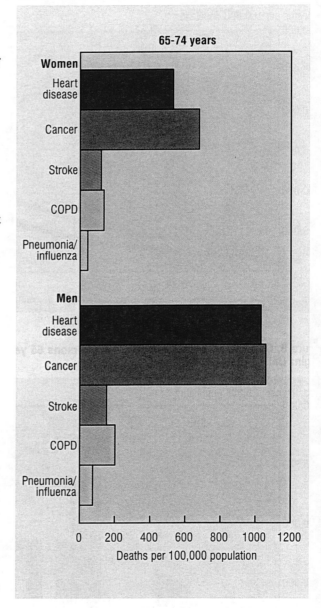

See notes on page 37.

Figure 9. Death rates for selected leading causes among persons 65 years of age and over by age and sex: United States, 1997—Continued

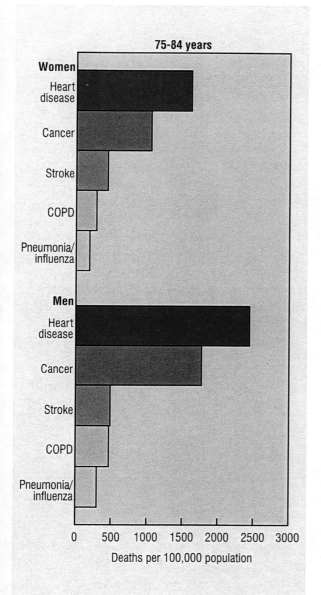

75-84 years

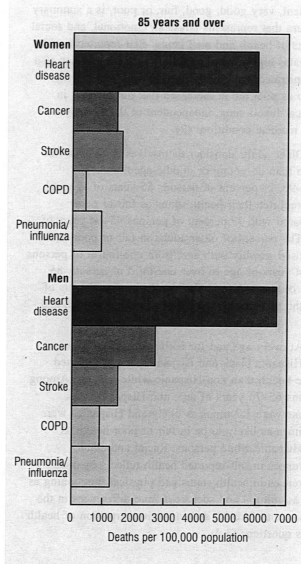

85 years and over

NOTES: COPD is chronic obstructive pulmonary diseases. For a description of *International Classification of Diseases* code numbers for causes of death, see Appendix II.

SOURCE: Centers for Disease Control and Prevention, National Center for Health Statistics, National Vital Statistics System. See related *Health, United States, 1999*, tables 33, 37–39, and 42.

Self-Reported Health

■ Self-assessed health, the reporting of health as excellent, very good, good, fair, or poor, is a summary measure that represents physical, emotional, and social aspects of health and well-being. Self-reported health correlates highly with mortality (1). Research has also demonstrated that elderly persons who report their health as poor are at increased risk for declines in physical functioning, independent of the severity of other medical conditions (2).

■ Older adults consider themselves to be in worse health than do young or middle-aged adults. In 1994–96, 28 percent of persons 65 years of age and over reported their health status as fair or poor compared with 17 percent of persons 45–64 years of age. The percent of older adults in fair or poor health increased steadily with age, from one-fourth of persons 65–74 years of age to over one-third of persons 85 years of age and over. The age pattern and levels of fair and poor health were similar among women and men.

■ At every age and for both men and women, non-Hispanic black and Hispanic persons reported worse health than non-Hispanic white persons. Among persons 65–74 years of age, non-Hispanic black persons were 1.7 times as likely and Hispanics were 1.4 times as likely to be in fair or poor health as non-Hispanic white persons. Racial and ethnic differences in self-reported health reflect objective differences in health status and physical functioning as well as cultural and socioeconomic differences in the assessment of health and in the interpretation of health status questions (3,4).

References

1. Idler EL, Benyamini Y. Self-reported health and mortality: A review of twenty-seven community studies. J Health Soc Behav 38:21–37. 1997.

2. Idler EL, Kasl SV. Self-ratings of health: Do they also predict change in functional ability? J Gerontol 50B(6):S344–53. 1995.

3. Coward RT, Peek CW, Henretta JC, et al. Race differences in the health of elders who live alone. J Aging Health 9(2): 147–70. 1997.

4. Krause NM, Jay GM. What do global self-rated health items measure? Med Care 32(9): 930–42. 1994.

Figure 10. Fair or poor health among persons 65 years of age and over by age, sex, race, and Hispanic origin: United States, 1994–96

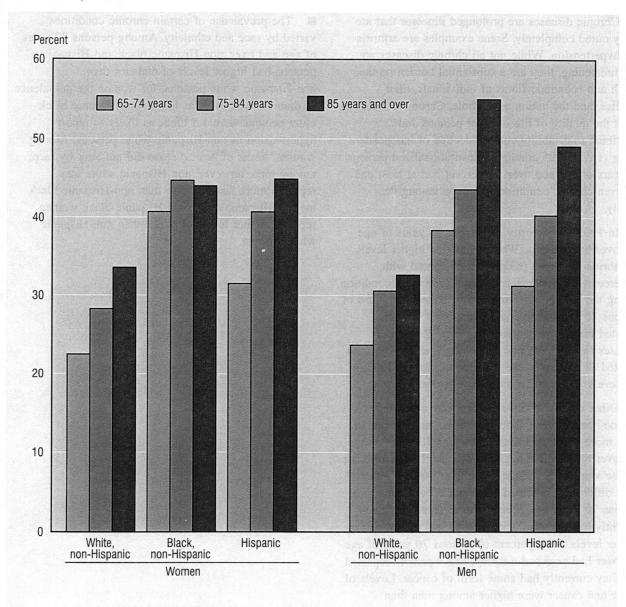

SOURCE: Centers for Disease Control and Prevention, National Center for Health Statistics, National Health Interview Survey. See related *Health, United States, 1999*, table 60.

Chronic Conditions

■ Chronic diseases are prolonged illnesses that are rarely cured completely. Some examples are arthritis and hypertension. While not all chronic diseases are life threatening, they are a substantial burden on the health and economic status of individuals, their families, and the nation as a whole. Chronic conditions affect the quality of life of older persons and contribute to disability and the decline of independent living (1). In 1995 among noninstitutionalized persons 70 years of age and over, 79 percent had at least one of seven chronic conditions common among the elderly.

■ In 1995 the majority of persons 70 years of age and over had arthritis. Women reported higher levels of arthritis than men (63 percent compared with 50 percent). Hypertension is also a prominent condition among the elderly, affecting approximately one-third of persons 70 years of age and over. Older women reported more hypertension than men. Respiratory illnesses (asthma, chronic bronchitis, and emphysema) affected 11 percent of the older population in 1995, and levels were similar among women and men.

■ Other chronic diseases suffered by older persons include heart disease, diabetes, stroke, and cancer. In 1995 more than one-fourth of persons 70 years of age and over reported having heart disease. Levels of heart disease were higher among men than women, although these differences declined with age. Eleven percent of persons 70 years of age and over reported that they currently had diabetes, with women and men reporting similar levels. Nine percent of persons 70 years of age and over had ever had a stroke, and 4 percent reported that they currently had some form of cancer. Levels of stroke and cancer were higher among men than women.

■ The prevalence of certain chronic conditions varied by race and ethnicity. Among persons 70 years of age and over, non-Hispanic black and Hispanic persons had higher levels of diabetes than non-Hispanic white persons; for women the prevalence of diabetes was twice as high. Non-Hispanic black older persons were 1.5 times as likely to report hypertension as non-Hispanic white persons. Among women, levels of heart disease did not vary by race; among men, however, non-Hispanic white men reported more heart disease than non-Hispanic black men or Hispanic men. Non-Hispanic black women reported higher levels of stroke than non-Hispanic white women.

Reference

1. Centers for Disease Control and Prevention. Unrealized prevention opportunities: Reducing the health and economic burden of chronic disease. Centers for Disease Control and Prevention, National Center for Chronic Disease Prevention and Health Promotion. 1997.

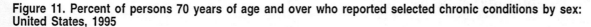

Figure 11. Percent of persons 70 years of age and over who reported selected chronic conditions by sex: United States, 1995

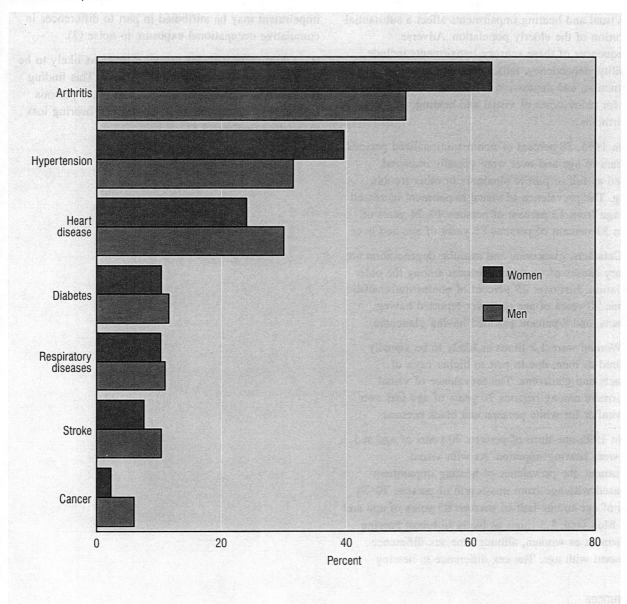

NOTES: Based on interviews conducted between October 1994 and March 1996 with noninstitutionalized persons. Percents are age adjusted. See Technical Notes for definitions of conditions and age adjustment procedures.

SOURCE: Centers for Disease Control and Prevention, National Center for Health Statistics, 1994 National Health Interview Survey, Second Supplement on Aging. See related figures 33 and 34 on cost of heart disease and cost of diabetes.

Health Status

Visual and Hearing Impairments

■ Visual and hearing impairments affect a substantial proportion of the elderly population. Adverse consequences of these sensory impairments include disability, dependency, falls, communication dysfunction, and depression (1). Effective treatments exist for many types of visual and hearing impairments.

■ In 1995, 18 percent of noninstitutionalized persons 70 years of age and over were visually impaired, defined as full or partial blindness or other trouble seeing. The prevalence of visual impairment increased with age from 13 percent of persons 70–74 years of age to 31 percent of persons 85 years of age and over.

■ Cataracts, glaucoma, and macular degeneration are primary causes of visual impairment among the older population. Just over 25 percent of noninstitutionalized persons 70 years of age and over reported having cataracts, and 8 percent reported having glaucoma.

■ Women were 1.2 times as likely to be visually impaired as men, due in part to higher rates of cataracts and glaucoma. The prevalence of visual impairment among persons 70 years of age and over was similar for white persons and black persons.

■ In 1995 one-third of persons 70 years of age and over were hearing impaired. As with visual impairment, the prevalence of hearing impairment increased with age from one-fourth of persons 70–74 years of age to one-half of persons 85 years of age and over. Men were 1.5 times as likely to report hearing impairment as women, although the sex difference decreased with age. The sex difference in hearing

impairment may be attributed in part to differences in cumulative occupational exposure to noise (2).

■ Older white persons were 1.8 times as likely to be hearing impaired as older black persons. This finding is consistent with studies that suggest black persons may be less susceptible to noise-induced hearing loss than white persons (3,4).

References

1. Lichtenstein MJ. Hearing and visual impairments. Clin Geriatr Med 8:173–82. 1992.

2. Wallhagen MI, Strawbridge WJ, Cohen RD, Kaplan GA. An increasing prevalence of hearing impairment and associated risk factors over three decades of the Alameda County study. AJPH 87(3):440-2. 1997.

3. Jerger J, Jerger S, Pepe P, Miller R. Race differences in susceptibility to noise-induced hearing loss. Am J Otol 7:425–9. 1986.

4. Henselman LW, Henderson D, Shadoan J, et al. Effects of noise exposure, race, and years of service on hearing in U.S. Army soldiers. Ear Hear 16:382–91. 1995.

Health Status

Figure 12. Prevalence of visual impairment among persons 70 years of age and over by age, sex, and race: United States, 1995

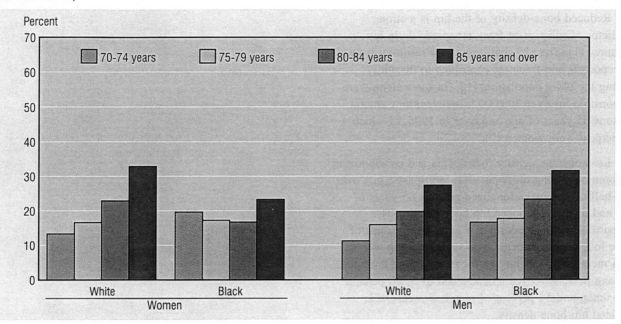

Figure 13. Prevalence of hearing impairment among persons 70 years of age and over by age, sex, and race: United States, 1995

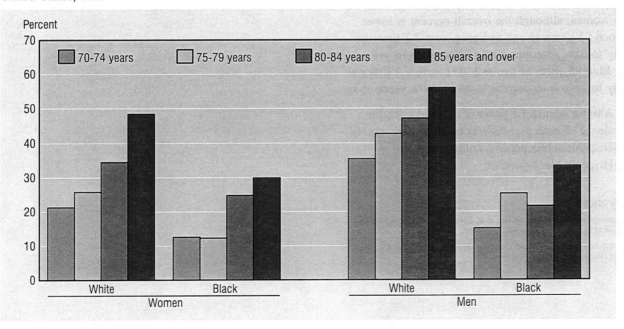

NOTES: Based on interviews conducted between October 1994 and March 1996 with noninstitutionalized persons. See Technical Notes for definitions of visual impairment and hearing impairment.

SOURCE: Centers for Disease Control and Prevention, National Center for Health Statistics, 1994 National Health Interview Survey, Second Supplement on Aging.

Health Status

Osteoporosis

■ Reduced bone density of the hip is a strong predictor of subsequent fractures, particularly hip fractures (1). The physical limitations resulting from osteoporosis and fractures contribute to disability among the older population. Hip fractures alone were responsible for over 300,000 hospitalizations among persons 65 years of age and over in 1996, of which 80 percent were women (2).

■ Loss of bone density (osteopenia and osteoporosis) is common among older persons. In 1988–94 just over one-half of noninstitutionalized persons 65 years of age and over had reduced hip bone density. The proportion with osteoporosis, a more severe form of bone loss than osteopenia, was higher among women than men and rose with age for both women and men. Among persons 85 years of age and over, 90 percent of women and 54 percent of men had measurable reduced hip bone density.

■ The prevalence of osteoporosis in the hip increases with age for both women and men. The percent with osteoporosis increases more steeply with age for men than women, although the overall percent is lower. Women 85 years of age and over were 2.7 times as likely to have osteoporosis as women 65–74 years of age. Men 85 years of age and over were 6.9 times as likely to have osteoporosis as men 65–74 years of age.

■ Among women 65 years of age and over, the prevalence of osteoporosis was twice as high among non-Hispanic white persons compared with non-Hispanic black persons.

References

1. Cummings SR, Black DM, Nevitt MC, et al. Bone density at various sites for prediction of hip fractures. Lancet 341:72–5. 1993.

2. Centers for Disease Control and Prevention, National Center for Health Statistics, National Hospital Discharge Survey. 1996.

Figure 14. Prevalence of reduced hip bone density among persons 65 years of age and over by age, sex, and severity: United States, 1988–94

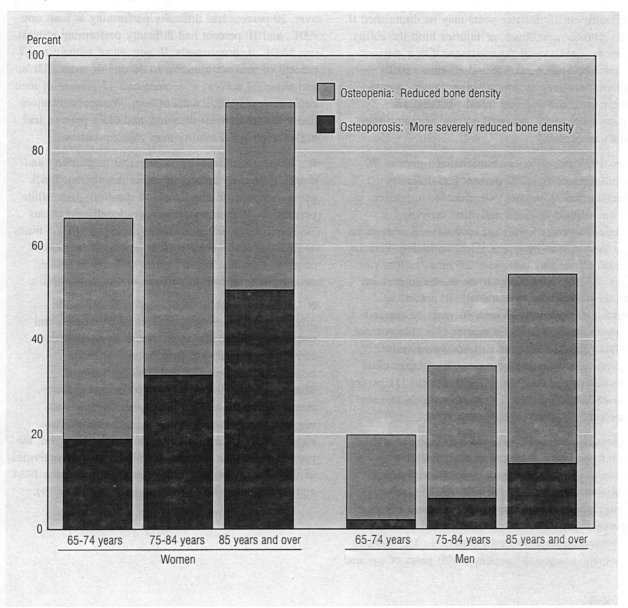

NOTES: Figures are based on the noninstitutionalized population. Osteopenia is defined as bone mineral density 1–2.5 standard deviations below the mean of non-Hispanic white women 20–29 years of age as measured in NHANES III; osteoporosis is defined as bone mineral density more than 2.5 standard deviations below the mean of non-Hispanic white women 20–29 years of age as measured in NHANES III. See Technical Notes for further discussion.

SOURCE: Centers for Disease Control and Prevention, National Center for Health Statistics, Third National Health and Nutrition Examination Survey.

Physical Functioning and Disability

■ Quality of life in later years may be diminished if illness, chronic conditions, or injuries limit the ability to care for oneself without assistance. Older persons maintain their independence and eliminate costly caregiving services by, among other things, shopping on their own, cooking their meals, bathing and dressing themselves, and walking and climbing stairs without assistance.

■ In 1995 among noninstitutionalized persons 70 years of age and over, 32 percent had difficulty performing and 25 percent were unable to perform at least one of nine physical activities. Activity limitations increased with age, and women were more likely than men to have a physical limitation. Persons 85 years of age and over were 2.6 times as likely as persons 70–74 years of age to be unable to perform physical activities. Approximately 18 percent of women and 12 percent of men 70 years of age and over were unable to walk a quarter of a mile without assistance. Similarly for other important physical activities, older women were more likely than older men to be unable to climb a flight of steps (11 percent compared with 6 percent), or stoop, crouch, or kneel (15 percent compared with 8 percent).

■ An indication of functional well-being is the ability to perform certain tasks of daily living. Researchers group these tasks into two categories: essential activities of daily living (ADL), such as bathing, eating, and dressing; and the more complex instrumental activities of daily living (IADL), such as making meals, shopping, or cleaning. In 1995 among the noninstitutionalized population 70 years of age and

over, 20 percent had difficulty performing at least one ADL, and 10 percent had difficulty performing at least one IADL. Approximately 10 percent of women and 7 percent of men were unable to do one or more ADL's, and about 23 percent of women and 13 percent of men could not do IADL's without help. Women were more likely than men to be disabled, and older persons had higher levels of disability than younger persons.

■ There are differences in physical functioning and disability by race among the older population. Black persons reported higher levels of disability than white persons. In 1995 among noninstitutionalized persons 70 years of age and over, black persons were 1.3 times as likely as white persons to be unable to do certain physical activities and 1.5 times as likely as white persons to be unable to perform one or more ADL's.

■ Between the mid-1980's and mid-1990's the proportion of noninstitutionalized older women and men who were unable to do one or more physical activities and unable to perform one or more instrumental activities of daily living declined. Moreover, disability appears to be declining more among women than men. This trend may provide important evidence of healthy aging, a result also supported by several other studies (1–3). However, the proportion of older persons unable to perform activities of daily living appears to have increased between 1984 and 1995, although the level remains quite low (4).

References

1. Crimmins E, Saito Y, Reynolds S. Further evidence on recent trends in the prevalence and incidence of disability among older Americans from two sources: The LSOA and the NHIS. J Gerontol 52B(2):S59–71. 1997.

2. Manton K, Corder L, Stallard E. Chronic disability trends in elderly United States populations: 1982–1994. Proceedings of the National Academy of Sciences: Medical Sciences, USA 94:2593–8. 1997.

3. Freedman V, Martin L. Changing patterns of functional limitation among the older American population. AJPH 88:1457-62. 1998.

4. Lentzner HR, Weeks JD, Feldman JJ. Changes in disability in the elderly population: Preliminary results from the Second Supplement on Aging. Paper presented at the annual meetings of the Population Association of America. Chicago: April 1998.

Figure 15. Percent of persons 70 years of age and over who have difficulty performing 1 or more physical activities, activities of daily living, and instrumental activities of daily living by age and sex: United States, 1995

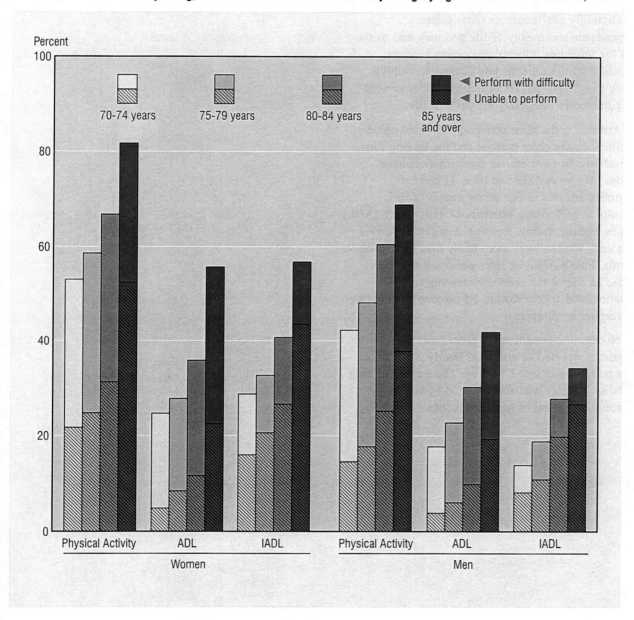

NOTES: Based on interviews conducted between October 1994 and March 1996 with noninstitutionalized persons. See Technical Notes for definitions of physical activities, activities of daily living (ADL) and instrumental activities of daily living (IADL).

SOURCE: Centers for Disease Control and Prevention, National Center for Health Statistics, 1994 National Health Interview Survey, Second Supplement on Aging.

Conditions Associated With Disability

■ Disability can reduce an older person's independence and quality of life and may lead to the need for formal or informal caregiving services. Chronic conditions are leading causes of disability among the elderly and result in many older persons being limited in their daily activities of life.

■ Arthritis is the most commonly reported chronic condition among older persons and the leading cause of disability. In 1995 among noninstitutionalized persons 70 years of age and over, 11 percent mentioned arthritis as one of the causes of their difficulty in performing activities of daily living (ADL) such as bathing, eating, dressing, and getting around the house. Women were more likely than men to report arthritis. Four percent of older persons listed heart disease as one of the conditions leading to their limitation, and approximately 2.5 percent listed stroke and respiratory diseases.

■ Nonspecific conditions or procedures are sometimes reported as disablers. Nearly 2 percent of older persons mentioned "old age" as a cause of their disability. Surgery was also reported by almost 2 percent as a cause of ADL limitations.

Figure 16. Percent of persons 70 years of age and over who report specific conditions as a cause of limitation in activities of daily living: United States, 1995

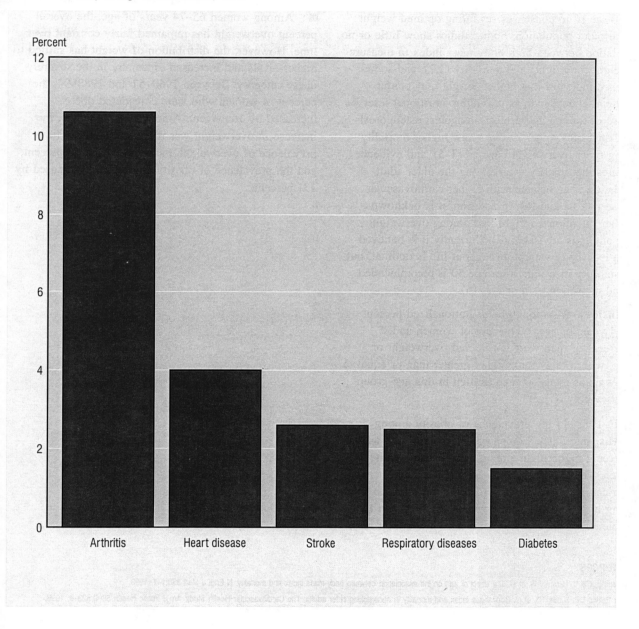

NOTES: Based on interviews conducted between October 1994 and March 1996 with noninstitutionalized persons. Conditions are reported by persons who had any difficulty performing one or more activities of daily living (ADL). Multiple conditions may be reported. See Technical Notes for definitions of respiratory diseases and ADL.

SOURCE: Centers for Disease Control and Prevention, National Center for Health Statistics, 1994 National Health Interview Survey, Second Supplement on Aging. See related figure 11 on chronic conditions and figure 15 on physical functioning and disability.

Overweight

■ There is no consensus regarding optimal weight for the older population. Some studies show little or no association between high body mass index (a measure of weight for height) and mortality (1,2), and some evidence indicates that higher weight may confer beneficial effects such as providing nutritional reserves in case of trauma and protection against osteoporosis (2). Conversely, other studies show higher mortality among older overweight persons (3–5), and evidence indicates that obesity even among the older adult population is associated with higher cardiovascular disease risk factors (6). In addition, it is unknown whether intentional weight loss among overweight older adults is advisable (7). Currently it is believed that a lean body weight throughout life is optimal, but that stability in weight after age 50 is recommended instead of weight gain or loss (6).

■ In 1988–94 among noninstitutionalized persons 65–74 years of age, 60 percent of women and 68 percent of men were considered overweight or obese, with a body mass index greater than or equal to 25. Twice as many women as men in this age group were severely obese.

■ In 1988–94 the prevalence of obesity among non-Hispanic black women 65–74 years of age was 63 percent higher than among non-Hispanic white women. The level of obesity among Mexican-American women was 28 percent higher than the level among non-Hispanic white women. Among men the prevalence of obesity was similar in the three groups.

■ Among women 65–74 years of age, the overall percent overweight has remained fairly constant over time. However, the distribution of weight has shifted to higher levels and increased especially in the severely obese category. Between 1960–62 and 1988–94, the percent of women who were considered obese increased by 16 percent. Among men, however, the increase in overweight was more substantial. The prevalence of overweight among men rose 43 percent, and the prevalence of obesity among men increased by 131 percent.

References

1. Stevens J, Cai J, Pamuk ER, et al. The effect of age on the association between body-mass index and mortality. N Engl J Med 338:1–7. 1998.

2. Diehr P, Bild DE, Harris TB, et al. Body mass index and mortality in nonsmoking older adults: The Cardiovascular Health Study. Am J Public Health 88(4):623–9. 1998.

3. Rumpel C, Harris TB, Madans J. Modification of the relationship between the Quetelet Index and mortality by weight-loss history among older women. Ann Epidemiol 3(4):343–50. 1993.

4. Harris TB, Ballard-Barbasch R, Madans J, et al. Overweight, weight loss and risk of coronary heart disease in older women. The NHANES I Epidemiologic Follow-up Study. Am J Epidemiol 137:1318–27. 1993.

5. Harris T, Cook EF, Garrison R, et al. Body mass index and mortality among nonsmoking older persons. The Framingham Heart Study. J Am Med Assoc 259(10):1520–4. 1988.

6. Harris TB, Savage PJ, Tell GS, et al. Carrying the burden of cardiovascular risk in old age: Associations of weight and weight change with prevalent cardiovascular disease, risk factors, and health status in the Cardiovascular Health Study. Am J Clin Nutr 66:837–44. 1997.

7. Lee I-M, Paffenbarger RS Jr. Is weight loss hazardous? Nutr Rev 54(4 Pt 2):S116–24. 1996.

Figure 17. Distribution of weight among persons 65–74 years of age by sex: United States, 1988–94

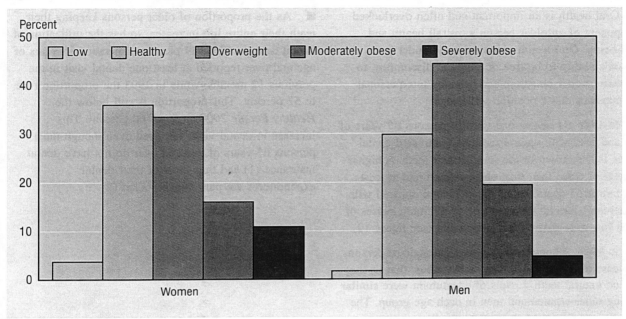

Figure 18. Prevalence of obesity among persons 65–74 years of age by sex: United States, 1960–94

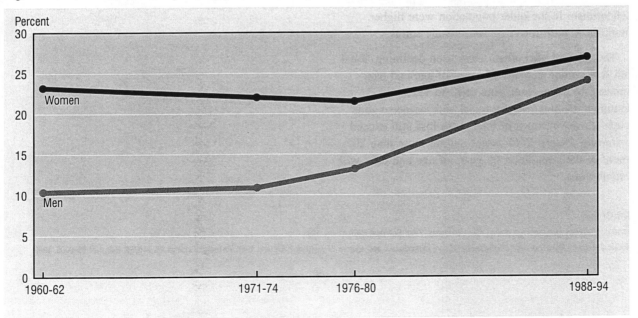

NOTES: Figures are based on the noninstitutionalized population. See Technical Notes for definitions of weight categories. Obesity is defined as a body mass index greater than or equal to 30 kilograms per meter squared.

SOURCES: Centers for Disease Control and Prevention, National Center for Health Statistics, National Health Examination Survey (1960–62), First National Health and Nutrition Examination Survey (1971–74), Second National Health and Nutrition Examination Survey (1976–80), and Third National Health and Nutrition Examination Survey (1988–94). See related *Health, United States, 1999*, table 70.

Oral Health

■ Oral health is an important and often overlooked component of an older person's overall health and well-being. Oral health problems may hinder a person's ability to be free of pain and discomfort, to maintain proper nutrition, and to enjoy interpersonal relationships and a positive self-image.

■ In 1988–94 nearly one-third of persons 65 years of age and over with natural teeth had untreated dental caries in the crown or the root of their teeth. A higher percent of older men than older women had at least one untreated dental caries (35 percent compared with 27 percent). Dental caries is one of the main causes of tooth loss among the older population (see figure 19).

■ In 1993, 30 percent of noninstitutionalized persons 65 years of age and over were edentulous, that is, they had no natural teeth. Levels of edentulism were similar among older women and men in each age group. The prevalence of total tooth loss was higher among non-Hispanic black persons than among non-Hispanic white persons and Hispanic persons. In addition, levels of edentulism in the older population were higher among those with lower socioeconomic status.

■ The rates of edentulism have been declining. Total tooth loss among persons 65 years of age and over decreased by 23 percent from 1983 to 1993. Edentulism declined for all racial and socioeconomic groups. However, rates of total tooth loss still exceed the *Healthy People 2000* target that no more than 20 percent of the population 65 years of age and over will be edentulous.

■ As the proportion of older persons keeping their teeth their entire life increases, so has the utilization of dental care. In 1983, 39 percent of persons 65 years of age and over reported at least one dental visit in the previous 12 months, while in 1993 the proportion rose to 52 percent. This proportion is still below the *Healthy People 2000* target of 60 percent. This increase in dental visits occurred even though most persons 65 years of age and over do not have dental insurance (1) and thus most of their dental expenditures are paid out-of-pocket (2).

References

1. Manski, RJ. Dental care coverage among older Americans. J Am Coll Dent 62(3):41–44. 1995.

2. Moeller J, Levy H. Dental services: A comparison of use, expenditures, and sources of payment, 1977 and 1987. Research Findings 26. AHCPR Pub. No. 96–0005. 1996.

Health Status

Figure 19. Percent with untreated dental caries among dentate persons 65 years of age and over by age and sex: United States, 1988–94

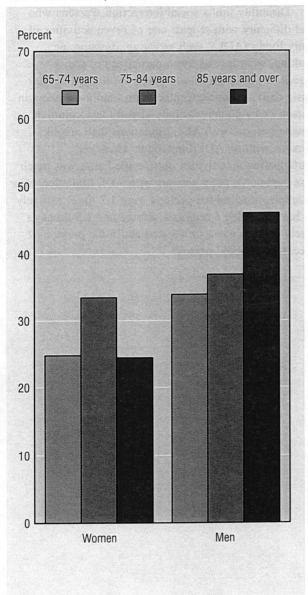

Figure 20. Prevalence of total tooth loss (edentulism) among persons 65 years of age and over by age: United States, 1983 and 1993

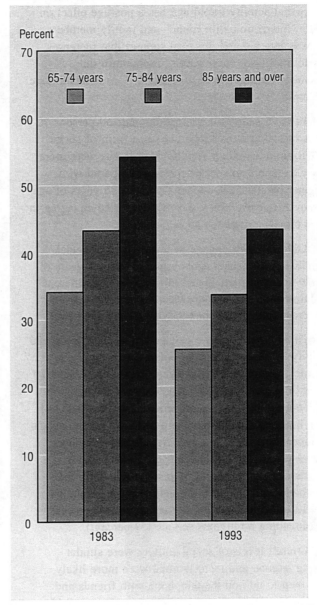

NOTES: Dental caries includes coronal and root caries. Dentate persons have at least one natural tooth. Figures are based on the noninstitutionalized population.

SOURCE: Centers for Disease Control and Prevention, National Center for Health Statistics, Third National Health and Nutrition Examination Survey.

NOTE: Figures are based on the noninstitutionalized population.

SOURCE: Centers for Disease Control and Prevention, National Center for Health Statistics, National Health Interview Survey.

Social Activities

■   Social activity in old age has a positive effect on health. Interaction with friends and family members offers emotional and practical support that increases the ability of an older person to remain in the community and decreases the use of formal health care services.

■   In 1995 nearly all noninstitutionalized persons 70 years of age and over reported some form of social activity in a 2-week period. Older persons were more likely to report no social activities compared with younger persons. Even among persons 85 years of age and over, however, only 4 percent reported engaging in none of seven common social activities.

■   Older persons engage in fewer types of social activities as they age. Among persons 70–74 years of age, 64 percent participated in five to seven different social activities in a 2-week period compared with 38 percent among persons 85 years of age and over.

■   Among persons who engaged in at least one social activity in a 2-week period, contact with family was the most common. Eighty-seven percent of persons 70 years of age and over had talked on the telephone at least once with family members who lived outside of their household, and 76 percent had seen noncoresident relatives. Social contact with friends and neighbors was also prevalent: 72 percent got together with friends or neighbors, and 81 percent talked on the telephone with a friend or neighbor. Other common activities included eating at a restaurant (65 percent) and attending a religious service (51 percent).

■   Overall levels of social activity were similar among women and men. Women were more likely than men to talk on the telephone with friends and neighbors, but women and men reported comparable levels of getting together socially.

■   Disability limits social interaction. Persons who had difficulty with at least one of seven activities of daily living (ADL), such as eating, dressing, or bathing, were less likely to participate in social activities than persons who were not limited in their basic daily activities. Contact with family members in person or by phone was only slightly less common among persons with ADL limitations than among persons with no ADL limitations. However, participation in activities outside the house was much less common among persons with ADL limitations. For example, nondisabled persons were 1.7 times as likely to have attended a religious service and 1.5 times as likely to have eaten in a restaurant in the previous 2 weeks as disabled persons.

Figure 21. Number of social activities in a 2-week period among persons 70 years of age and over by age and sex: United States, 1995

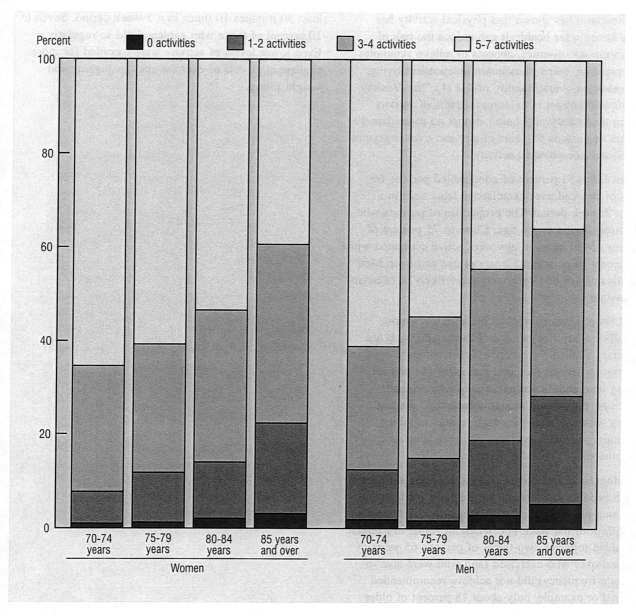

NOTES: Based on interviews conducted between October 1994 and March 1996 with noninstitutionalized persons. See Technical Notes for definitions of social activities.

SOURCE: Centers for Disease Control and Prevention, National Center for Health Statistics, 1994 National Health Interview Survey, Second Supplement on Aging.

Health Status

Exercise

■ Research has shown that physical activity has many benefits for health. It can reduce the risk of certain chronic diseases, appears to relieve symptoms of depression, helps to maintain independent living, and enhances overall quality of life (1). The *Healthy People 2000* target is to increase levels of activity among the elderly population so that no more than 22 percent of persons 65 years of age and over engage in no leisure-time physical activity.

■ In 1995, 71 percent of nondisabled persons 65 years of age and over exercised at least once in a recent 2-week period. The proportion of persons who exercised declined with age. Close to 75 percent of persons 65–74 years of age were active compared with 60 percent of persons 85 years of age and over. Men 65 years of age and over were more likely to exercise than women.

■ Less strenuous forms of exercise were most prevalent. Sixty-five percent of those who were not sedentary walked for exercise. Other common light and moderate activities included gardening (54 percent among men and 38 percent among women) and stretching (26 percent among men and 32 percent among women). Activities such as stair climbing, swimming, aerobics, and cycling were less frequently undertaken.

■ Regular exercise is important to obtain substantial health benefits. The recommended level for light to moderate physical activity is 30 minutes each time on most days of the week (1). When all forms of exercise are added together, two-thirds of persons 65 years of age and over who exercised (and who were able to estimate frequency) did not achieve recommended levels. For example, only about 18 percent of older men and women who walked for exercise did so for at least 30 minutes 10 times in a 2-week period. Seven to 10 percent of those who gardened did so regularly. Even lower levels of activity were recorded for more challenging forms of exercise such as jogging and weight lifting.

Reference

1. U.S. Department of Health and Human Services. Physical activity and health: A report of the surgeon general. Atlanta, GA: U.S. Department of Health and Human Services, Centers for Disease Control and Prevention, National Center for Chronic Disease Prevention and Health Promotion. 1996.

Figure 22. Percent who exercise and selected type of exercise among persons 65 years of age and over by sex: United States, 1995

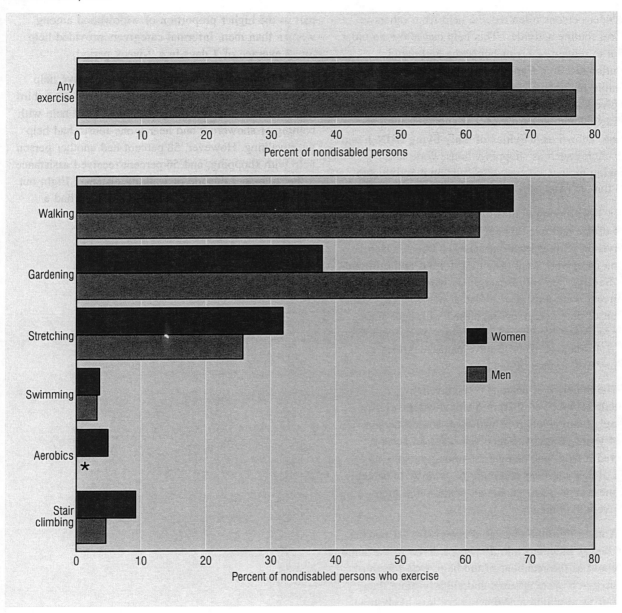

* The number of men 65 years of age and over who participated in aerobic exercise was too small to calculate reliable rates.

NOTES: Figures are based on the noninstitutionalized population. Percents are age adjusted. Exercise is defined as doing at least 1 of 20 exercises, sports, or physically active hobbies at least once within a 2-week period. The percent engaging in a specific activity is calculated among persons who engage in any exercise. See Technical Notes for list of activities.

SOURCE: Centers for Disease Control and Prevention, National Center for Health Statistics, National Health Interview Survey.

Caregivers

■ Older persons often receive help from others to perform routine activities. This help can allow an older person to remain in his or her home and avoid institutionalization. Caregivers who provide help may be family members, friends, or paid employees. Caregivers provide assistance with a variety of activities including basic needs such as dressing and bathing, known as activities of daily living (ADL), and other chores such as shopping, housework, and managing money, known as instrumental activities of daily living (IADL).

■ In 1995 among noninstitutionalized persons 70 years of age and over, 34 percent received help or supervision with at least one ADL or IADL. Over 12 million caregivers were providing formal and informal care. Seventy percent of caregivers were women, and 73 percent were unpaid or informal helpers. The percent of paid caregivers increased with age: among those receiving help, persons 85 years of age and over were 1.4 times as likely to have paid caregivers as persons 70–74 years of age.

■ The majority of persons receiving help (56 percent) received it from a single caregiver. The number of caregivers rose with age: among persons 70–74 years of age who received help, 63 percent received it from one caregiver. Among persons 85 years of age and over receiving help, only 44 percent had one caregiver. At each age, women had more caregivers than men.

■ Among informal or unpaid caregivers, 91 percent were family members and 51 percent lived in the same household as the recipient of the help. One-fourth of the caregivers were spouses and slightly more than one-half were children. Women were less likely than men to receive care from their spouses, due in large part to the higher proportion of widowhood among women than men. Informal caregivers provided help on an average of 7 days in a 2-week period.

■ Older persons were more likely to receive help from caregivers for IADL's than for ADL's. One-third of persons who received any assistance, had help with bathing or showering and nearly one-fourth had help with walking. However, 58 percent had another person help with shopping, and 56 percent received assistance to get to places outside of walking distance. Eight out of ten older persons who received any help had a caregiver help with heavy housework.

Figure 23. Number of caregivers providing assistance with activities of daily living or instrumental activities of daily living to persons 70 years of age and over by age and sex: United States, 1995

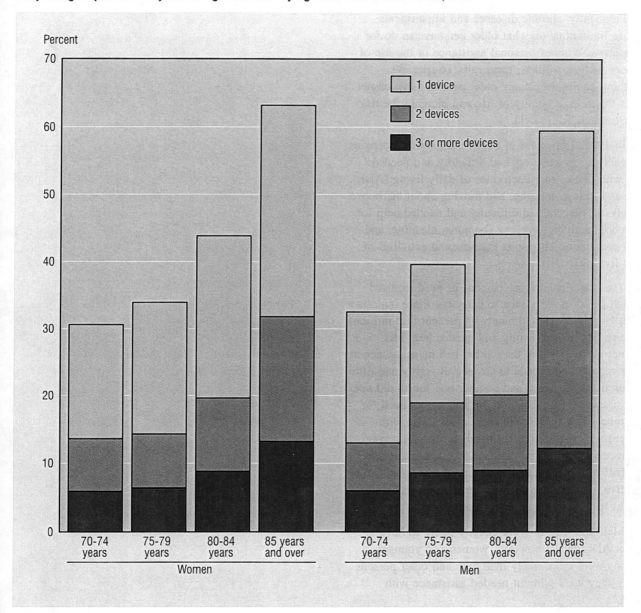

NOTES: Based on interviews conducted between October 1994 and March 1996 with noninstitutionalized persons. Caregivers provide help or supervision with at least one activity of daily living (ADL) or instrumental activity of daily living (IADL). See Technical Notes for definitions of ADL and IADL.

SOURCE: Centers for Disease Control and Prevention, National Center for Health Statistics, 1994 National Health Interview Survey, Second Supplement on Aging.

Health Care Access and Utilization

Unmet Needs

■ Frequently, chronic diseases and impairments impose limitations on what older persons can do for themselves. Without personal assistance or the use of devices such as walkers, hand rails, or special breathing equipment, many older persons have unmet needs that reduce quality of life and increase the risk of institutionalization (1).

■ In 1995, 14 percent of noninstitutionalized persons 70 years of age and over had difficulty and needed help with one or more activities of daily living (ADL), such as bathing, dressing, and moving about the house. Twenty-six percent had difficulty and needed help for household activities such as shopping, cleaning, and meal preparation known as instrumental activities of daily living (IADL).

■ The majority of older persons in need received enough personal assistance to carry out these important tasks. However, approximately 44 percent (1.4 million) of those who had difficulty and needed help had "unmet needs," that is they either had no assistance at all or required additional assistance. Roughly one-fifth had unmet ADL needs and another one-fourth did not need assistance with ADL's, but had unmet need for assistance with IADL's. In most cases those with unmet needs required direct hands-on help. Lacking the necessary assistance with ADL's, approximately one-half of those in need experienced a serious negative consequence such as burns from bath water, weight loss, or being chair- or bed-bound.

■ Men and women were equally likely to have unmet ADL needs; however, women and younger persons were more likely than men and older persons to say they went without needed assistance with IADL's.

Reference

1. Allen SM, Mor V. The prevalence and consequences of unmet need: Contrasts between older and younger adults with disability. Med Care. 35(11):1132–48. 1997.

Figure 24. Percent with unmet needs among persons 70 years of age and over who need help with 1 or more activities of daily living or instrumental activities of daily living by age and sex: United States, 1995

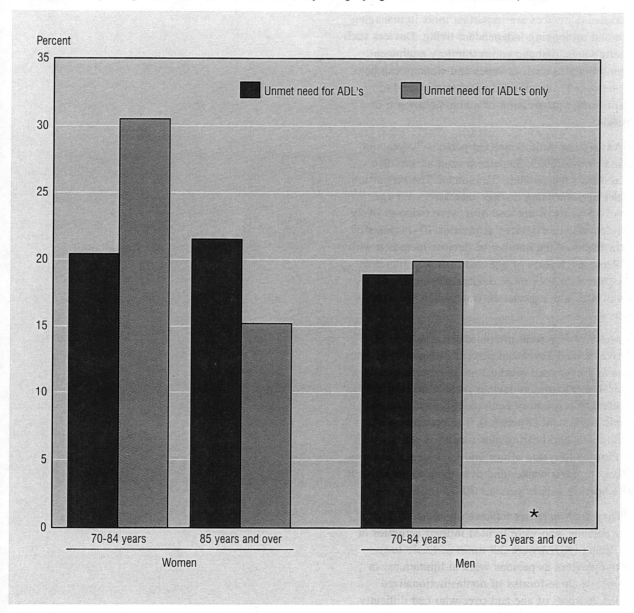

* The number of men 85 years of age and over with unmet needs was too small to calculate reliable rates.

NOTES: Based on interviews conducted between October 1994 and March 1996 with noninstitutionalized persons. See Technical Notes for definitions of activities of daily living (ADL) and instrumental activities of daily living (IADL). Persons with unmet ADL needs may also have unmet IADL needs.

SOURCE: Centers for Disease Control and Prevention, National Center for Health Statistics, 1994 National Health Interview Survey, Second Supplement on Aging.

Assistive Devices

■ Assistive devices are important tools in managing health and prolonging independent living. Devices such as hearing aids, diabetic and respiratory equipment, and mobility aids such as canes and walkers can help older persons to remain in the community and to prevent further progression of a chronic disease or condition.

■ Among noninstitutionalized persons 70 years of age and over in 1995, 39 percent used an assistive device during the previous 12 months. The proportion of older persons using devices increased with age. Persons 85 years of age and over were twice as likely to rely on assistive devices as persons 70–74 years of age. In addition, the number of devices increased with age. Persons 85 years of age and over were twice as likely to use three or more devices as persons 70–74 years of age. The age pattern was similar for women and men.

■ Mobility aids were the most common type of assistive device. Seventeen percent of persons 70 years of age and over used a cane, and 10 percent used a walker. Other common devices include hearing aids (11 percent), respiratory equipment (8 percent), and diabetic equipment (7 percent). The prevalence of mobility aids and hearing aids increased sharply with age. Persons 85 years of age and over were five times as likely to use a walker and over three times as likely to use hearing aids as persons 70–74 years of age.

■ Disability increases reliance on assistive devices. Older persons who were limited in their activities of daily living (ADL) were 2.8 times as likely to use assistive devices as persons without limitations. In 1995 nearly three-fourths of noninstitutionalized persons 70 years of age and over who had difficulty with these activities used at least one assistive device in the previous 12 months. Four out of ten persons with at least one ADL limitation reported using a cane and three out of ten used a walker.

Figure 25. Assistive devices used among persons 70 years of age and over by age and sex: United States, 1995

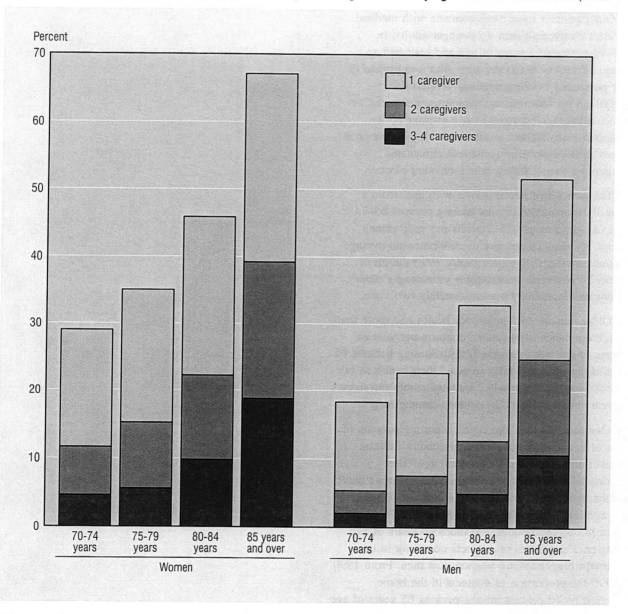

NOTES: Based on interviews conducted between October 1994 and March 1996 with noninstitutionalized persons. See Technical Notes for definitions of assistive devices.

SOURCE: Centers for Disease Control and Prevention, National Center for Health Statistics, 1994 National Health Interview Survey, Second Supplement on Aging.

Physician Contacts

■ Older persons have more contacts with medical providers on average than do younger adults. In 1994–96 persons 65 years of age and over had an average of 11.4 contacts per year with a physician or other personnel working under a physician's supervision for examination, diagnosis, treatment, or advice. Adults 45–64 years of age averaged 7.2 contacts per year. These contacts were by phone or at doctors' offices, hospital outpatient clinics and emergency rooms, clinics, home, or other places.

■ The number of contacts rose with age, from a mean of 10 contacts per year among persons 65–74 years of age to nearly 15 contacts per year among persons 85 years of age and over. Women on average had more contacts than men. Since 1990 the mean number of physician contacts per year among older persons has increased by approximately two visits.

■ Older persons in fair or poor health had more than twice the number of physician contacts per year as persons in good to excellent health. Among persons 85 years of age and over who reported their health as fair or poor, women had nearly 27 contacts with physicians per year compared with 20 contacts among men.

■ One-half of physician contacts among persons 65 years of age and over occurred in doctors' offices; however, this percent declined with age. The proportion of outpatient medical contacts among older persons that occurred in the home increased sharply with age from 10 percent among persons 65–74 years of age to 38 percent among persons 85 years of age and over. The percent of contacts occurring in the home was higher among women than men. From 1990 to 1996 the proportion of contacts in the home increased by 63 percent among persons 65 years of age and over. This trend probably reflects the increased use of home health care services among the elderly.

Figure 26. Place of ambulatory physician contacts among persons 65 years of age and over by age and sex: United States, 1994–96

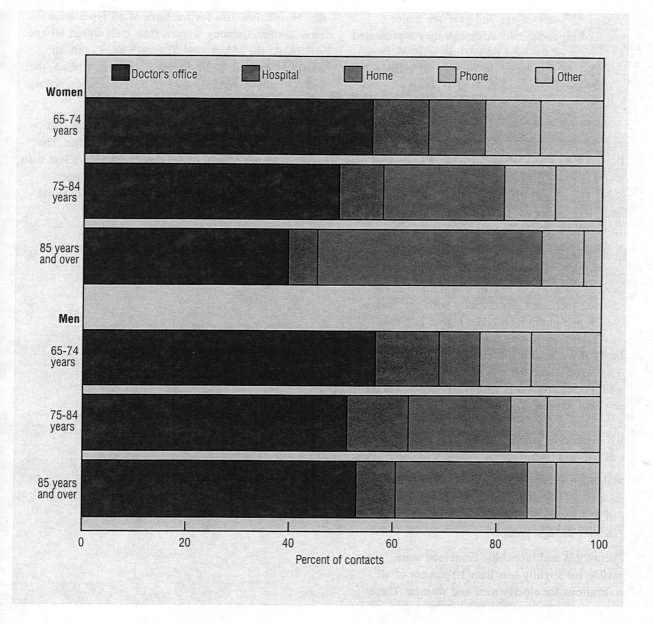

NOTES: Figures are based on the noninstitutionalized population. Physician contacts include contact with other medical personnel working under a physician's supervision and do not include contacts during overnight hospital stays. Persons with unknown place of contact are excluded from calculations. See Appendix II for definitions.

SOURCE: Centers for Disease Control and Prevention, National Center for Health Statistics, National Health Interview Survey. See related *Health, United States, 1999*, tables 75–77.

Inpatient Health Care

■ Persons 65 years of age and over are major consumers of inpatient care. Although they represented only 13 percent of the total population in 1996, they accounted for 38 percent of the roughly 31 million patient discharges from non-Federal short-stay hospitals. Moreover, the average length of stay for older persons exceeds that for younger adults.

■ Hospitalizations increased with age. Compared with those 65–74 years of age, persons 85 years of age and over had more than twice the rate of hospital discharge. The overall discharge rate for all diagnoses combined was higher for men than for women within each of the three age groups.

■ Heart disease was the most common cause for hospitalization as determined by the first-listed discharge diagnosis. The rate of hospitalization for heart disease increased substantially with age, and within each age group men had a higher rate than women. Patient discharges from stroke, the other major circulatory disease, also increased with age. Except at the oldest ages where the rate was nearly the same for men and women, discharges from stroke were higher for men than women. Combined heart disease and stroke accounted for more than one-fourth of all hospital discharges among elderly men and women 85 years of age and over.

■ Malignant neoplasms accounted for approximately 6 percent of all hospital discharges among persons 65 years of age and over, and the rate remained relatively stable across the age groups.

■ Pneumonia and bronchitis combined were responsible for slightly less than 10 percent of all hospitalizations for elderly men and women. These rates increased rapidly with age, and the combined rate for these two diseases was about twice as high for men as women among persons 85 years of age and over.

■ Hospitalizations for fractures of all types were more common among women than men within all age groups. At the oldest ages, fractures accounted for nearly 10 percent of all discharges among women, the second most important cause of hospitalization among the listed diagnoses.

■ Hospital stays for persons 65 years of age and over were shorter in 1996 than a decade earlier. The average length of stay of 6.5 days was 2 days less than in 1986. Similar trends were evident for younger (65–74 years of age) and older (75 years of age and over) persons.

Figure 27. Hospital discharge rates in non-Federal short-stay hospitals for selected first-listed diagnoses among persons 65 years of age and over by age and sex: United States, 1996

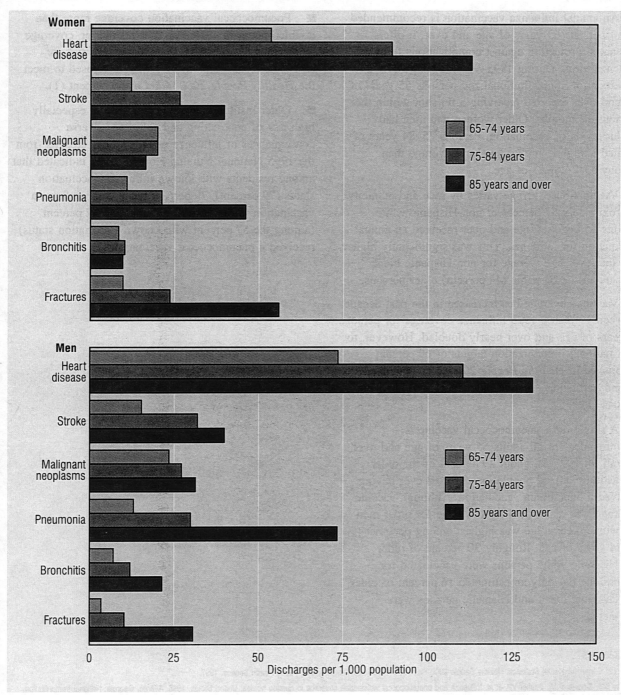

NOTES: For a description of the *International Classification of Diseases* code numbers for diagnoses, see Appendix II. Rates are based on the civilian population as of July 1, 1996.

SOURCE: Centers for Disease Control and Prevention, National Center for Health Statistics, National Hospital Discharge Survey. See related *Health, United States, 1999*, tables 90–93.

Influenza and Pneumococcal Vaccinations

■ An annual influenza vaccination is recommended for all persons 65 years of age and over; it offers substantial protection against complications from the influenza virus. During 1993–95 an average of 55 percent of noninstitutionalized persons 65 years of age and over reported receiving a flu shot within the previous 12 months. Older women and men had similar levels of vaccination. Persons 75–84 years of age had a slightly higher level of coverage than persons 65–74 years of age.

■ Vaccination coverage varies by race and ethnicity. Approximately 57 percent of non-Hispanic white persons 65 years of age and over received an annual vaccination for influenza. This was significantly higher than the level of coverage for non-Hispanic black (36 percent) or Hispanic (44 percent) older persons.

■ Vaccine coverage has increased in the past decade. Between 1989 and 1995 influenza coverage for persons 65 years of age and over nearly doubled. However, to meet national immunization targets of 60 percent established in *Healthy People 2000*, coverage needs to expand particularly among older black and Hispanic persons (1).

■ A single-dose pneumococcal vaccine is recommended for all adults 65 years of age and over. Overall, in 1993–95 about 29 percent of the older noninstitutionalized population reported ever having received a pneumonia vaccination. Although vaccine coverage was approximately the same for older men and women, coverage was highest among persons 75–84 years of age. Roughly 30 percent of older non-Hispanic white persons were vaccinated for pneumonia, but only an estimated 16 percent of older non-Hispanic black and Hispanic persons were vaccinated.

■ Pneumococcal vaccination coverage more than doubled between 1989 and 1995. However, coverage among older persons, who are at greatest risk for adverse effects, needs to be greatly increased to meet the *Healthy People 2000* target of 60 percent (1).

■ Older institutionalized persons are at especially high risk of contracting and suffering adverse consequences of influenza or pneumonia. Results from the 1995 National Nursing Home Survey indicated that among residents with known influenza vaccination status (79 percent), 79 percent received an influenza vaccination in the past 12 months, and 42 percent (among the 57 percent with known vaccination status) received a pneumococcal vaccination (2).

References

1. National Center for Health Statistics. Healthy People 2000 Review, 1997. Hyattsville, Maryland: Public Health Service. 1997.

2. Greby SM, Singleton JA, Sneller VP, et al. Influenza and pneumococcal vaccination coverage in nursing homes, United States, 1995. Atlanta, Georgia: National Immunization Program, Centers for Disease Control and Prevention. 1998.

Figure 28. Percent vaccinated against influenza and pneumococcal disease among persons 65 years of age and over by race and Hispanic origin: United States, 1993–95

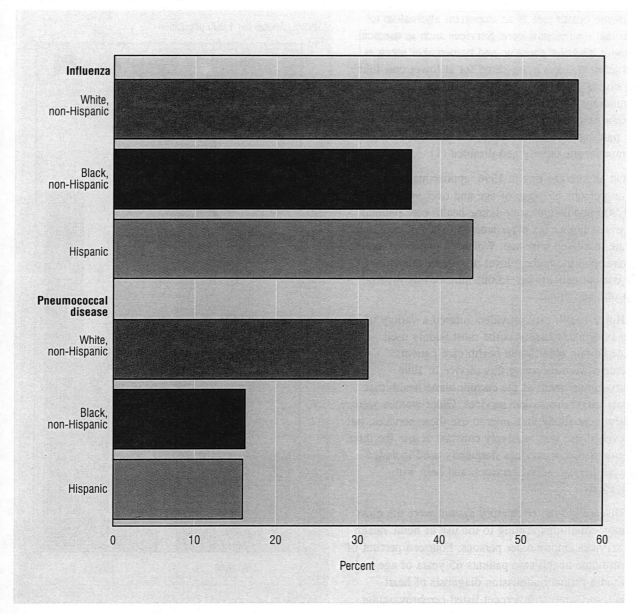

NOTES: Figures are based on the noninstitutionalized population. For influenza, the percent vaccinated consists of persons who reported having a flu shot during the past 12 months. For pneumococcal disease, the percent is persons who reported ever having a pneumonia vaccination.

SOURCE: Centers for Disease Control and Prevention, National Center for Health Statistics, National Health Interview Survey.

Health Care Access and Utilization

Home Health Care

■ Home health care is an important alternative to traditional institutional care. Services such as medical treatment, physical therapy, and homemaker services often allow patients to be cared for at lower cost than a nursing home or hospital and in the familiar surroundings of their home. In 1996 nearly one-half of all home health care expenditures in the United States were paid by Medicare, the Federal health insurance program for the elderly and disabled (1).

■ On an average day in 1996, approximately 1.7 million persons 65 years of age and over, roughly 51 per 1,000 population, were home health care patients. Usage was higher for older women than for men, and the rate increased with age. Women 85 years of age and over had the highest level of current utilization, (130 current patients per 1,000) followed by men in this same age group.

■ Home health care providers offered a variety of services. Nursing care was the most widely used service among older home health care patients; 85 percent were receiving this service in 1996. Twenty-nine percent of the current home health care patients used homemaker services. Older women were slightly more likely than men to use these services, but the level of use was relatively constant across the three age groups. Other services frequently used included physical therapy, social services, and help with medications.

■ Diseases of the circulatory system were the most common conditions leading to the use of home health care services among older persons. Fourteen percent of current home health care patients 65 years of age and over had a primary admission diagnosis of heart disease, and another 9 percent listed cerebrovascular diseases. Respiratory diseases and diabetes, accounting for about 9 percent each, were also common conditions. Fractures were the primary admission diagnosis for approximately 4 percent of elderly home health care patients, with women patients having twice the rate of fractures as men.

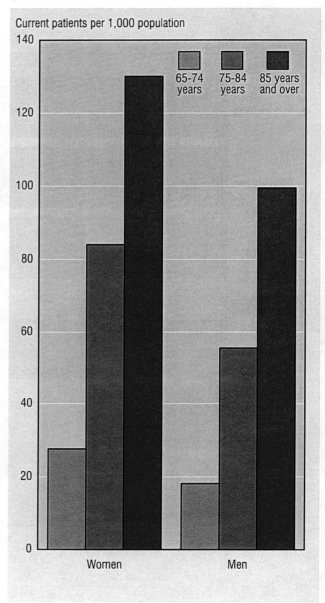

Figure 29. Home health care patients among persons 65 years of age and over by age and sex: United States, 1996

Current patients per 1,000 population

Legend: 65-74 years | 75-84 years | 85 years and over

NOTES: Age is defined as age at interview. See Technical Notes for details on calculations. Rates are based on the civilian population as of July 1, 1996. See Appendix II for definition of home health care.

SOURCE: Centers for Disease Control and Prevention, National Center for Health Statistics, National Home and Hospice Care Survey.

Reference

1. Levit KR, Lazenby HC, Braden BR, et al. National Health Expenditures, 1996. Health Care Financing Rev 19(1):161–200. 1997.

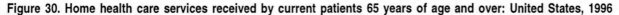

Figure 30. Home health care services received by current patients 65 years of age and over: United States, 1996

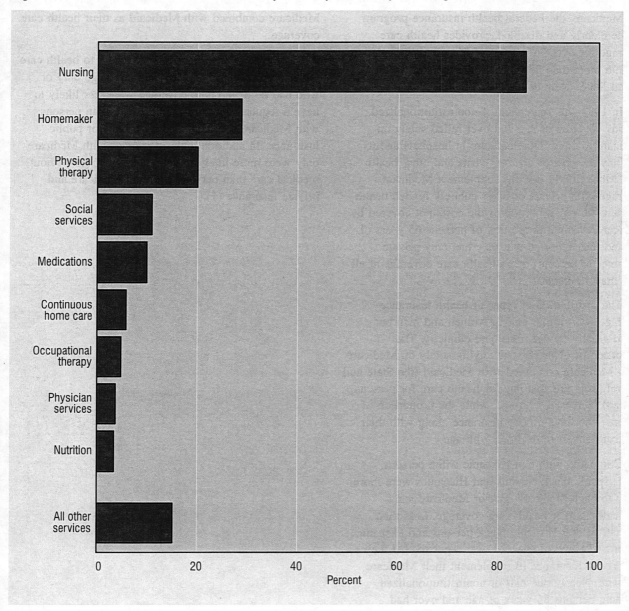

NOTE: Home health care patients may receive one or more services per visit.

SOURCE: Centers for Disease Control and Prevention, National Center for Health Statistics, National Home and Hospice Care Survey.

Health Insurance

■ Medicare, the Federal health insurance program for the elderly and disabled, provides health care coverage for over 96 percent of the elderly population. In 1996 more than 33 million older persons in the United States were covered by Medicare.

■ In 1994–96, 16 percent of noninstitutionalized persons 65 years of age and over relied solely on Medicare to cover inpatient care in hospitals and to help pay the cost of doctors' visits and other health care. Most elderly persons supplement Medicare coverage with private or other publicly funded health insurance to pay a portion of the costs not covered by Medicare. A small proportion of persons 65 years of age and over reported that they had only private insurance (3 percent) or no health care coverage at all (less than 1 percent).

■ The distribution of types of health insurance coverage was similar among women and men but varied greatly by age, race, and ethnicity. The proportion of older persons relying solely on Medicare or on Medicare combined with Medicaid (the State and Federal programs that pay for health care for persons in need) increased with age, while the proportion of persons who have private insurance along with their Medicare coverage declined with age.

■ Compared with non-Hispanic white persons, non-Hispanic black persons and Hispanics were more likely to have Medicare only or Medicare and Medicaid as their health care coverage. Less than one-half of non-Hispanic black persons and Hispanic persons 65 years of age and over reported that they had private insurance to supplement their Medicare coverage. Nearly one-half of noninstitutionalized Hispanic persons 85 years of age and over had

Medicare combined with Medicaid as their health care coverage.

■ The type of insurance affects access to health care. Older persons who had Medicare coverage only or who had no health care coverage were less likely to have a regular source of medical care than persons with Medicare supplemented by private or public insurance. In addition, elderly persons with Medicare only were more likely to delay care or to go without medical care than persons who had Medicare and private insurance (1).

Reference

1. Cohen RA, Bloom B, Simpson G, Parsons PE. Access to health care part 3: Older adults. National Center for Health Statistics. Vital Health Stat 10(198). 1997.

Figure 31. Health insurance coverage among persons 65 ~~years of age and over~~ by age, race, Hispanic origin, and type of insurance: United States, 1994–96

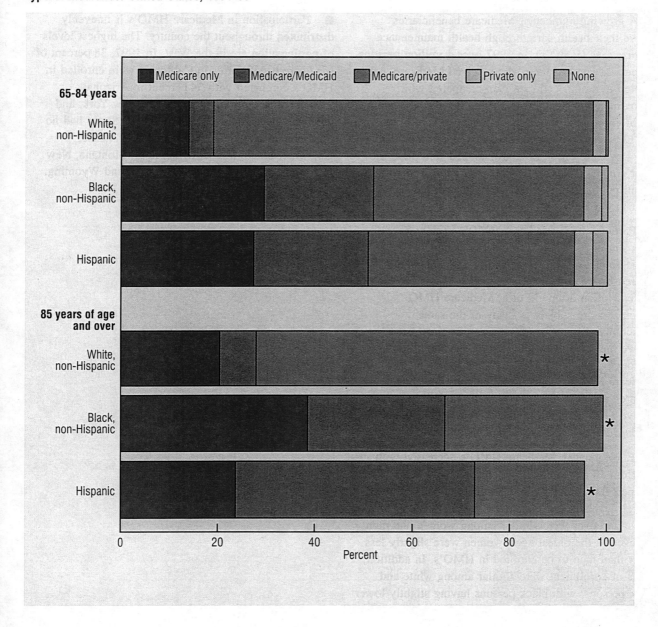

* The number of persons 85 years of age and over with private health insurance only or with no health insurance was too small to calculate reliable rates.

NOTES: Figures are based on the noninstitutionalized population. Figures exclude persons with unknown health insurance coverage. The category Medicare/Medicaid can include other public health insurance programs. The category Medicare/private includes a small number of persons who reported that they had Medicaid in addition to Medicare and private health insurance.

SOURCE: Centers for Disease Control and Prevention, National Center for Health Statistics, National Health Interview Survey. See related *Health, United States, 1999*, table 130.

Medicare Health Maintenance Organization Enrollment

■ A growing number of Medicare beneficiaries receive their health care through health maintenance organizations (HMO's). In 1997 over 4 million persons 65 years of age and over who received Medicare were enrolled in a managed care plan compared with approximately one million in 1985. In 1997 the overall rate of enrollment in Medicare managed care plans was 12 percent among persons 65 years of age and over. Levels of enrollment in managed care plans are lower among Medicare beneficiaries compared with the overall population, but the rate of growth has been faster in the 1990's.

■ Participants in Medicare HMO's usually have lower out-of-pocket costs for services covered by Medicare and often receive additional benefits not covered by traditional fee-for-service Medicare, such as prescription drugs. In turn, Medicare HMO participants are subject to many of the same restrictions of other managed care plans and usually receive their health care through a specific clinic or network of providers. Research has shown that Medicare HMO enrollees are generally healthier, younger, and less likely to be institutionalized or to receive Medicaid than Medicare beneficiaries who are not enrolled in managed care plans (1).

■ Enrollment in Medicare HMO's decreased with age from 13 percent among persons 65–74 years of age to 9 percent among persons 85 years of age and over. Overall levels of enrollment among persons 65 years of age and over were similar among women and men; however, at the oldest ages, women were slightly less likely than men to be enrolled in HMO's. In addition, levels of enrollment were similar among white and black persons, with black persons having slightly lower rates of participation in Medicare HMO's at the oldest ages.

■ Participation in Medicare HMO's is unevenly distributed throughout the country. The highest levels of participation are in the West. In 1997, 38 percent of Medicare beneficiaries in California were enrolled in HMO's compared with 34 percent in Arizona, 22 percent in Florida, 13 percent in New York, and 2 percent in Indiana. The following 10 States had no Medicare managed care plans in 1997: Alaska, Delaware, Idaho, Maine, Mississippi, Montana, New Hampshire, South Dakota, Tennessee, and Wyoming.

Reference

1. Zarabozo C, Taylor C, Hicks J. Medicare managed care: Numbers and trends. Health Care Financing Rev 17(3):243–61. 1996.

Figure 32. Percent of Medicare enrollees in health maintenance organizations by State: United States, 1997

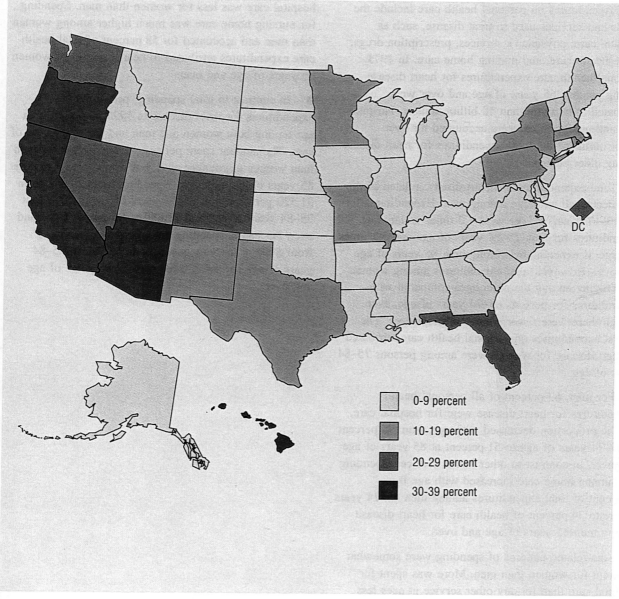

DC

Legend:
- 0-9 percent
- 10-19 percent
- 20-29 percent
- 30-39 percent

NOTES: Data as of January 1997. Figure includes Medicare beneficiaries less than 65 years of age. Persons 65 years of age and over are 87 percent of all Medicare enrollees and 95 percent of Medicare HMO enrollees.

SOURCE: Health Care Financing Administration/OMC/BDMS. See related *Health, United States, 1999*, table 143.

Health and Aging

Cost of Heart Disease

■   Expenditures on personal health care include the goods and services used to treat disease, such as hospital care, physician's services, prescription drugs, home health care, and nursing home care. In 1995 personal health care expenditures for heart disease among persons 65 years of age and over were estimated to be more than 58 billion dollars. Hospital care and nursing home care accounted for over three-fourths of the total expenditures for heart disease among older persons.

■   Total expenditures for heart disease-related health care decreased with age among men. Expenditures for men 65–74 years of age were 1.3 times as large as expenditures for men 75–84 years of age and 3.2 times as large as expenditures among men 85 years of age and over. However, total expenditures among women were higher among the older ages compared with expenditures for persons 65–74 years of age, even though there were fewer women at older ages. The largest expenditures on personal health care attributed to heart disease for women were among persons 75–84 years of age.

■   For men, 69 percent of all personal health expenditures for heart disease were for hospital care, but the proportion decreased with age, from 75 percent at 65–74 years of age to 51 percent at 85 years of age and over. In contrast to other health services, spending for nursing home care increased with age from 3 percent of total expenditures among men 65–74 years of age to 34 percent of health care for heart disease among men 85 years of age and over.

■   Age-related patterns of spending were somewhat different for women than men. More was spent for hospital care than for any other service at ages less than 85 years, but the proportion of total spending for hospital care was less for women than men. Spending for nursing home care was much higher among women than men and accounted for 58 percent of total health care expenditures attributed to heart disease for women 85 years of age and over.

■   In contrast to total spending, per capita expenditures for heart disease in 1995 increased with age among both women and men and for every type of care. The amount spent per person was higher for men than women at younger ages, but women spent more at 85 years of age and over. Spending by men rose from $1,520 per person at 65–74 years of age to $2,290 at 75–84 years of age and $3,850 at 85 years of age and over. Per capita spending among women increased from $790 at the youngest ages to $1,770 at 75–84 years of age and $4,220 for persons 85 years of age and over.

Figure 33. Estimated amount of personal health care expenditures attributed to heart disease among persons 65 years of age and over by age, sex, and type of health service: United States, 1995

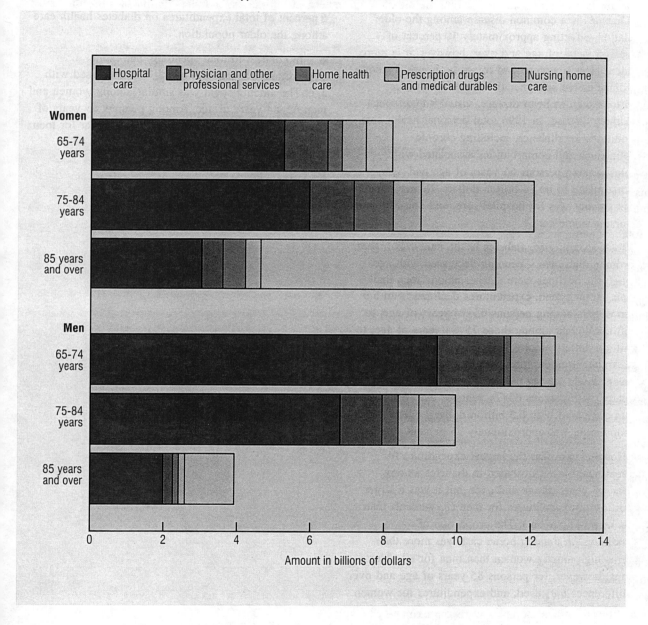

NOTE: Cost estimates are calculated from first-listed diagnoses of heart disease only.

SOURCE: Hodgson TA, Cohen AJ. Medical care expenditures for selected circulatory diseases: Opportunities for reducing national health expenditures. Med Care. Forthcoming.

Cost of Diabetes

■ Diabetes is a common disease among the older population, affecting approximately 10 percent of persons 65 years of age and over; however, it is more prevalent among women and minority groups. Persons with diabetes are at higher risk for other chronic conditions such as heart disease, visual impairments, and kidney disease. In 1995 total personal health care expenditures for diabetes, including chronic complications and comorbidities associated with diabetes, among persons 65 years of age and over, were estimated to be 26 billion dollars. Nearly one-half of this amount was for hospital care, and one-fifth was for nursing home care.

■ Total spending on diabetes health care was higher for women than men. Spending decreased with age, although the declines were steeper among men than women. Among men, expenditures declined from 5.6 billion dollars among persons 65–74 years of age, to 3.5 billion dollars among those 75–84 years of age, to 1.5 billion dollars among those 85 years of age and over. Among women, total spending was only 6 percent lower among persons 75–84 years of age compared with persons 65–74 years of age (6.1 billion dollars compared with 6.5 billion dollars) even though the population was approximately 35 percent smaller.

■ Hospital care was the largest expenditure for personal health care attributed to diabetes among persons 65 years of age and over, but it was a larger proportion of expenditures for men (53 percent) than for women (41 percent). The proportion of expenditures on nursing home care was more than twice as high among women than men for all older persons; however, for persons 85 years of age and over the differences narrowed, and expenditures for women were 1.5 times as large as those for men. Prescription drugs and other medical durables were approximately

6 percent of total expenditures on diabetes health care among the older population.

■ In contrast to total spending, per capita expenditures for diabetes health care increased with age. The amount spent was similar among women and men 65–84 years of age. Among persons 85 years of age and over, per capita spending was higher for men ($1,430) than for women ($1,170).

Figure 34. Estimated amount of personal health care expenditures attributed to diabetes among persons 65 years of age and over by age, sex, and type of health service: United States, 1995

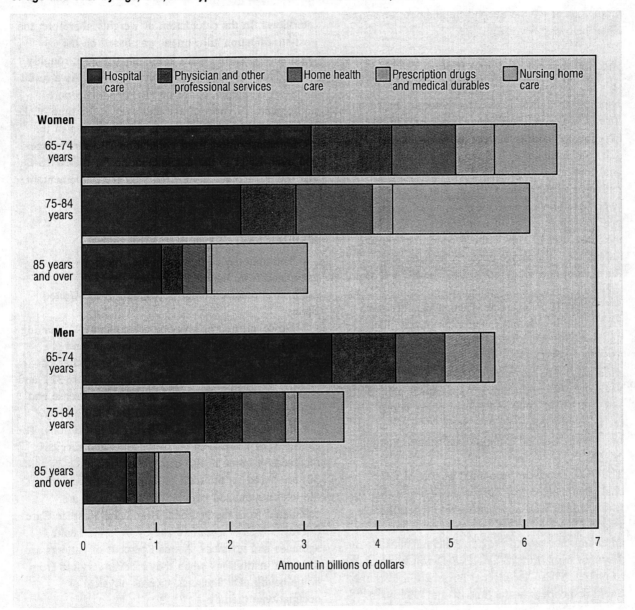

NOTE: Cost estimates are calculated from first-listed diagnoses of diabetes, chronic complications and other unrelated diagnoses attributed to diabetes, and certain comorbidities among persons with diabetes.

SOURCE: Hodgson TA, Cohen AJ. Medical care expenditures for diabetes, its chronic complications and comorbidities. Prev Med. Forthcoming.

Health and Aging

Data Sources

Appendix I describes the data sources used in the chartbook except for the Second Supplement on Aging described below.

Second Supplement on Aging (figures 11–13, 15 and 16, 21, 23–25)

Nine of the figures in the chartbook are based on data from the Second Supplement on Aging to the 1994 National Health Interview Survey (SOA II). The SOA II, conducted by NCHS with the support of the National Institute on Aging, is a survey of 9,447 noninstitutionalized persons 70 years of age and over who were interviewed originally as part of the 1994 National Health Interview Survey (NHIS). The SOA II includes measures of health and functioning, chronic conditions, use of assistive devices, housing and long-term care, and social activities. The SOA II was designed to replicate the Supplement on Aging (SOA) to the 1984 NHIS to examine whether changes have occurred in the health and functioning of the older population between the mid-1980's and the mid-1990's. The SOA served as the baseline for the Longitudinal Study on Aging (LSOA), which followed the original 1984 cohort through subsequent interviews in 1986, 1988, and 1990 and is continuing with passive mortality followup. The SOA II serves as the baseline for the Second Longitudinal Study on Aging (LSOA II).

The SOA II was implemented as part of the National Health Interview Survey on Disability (NHIS-D), which was designed to help researchers understand disability, to estimate the prevalence of certain conditions, and to provide baseline statistics on the effects of disabilities. The NHIS-D was conducted in two phases. Phase 1 collected information from the household respondent at the time of the 1994 NHIS core interview and was used as a screening instrument for Phase 2. The screening criteria were broadly defined, and more than 50 percent of persons 70 years of age and over were included in the Phase 2 NHIS-D interviews. Persons 70 years of age and over who were not included in Phase 2 NHIS-D received the SOA II survey instrument, which was a subset of questions from the NHIS-D.

While the 1994 NHIS core and NHIS-D Phase 1 interviews took place in 1994, Phase 2 was conducted as a followup survey, 7–17 months after the core interviews. In the calculation of weights, therefore, the post-stratification adjustment was based on the population control counts from July 1, 1995, roughly the midpoint of the Phase 2 survey period. As a result, the SOA II sample, based on all 1994 NHIS core participants 70 years of age and over at the time of the Phase 2 NHIS-D interviews, is representative of the 1995 noninstitutionalized population 70 years of age and over. Refer to the documentation for the NHIS-D and the SOA II for more details on the implementation of the surveys (1,2).

Institutionalized Population

The majority of figures in the chartbook are calculated from data that represent the noninstitutionalized older population in the United States.

However, figures on population (figure 1), nursing home residence (figure 3), life expectancy and mortality (figures 5–9), rates of hospital discharges (figure 27), Medicare HMO enrollment (figure 32), and cost of health care expenditures for heart disease and diabetes (figures 33 and 34) cover the total elderly population, including persons living in institutions. The estimates of home health care patients and services received by home health care patients (figures 29 and 30) are based on the total older population including the institutionalized population. These rates are calculated from the National Home and Hospice Care Survey, which is a sample survey of home health agencies and hospices. A small percent of patients are living in institutions when they receive services from home health care agencies such as physical or occupational therapy.

Age Adjustment

The age distribution of older women and men is different: among persons 65 years of age and over, the average woman is older than the average man. Consequently, comparing rates for women and men among the total older population may confound differences in rates with differences in age composition.

In general, the chartbook presents rates by sex and at least three age groups. When data are presented for the total older population (65 years of age and over or 70 years of age and over) and sex differences are highlighted, the rates are age adjusted. Appendix II describes the age adjustment procedures and the source of the standard population. The prevalence of chronic conditions (figure 11) is age adjusted using four age groups (70–74 years, 75–79 years, 80–84 years, and 85 years and over). Rates of exercise (figure 22) are age adjusted using three age groups (65–74 years, 75–84 years, and 85 years and over).

Race and Ethnicity

The focus of the chartbook is age and sex differences in the health of the older population. Depending on the variable of interest, some data sources did not have sufficient numbers of observations to allow calculation of reliable estimates of the older population by race and ethnicity. When race and ethnicity differences are presented, data are shown for white and black persons or for non-Hispanic white, non-Hispanic black, and Hispanic persons, except for the figure on deaths from all causes (figure 8).

Death rates for all causes (figure 8) are presented for five groups: white persons, black persons, Hispanic persons, Asians or Pacific Islanders, and American Indians or Alaska Natives.

Among persons 65–74 and 75–84 years of age, the death rates for Hispanics, Asians or Pacific Islanders, and American Indians or Alaska Natives were lower than the death rates for white persons; in addition, the death rates for black persons were higher than the rates for white persons. Among persons 85 years of age and over, white persons had higher death rates than other groups.

There are various explanations for the race and ethnicity patterns of mortality among the older population. Inconsistency in the reporting of race and ethnicity in vital statistics (the source of numerators for death rates) and in census data (the source of denominators for death rates) is one explanation. Death rates will be underestimated if persons who are identified as Asian, American Indian, or Hispanic in data from the Census Bureau are reported as white or non-Hispanic on death certificates.

Among Hispanics and Asians or Pacific Islanders, many of whom are foreign born, the "healthy migrant" effect may be operating. Immigration is a selective process, and immigrants are usually healthier than people who do not migrate. In addition, if foreign-born persons return to their homeland to die, then death rates will be underestimated because their deaths will not be counted in U.S. vital statistics (3). These broad racial and ethnic categories include native-born persons and immigrants from many different countries and diverse backgrounds. The overall death rate may obscure differences in health and mortality between subgroups of these populations.

Death rates for American Indians and Alaska Natives are regarded as understated because population estimates between 1980 and 1990 increased by 45 percent, in part due to more people identifying themselves as American Indian and because there is evidence that American Indians are underreported on death certificates (4).

The racial "crossover" in mortality, with younger black persons having higher death rates than younger white persons, but older black persons having lower death rates, is a subject of debate. Some research shows that age misreporting may have artificially depressed death rates; however, other research has suggested that black persons who survive to the oldest ages may be healthier than white persons and have lower mortality rates (5,6).

Other Measures and Methods

Living Arrangements (figure 2)

The categories of living arrangements were computed from data on family status and marital status. Persons living "with spouse" may also be living with other relatives or nonrelatives. The category "with other relatives" does not include persons living with a spouse. Persons living "with nonrelatives" does not include persons living with spouses or other relatives.

Health and Aging ....

Technical Notes

Life Expectancy (figures 5 and 6)

In figure 5 the estimates of life expectancy at age 85 for the years 1950–90 are based on death rates calculated from 3 years of data. The denominator of the rate is the population from the decennial census (1950, 1960, 1970, 1980, and 1990). The numerator is the deaths occurring in the decennial census year and the 2 surrounding years (1949–51, 1959–61, 1969–71, 1979–81, and 1989–91).

Beginning in 1997 life table methodology was revised to construct complete life tables by single years of age that extend to age 100. Previously, abridged life tables were constructed for 5-year age groups ending with the age group 85 years and over. In the revised methodology, Medicare data are used to adjust estimates of life expectancy at ages 85–100. Some of the increase in life expectancy from 1996 to 1997 may be due to the change in methodology. The race differences in life expectancy at the oldest ages are also affected by this change. See the forthcoming Vital and Health Statistics report for further discussion (7).

Chronic Conditions (figure 11)

Estimates of the prevalence of chronic conditions are based on self-reports in the Second Supplement on Aging. Respondents were asked whether they "ever had" various conditions common among older persons. For certain conditions, the respondents were asked a followup question about whether they "still had" the condition. The estimates of heart disease prevalence are based on persons who said they ever had heart disease, including coronary heart disease, angina, heart attack or myocardial infarction, or any other heart disease. The estimates of the prevalence of respiratory diseases are based on persons who said they "still had" chronic bronchitis, emphysema, or asthma. Estimates of cancer prevalence are calculated from persons who reported that they "still had" cancer of any kind. Arthritis prevalence was estimated from persons who reported they "ever had" arthritis. Estimates of hypertension and diabetes were based on persons who reported that they "still had" the condition. The prevalence of hypertension in figure 11,

based on self-reports in the Second Supplement on Aging, differs from estimates based on NHANES III, which were measured in physical examinations. (See *Health, United States, 1999*, table 68.)

Visual and Hearing Impairments (figures 12 and 13)

The prevalence of visual and hearing impairment is based on self-reports in the Second Supplement on Aging in response to several questions. Visual impairment is defined as blindness in one or both eyes or any other trouble seeing with one or both eyes even when wearing glasses. Hearing impairment is defined as deafness in one or both ears or any other trouble hearing with one or both ears.

Osteoporosis (reduced hip bone density) (figure 14)

The definitions of osteoporosis and osteopenia are based on diagnostic criteria proposed by the World Health Organization (8,9). Estimates are based on the total femur region.

There is no consensus at this time concerning the definition of low bone density in men. The estimates of osteopenia and osteoporosis for men in figure 14 are made by comparing their levels of bone mineral density to the values for non-Hispanic white women 20–29 years of age as measured in NHANES III.

Using the bone mineral density values of young white women as the cutoff point for diagnosing osteoporosis in men gives a conservative estimate of the prevalence of this condition in men, since white women have the lowest values of bone mineral density (10).

Physical Functioning and Disability (figure 15)

Limitation in physical activities, activities of daily living, and instrumental activities of daily living are based on self-reports in the Second Supplement on Aging.

Nine physical activities are measured in figure 15: walking for a quarter of a mile; walking up 10 steps without resting; standing or being on one's feet for about 2 hours; sitting for about 2 hours; stooping, crouching, or kneeling; reaching up over one's head; reaching out (as if to shake someone's hand); using one's fingers to grasp or handle; and lifting or carrying something as heavy as 10 pounds.

To determine severity of limitations in physical activities, respondents in SOA II were asked a series of questions. The first question was "By yourself and not using aids, do you have any difficulty (name of activity)?" Persons who answered "yes" to this question were then asked, "How much difficulty do you have (name of activity), some, a lot, or are you unable to do it?" The category "perform with difficulty" in figure 15 consists of persons who reported that they had "some" or "a lot" of difficulty.

ADL and IADL

Researchers group the important tasks of daily living into two categories frequently referred to in this chartbook:

■ ADL - activities of daily living. ADL's include seven activities: bathing or showering; dressing; eating; getting in and out of bed or chairs; walking; getting outside; and using the toilet, including getting to the toilet.

■ IADL - instrumental activities of daily living. IADL's include six activities: preparing one's own meals; shopping for groceries and personal items such as toilet items or medicines; managing one's money, such as keeping track of expenses or paying bills; using the telephone; doing heavy housework, like scrubbing floors or washing windows; and doing light housework, like doing dishes, straightening up, or light cleaning.

To determine severity of limitations in activities of daily living and instrumental activities of daily living, respondents in SOA II were asked a series of questions. The first question was: "Because of a health or physical problem, do you have any difficulty (name of activity)? Persons who answered "yes" to this question were then asked, "By yourself (and without using special equipment), how much difficulty do you have (name of activity), some, a lot, or are you unable to do it?" The category "perform with difficulty" in

figure 15 consists of persons who reported that they had "some" or "a lot" of difficulty.

Conditions Associated with Disability (figure 16)

In SOA II, persons who had any difficulty with one or more activities of daily living were asked, "What condition causes the trouble in (list of activities previously mentioned)?" Respondents could name up to five conditions. In figure 16 the percent and rank-order of conditions are computed from all conditions mentioned.

The category of respiratory diseases includes asthma, bronchitis, emphysema, influenza, pneumonia, and other respiratory, lung, or breathing problems.

Overweight (figures 17 and 18)

The categories of weight distribution reflect current Federal guidelines for overweight and obesity (11). The categories are based on body mass index (BMI), a measure of weight for height (kilograms per meter squared). Low weight is defined as a BMI less than 19. Healthy weight is a BMI of 19–24.99. Overweight is a BMI of 25–29.99. Moderately obese is a BMI of 30–34.99, and severely obese is a BMI greater than or equal to 35.

Oral Health (figures 19 and 20)

In 1993 estimates of edentulism are based on data from the *1993 Healthy People 2000 Supplement* to the National Health Interview Survey. This supplement was administered to one adult sample person per family in the second half of the year. Respondents were asked two questions concerning loss of natural teeth: if they had lost all of their upper natural teeth and if they had lost all of their lower natural teeth.

Estimates of edentulism in 1983 are based on data from the 1983 NHIS core interview that obtained information on all household members. One question asked respondents if they had lost all of their natural teeth.

Health and Aging ....

Technical Notes

Social Activity (figure 21)

Social activity, estimated from the Second Supplement on Aging, is defined as doing at least one of the seven following activities at least once in a 2-week period: getting together with friends or neighbors; talking with friends or neighbors on the telephone; getting together with any relatives not including those living with the respondent; talking with any relatives on the telephone not including those living with the respondent; going to church, temple, or another place of worship for services or other activities; going to a show or movie, sports event, club meeting, class, or other group event; and going out to eat at a restaurant.

Exercise (figure 22)

Estimates of exercise are based on data from the *1995 Healthy People 2000 Supplement* to the National Health Interview Survey. This supplement was administered to one adult sample person per family in one-half of the households in the 1995 NHIS core. Persons who were physically handicapped, as determined by the interviewer, were not asked questions regarding specific types of exercise and were excluded from the calculations.

Exercise is defined as doing at least 1 of the following 20 exercises, sports, or physically active hobbies at least once within a 2-week period: walking for exercise; gardening or yard work; stretching exercises; weightlifting or other exercises to increase muscle strength; jogging or running; aerobics or aerobic dancing; riding a bicycle or exercise bike; stair climbing for exercise; swimming for exercise; playing tennis; playing golf; bowling; playing baseball or softball; playing handball, racquetball, or squash; skiing; playing basketball; playing volleyball; playing soccer; playing football; or other exercises, sports, or physically active hobbies not mentioned above.

Caregivers (figure 23)

In the Second Supplement on Aging, respondents could name a maximum of four persons who provided help with activities of daily living (ADL) or instrumental activities of daily living (IADL). See notes for figure 15 above for definitions of ADL and IADL.

Assistive Devices (figure 25)

The use of assistive devices in the Second Supplement on Aging was defined as using any of the following medical devices or supplies in the 12 months before the interview: tracheotomy tube; respirator; ostomy bag; catheterization equipment; glucose monitor; diabetic equipment or supplies; inhaler; nebulizer; hearing aid; crutches; cane; walker; wheelchair; scooter; or feeding tube. Use of respiratory equipment was defined as using a respirator, inhaler, or nebulizer. Use of diabetic equipment was defined as using a glucose monitor or other diabetic equipment and supplies.

Influenza and Pneumonia (figure 28)

Estimates of influenza and pneumonia vaccinations are based on data from the *Healthy People 2000 Supplement* to the 1993–95 National Health Interview Surveys (NHIS). In 1994–95, this supplement was administered to one adult sample person per family in one-half of the households in the NHIS core. In 1993 the supplement was administered to one adult sample person per family in the second half of the year.

Home Health Care (figures 29 and 30)

Rates of home health care patients per 1,000 population are based on age at interview, calculated from date of birth and date of interview. Persons with missing date of birth information were excluded from calculations.

References

1. National Center for Health Statistics. Data file documentation, National Health Interview Survey, Second Supplement on Aging, 1994 (machine readable data file and documentation). Hyattsville, Maryland. 1998.

2. National Center for Health Statistics. Data file documentation, National Health Interview Survey of Disability, Phase 1, 1995 (machine readable data file and documentation). Hyattsville, Maryland. 1998.

3. Elo IT, Preston SH. Racial and ethnic differences in mortality at older ages. In: Martin LG, Soldo BJ eds. Racial and ethnic differences in the health of older Americans. Washington: National Academy Press 10–42. 1997.

4. Sorlie PD, Rogot E, Johnson NJ. Validity of demographic characteristics on the death certificate. Epidemiology 3(2):181–4. 1992.

5. Preston SH, Elo IT, Rosenwaike I, Hill M. African-American mortality at older ages: Results of a matching study. Demography 33(2):193–209. 1996.

6. Manton KC, Stallard E, Wing S. Analyses of black and white differentials in the age trajectory of mortality in two closed cohort studies. Stat Med 10:1043–59. 1991.

7. Anderson RN. A methodology for constructing complete life tables for the United States. National Center for Health Statistics. Vital and Health Stat (in preparation).

8. Kanis JL, Melton LJ, Christiansen C, et al. The diagnosis of osteoporosis. J Bone Miner Res 9:1137–41. 1994.

9. World Health Organization. Assessment of fracture risk and its application to screening for postmenopausal osteoporosis. Technical Report Series no. 842. WHO, Geneva, Switzerland. 1994.

10. Looker AC, Orwoll ES, Johnston Jr. CC, et al. Prevalence of low femoral bone density in older U.S. adults from NHANES III. J Bone Miner Res 12(11):1761–8. 1997.

11. Report of the dietary guidelines advisory committee on the dietary guidelines for Americans, 1995 to the Secretary of Health and Human Services and the Secretary of Agriculture. U.S. Department of Agriculture, Agricultural Research Service. 1995.

Data Tables for Figures 1–34 ....

Figure 1. Population 65 years of age and over

Year	65 years and over	85 years and over
	Number in millions	
1950	12.2	0.6
1960	16.6	0.9
1970	20.1	1.5
1980	25.5	2.2
1990	31.1	3.0
2000	34.7	4.3
2010	39.4	5.7
2020	53.2	6.5
2030	69.4	8.5

Figure 2. Living arrangements of persons 65 years of age and over

Age and type of arrangement	Women	Men
	Percent	
65–74 years		
Living alone	32.1	14.6
Living with spouse	51.1	76.8
Living with other relatives	14.8	5.7
Living with nonrelatives only	2.0	2.9
75–84 years		
Living alone	50.0	19.6
Living with spouse	31.5	68.2
Living with other relatives	16.9	9.7
Living with nonrelatives only	1.7	2.5
85 years and over		
Living alone	58.6	29.2
Living with spouse	10.7	46.0
Living with other relatives	28.4	17.5
Living with nonrelatives only	2.3	7.3

Figure 3. Nursing home residents among persons 65 years of age and over

Sex and age	Residents per 1,000 population			
	White		Black	
	Rate	SE	Rate	SE
Women				
65 years and over ...	55.5	0.7	54.7	3.3
65–74 years........	11.1	0.5	18.1	1.9
75–84 years........	51.9	1.3	62.6	5.8
85 years and over ...	222.5	4.3	203.3	15.9
Men				
65 years and over ...	25.3	0.7	41.1	3.1
65–74 years........	8.6	0.5	20.7	2.4
75–84 years........	32.6	1.3	57.3	6.5
85 years and over ...	117.3	5.1	144.3	18.4

Figure 4. Percent in poverty among persons 65 years of age and over

Race, Hispanic origin, and sex	Percent
White:	
Women	11.5
Men	5.6
Black:	
Women	28.8
Men	21.8
Hispanic:	
Women	26.3
Men	20.3

Figure 5. Life expectancy at birth, age 65, and age 85

Year	At birth		At age 65		At age 85	
	Women	Men	Women	Men	Women	Men
1950	71.1	65.6	15.0	12.8	4.9	4.4
1960	73.1	66.6	15.8	12.8	4.7	4.4
1970	74.7	67.1	17.0	13.1	5.6	4.7
1980	77.4	70.0	18.3	14.1	6.4	5.1
1990	78.8	71.8	18.9	15.1	6.7	5.3
1992	79.1	72.3	19.2	15.4	6.6	5.3
1993	78.8	72.2	18.9	15.3	6.4	5.2
1994	79.0	72.4	19.0	15.5	6.4	5.2
1995	78.9	72.5	18.9	15.6	6.3	5.2
1996	79.1	73.1	19.0	15.7	6.4	5.4
1997	79.4	73.6	19.2	15.9	6.6	5.5

Figure 6. Life expectancy at birth, age 65, and age 85 by sex and race

Sex and age	White	Black
Women		
At birth	79.9	74.7
At age 65	19.3	17.6
At age 85	6.6	6.7
Men		
At birth	74.3	67.2
At age 65	16.0	14.2
At age 85	5.4	5.7

Data Tables for Figures 1–34 ....

Figure 7. Death rates for all causes among persons 65 years of age and over

Age	Women	Men
65–69 years....................................	1,530.1	2,556.7
70–74 years....................................	2,425.5	3,948.9
75–79 years....................................	3,763.5	5,831.3
80–84 years....................................	6,325.2	9,320.0
85–89 years....................................	11,202.6	15,261.7
90–94 years....................................	17,572.2	21,365.9
95 years and over	25,556.3	26,078.3

Figure 8. Death rates for all causes among persons 65 years of age and over

Sex and age	White	Black	Asian or Pacific Islander	American Indian or Alaska Native	Hispanic
Women					
65–74 years..........................	1,900.5	2,739.7	1,117.3	1,920.5	1,381.9
75–84 years..........................	4,786.3	5,669.3	3,052.1	3,531.6	3,220.5
85 years and over	14,681.4	13,701.7	8,414.1	5,773.6	8,708.6
Men					
65–74 years..........................	3,122.7	4,298.3	1,892.6	2,847.2	2,251.7
75–84 years..........................	7,086.0	8,296.3	4,749.1	4,796.3	4,750.3
85 years and over	17,767.1	16,083.5	11,796.3	7,888.1	10,487.1

Figure 9. Death rates for selected leading causes among persons 65 years of age and over

Age and sex	Heart disease	Cancer	Stroke	Chronic obstructive pulmonary disease	Pneumonia/ influenza
65–74 years					
Women	529.4	676.8	120.1	136.1	42.9
Men	1,031.1	1,058.4	153.1	201.3	74.3
75–84 years					
Women	1,616.6	1,050.6	444.4	287.6	189.3
Men	2,443.6	1,770.2	488.7	469.6	301.6
85 years and over					
Women	6,013.7	1,439.2	1,618.4	424.5	933.7
Men	6,658.5	2,712.5	1,500.7	902.8	1,250.5

Figure 10. Fair or poor health among persons 65 years of age and over

Sex, race, and Hispanic origin	65 years and over		65–74 years		75–84 years		85 years and over	
	Percent	SE	Percent	SE	Percent	SE	Percent	SE
Women								
Non-Hispanic white	25.7	0.4	22.5	0.5	28.3	0.7	33.6	1.3
Non-Hispanic black	42.2	1.3	40.7	1.6	44.7	2.1	44.0	3.8
Hispanic	35.4	1.6	31.5	1.8	40.7	3.0	44.9	4.7
All races	27.6	0.4	24.8	0.5	30.2	0.6	34.9	1.2
Men								
Non-Hispanic white	26.5	0.5	23.7	0.6	30.6	0.8	32.7	1.9
Non-Hispanic black	40.7	1.6	38.4	1.9	43.6	2.8	55.0	6.1
Hispanic	34.6	1.8	31.3	2.0	40.3	4.0	49.1	7.6
All races	28.0	0.4	25.4	0.5	31.7	0.8	35.0	1.8

SE Standard error.

Figure 11. Percent of persons 70 years of age and over who reported selected chronic conditions

Chronic condition	Women		Men	
	Percent	SE	Percent	SE
Arthritis	63.3	0.8	49.5	0.9
Hypertension	39.6	0.7	31.5	0.8
Heart disease	24.1	0.6	30.0	0.8
Diabetes	10.4	0.4	11.6	0.5
Respiratory diseases	10.3	0.4	11.0	0.5
Stroke	7.6	0.4	10.4	0.6
Cancer	2.3	0.2	6.0	0.4

SE Standard error.

Figure 12. Prevalence of visual impairment among persons 70 years of age and over

Race and age	Women		Men	
	Percent	SE	Percent	SE
White:				
70 years and over	19.0	0.7	15.6	0.7
70–74 years	13.3	0.8	11.2	0.9
75–79 years	16.6	1.1	15.9	1.3
80–84 years	22.9	1.4	19.7	1.7
85 years and over	32.9	1.9	27.4	2.4
Black:				
70 years and over	18.8	1.8	19.7	2.7
70–74 years	19.6	2.9	16.6	4.6
75–79 years	17.2	2.9	17.7	3.4
80–84 years	16.7	3.8	23.3	5.7
85 years and over	23.3	4.4	31.6	9.0

SE Standard error.

Data Tables for Figures 1–34

Figure 13. Prevalence of hearing impairment among persons 70 years of age and over

Race and age	Women Percent	Women SE	Men Percent	Men SE
White:				
70 years and over	29.2	0.8	41.6	1.0
70–74 years	21.3	1.1	35.4	1.4
75–79 years	25.8	1.1	42.7	1.8
80–84 years	34.5	1.6	47.1	2.3
85 years and over	48.4	2.0	55.9	2.9
Black:				
70 years and over	17.3	1.5	21.2	2.2
70–74 years	12.6	2.1	15.1	3.3
75–79 years	12.3	2.5	25.3	4.1
80–84 years	24.8	3.8	21.6	6.4
85 years and over	29.9	4.9	33.3	7.6

SE Standard error.

Figure 14. Prevalence of reduced hip bone density among persons 65 years of age and over

Age	Women Osteoporosis Percent	Women Osteoporosis SE	Women Osteopenia Percent	Women Osteopenia SE	Men Osteoporosis Percent	Men Osteoporosis SE	Men Osteopenia Percent	Men Osteopenia SE
65 years and over	26.1	1.6	45.9	1.5	3.8	0.7	21.8	1.5
65–74 years.	19.0	2.0	46.9	2.1	2.0	0.6	17.9	1.6
75–84 years.	32.5	2.1	45.8	2.2	6.4	1.4	28.0	2.6
85 years and over	50.5	3.5	39.6	3.1	13.7	3.0	40.2	4.4

SE Standard error.

Figure 15. Percent of persons 70 years of age and over who have difficulty performing 1 or more physical activities, activities of daily living, and instrumental activities of daily living

Sex	70 years and over Percent	70 years and over SE	70–74 years Percent	70–74 years SE	75–79 years Percent	75–79 years SE	80–84 years Percent	80–84 years SE	85 years and over Percent	85 years and over SE
Women					Perform with difficulty					
Physical activity	32.5	0.8	31.3	1.2	33.9	1.3	35.3	1.7	29.1	1.7
ADL	22.2	0.7	19.6	1.0	19.0	1.0	23.9	1.3	32.9	1.9
IADL	12.8	0.5	12.5	0.8	12.0	1.0	14.1	1.3	13.2	1.2
Men										
Physical activity	30.1	0.7	27.7	1.1	30.3	1.4	35.3	1.8	30.9	2.4
ADL	16.6	0.7	13.8	0.9	16.6	1.1	20.2	1.6	22.6	2.2
IADL	6.9	0.5	5.6	0.6	8.0	0.9	7.9	1.1	7.6	1.4
Women					Unable to perform					
Physical activity	28.9	0.8	21.7	1.0	24.7	1.2	31.2	1.5	52.5	2.0
ADL	9.9	0.4	4.9	0.5	8.5	0.9	11.8	1.0	22.6	1.5
IADL	23.4	0.7	16.0	0.9	20.6	1.1	26.5	1.4	43.6	2.1
Men										
Physical activity	19.6	0.7	14.6	0.9	17.7	1.2	25.1	1.9	37.8	2.4
ADL	7.1	0.4	3.9	0.5	6.1	0.7	9.9	1.2	19.3	2.2
IADL	12.8	0.6	8.2	0.8	10.9	0.9	19.8	1.7	26.5	2.5

SE Standard error.

Figure 16. Percent of persons 70 years of age and over who report specific conditions as a cause of limitation in activities of daily living

Type of condition	Percent
Arthritis	10.6
Heart disease	4.0
Stroke	2.6
Respiratory	2.5
Diabetes	1.5

Figure 17. Distribution of weight among persons 65–74 years of age

Body mass index	Classification	Women	Men
Less than 19	Low	3.7	1.7
19–24.99	Healthy	36.0	29.8
25–29.9	Overweight	33.5	44.4
30–34.9	Moderately obese	16.0	19.4
35 and over	Severely obese	10.9	4.6

Figure 18. Prevalence of obesity among persons 65–74 years of age

Sex	1960–62 NHES	1971–74 NHANES I	1976–80 NHANES II	1988–94 NHANES III
Women	23.2	22.0	21.5	26.9
Men	10.4	10.9	13.2	24.1

Figure 19. Percent with untreated dental caries among dentate persons 65 years of age and over

Age	Women Percent	SE	Men Percent	SE
65 years and over	27.5	1.8	35.2	1.9
65–74 years	24.7	2.0	33.9	2.3
75–84 years	33.5	2.5	37.0	2.8
85 years and over	24.4	3.8	46.0	6.0

SE Standard error.

Figure 20. Prevalence of total tooth loss (edentulism) among persons 65 years of age and over

Age	1983 Percent	SE	1993 Percent	SE
65 years and over	38.4	0.6	29.5	1.0
65–74 years	34.1	0.7	25.5	1.1
75–84 years	43.4	1.0	33.6	1.6
85 years and over	54.2	1.8	43.5	4.2

SE Standard error.

Data Tables for Figures 1–34 ....

Figure 21. Number of social activities in a 2-week period among persons 70 years of age and over

Age and number of activities	Women		Men	
	Percent	SE	Percent	SE
70 years and over				
0 activities	1.6	0.2	2.4	0.2
1–2 activities	10.7	0.5	13.5	0.6
3–4 activities	29.8	0.7	30.3	0.9
5–7 activities	57.9	0.8	53.8	1.0
70–74 years				
0 activities	1.0	0.2	1.9	0.3
1–2 activities	6.8	0.5	10.5	1.0
3–4 activities	26.8	1.1	26.3	1.2
5–7 activities	65.4	1.2	61.2	1.4
75–79 years				
0 activities	1.3	0.3	1.7	0.4
1–2 activities	10.5	0.9	13.3	1.1
3–4 activities	27.5	1.2	30.3	1.4
5–7 activities	60.7	1.4	54.7	1.8
80–84 years				
0 activities	2.1	0.5	2.9	0.7
1–2 activities	11.9	1.1	15.9	1.4
3–4 activities	32.5	1.5	36.7	1.7
5–7 activities	53.5	1.5	44.5	1.8
85 years and over				
0 activities	3.1	0.7	5.3	1.2
1–2 activities	19.2	1.4	23.0	2.1
3–4 activities	38.3	1.9	35.9	2.5
5–7 activities	39.4	1.8	35.9	2.8

SE Standard error.

Figure 22. Percent who exercise and selected type of exercise among persons 65 years of age and over

Type of exercise	Women		Men	
	Percent	SE	Percent	SE
Any exercise	67.0	1.3	77.0	1.3
Walking	67.3	1.5	62.1	1.8
Gardening	37.9	1.7	54.0	2.0
Stretching	31.9	1.5	25.7	1.6
Swimming	3.6	0.6	3.2	0.6
Aerobics	4.9	0.7	*	*
Stair climbing	9.2	1.0	4.6	0.8

SE Standard error.
* Number in this category is too small to calculate reliable rates.

Figure 23. Number of caregivers providing assistance with activities of daily living or instrumental activities of daily living to persons 70 years of age and over

	1 caregiver		2 caregivers		3–4 caregivers	
Sex and age	Percent	SE	Percent	SE	Percent	SE
Women						
70 years and over	20.8	0.6	10.8	0.5	7.9	0.5
70–74 years................................	17.4	0.9	7.0	0.6	4.6	0.5
75–79 years................................	19.8	1.0	9.6	0.8	5.6	0.7
80–84 years................................	23.6	1.4	12.4	1.0	9.8	0.9
85 years and over	27.9	1.7	20.5	1.6	18.7	1.6
Men						
70 years and over	16.2	0.6	5.4	0.4	3.8	0.3
70–74 years................................	12.9	0.9	3.3	0.5	2.1	0.4
75–79 years................................	15.1	1.1	4.3	0.6	3.3	0.6
80–84 years................................	20.2	1.6	7.7	1.0	5.0	0.8
85 years and over	26.9	2.5	14.1	1.8	10.7	1.7

SE Standard error.

Figure 24. Percent with unmet needs among persons 70 years of age and over who need help with 1 or more activities of daily living or instrumental activities of daily living

	Unmet need ADL's		Unmet need IADL's only	
Sex and age	Percent	SE	Percent	SE
Women				
70–84 years................................	20.4	1.7	30.5	1.8
85 years and over	21.5	2.3	15.2	2.0
Men				
70–84 years................................	18.9	2.3	19.9	2.4
85 years and over	*	*	*	*

ADL's Activities of daily living.
IADL's Instrumental activities of daily living.
SE Standard error.
* Number in this category is too small to calculate reliable rates.

Data Tables for Figures 1–34 ....

Figure 25. Assistive devices used among persons 70 years of age and over

Age and number of devices	Women		Men	
	Percent	SE	Percent	SE
70 years and over				
1 device	21.2	0.6	21.5	0.7
2 devices.................	10.1	0.5	10.1	0.5
3 or more devices...........	7.8	0.3	8.3	0.5
70–74 years				
1 device	17.0	0.8	19.5	1.1
2 devices.................	7.6	0.6	7.1	0.7
3 or more devices...........	6.0	0.5	6.5	0.6
75–79 years				
1 device	19.5	1.1	20.7	1.2
2 devices.................	8.0	0.7	10.9	1.0
3 or more devices...........	6.4	0.6	8.8	0.9
80–84 years				
1 device	23.8	1.4	24.4	1.7
2 devices.................	11.4	1.1	10.9	1.2
3 or more devices...........	8.9	0.8	9.1	1.2
85 years and over				
1 device	31.7	1.8	27.5	2.5
2 devices.................	18.5	1.6	19.2	2.1
3 or more devices...........	13.5	1.2	13.3	1.8

SE Standard error.

Figure 26. Place of ambulatory physician contacts among persons 65 years of age and over

Sex and age	Place of contact									
	Doctor's office		Hospital		Home		Phone		Other	
	Percent	SE	Percent	SE	Percent	SE	Percent	SE	Percent	SE
Women										
65 years and over	51.1	1.3	9.2	0.5	19.8	1.5	10.0	0.6	9.9	0.7
65–74 years...............	55.5	1.6	10.8	0.7	10.9	1.6	10.7	0.8	12.1	1.0
75–84 years...............	49.3	1.8	8.4	0.7	23.3	2.3	9.9	0.9	9.1	0.9
85 years and over	39.6	2.9	5.7	1.0	43.1	3.9	8.1	1.2	3.5	0.6
Men										
65 years and over	54.3	1.6	11.7	0.8	13.5	1.9	8.6	0.6	11.9	0.8
65–74 years...............	56.5	1.7	12.3	0.9	7.9	1.5	10.0	0.8	13.5	1.2
75–84 years...............	51.1	3.1	11.8	1.6	19.7	4.0	7.1	0.8	10.3	1.3
85 years and over	53.0	4.4	7.6	2.2	25.5	4.8	5.6	1.3	8.4	1.9

SE Standard error.

Figure 27. Hospital discharge rates in non-Federal short-stay hospitals for selected first-listed diagnoses among persons 65 years of age and over

	Women			Men		
Diagnosis	65–74 years	75–84 years	85 years and over	65–74 years	75–84 years	85 years and over
All diagnoses	246.6	395.3	565.3	270.6	441.3	624.7
Heart Disease	53.4	89.1	112.7	73.5	110.3	131.0
Stroke	12.0	26.4	39.5	15.3	31.9	39.8
Malignant neoplasms	19.8	19.8	16.3	23.5	27.2	31.3
Pneumonia	10.8	21.1	46.0	13.0	29.9	73.3
Bronchitis	8.4	10.2	9.6	7.1	12.0	21.4
Fractures	9.7	23.6	55.9	3.5	10.3	30.6

Figure 28. Percent vaccinated against influenza and pneumococcal disease among persons 65 years of age and over

	Influenza		Pneumococcal disease	
Race and Hispanic origin	Percent	SE	Percent	SE
White, non-Hispanic	56.8	0.6	31.2	0.7
Black, non-Hispanic	36.4	1.5	16.2	1.4
Hispanic	44.0	3.2	15.9	1.7

SE Standard error.

Figure 29. Home health care patients among persons 65 years of age and over

Sex	65 years and over	65–74 years	75–84 years	85 years and over
	Patients per 1,000 population			
Women	61.1	27.6	84.1	130.1
Men	36.5	18.2	55.4	99.5

Figure 30. Home health care services received by current patients 65 years of age and over

Type of service	Percent receiving service
Nursing	85.3
Homemaker	28.7
Physical therapy	20.0
Social services	10.9
Medications	9.9
Continuous home care	5.8
Occupational therapy	4.8
Physician services	3.7
Nutrition	3.4
All other services	15.1

Data Tables for Figures 1–34 ....

Figure 31. Health insurance coverage among persons 65 years of age and over

Age, race, and Hispanic origin	Medicare only		Medicare/Medicaid		Medicare/private		Private only		None	
	Percent	SE	Percent	SE	Percent	SE	Percent	SE	Percent	SE
65–84 years										
White, non-Hispanic	13.9	0.9	5.1	0.3	77.9	1.0	2.7	0.2	0.5	0.1
Black, non-Hispanic	29.5	1.7	22.4	1.2	43.2	1.9	3.6	0.6	1.3	0.3
Hispanic	27.3	2.5	23.5	1.9	42.4	2.9	3.8	0.8	3.0	0.5
85 years of age and over										
White, non-Hispanic	20.4	1.4	7.5	0.8	70.2	1.6	*	*	*	*
Black, non-Hispanic	38.6	4.5	28.1	3.3	32.5	4.8	*	*	*	*
Hispanic	23.7	5.6	49.2	5.7	22.6	4.4	*	*	*	*

SE Standard error.
* Number in this category is too small to calculate reliable rates.

Figure 32. Percent of Medicare enrollees in health maintenance organizations

State	Percent	State	Percent
New England		**East South Central**	
Maine........................	0	Kentucky	1
New Hampshire	0	Tennessee	0
Vermont........................	1	Alabama...........................	3
Massachusetts	16	Mississippi	0
Rhode Island	15	**West South Central**	
Connecticut	5	Arkansas	1
Middle Atlantic		Louisiana	9
New York.......................	13	Oklahoma..........................	6
New Jersey	7	Texas.............................	11
Pennsylvania	17	**Mountain**	
East North Central		Montana...........................	0
Ohio...........................	6	Idaho.............................	0
Indiana.........................	2	Wyoming	0
Illinois	9	Colorado	26
Michigan........................	1	New Mexico	17
Wisconsin.......................	2	Arizona	34
West North Central		Utah..............................	17
Minnesota.......................	18	Nevada	20
Iowa...........................	2	**Pacific**	
Missouri........................	10	Washington........................	20
North Dakota	1	Oregon............................	37
South Dakota	0	California..........................	38
Nebraska	3	Alaska	0
Kansas.........................	3	Hawaii	33
South Atlantic			
Delaware	0		
Maryland	8		
District of Columbia..............	21		
Virginia.........................	1		
West Virginia	2		
North Carolina...................	1		
South Carolina	1		
Georgia	1		
Florida.........................	22		

Figure 33. Estimated amount of personal health care expenditures attributed to heart disease among persons 65 years of age and over

Type of Health Service	Women				Men			
	65 years and over	65–74 years	75–84 years	85 years and over	65 years and over	65–74 years	75–84 years	85 years and over
	Amount in billions							
All personal health care.................	31.2	8.2	12.0	11.0	26.5	12.6	9.9	3.9
Hospital care.........................	14.2	5.2	5.9	3.0	18.2	9.4	6.8	2.0
Physician and other professional services....	3.0	1.2	1.2	0.6	3.2	1.8	1.1	0.3
Home health care....................	2.1	0.4	1.1	0.6	0.8	0.2	0.4	0.2
Prescription drugs and medical durables.....	1.8	0.7	0.8	0.4	1.6	0.9	0.6	0.2
Nursing home care...................	10.2	0.7	3.1	6.4	2.7	0.4	1.0	1.3

Figures may not sum to totals due to rounding.

Figure 34. Estimated amount of personal health care expenditures attributed to diabetes among persons 65 years and over

Type of Health Service	Women				Men			
	65 years and over	65–74 years	75–84 years	85 years and over	65 years and over	65–74 years	75–84 years	85 years and over
	Amount in billions							
All personal health care.................	15.6	6.5	6.1	3.1	10.6	5.6	3.5	1.5
Hospital care.........................	6.4	3.1	2.2	1.1	5.6	3.4	1.7	0.6
Physician and other professional services....	2.1	1.1	0.7	0.3	1.5	0.9	0.5	0.1
Home health care....................	2.2	0.9	1.0	0.3	1.5	0.7	0.6	0.3
Prescription drugs and medical durables.....	0.9	0.5	0.3	0.1	0.7	0.5	0.2	0.1
Nursing home care...................	4.0	0.8	1.9	1.3	1.2	0.2	0.6	0.4

Figures may not sum to totals due to rounding.

List of Detailed Tables ....

List of Detailed Tables ....

Table 1 (page 1 of 2). Resident population, according to age, sex, detailed race, and Hispanic origin: United States, selected years 1950–97

[Data are based on decennial census updated by data from multiple sources]

Sex, race, Hispanic origin, and year	Total resident population	Under 1 year	1–4 years	5–14 years	15–24 years	25–34 years	35–44 years	45–54 years	55–64 years	65–74 years	75–84 years	85 years and over
All persons						Number in thousands						
1950	150,697	3,147	13,017	24,319	22,098	23,759	21,450	17,343	13,370	8,340	3,278	577
1960	179,323	4,112	16,209	35,465	24,020	22,818	24,081	20,485	15,572	10,997	4,633	929
1970	203,212	3,485	13,669	40,746	35,441	24,907	23,088	23,220	18,590	12,435	6,119	1,511
1980	226,546	3,534	12,815	34,942	42,487	37,082	25,634	22,800	21,703	15,580	7,729	2,240
1990	248,710	3,946	14,812	35,095	37,013	43,161	37,435	25,057	21,113	18,045	10,012	3,021
1996	265,284	3,769	15,516	38,422	36,221	40,368	43,393	32,370	21,361	18,669	11,430	3,762
1997	267,636	3,797	15,353	38,778	36,580	39,610	43,998	33,633	21,813	18,499	11,706	3,871
Male												
1950	74,833	1,602	6,634	12,375	10,918	11,597	10,588	8,655	6,697	4,024	1,507	237
1960	88,331	2,090	8,240	18,029	11,906	11,179	11,755	10,093	7,537	5,116	2,025	362
1970	98,912	1,778	6,968	20,759	17,551	12,217	11,231	11,199	8,793	5,437	2,436	542
1980	110,053	1,806	6,556	17,855	21,418	18,382	12,570	11,009	10,152	6,757	2,867	682
1990	121,239	2,018	7,581	17,971	18,915	21,564	18,510	12,232	9,955	7,907	3,745	841
1996	129,810	1,928	7,940	19,681	18,618	20,191	21,569	15,837	10,166	8,325	4,486	1,070
1997	131,018	1,943	7,858	19,861	18,806	19,810	21,883	16,457	10,390	8,269	4,629	1,112
Female												
1950	75,864	1,545	6,383	11,944	11,181	12,162	10,863	8,688	6,672	4,316	1,771	340
1960	90,992	2,022	7,969	17,437	12,114	11,639	12,326	10,393	8,036	5,881	2,609	567
1970	104,300	1,707	6,701	19,986	17,890	12,690	11,857	12,021	9,797	6,998	3,683	969
1980	116,493	1,727	6,259	17,087	21,068	18,700	13,065	11,791	11,551	8,825	4,862	1,559
1990	127,471	1,928	7,231	17,124	18,098	21,596	18,925	12,824	11,158	10,139	6,267	2,180
1996	135,474	1,841	7,577	18,741	17,604	20,177	21,825	16,533	11,195	10,345	6,944	2,692
1997	136,618	1,854	7,495	18,917	17,774	19,799	22,115	17,176	11,422	10,230	7,077	2,759
White male												
1950	67,129	1,400	5,845	10,860	9,689	10,430	9,529	7,836	6,130	3,736	1,406	218
1960	78,367	1,784	7,065	15,659	10,483	9,940	10,564	9,114	6,850	4,702	1,875	331
1970	86,721	1,501	5,873	17,667	15,232	10,775	9,979	10,090	7,958	4,916	2,243	487
1980	94,924	1,485	5,397	14,764	18,110	15,928	11,005	9,771	9,149	6,095	2,600	621
1990	102,143	1,604	6,071	14,467	15,389	18,071	15,819	10,624	8,813	7,127	3,397	760
1996	108,052	1,546	6,294	15,622	14,910	16,587	18,128	13,649	8,864	7,419	4,076	959
1997	108,893	1,549	6,240	15,727	15,057	16,209	18,355	14,158	9,047	7,349	4,204	998
White female												
1950	67,813	1,341	5,599	10,431	9,821	10,851	9,719	7,868	6,168	4,031	1,669	314
1960	80,465	1,714	6,795	15,068	10,596	10,204	11,000	9,364	7,327	5,428	2,441	527
1970	91,028	1,434	5,615	16,912	15,420	11,004	10,349	10,756	8,853	6,366	3,429	890
1980	99,788	1,410	5,121	14,048	17,643	15,887	11,227	10,282	10,324	7,950	4,457	1,440
1990	106,561	1,524	5,762	13,706	14,599	17,757	15,834	10,946	9,698	9,048	5,687	2,001
1996	111,696	1,469	5,980	14,816	13,937	16,230	17,953	13,946	9,551	9,093	6,273	2,447
1997	112,441	1,472	5,924	14,926	14,064	15,857	18,161	14,456	9,728	8,961	6,388	2,507
Black male												
1950	7,300	- - -	- - -	1,442	1,162	1,105	1,003	772	460	299	- - -	- - -
1960	9,114	281	1,082	2,185	1,305	1,120	1,086	891	617	382	137	29
1970	10,748	245	975	2,784	2,041	1,226	1,084	979	739	461	169	46
1980	12,612	270	970	2,618	2,813	1,974	1,238	1,026	855	568	228	53
1990	14,420	322	1,164	2,700	2,669	2,592	1,962	1,175	878	614	277	66
1996	15,903	277	1,218	3,044	2,756	2,565	2,485	1,545	937	682	311	83
1997	16,121	282	1,185	3,090	2,790	2,551	2,548	1,622	960	690	319	86
Black female												
1950	7,745	- - -	- - -	1,446	1,300	1,260	1,112	796	443	322	- - -	- - -
1960	9,758	283	1,085	2,191	1,404	1,300	1,229	974	663	430	160	38
1970	11,832	243	970	2,773	2,196	1,456	1,309	1,134	868	582	230	71
1980	14,071	267	953	2,583	2,942	2,272	1,490	1,260	1,061	777	360	106
1990	16,063	316	1,137	2,641	2,700	2,905	2,279	1,416	1,135	884	495	156
1996	17,600	270	1,185	2,953	2,741	2,847	2,830	1,864	1,221	951	535	203
1997	17,826	274	1,151	2,995	2,771	2,827	2,892	1,956	1,253	958	544	207

See notes at end of table.

Table 1 (page 2 of 2). Resident population, according to age, sex, detailed race, and Hispanic origin: United States, selected years 1950–97

[Data are based on decennial census updated by data from multiple sources]

Sex, race, Hispanic origin, and year	Total resident population	Under 1 year	1–4 years	5–14 years	15–24 years	25–34 years	35–44 years	45–54 years	55–64 years	65–74 years	75–84 years	85 years and over
American Indian or Alaska Native male						Number in thousands						
1980	702	17	60	153	164	114	75	53	37	22	9	2
1990	1,024	24	88	206	192	183	140	86	55	32	13	3
1996	1,136	20	82	236	203	192	168	110	63	39	18	5
1997	1,153	21	81	237	206	193	172	115	65	39	19	6
American Indian or Alaska Native female												
1980	718	16	57	149	158	118	79	57	41	26	12	4
1990	1,041	24	85	200	178	186	148	92	61	41	21	6
1996	1,152	20	80	228	195	182	174	118	71	47	26	11
1997	1,169	20	79	229	200	181	177	122	73	48	27	12
Asian or Pacific Islander male												
1980	1,814	35	129	321	334	367	252	159	110	72	29	6
1990	3,652	68	258	598	665	718	588	347	208	133	57	12
1996	4,719	86	346	779	749	849	788	532	302	185	82	22
1997	4,851	91	352	808	753	858	808	562	319	190	87	23
Asian or Pacific Islander female												
1980	1,915	34	127	307	325	423	269	193	126	70	33	9
1990	3,805	65	247	578	621	749	664	371	264	166	65	17
1996	5,024	83	332	743	731	918	867	605	352	254	110	31
1997	5,182	88	340	767	740	934	886	642	369	264	118	33
Hispanic male												
1980	7,280	187	661	1,530	1,646	1,255	761	570	364	201	86	19
1990	11,388	279	980	2,128	2,376	2,310	1,471	818	551	312	131	32
1996	14,519	343	1,334	2,658	2,677	2,779	2,164	1,212	683	439	179	51
1997	15,074	354	1,363	2,786	2,764	2,824	2,281	1,292	711	454	192	54
Hispanic female												
1980	7,329	181	634	1,482	1,547	1,249	805	615	411	257	116	30
1990	10,966	268	939	2,039	2,028	2,073	1,448	868	632	403	209	59
1996	13,750	326	1,269	2,534	2,298	2,373	2,016	1,242	769	549	275	99
1997	14,274	336	1,294	2,657	2,387	2,408	2,111	1,319	801	567	289	106
Non-Hispanic White male												
1980	88,035	1,308	4,773	13,318	16,555	14,739	10,285	9,229	8,802	5,906	2,519	603
1990	91,743	1,351	5,181	12,525	13,219	15,967	14,481	9,875	8,303	6,837	3,275	729
1996	94,799	1,232	5,075	13,216	12,455	14,049	16,160	12,542	8,237	7,012	3,909	911
1997	95,127	1,225	4,995	13,202	12,522	13,628	16,280	12,979	8,394	6,930	4,025	947
Non-Hispanic White female												
1980	92,872	1,240	4,522	12,647	16,185	14,711	10,468	9,700	9,935	7,708	4,345	1,411
1990	96,557	1,280	4,909	11,846	12,749	15,872	14,520	10,153	9,116	8,674	5,491	1,945
1996	99,179	1,171	4,821	12,521	11,843	14,075	16,125	12,817	8,848	8,587	6,017	2,353
1997	99,444	1,165	4,742	12,517	11,889	13,669	16,246	13,256	8,996	8,439	6,119	2,407

- - - Data not available.

NOTES: The race groups, white, black, American Indian or Alaska Native, and Asian or Pacific Islander, include persons of Hispanic and non-Hispanic origin. Conversely, persons of Hispanic origin may be of any race. Population figures are census counts as of April 1 for 1950, 1960, 1970, 1980, and 1990 and estimates as of July 1 for other years. See Appendix I, Department of Commerce. Populations for age groups may not sum to the total due to rounding. Although population figures are shown rounded to the nearest 1,000, calculations of birth rates and death rates shown in this volume are based on unrounded population figures for decennial years and starting with data year 1992. See Appendix II, Rate. Data for additional years are available (see Appendix III).

SOURCES: U.S. Bureau of the Census: 1950 Nonwhite Population by Race. Special Report P-E, No. 3B. Washington. U.S. Government Printing Office, 1951; U.S. Census of Population: 1960, Number of Inhabitants, PC(1)-A1, United States Summary, 1964; 1970, Number of Inhabitants, Final Report PC(1)-A1, United States Summary, 1971; U.S. population estimates, by age, sex, race, and Hispanic origin: 1980 to 1991. Current Population Reports. Series P–25, No. 1095. Washington. U.S. Government Printing Office, Feb. 1993; U.S. resident population—estimates by age, sex, race, and Hispanic origin (consistent with the 1990 Census, as enumerated): 1992. Census files RESP0792 in PPL–21, series 1294. 1993; July 1, 1993. RES0793. 1994; July 1, 1994. RESD0794. 1995; July 1, 1995. RESD0795. 1996; July 1, 1996. NESTV96 in PPL-57. 1997; July 1, 1997. NESTV97 in PPL–91R. 1998.

Table 2. Persons and families below poverty level, according to selected characteristics, race, and Hispanic origin: United States, selected years 1973–97

[Data are based on household interviews of the civilian noninstitutionalized population]

Selected characteristics, race, and Hispanic origin	1973	1980	1985	1990	1991	1992	1993	1994	1995	1996	1997
All persons					Percent below poverty						
All races	11.1	13.0	14.0	13.5	14.2	14.8	15.1	14.5	13.8	13.7	13.3
White	8.4	10.2	11.4	10.7	11.3	11.9	12.2	11.7	11.2	11.2	11.0
Black	31.4	32.5	31.3	31.9	32.7	33.4	33.1	30.6	29.3	28.4	26.5
Asian or Pacific Islander	- - -	- - -	- - -	12.2	13.8	12.7	15.3	14.6	14.6	14.5	14.0
Hispanic origin.	21.9	25.7	29.0	28.1	28.7	29.6	30.6	30.7	30.3	29.4	27.1
Mexican.	- - -	- - -	28.8	28.1	29.5	30.1	31.6	32.3	31.2	31.0	27.9
Puerto Rican	- - -	- - -	43.3	40.6	39.4	36.5	38.4	36.0	38.1	35.7	34.2
White, non-Hispanic	- - -	- - -	- - -	8.8	9.4	9.6	9.9	9.4	8.5	8.6	8.6
Related children under 18 years of age in families											
All races	14.2	17.9	20.1	19.9	21.1	21.6	22.0	21.2	20.2	19.8	19.2
White	9.7	13.4	15.6	15.1	16.1	16.5	17.0	16.3	15.5	15.5	15.4
Black	40.6	42.1	43.1	44.2	45.6	46.3	45.9	43.3	41.5	39.5	36.8
Asian or Pacific Islander.	- - -	- - -	- - -	17.0	17.1	16.0	17.6	17.9	18.6	19.1	19.9
Hispanic origin.	27.8	33.0	39.6	37.7	39.8	39.0	39.9	41.1	39.3	39.9	36.4
Mexican.	- - -	- - -	37.4	35.5	38.9	38.2	39.5	41.8	39.3	40.7	35.8
Puerto Rican	- - -	- - -	58.6	56.7	57.7	52.2	53.8	50.5	53.2	49.4	49.1
White, non-Hispanic	- - -	- - -	- - -	11.6	12.4	12.4	12.8	11.8	10.6	10.4	10.7
Related children under 18 years of age in families with female householder and no spouse present											
All races	- - -	50.8	53.6	53.4	55.5	54.3	53.7	52.9	50.3	49.3	49.0
White	- - -	41.6	45.2	45.9	47.1	45.3	45.6	45.7	42.5	43.1	44.3
Black	- - -	64.8	66.9	64.7	68.2	67.1	65.9	63.2	61.6	58.2	55.3
Asian or Pacific Islander	- - -	- - -	- - -	32.2	31.9	43.5	32.2	36.8	42.4	48.8	58.3
Hispanic origin.	- - -	65.0	72.4	68.4	68.6	65.7	66.1	68.3	65.7	67.4	62.8
Mexican.	- - -	- - -	64.4	62.4	66.6	63.5	64.6	69.5	65.9	68.1	62.2
Puerto Rican	- - -	- - -	85.4	82.7	83.3	74.1	73.4	73.6	79.6	76.6	71.0
White, non-Hispanic	- - -	- - -	- - -	39.6	41.0	39.6	39.0	38.0	33.5	34.9	37.2
All persons					Number below poverty in thousands						
All races	22,973	29,272	33,064	33,585	35,708	38,014	39,265	38,059	36,425	36,529	35,574
White	15,142	19,699	22,860	22,326	23,747	25,259	26,226	25,379	24,423	24,650	24,396
Black	7,388	8,579	8,926	9,837	10,242	10,827	10,877	10,196	9,872	9,694	9,116
Asian or Pacific Islander	- - -	- - -	- - -	858	996	985	1,134	974	1,411	1,454	1,468
Hispanic origin.	2,366	3,491	5,236	6,006	6,339	7,592	8,126	8,416	8,574	8,697	8,308
Mexican.	- - -	- - -	3,220	3,764	4,149	4,404	5,373	5,781	5,608	5,815	5,509
Puerto Rican	- - -	- - -	1,011	966	924	874	1,061	981	1,183	1,116	1,059
White, non-Hispanic	- - -	- - -	- - -	16,622	17,741	18,202	18,882	18,110	16,267	16,462	16,491
Related children under 18 years of age in families											
All races	9,453	11,114	12,483	12,715	13,658	14,521	14,961	14,610	13,999	13,764	13,422
White	5,462	6,817	7,838	7,696	8,316	8,752	9,123	8,826	8,474	8,488	8,441
Black	3,822	3,906	4,057	4,412	4,637	5,015	5,030	4,787	4,644	4,411	4,116
Asian or Pacific Islander	- - -	- - -	- - -	356	348	352	358	308	532	553	608
Hispanic origin.	1,364	1,718	2,512	2,750	2,977	3,440	3,666	3,956	3,938	4,090	3,865
Mexican.	- - -	- - -	1,589	1,733	2,004	2,019	2,520	2,805	2,655	2,853	2,666
Puerto Rican	- - -	- - -	535	490	475	457	537	485	610	545	519
White, non-Hispanic	- - -	- - -	- - -	5,106	5,497	5,558	5,819	5,404	4,745	4,656	4,759
Related children under 18 years of age in families with female householder and no spouse present											
All races	- - -	5,866	6,716	7,363	8,065	8,032	8,503	8,427	8,364	7,990	7,928
White	- - -	2,813	3,372	3,597	3,941	3,783	4,102	4,099	4,051	4,029	4,186
Black	- - -	2,944	3,181	3,543	3,853	3,967	4,104	3,935	3,954	3,619	3,402
Asian or Pacific Islander	- - -	- - -	- - -	80	81	103	72	59	145	167	200
Hispanic origin.	- - -	809	1,247	1,314	1,398	1,289	1,673	1,804	1,872	1,779	1,758
Mexican.	- - -	- - -	553	615	785	679	890	1,054	1,056	948	991
Puerto Rican	- - -	- - -	449	382	369	363	430	394	459	444	392
White, non-Hispanic	- - -	- - -	- - -	2,411	2,661	2,588	2,636	2,563	2,299	2,419	2,551

- - - Data not available.

NOTES: The race groups white, black, and Asian include persons of Hispanic and non-Hispanic origin; persons of Hispanic origin may be of any race. Poverty status is based on family income and family size using Bureau of the Census poverty thresholds. See Appendix II. In 1989, 31.2 percent of the American Indian population in the United States, or 585,000 persons, were below the poverty threshold, based on 1989 income data from the 1990 decennial census (U.S. Bureau of the Census, 1990 Census of Population, *Characteristics of American Indians by Tribe and Language*, 1990 CP–3–7). Data for additional years are available (see Appendix III).

SOURCE: U.S. Bureau of the Census. Dalaker J and Naifeh M. Poverty in the United States: 1997. Current population reports, series P–60, no 201. Washington: U.S. Government Printing Office. 1998; unpublished data.

Table 3 (page 1 of 2). Crude birth rates, fertility rates, and birth rates by age of mother, according to detailed race and Hispanic origin: United States, selected years 1950–97

[Data are based on the National Vital Statistics System]

Race of mother, Hispanic origin of mother, and year	Crude birth rate[1]	Fertility rate[2]	10–14 years	15–19 years Total	15–17 years	18–19 years	20–24 years	25–29 years	30–34 years	35–39 years	40–44 years	45–49 years[3]
All races					Live births per 1,000 women							
1950	24.1	106.2	1.0	81.6	40.7	132.7	196.6	166.1	103.7	52.9	15.1	1.2
1960	23.7	118.0	0.8	89.1	43.9	166.7	258.1	197.4	112.7	56.2	15.5	0.9
1970	18.4	87.9	1.2	68.3	38.8	114.7	167.8	145.1	73.3	31.7	8.1	0.5
1980	15.9	68.4	1.1	53.0	32.5	82.1	115.1	112.9	61.9	19.8	3.9	0.2
1985	15.8	66.3	1.2	51.0	31.0	79.6	108.3	111.0	69.1	24.0	4.0	0.2
1990	16.7	70.9	1.4	59.9	37.5	88.6	116.5	120.2	80.8	31.7	5.5	0.2
1991	16.3	69.6	1.4	62.1	38.7	94.4	115.7	118.2	79.5	32.0	5.5	0.2
1992	15.9	68.9	1.4	60.7	37.8	94.5	114.6	117.4	80.2	32.5	5.9	0.3
1993	15.5	67.6	1.4	59.6	37.8	92.1	112.6	115.5	80.8	32.9	6.1	0.3
1994	15.2	66.7	1.4	58.9	37.6	91.5	111.1	113.9	81.5	33.7	6.4	0.3
1995	14.8	65.6	1.3	56.8	36.0	89.1	109.8	112.2	82.5	34.3	6.6	0.3
1996	14.7	65.3	1.2	54.4	33.8	86.0	110.4	113.1	83.9	35.3	6.8	0.3
1997	14.5	65.0	1.1	52.3	32.1	83.6	110.4	113.8	85.3	36.1	7.1	0.4
Race of child:[4] White												
1950	23.0	102.3	0.4	70.0	31.3	120.5	190.4	165.1	102.6	51.4	14.5	1.0
1960	22.7	113.2	0.4	79.4	35.5	154.6	252.8	194.9	109.6	54.0	14.7	0.8
1970	17.4	84.1	0.5	57.4	29.2	101.5	163.4	145.9	71.9	30.0	7.5	0.4
1980	14.9	64.7	0.6	44.7	25.2	72.1	109.5	112.4	60.4	18.5	3.4	0.2
Race of mother:[5] White												
1980	15.1	65.6	0.6	45.4	25.5	73.2	111.1	113.8	61.2	18.8	3.5	0.2
1985	15.0	64.1	0.6	43.3	24.4	70.4	104.1	112.3	69.9	23.3	3.7	0.2
1990	15.8	68.3	0.7	50.8	29.5	78.0	109.8	120.7	81.7	31.5	5.2	0.2
1991	15.4	67.0	0.8	52.8	30.7	83.5	109.0	118.8	80.5	31.8	5.2	0.2
1992	15.0	66.5	0.8	51.8	30.1	83.8	108.2	118.4	81.4	32.2	5.7	0.2
1993	14.7	65.4	0.8	51.1	30.3	82.1	106.9	116.6	82.1	32.7	5.9	0.3
1994	14.4	64.9	0.8	51.1	30.7	82.1	106.2	115.5	83.2	33.7	6.2	0.3
1995	14.2	64.4	0.8	50.1	30.0	81.2	106.3	114.8	84.6	34.5	6.4	0.3
1996	14.1	64.3	0.8	48.1	28.4	78.4	107.2	116.1	86.3	35.6	6.7	0.3
1997	13.9	63.9	0.7	46.3	27.1	75.9	106.7	116.6	87.8	36.4	6.9	0.4
Race of child:[4] Black												
1960	31.9	153.5	4.3	156.1	- - -	- - -	295.4	218.6	137.1	73.9	21.9	1.1
1970	25.3	115.4	5.2	140.7	101.4	204.9	202.7	136.3	79.6	41.9	12.5	1.0
1980	22.1	88.1	4.3	100.0	73.6	138.8	146.3	109.1	62.9	24.5	5.8	0.3
Race of mother:[5] Black												
1980	21.3	84.9	4.3	97.8	72.5	135.1	140.0	103.9	59.9	23.5	5.6	0.3
1985	20.4	78.8	4.5	95.4	69.3	132.4	135.0	100.2	57.9	23.9	4.6	0.3
1990	22.4	86.8	4.9	112.8	82.3	152.9	160.2	115.5	68.7	28.1	5.5	0.3
1991	21.9	85.2	4.8	115.5	84.1	158.6	160.9	113.1	67.7	28.3	5.5	0.2
1992	21.3	83.2	4.7	112.4	81.3	157.9	158.0	111.2	67.5	28.8	5.6	0.2
1993	20.5	80.5	4.6	108.6	79.8	151.9	152.6	108.4	67.3	29.2	5.9	0.3
1994	19.5	76.9	4.6	104.5	76.3	148.3	146.0	104.0	65.8	28.9	5.9	0.3
1995	18.2	72.3	4.2	96.1	69.7	137.1	137.1	98.6	64.0	28.7	6.0	0.3
1996	17.8	70.7	3.6	91.4	64.7	132.5	136.8	98.2	63.3	29.1	6.1	0.3
1997	17.7	70.7	3.3	88.2	60.8	130.1	139.0	99.5	64.3	29.7	6.5	0.3
American Indian or Alaska Native mothers[5]												
1980	20.7	82.7	1.9	82.2	51.5	129.5	143.7	106.6	61.8	28.1	8.2	*
1985	19.8	78.6	1.7	79.2	47.7	124.1	139.1	109.6	62.6	27.4	6.0	*
1990	18.9	76.2	1.6	81.1	48.5	129.3	148.7	110.3	61.5	27.5	5.9	*
1991	18.3	75.1	1.6	85.0	52.7	134.3	144.9	106.9	61.9	27.2	5.9	0.4
1992	18.4	75.4	1.6	84.4	53.8	132.6	145.5	109.4	63.0	28.0	6.1	*
1993	17.8	73.4	1.4	83.1	53.7	130.7	139.8	107.6	62.8	27.6	5.9	*
1994	17.1	70.9	1.9	80.8	51.3	130.3	134.2	104.1	61.2	27.5	5.9	0.4
1995	16.6	69.1	1.8	78.0	47.8	130.7	132.5	98.4	62.2	27.7	6.1	*
1996	16.6	68.7	1.7	73.9	46.4	122.3	133.9	98.5	63.2	28.5	6.3	*
1997	16.6	69.1	1.7	71.8	45.3	117.6	134.9	100.8	64.2	29.3	6.4	0.4

See footnotes at end of table.

[Data are based on the National Vital Statistics System]

Race of mother, Hispanic origin of mother, and year	Crude birth rate[1]	Fertility rate[2]	Age of mother									
			10–14 years	15–19 years			20–24 years	25–29 years	30–34 years	35–39 years	40–44 years	45–49 years[3]
				Total	15–17 years	18–19 years						
Asian or Pacific Islander mothers[5]			Live births per 1,000 women									
1980	19.9	73.2	0.3	26.2	12.0	46.2	93.3	127.4	96.0	38.3	8.5	0.7
1985	18.7	68.4	0.4	23.8	12.5	40.8	83.6	123.0	93.6	42.7	8.7	1.2
1990	19.0	69.6	0.7	26.4	16.0	40.2	79.2	126.3	106.5	49.6	10.7	1.1
1991	18.2	67.6	0.8	27.4	16.1	43.1	75.2	123.2	103.3	49.0	11.2	1.1
1992	18.0	67.2	0.7	26.6	15.2	43.1	74.6	121.0	103.0	50.6	11.0	0.9
1993	17.7	66.7	0.6	27.0	16.0	43.3	73.3	119.9	103.9	50.2	11.3	0.9
1994	17.5	66.8	0.7	27.1	16.1	44.1	73.1	118.6	105.2	51.3	11.6	1.0
1995	17.3	66.4	0.7	26.1	15.4	43.4	72.4	113.4	106.9	52.4	12.1	0.8
1996	17.0	65.9	0.6	24.6	14.9	40.4	70.7	111.2	109.2	52.2	12.2	0.8
1997	16.9	66.3	0.5	23.7	14.3	39.3	70.5	113.2	110.3	54.1	11.9	0.9
Hispanic mothers[5,6,7]												
1980	23.5	95.4	1.7	82.2	52.1	126.9	156.4	132.1	83.2	39.9	10.6	0.7
1990	26.7	107.7	2.4	100.3	65.9	147.7	181.0	153.0	98.3	45.3	10.9	0.7
1991	26.7	108.1	2.4	106.7	70.6	158.5	186.3	152.8	96.1	44.9	10.7	0.6
1992	26.5	108.6	2.6	107.1	71.4	159.7	190.6	154.4	96.8	45.6	10.9	0.6
1993	26.0	106.9	2.7	106.8	71.7	159.1	188.3	154.0	96.4	44.7	10.6	0.6
1994	25.5	105.6	2.7	107.7	74.0	158.0	188.2	153.2	95.4	44.3	10.7	0.6
1995	25.2	105.0	2.7	106.7	72.9	157.9	188.5	153.8	95.9	44.9	10.8	0.6
1996	24.8	104.9	2.6	101.8	69.0	151.1	189.5	161.0	98.1	45.1	10.8	0.6
1997	24.2	102.8	2.3	97.4	66.3	144.3	184.2	161.7	97.9	45.0	10.8	0.6
White, non-Hispanic mothers[5,6,7]												
1980	14.2	62.4	0.4	41.2	22.4	67.7	105.5	110.6	59.9	17.7	3.0	0.1
1990	14.4	62.8	0.5	42.5	23.2	66.6	97.5	115.3	79.4	30.0	4.7	0.2
1991	13.9	61.0	0.5	43.4	23.6	70.5	94.2	110.9	76.5	29.6	4.6	0.2
1992	13.5	60.2	0.5	41.7	22.7	69.8	93.9	111.5	78.7	30.5	5.1	0.2
1993	13.1	59.0	0.5	40.7	22.7	67.7	90.8	107.6	78.0	30.4	5.2	0.2
1994	12.8	58.3	0.5	40.4	22.8	67.4	90.9	107.9	80.7	32.1	5.7	0.2
1995	12.6	57.6	0.4	39.3	22.0	66.1	90.0	106.5	82.0	32.9	5.9	0.3
1996	12.4	57.3	0.4	37.6	20.6	63.7	90.1	107.0	83.5	34.0	6.2	0.3
1997	12.2	57.0	0.4	36.0	19.4	61.9	89.8	107.2	85.2	34.9	6.4	0.3

- - - Data not available.
* Based on fewer than 20 births.
[1] Live births per 1,000 population.
[2] Total number of live births regardless of age of mother per 1,000 women 15–44 years of age.
[3] Starting in 1997 data are for live births to mothers 45–54 years of age per 1,000 women 45–49 years of age (see Appendix I, National Vital Statistics System).
[4] Live births are tabulated by race of child.
[5] Live births are tabulated by race and/or Hispanic origin of mother.
[6] Trend data for Hispanics and non-Hispanics are affected by expansion of the reporting area for an Hispanic-origin item on the birth certificate and by immigration. These two factors affect numbers of events, composition of the Hispanic population, and maternal and infant health characteristics. The number of States in the reporting area increased from 22 in 1980, to 23 and the District of Columbia (DC) in 1983–87, 30 and DC in 1988, 47 and DC in 1989, 48 and DC in 1990, 49 and DC in 1991–92, and 50 and DC in 1993 and later years (see Appendix I, National Vital Statistics System).
[7] Rates in 1985 were not calculated because estimates for the Hispanic and non-Hispanic populations were not available.

NOTES: Data are based on births adjusted for underregistration for 1950 and on registered births for all other years. Beginning in 1970, births to persons who were not residents of the 50 States and the District of Columbia are excluded. The race groups, white, black, American Indian or Alaska Native, and Asian or Pacific Islander, include persons of Hispanic and non-Hispanic origin. Conversely, persons of Hispanic origin may be of any race. Data for additional years are available (see Appendix III).

SOURCES: Centers for Disease Control and Prevention, National Center for Health Statistics: Ventura SJ, Martin JA, Curtin SC, Mathews TJ. Births: Final data for 1997. National vital statistics reports; vol 48, no 18. Hyattsville, Maryland: 1999; for age-specific birth rates for 1950–80 see table 1–9 in *Vital statistics of the United States, vol I, natality, 1990*. Washington: Public Health Service, 1994; Ventura SJ. Births of Hispanic parentage, 1980 and 1985. Monthly vital statistics report; vol 32 no 6 and vol 36 no 11, suppl. Public Health Service. Hyattsville, Maryland. 1983 and 1988; Vital statistics of the United States, 1992, vol I, natality, Washington: Public Health Service. 1996.

Table 4. Women 15–44 years of age who have not had at least 1 live birth, by age: United States, selected years 1960–97

[Data are based on the National Vital Statistics System]

Year[1]	15–19 years	20–24 years	25–29 years	30–34 years	35–39 years	40–44 years
	Percent of women					
1960.	91.4	47.5	20.0	14.2	12.0	15.1
1965.	92.7	51.4	19.7	11.7	11.4	11.0
1970.	93.0	57.0	24.4	11.8	9.4	10.6
1975.	92.6	62.5	31.1	15.2	9.6	8.8
1980.	93.4	66.2	38.9	19.7	12.5	9.0
1985.	93.7	67.7	41.5	24.6	15.4	11.7
1986.	93.8	68.0	42.0	25.1	16.1	12.2
1987.	93.8	68.2	42.5	25.5	16.9	12.6
1988.	93.8	68.4	43.0	25.7	17.7	13.0
1989.	93.7	68.4	43.3	25.9	18.2	13.5
1990.	93.3	68.3	43.5	25.9	18.5	13.9
1991.	93.0	67.9	43.6	26.0	18.7	14.5
1992.	92.7	67.3	43.7	26.0	18.8	15.2
1993.	92.6	66.7	43.8	26.1	18.8	15.8
1994.	92.6	66.1	43.9	26.2	18.7	16.2
1995.	92.5	65.5	44.0	26.2	18.6	16.5
1996.	92.5	65.0	43.8	26.2	18.5	16.6
1997.	92.8	64.9	43.5	26.2	18.4	16.6

[1]As of January 1.

NOTES: Data are based on cohort fertility. See Appendix II, Cohort fertility. Percents are derived from the cumulative childbearing experience of cohorts of women, up to the ages specified. Data on births are adjusted for underregistration and population estimates are corrected for underregistration and misstatement of age. Beginning in 1970 births to persons who were not residents of the 50 States and the District of Columbia are excluded.

SOURCE: Centers for Disease Control and Prevention, National Center for Health Statistics. *Vital statistics of the United States, vol I, 1997 natality*, table 1–17. Washington, in preparation.

Table 5. Live births, according to detailed race of mother and Hispanic origin of mother: United States, selected years 1970–97

[Data are based on the National Vital Statistics System]

Race of mother and Hispanic origin of mother	1970	1975	1980	1985	1990	1994	1995	1996	1997
					Total number of live births				
All races	3,731,386	3,144,198	3,612,258	3,760,561	4,158,212	3,952,767	3,899,589	3,891,494	3,880,894
White	3,109,956	2,576,818	2,936,351	3,037,913	3,290,273	3,121,004	3,098,885	3,093,057	3,072,640
Black	561,992	496,829	568,080	581,824	684,336	636,391	603,139	594,781	599,913
American Indian or Alaska Native	22,264	22,690	29,389	34,037	39,051	37,740	37,278	37,880	38,572
Asian or Pacific Islander	- - -	- - -	74,355	104,606	141,635	157,632	160,287	165,776	169,769
Chinese	7,044	7,778	11,671	16,405	22,737	26,578	27,380	28,500	28,434
Japanese	7,744	6,725	7,482	8,035	8,674	9,230	8,901	8,902	8,890
Filipino	8,066	10,359	13,968	20,058	25,770	30,495	30,551	31,106	31,501
Hawaiian and part Hawaiian	- - -	- - -	4,669	4,938	6,099	5,955	5,787	5,907	5,687
Other Asian or Pacific Islander	- - -	- - -	36,565	55,170	78,355	85,374	87,668	91,361	95,257
Hispanic origin (selected States)[1,2]	- - -	- - -	307,163	372,814	595,073	665,026	679,768	701,339	709,767
Mexican	- - -	- - -	215,439	242,976	385,640	454,536	469,615	489,666	499,024
Puerto Rican	- - -	- - -	33,671	35,147	58,807	57,240	54,824	54,863	55,450
Cuban	- - -	- - -	7,163	10,024	11,311	11,889	12,473	12,613	12,887
Central and South American	- - -	- - -	21,268	40,985	83,008	93,485	94,996	97,888	97,405
Other and unknown Hispanic	- - -	- - -	29,622	43,682	56,307	47,876	47,860	46,309	45,001
White, non-Hispanic (selected States)[1]	- - -	- - -	1,245,221	1,394,729	2,626,500	2,438,855	2,382,638	2,358,989	2,333,363
Black, non-Hispanic (selected States)[1]	- - -	- - -	299,646	336,029	661,701	619,198	587,781	578,099	581,431

- - - Data not available.

[1]Trend data for Hispanics and non-Hispanics are affected by expansion of the reporting area for an Hispanic-origin item on the birth certificate and by immigration. These two factors affect numbers of events, composition of the Hispanic population, and maternal and infant health characteristics. The number of States in the reporting area increased from 22 in 1980, to 23 and the District of Columbia (DC) in 1983–87, 30 and DC in 1988, 47 and DC in 1989, 48 and DC in 1990, 49 and DC in 1991–92, and 50 and DC in 1993 and later years (see Appendix I, National Vital Statistics System).
[2]Includes mothers of all races.

NOTES: The race groups, white, black, American Indian or Alaska Native, and Asian or Pacific Islander, include persons of Hispanic and non-Hispanic origin. Conversely, persons of Hispanic origin may be of any race. Data for additional years are available (see Appendix III).

SOURCES: Centers for Disease Control and Prevention, National Center for Health Statistics. Data computed by the Division of Health and Utilization Analysis from data compiled by the Division of Vital Statistics; Ventura SJ, Martin JA, Curtin SC, Mathews TJ. Births: Final data for 1997. National vital statistics reports; vol 48, no 18. Hyattsville, Maryland: 1999; Report of final natality statistics, for each data year 1970–96. Monthly vital statistics report. Hyattsville, Maryland.

Table 6. Prenatal care for live births, according to detailed race of mother and Hispanic origin of mother: United States, selected years 1970–97

[Data are based on the National Vital Statistics System]

Prenatal care, race of mother, and Hispanic origin of mother	1970	1975	1980	1985	1990	1991	1992	1993	1994	1995	1996	1997
Prenatal care began during 1st trimester						Percent of live births[1]						
All races	68.0	72.4	76.3	76.2	75.8	76.2	77.7	78.9	80.2	81.3	81.9	82.5
White	72.3	75.8	79.2	79.3	79.2	79.5	80.8	81.8	82.8	83.6	84.0	84.7
Black	44.2	55.5	62.4	61.5	60.6	61.9	63.9	66.0	68.3	70.4	71.4	72.3
American Indian or Alaska Native	38.2	45.4	55.8	57.5	57.9	59.9	62.1	63.4	65.2	66.7	67.7	68.1
Asian or Pacific Islander	- - -	- - -	73.7	74.1	75.1	75.3	76.6	77.6	79.7	79.9	81.2	82.1
Chinese	71.8	76.7	82.6	82.0	81.3	82.3	83.8	84.6	86.2	85.7	86.8	87.4
Japanese	78.1	82.7	86.1	84.7	87.0	87.7	88.2	87.2	89.2	89.7	89.3	89.3
Filipino	60.6	70.6	77.3	76.5	77.1	77.1	78.7	79.3	81.3	80.9	82.5	83.3
Hawaiian and part Hawaiian	- - -	- - -	68.8	67.7	65.8	68.1	69.9	70.6	77.0	75.9	78.5	78.0
Other Asian or Pacific Islander	- - -	- - -	67.4	69.9	71.9	71.9	72.8	74.4	76.2	77.0	78.4	79.7
Hispanic origin (selected States)[2,3]	- - -	- - -	60.2	61.2	60.2	61.0	64.2	66.6	68.9	70.8	72.2	73.7
Mexican	- - -	- - -	59.6	60.0	57.8	58.7	62.1	64.8	67.3	69.1	70.7	72.1
Puerto Rican	- - -	- - -	55.1	58.3	63.5	65.0	67.8	70.0	71.7	74.0	75.0	76.5
Cuban	- - -	- - -	82.7	82.5	84.8	85.4	86.8	88.9	90.1	89.2	89.2	90.4
Central and South American	- - -	- - -	58.8	60.6	61.5	63.4	66.8	68.7	71.2	73.2	75.0	76.9
Other and unknown Hispanic	- - -	- - -	66.4	65.8	66.4	65.6	68.0	70.0	72.1	74.3	74.6	76.0
White, non-Hispanic (selected States)[2]	- - -	- - -	81.2	81.4	83.3	83.7	84.9	85.6	86.5	87.1	87.4	87.9
Black, non-Hispanic (selected States)[2]	- - -	- - -	60.7	60.1	60.7	61.9	64.0	66.1	68.3	70.4	71.5	72.3
Prenatal care began during 3d trimester or no prenatal care												
All races	7.9	6.0	5.1	5.7	6.1	5.8	5.2	4.8	4.4	4.2	4.0	3.9
White	6.3	5.0	4.3	4.8	4.9	4.7	4.2	3.9	3.6	3.5	3.3	3.2
Black	16.6	10.5	8.9	10.2	11.3	10.7	9.9	9.0	8.2	7.6	7.3	7.3
American Indian or Alaska Native	28.9	22.4	15.2	12.9	12.9	12.2	11.0	10.3	9.8	9.5	8.6	8.6
Asian or Pacific Islander	- - -	- - -	6.5	6.5	5.8	5.7	4.9	4.6	4.1	4.3	3.9	3.8
Chinese	6.5	4.4	3.7	4.4	3.4	3.4	2.9	2.9	2.7	3.0	2.5	2.4
Japanese	4.1	2.7	2.1	3.1	2.9	2.5	2.4	2.8	1.9	2.3	2.2	2.7
Filipino	7.2	4.1	4.0	4.8	4.5	5.0	4.3	4.0	3.6	4.1	3.3	3.3
Hawaiian and part Hawaiian	- - -	- - -	6.7	7.4	8.7	7.5	7.0	6.7	4.7	5.1	5.0	5.4
Other Asian or Pacific Islander	- - -	- - -	9.3	8.2	7.1	6.8	5.9	5.4	4.8	5.0	4.6	4.4
Hispanic origin (selected States)[2,3]	- - -	- - -	12.0	12.4	12.0	11.0	9.5	8.8	7.6	7.4	6.7	6.2
Mexican	- - -	- - -	11.8	12.9	13.2	12.2	10.5	9.7	8.3	8.1	7.2	6.7
Puerto Rican	- - -	- - -	16.2	15.5	10.6	9.1	8.0	7.1	6.5	5.5	5.7	5.4
Cuban	- - -	- - -	3.9	3.7	2.8	2.4	2.1	1.8	1.6	2.1	1.6	1.5
Central and South American	- - -	- - -	13.1	12.5	10.9	9.5	7.9	7.3	6.5	6.1	5.5	5.0
Other and unknown Hispanic	- - -	- - -	9.2	9.4	8.5	8.2	7.5	7.0	6.2	6.0	5.9	5.3
White, non-Hispanic (selected States)[2]	- - -	- - -	3.5	4.0	3.4	3.2	2.8	2.7	2.5	2.5	2.4	2.4
Black, non-Hispanic (selected States)[2]	- - -	- - -	9.7	10.9	11.2	10.7	9.8	9.0	8.2	7.6	7.3	7.3

- - - Data not available.

[1]Excludes live births for whom trimester when prenatal care began is unknown.

[2]Trend data for Hispanics and non-Hispanics are affected by expansion of the reporting area for an Hispanic-origin item on the birth certificate and by immigration. These two factors affect numbers of events, composition of the Hispanic population, and maternal and infant health characteristics. The number of States in the reporting area increased from 22 in 1980, to 23 and the District of Columbia (DC) in 1983–87, 30 and DC in 1988, 47 and DC in 1989, 48 and DC in 1990, 49 and DC in 1991–92, and 50 and DC in 1993 and later years (see Appendix I, National Vital Statistics System).

[3]Includes mothers of all races.

NOTES: Data for 1970 and 1975 exclude births that occurred in States not reporting prenatal care (see Appendix I). The race groups, white, black, American Indian or Alaska Native, and Asian or Pacific Islander, include persons of Hispanic and non-Hispanic origin. Conversely, persons of Hispanic origin may be of any race. Data for additional years are available (see Appendix III).

SOURCES: Centers for Disease Control and Prevention, National Center for Health Statistics. Data computed by the Division of Health and Utilization Analysis from data compiled by the Division of Vital Statistics; Ventura SJ, Martin JA, Curtin SC, Mathews TJ. Births: Final data for 1997. National vital statistics reports; vol 48, no 18. Hyattsville, Maryland: 1999; Report of final natality statistics, for each data year 1970–96. Monthly vital statistics report. Hyattsville, Maryland.

Table 7. Teenage childbearing, according to detailed race of mother and Hispanic origin of mother: United States, selected years 1970–97

[Data are based on the National Vital Statistics System]

Maternal age, race of mother, and Hispanic origin of mother	1970	1975	1980	1985	1990	1991	1992	1993	1994	1995	1996	1997
Age of mother under 18 years						Percent of live births						
All races	6.3	7.6	5.8	4.7	4.7	4.9	4.9	5.1	5.3	5.3	5.1	4.9
White	4.8	6.0	4.5	3.7	3.6	3.8	3.9	4.0	4.2	4.3	4.2	4.1
Black	14.8	16.3	12.5	10.6	10.1	10.3	10.3	10.6	10.8	10.8	10.3	9.7
American Indian or Alaska Native	7.5	11.2	9.4	7.6	7.2	7.9	8.0	8.4	8.7	8.7	8.7	8.6
Asian or Pacific Islander	---	---	1.5	1.6	2.1	2.1	2.0	2.1	2.2	2.2	2.1	2.0
Chinese	1.1	0.4	0.3	0.3	0.4	0.3	0.3	0.3	0.3	0.3	0.3	0.3
Japanese	2.0	1.7	1.0	0.9	0.8	1.0	0.9	0.9	0.9	0.8	0.9	0.8
Filipino	3.7	2.4	1.6	1.6	2.0	2.0	1.9	2.0	2.2	2.2	2.1	2.1
Hawaiian and part Hawaiian	---	---	6.6	5.7	6.5	6.8	7.0	7.1	8.0	7.6	6.8	6.7
Other Asian or Pacific Islander	---	---	1.2	1.8	2.4	2.4	2.3	2.5	2.5	2.5	2.5	2.3
Hispanic origin (selected States)[1,2]	---	---	7.4	6.4	6.6	6.9	7.1	7.2	7.6	7.6	7.3	7.2
Mexican	---	---	7.7	6.9	6.9	7.2	7.3	7.5	7.9	8.0	7.7	7.6
Puerto Rican	---	---	10.0	8.5	9.1	9.5	9.6	10.2	10.8	10.8	10.2	9.5
Cuban	---	---	3.8	2.2	2.7	2.6	2.5	2.5	3.0	2.8	2.8	2.7
Central and South American	---	---	2.4	2.4	3.2	3.5	3.6	3.8	4.0	4.1	4.0	3.9
Other and unknown Hispanic	---	---	6.5	7.0	8.0	8.3	8.9	9.4	9.4	9.0	8.8	8.9
White, non-Hispanic (selected States)[1]	---	---	4.0	3.2	3.0	3.1	3.1	3.2	3.4	3.4	3.3	3.2
Black, non-Hispanic (selected States)[1]	---	---	12.7	10.7	10.2	10.3	10.4	10.6	10.9	10.8	10.4	9.8
Age of mother 18–19 years												
All races	11.3	11.3	9.8	8.0	8.1	8.1	7.8	7.8	7.9	7.9	7.9	7.8
White	10.4	10.3	9.0	7.1	7.3	7.2	7.0	7.0	7.1	7.2	7.2	7.1
Black	16.6	16.9	14.5	12.9	13.0	12.8	12.4	12.1	12.3	12.4	12.5	12.5
American Indian or Alaska Native	12.8	15.2	14.6	12.4	12.3	12.4	11.9	11.9	12.3	12.7	12.3	12.2
Asian or Pacific Islander	---	---	3.9	3.4	3.7	3.7	3.6	3.6	3.5	3.5	3.2	3.2
Chinese	3.9	1.7	1.0	0.6	0.8	0.8	0.7	0.7	0.7	0.6	0.6	0.6
Japanese	4.1	3.3	2.3	1.9	2.0	1.7	1.7	1.8	1.9	1.7	1.6	1.5
Filipino	7.1	5.0	4.0	3.7	4.1	4.0	3.7	3.8	3.8	4.1	4.0	3.8
Hawaiian and part Hawaiian	---	---	13.3	12.3	11.9	11.3	11.4	11.3	11.6	11.5	11.6	11.9
Other Asian or Pacific Islander	---	---	3.8	3.5	3.9	4.1	4.1	4.0	3.9	3.8	3.4	3.3
Hispanic origin (selected States)[1,2]	---	---	11.6	10.1	10.2	10.3	10.1	10.1	10.2	10.3	10.1	9.8
Mexican	---	---	12.0	10.6	10.7	10.9	10.7	10.7	10.7	10.8	10.5	10.2
Puerto Rican	---	---	13.3	12.4	12.6	12.2	11.8	12.1	12.4	12.7	13.0	12.7
Cuban	---	---	9.2	4.9	5.0	4.5	4.6	4.3	4.3	4.9	4.9	4.7
Central and South American	---	---	6.0	5.8	5.9	6.0	5.9	6.1	6.4	6.5	6.5	6.5
Other and unknown Hispanic	---	---	10.8	10.5	11.1	11.4	11.1	11.6	11.4	11.1	11.1	10.9
White, non-Hispanic (selected States)[1]	---	---	8.5	6.6	6.6	6.5	6.3	6.2	6.3	6.4	6.4	6.3
Black, non-Hispanic (selected States)[1]	---	---	14.7	12.9	13.0	12.9	12.5	12.2	12.4	12.4	12.6	12.6

- - - Data not available.

[1]Trend data for Hispanics and non-Hispanics are affected by expansion of the reporting area for an Hispanic-origin item on the birth certificate and by immigration. These two factors affect numbers of events, composition of the Hispanic population, and maternal and infant health characteristics. The number of States in the reporting area increased from 22 in 1980, to 23 and the District of Columbia (DC) in 1983–87, 30 and DC in 1988, 47 and DC in 1989, 48 and DC in 1990, 49 and DC in 1991–92, and 50 and DC in 1993 and later years (see Appendix I, National Vital Statistics System).
[2]Includes mothers of all races.

NOTES: The race groups, white, black, American Indian or Alaska Native, and Asian or Pacific Islander, include persons of Hispanic and non-Hispanic origin. Conversely, persons of Hispanic origin may be of any race. Data for additional years are available (see Appendix III).

SOURCES: Centers for Disease Control and Prevention, National Center for Health Statistics. Data computed by the Division of Health and Utilization Analysis from data compiled by the Division of Vital Statistics; Ventura SJ, Martin JA, Curtin SC, Mathews TJ. Births: Final data for 1997. National vital statistics reports; vol 48, no 18. Hyattsville, Maryland: 1999; Report of final natality statistics, for each data year 1970–96. Monthly vital statistics report. Hyattsville, Maryland.

Table 8. Nonmarital childbearing according to detailed race of mother, Hispanic origin of mother, and maternal age and birth rates for unmarried women by race of mother and Hispanic origin of mother:United States, selected years 1970–97

[Data are based on the National Vital Statistics System]

Race of mother, Hispanic origin of mother, and maternal age	1970	1975	1980	1985	1990	1991	1992	1993	1994	1995	1996	1997
					Percent of live births to unmarried mothers							
All races	10.7	14.3	18.4	22.0	28.0	29.5	30.1	31.0	32.6	32.2	32.4	32.4
White	5.5	7.1	11.2	14.7	20.4	21.8	22.6	23.6	25.4	25.3	25.7	25.8
Black	37.5	49.5	56.1	61.2	66.5	67.9	68.1	68.7	70.4	69.9	69.8	69.2
American Indian or Alaska Native	22.4	32.7	39.2	46.8	53.6	55.3	55.3	55.8	57.0	57.2	58.0	58.7
Asian or Pacific Islander	- - -	- - -	7.3	9.5	13.2	13.9	14.7	15.7	16.2	16.3	16.7	15.6
Chinese	3.0	1.6	2.7	3.0	5.0	5.5	6.1	6.7	7.2	7.9	9.2	6.5
Japanese	4.6	4.6	5.2	7.9	9.6	9.8	9.8	10.0	11.2	10.8	11.4	10.1
Filipino	9.1	6.9	8.6	11.4	15.9	16.8	16.8	17.7	18.5	19.5	19.4	19.5
Hawaiian and part Hawaiian	- - -	- - -	32.9	37.3	45.0	45.0	45.7	47.8	48.6	49.0	49.9	49.1
Other Asian or Pacific Islander	- - -	- - -	5.4	8.5	12.6	13.5	14.9	16.1	16.4	16.2	16.5	15.6
Hispanic origin (selected States)[1,2]	- - -	- - -	23.6	29.5	36.7	38.5	39.1	40.0	43.1	40.8	40.7	40.9
Mexican	- - -	- - -	20.3	25.7	33.3	35.3	36.3	37.0	40.8	38.1	37.9	38.9
Puerto Rican	- - -	- - -	46.3	51.1	55.9	57.5	57.5	59.4	60.2	60.0	60.7	59.4
Cuban	- - -	- - -	10.0	16.1	18.2	19.5	20.2	21.0	22.9	23.8	24.7	24.4
Central and South American	- - -	- - -	27.1	34.9	41.2	43.1	43.9	45.2	45.9	44.1	44.1	41.8
Other and unknown Hispanic	- - -	- - -	22.4	31.1	37.2	37.9	37.6	38.7	43.5	44.0	43.5	43.6
White, non-Hispanic (selected States)[1]	- - -	- - -	9.6	12.4	16.9	18.0	18.5	19.5	20.8	21.2	21.5	21.5
Black, non-Hispanic (selected States)[1]	- - -	- - -	57.3	62.1	66.7	68.2	68.3	68.9	70.7	70.0	70.0	69.4
					Number of live births, in thousands							
Live births to unmarried mothers	399	448	666	828	1,165	1,214	1,225	1,240	1,290	1,254	1,260	1,257
Maternal age					Percent distribution of live births to unmarried mothers							
Under 20 years	50.1	52.1	40.8	33.8	30.9	30.4	29.8	29.7	30.5	30.9	30.4	30.7
20–24 years	31.8	29.9	35.6	36.3	34.7	35.4	35.6	35.4	34.8	34.5	34.2	34.9
25 years and over	18.1	18.0	23.5	29.9	34.4	34.3	34.6	34.9	34.6	34.7	35.3	34.4
					Live births per 1,000 unmarried women 15–44 years of age[3]							
All races and origins	26.4	24.5	29.4	32.8	43.8	45.2	45.2	45.3	46.9	45.1	44.8	44.0
White[4]	13.9	12.4	18.1	22.5	32.9	34.6	35.2	35.9	38.3	37.5	37.6	37.0
Black[4]	95.5	84.2	81.1	77.0	90.5	89.5	86.5	84.0	82.1	75.9	74.4	73.4
Hispanic origin (selected States)[1,2]	- - -	- - -	- - -	- - -	89.6	93.7	95.3	95.2	101.2	95.0	93.2	91.4
White, non-Hispanic	- - -	- - -	- - -	- - -	- - -	- - -	- - -	- - -	28.5	28.2	28.3	27.0

- - - Data not available.

[1]Trend data for Hispanics and non-Hispanics are affected by expansion of the reporting area for an Hispanic-origin item on the birth certificate and by immigration. These two factors affect numbers of events, composition of the Hispanic population, and maternal and infant health characteristics. The number of States in the reporting area increased from 22 in 1980, to 23 and the District of Columbia (DC) in 1983–87, 30 and DC in 1988, 47 and DC in 1989, 48 and DC in 1990, 49 and DC in 1991–92, and 50 and DC in 1993 and later years (see Appendix I, National Vital Statistics System).
[2]Includes mothers of all races.
[3]Rates computed by relating births to unmarried mothers, regardless of age of mother, to unmarried women 15–44 years of age.
[4]For 1970 and 1975, birth rates are by race of child.

NOTES: National estimates for 1970 and 1975 for unmarried mothers based on births occurring in States reporting marital status of mother (see Appendix I, National Vital Statistics System). The race groups, white, black, American Indian or Alaska Native, and Asian or Pacific Islander, include persons of Hispanic and non-Hispanic origin. Conversely, persons of Hispanic origin may be of any race. In 1995 procedures implemented in California to more accurately identify the marital status of Hispanic mothers account for some of the decline in measures of nonmarital childbearing for women of all races, white women, and Hispanic women between 1994 and 1995. Data for additional years are available (see Appendix III).

SOURCES: Centers for Disease Control and Prevention, National Center for Health Statistics. Data computed by the Division of Health and Utilization Analysis from data compiled by the Division of Vital Statistics; Ventura SJ, Martin JA, Curtin SC, Mathews TJ. Births: Final data for 1997. National vital statistics reports; vol 48, no 18. Hyattsville, Maryland: 1999; Ventura SJ. Births to unmarried mothers: United States, 1980–92. Vital Health Stat 21(53). 1995; Report of final natality statistics, for each data year 1993–96. Monthly vital statistics report. Hyattsville, Maryland.

Table 9. Maternal education for live births, according to detailed race of mother and Hispanic origin of mother: United States, selected years 1970–97

[Data are based on the National Vital Statistics System]

Mother's education, race of mother, and Hispanic origin of mother	1970	1975	1980	1985	1990	1991	1992	1993	1994	1995	1996	1997
Less than 12 years of education					Percent of live births[1]							
All races	30.8	28.6	23.7	20.6	23.8	23.9	23.6	23.3	22.9	22.6	22.4	22.1
White	27.1	25.1	20.8	17.8	22.4	22.5	22.3	22.0	21.7	21.6	21.6	21.3
Black	51.2	45.3	36.4	32.6	30.2	30.4	30.0	29.8	29.3	28.7	28.2	27.6
American Indian or Alaska Native	60.5	52.7	44.2	39.0	36.4	36.3	35.9	34.8	34.0	33.0	33.0	32.8
Asian or Pacific Islander	- - -	- - -	21.0	19.4	20.0	19.7	19.0	18.1	17.4	16.1	15.0	14.0
Chinese	23.0	16.5	15.2	15.5	15.8	15.7	15.2	14.3	13.7	12.9	12.8	12.3
Japanese	11.8	9.1	5.0	4.8	3.5	3.0	2.4	2.6	2.8	2.6	2.7	2.3
Filipino	26.4	22.3	16.4	13.9	10.3	10.1	9.3	8.8	8.9	8.0	7.4	7.3
Hawaiian and part Hawaiian	- - -	- - -	20.7	18.7	19.3	19.4	18.6	17.3	18.5	17.6	16.9	16.8
Other Asian or Pacific Islander	- - -	- - -	27.6	24.3	26.8	26.0	25.7	24.6	23.3	21.2	19.4	17.8
Hispanic origin (selected States)[2,3]	- - -	- - -	51.1	44.5	53.9	54.3	54.1	53.4	52.7	52.1	51.4	50.3
Mexican	- - -	- - -	62.8	59.0	61.4	61.7	61.3	60.4	59.5	58.6	57.7	56.3
Puerto Rican	- - -	- - -	55.3	46.6	42.7	41.9	41.0	40.3	39.6	38.6	38.1	37.1
Cuban	- - -	- - -	24.1	21.1	17.8	16.7	15.6	14.6	15.0	14.4	14.5	13.7
Central and South American	- - -	- - -	41.2	37.0	44.2	44.5	43.6	43.0	42.0	41.7	40.8	39.6
Other and unknown Hispanic	- - -	- - -	40.1	36.5	33.3	34.4	34.7	33.9	33.9	33.8	33.0	32.8
White, non-Hispanic (selected States)[2]	- - -	- - -	18.3	15.8	15.2	15.0	14.5	14.0	13.5	13.3	13.0	12.9
Black, non-Hispanic (selected States)[2]	- - -	- - -	37.4	33.5	30.0	30.3	29.8	29.6	29.1	28.6	28.0	27.5
16 years or more of education												
All races	8.6	11.4	14.0	16.7	17.5	18.1	18.9	19.5	20.4	21.4	22.1	22.8
White	9.6	12.7	15.5	18.6	19.3	19.9	20.7	21.4	22.2	23.1	23.9	24.6
Black	2.8	4.3	6.2	7.0	7.2	7.3	7.8	8.2	8.7	9.5	10.0	10.5
American Indian or Alaska Native	2.7	2.2	3.5	3.7	4.4	4.0	4.7	5.5	5.7	6.2	6.3	6.8
Asian or Pacific Islander	- - -	- - -	30.8	30.3	31.0	31.8	32.5	33.0	33.9	35.0	36.2	38.0
Chinese	34.0	37.8	41.5	35.2	40.3	41.7	44.0	45.7	46.6	49.0	49.1	51.1
Japanese	20.7	30.6	36.8	38.1	44.1	45.0	46.6	46.3	45.2	46.2	46.8	48.3
Filipino	28.1	36.6	37.1	35.2	34.5	34.1	35.8	36.1	36.6	36.7	38.0	38.6
Hawaiian and part Hawaiian	- - -	- - -	7.9	6.5	6.8	6.7	8.0	8.5	8.9	9.7	11.3	11.0
Other Asian or Pacific Islander	- - -	- - -	29.2	30.2	27.3	28.6	28.0	28.1	29.4	30.5	32.2	34.4
Hispanic origin (selected States)[2,3]	- - -	- - -	4.2	6.0	5.1	5.2	5.4	5.5	5.8	6.1	6.4	6.7
Mexican	- - -	- - -	2.2	3.0	3.3	3.3	3.5	3.5	3.8	4.0	4.2	4.5
Puerto Rican	- - -	- - -	3.0	4.6	6.5	6.8	7.3	7.5	8.1	8.7	8.9	9.2
Cuban	- - -	- - -	11.6	15.0	20.4	21.9	22.5	24.3	24.8	26.5	27.0	27.8
Central and South American	- - -	- - -	6.1	8.1	8.6	9.1	9.2	9.4	9.8	10.3	11.2	11.9
Other and unknown Hispanic	- - -	- - -	5.5	7.2	8.5	8.2	8.5	9.2	9.8	10.5	11.1	11.7
White, non-Hispanic (selected States)[2]	- - -	- - -	16.4	19.3	22.6	23.3	24.4	25.3	26.5	27.7	28.8	29.7
Black, non-Hispanic (selected States)[2]	- - -	- - -	5.7	6.7	7.3	7.3	7.8	8.2	8.7	9.5	10.0	10.6

- - - Data not available.

[1]Excludes live births for whom education of mother is unknown.

[2]Trend data for Hispanics and non-Hispanics are affected by expansion of the reporting area for an Hispanic-origin item on the birth certificate and by immigration. These two factors affect numbers of events, composition of the Hispanic population, and maternal and infant health characteristics. Data shown only for States with an Hispanic-origin item and education of mother item on their birth certificates. The number of States reporting both items increased from 20 in 1980, to 21 and the District of Columbia (DC) in 1983–87, 26 and DC in 1988, 45 and DC in 1989, 47 and DC in 1990–91, 49 and DC in 1992, and 50 and DC in 1993 and later years (see Appendix I, National Vital Statistics System).

[3]Includes mothers of all races.

NOTES: Excludes births that occurred in States not reporting education (see Appendix I). The race groups, white, black, American Indian or Alaska Native, and Asian or Pacific Islander, include persons of Hispanic and non-Hispanic origin. Conversely, persons of Hispanic origin may be of any race. Maternal education groups shown in this table generally represent the group at highest risk for unfavorable birth outcomes (less than 12 years of education) and the group at lowest risk (16 years or more of education). Data for additional years are available (see Appendix III).

SOURCE: Centers for Disease Control and Prevention, National Center for Health Statistics. Data computed by the Division of Health and Utilization Analysis from data compiled by the Division of Vital Statistics.

Table 10. Mothers who smoked cigarettes during pregnancy, according to mother's detailed race, Hispanic origin, age, and educational attainment: Selected States, 1989–97

[Data are based on the National Vital Statistics System]

Characteristic of mother	1989	1990	1991	1992	1993	1994	1995	1996	1997
Race of mother[1]				Percent of mothers who smoked[2]					
All races	19.5	18.4	17.8	16.9	15.8	14.6	13.9	13.6	13.2
White	20.4	19.4	18.8	17.9	16.8	15.6	15.0	14.7	14.3
Black	17.1	15.9	14.6	13.8	12.7	11.4	10.6	10.2	9.7
American Indian or Alaska Native	23.0	22.4	22.6	22.5	21.6	21.0	20.9	21.3	20.8
Asian or Pacific Islander[3]	5.7	5.5	5.2	4.8	4.3	3.6	3.4	3.3	3.2
Chinese	2.7	2.0	1.9	1.7	1.1	0.9	0.8	0.7	1.0
Japanese	8.2	8.0	7.5	6.6	6.7	5.4	5.2	4.8	4.7
Filipino	5.1	5.3	5.3	4.8	4.3	3.7	3.4	3.5	3.4
Hawaiian and part Hawaiian	19.3	21.0	19.4	18.5	17.2	16.0	15.9	15.3	15.8
Other Asian or Pacific Islander	4.2	3.8	3.8	3.6	3.2	2.9	2.7	2.7	2.5
Hispanic origin and race of mother[4]									
Hispanic origin	8.0	6.7	6.3	5.8	5.0	4.6	4.3	4.3	4.1
Mexican	6.3	5.3	4.8	4.3	3.7	3.4	3.1	3.1	2.9
Puerto Rican . . . . : . .	14.5	13.6	13.2	12.7	11.2	10.9	10.4	11.0	11.0
Cuban	6.9	6.4	6.2	5.9	5.0	4.8	4.1	4.7	4.2
Central and South American	3.6	3.0	2.8	2.6	2.3	1.8	1.8	1.8	1.8
Other and unknown Hispanic	12.1	10.8	10.7	10.1	9.3	8.1	8.2	9.1	8.5
White, non-Hispanic	21.7	21.0	20.5	19.7	18.6	17.7	17.1	16.9	16.5
Black, non-Hispanic	17.2	15.9	14.6	13.8	12.7	11.5	10.6	10.3	9.8
Age of mother[1]									
Under 15 years	7.7	7.5	7.6	6.9	7.0	6.7	7.3	7.7	8.1
15–19 years	22.2	20.8	19.7	18.6	17.5	16.7	16.8	17.2	17.6
15–17 years	19.0	17.6	16.6	15.6	14.8	14.4	14.6	15.4	15.5
18–19 years	23.9	22.5	21.5	20.3	19.1	18.1	18.1	18.3	18.8
20–24 years	23.5	22.1	21.2	20.3	19.2	17.8	17.1	16.8	16.6
25–29 years	19.0	18.0	17.2	16.1	14.8	13.5	12.8	12.3	11.8
30–34 years	15.7	15.3	15.1	14.5	13.4	12.3	11.4	10.9	10.0
35–39 years	13.6	13.3	13.3	13.4	12.8	12.2	12.0	11.7	11.1
40–49 years	13.2	12.3	11.9	11.6	11.0	10.3	10.1	10.1	10.1
Education of mother[5]				Percent of mothers 20 years of age and over who smoked[2]					
0–8 years	18.9	17.5	16.8	15.5	13.9	12.1	11.0	10.3	9.9
9–11 years	42.2	40.5	39.1	37.8	36.1	33.6	32.0	31.1	30.2
12 years	22.8	21.9	21.2	20.7	19.9	18.7	18.3	18.0	17.5
13–15 years	13.7	12.8	12.5	12.1	11.4	10.8	10.6	10.4	9.9
16 years or more	5.0	4.5	4.2	3.9	3.1	2.8	2.7	2.6	2.4

[1]Includes data for 43 States and the District of Columbia (DC) in 1989, 45 States and DC in 1990, 46 States and DC in 1991–93, and 46 States, DC, and New York City (NYC) in 1994–97. Excludes data for California, Indiana, New York (but includes NYC in 1994–97), and South Dakota (1989–97), Oklahoma (1989–90), and Louisiana and Nebraska (1989), which did not require the reporting of mother's tobacco use during pregnancy on the birth certificate (see Appendix I).
[2]Excludes live births for whom smoking status of mother is unknown.
[3]Maternal tobacco use during pregnancy was not reported on the birth certificates of California and New York, which during 1989–91 together accounted for 43–6ε percent of the births in each Asian subgroup (except Hawaiian).
[4]Includes data for 42 States and DC in 1989, 44 States and DC in 1990, 45 States and DC in 1991–92, 46 States and DC in 1993, and 46 States, DC, and NYC in 1994–97. Excludes data for California, Indiana, New York (but includes NYC in 1994–97), and South Dakota (1989–97), New Hampshire (1989–92), Oklahoma (1989–90), and Louisiana and Nebraska (1989), which did not require the reporting of either Hispanic origin of mother or tobacco use during pregnancy on the birth certificate (see Appendix I).
[5]Includes data for 42 States and DC in 1989, 44 States and DC in 1990, 45 States and DC in 1991, 46 States and DC in 1992–93, and 46 States, DC, and NYC in 1994–97. Excludes data for California, Indiana, New York (but includes NYC in 1994–97), and South Dakota (1989–97), Washington (1989–91), Oklahoma (1989–90), and Louisiana and Nebraska (1989), which did not require the reporting of either mother's education or tobacco use during pregnancy on the birth certificate (see Appendix I).

NOTES: The race groups, white, black, American Indian or Alaska Native, and Asian or Pacific Islander, include persons of Hispanic and non-Hispanic origin. Conversely, persons of Hispanic origin may be of any race.

SOURCES: Centers for Disease Control and Prevention, National Center for Health Statistics. Data computed by the Division of Health and Utilization Analysis from data compiled by the Division of Vital Statistics; Ventura SJ, Martin JA, Curtin SC, Mathews TJ. Births: Final data for 1997. National vital statistics reports; vol 48, no 18. Hyattsville, Maryland: 1999; Report of final natality statistics, for each data year 1989–96. Monthly vital statistics report. Hyattsville, Maryland.

Table 11. Low-birthweight live births, according to mother's detailed race, Hispanic origin, and smoking status: United States, selected years 1970–97

[Data are based on the National Vital Statistics System]

Birthweight, race of mother, Hispanic origin of mother, and smoking status of mother	1970	1975	1980	1985	1990	1991	1992	1993	1994	1995	1996	1997
Low birthweight (less than 2,500 grams)					Percent of live births[1]							
All races	7.93	7.38	6.84	6.75	6.97	7.12	7.08	7.22	7.28	7.32	7.39	7.51
White	6.85	6.27	5.72	5.65	5.70	5.80	5.80	5.98	6.11	6.22	6.34	6.46
Black	13.90	13.19	12.69	12.65	13.25	13.55	13.31	13.34	13.24	13.13	13.01	13.01
American Indian or Alaska Native	7.97	6.41	6.44	5.86	6.11	6.15	6.22	6.42	6.45	6.61	6.49	6.75
Asian or Pacific Islander	---	---	6.68	6.16	6.45	6.54	6.57	6.55	6.81	6.90	7.07	7.23
Chinese	6.67	5.29	5.21	4.98	4.69	5.10	4.98	4.91	4.76	5.29	5.03	5.06
Japanese	9.03	7.47	6.60	6.21	6.16	5.90	7.00	6.53	6.91	7.26	7.27	6.82
Filipino	10.02	8.08	7.40	6.95	7.30	7.31	7.43	6.99	7.77	7.83	7.92	8.33
Hawaiian and part Hawaiian	---	---	7.23	6.49	7.24	6.73	6.89	6.76	7.20	6.84	6.77	7.20
Other Asian or Pacific Islander	---	---	6.83	6.19	6.65	6.74	6.68	6.89	7.06	7.05	7.42	7.54
Hispanic origin (selected States)[2,3]	---	---	6.12	6.16	6.06	6.15	6.10	6.24	6.25	6.29	6.28	6.42
Mexican	---	---	5.62	5.77	5.55	5.60	5.61	5.77	5.80	5.81	5.86	5.97
Puerto Rican	---	---	8.95	8.69	8.99	9.42	9.19	9.23	9.13	9.41	9.24	9.39
Cuban	---	---	5.62	6.02	5.67	5.57	6.10	6.18	6.27	6.50	6.46	6.78
Central and South American	---	---	5.76	5.68	5.84	5.87	5.77	5.94	6.02	6.20	6.03	6.26
Other and unknown Hispanic	---	---	6.96	6.83	6.87	7.25	7.24	7.51	7.54	7.55	7.68	7.93
White, non-Hispanic (selected States)[2]	---	---	5.67	5.60	5.61	5.72	5.73	5.92	6.06	6.20	6.36	6.47
Black, non-Hispanic (selected States)[2]	---	---	12.71	12.61	13.32	13.62	13.40	13.43	13.34	13.21	13.12	13.11
Cigarette smoker[4]	---	---	---	---	11.25	11.41	11.49	11.84	12.28	12.18	12.13	12.06
Nonsmoker[4]	---	---	---	---	6.14	6.36	6.35	6.56	6.71	6.79	6.91	7.07
Very low birthweight (less than 1,500 grams)												
All races	1.17	1.16	1.15	1.21	1.27	1.29	1.29	1.33	1.33	1.35	1.37	1.42
White	0.95	0.92	0.90	0.94	0.95	0.96	0.96	1.01	1.02	1.06	1.09	1.13
Black	2.40	2.40	2.48	2.71	2.92	2.96	2.96	2.96	2.96	2.97	2.99	3.04
American Indian or Alaska Native	0.98	0.95	0.92	1.01	1.01	1.07	0.95	1.05	1.10	1.10	1.21	1.19
Asian or Pacific Islander	---	---	0.92	0.85	0.87	0.85	0.91	0.86	0.93	0.91	0.99	1.05
Chinese	0.80	0.52	0.66	0.57	0.51	0.65	0.67	0.63	0.58	0.67	0.64	0.74
Japanese	1.48	0.89	0.94	0.84	0.73	0.62	0.85	0.74	0.92	0.87	0.81	0.78
Filipino	1.08	0.93	0.99	0.86	1.05	0.97	1.05	0.95	1.19	1.13	1.20	1.29
Hawaiian and part Hawaiian	---	---	1.05	1.03	0.97	1.02	1.02	1.14	1.20	0.94	0.97	1.41
Other Asian or Pacific Islander	---	---	0.96	0.91	0.92	0.87	0.93	0.89	0.93	0.91	1.04	1.07
Hispanic origin (selected States)[2,3]	---	---	0.98	1.01	1.03	1.02	1.04	1.06	1.08	1.11	1.12	1.13
Mexican	---	---	0.92	0.97	0.92	0.92	0.94	0.97	0.99	1.01	1.01	1.02
Puerto Rican	---	---	1.29	1.30	1.62	1.66	1.70	1.66	1.63	1.79	1.70	1.85
Cuban	---	---	1.02	1.18	1.20	1.15	1.24	1.23	1.31	1.19	1.35	1.36
Central and South American	---	---	0.99	1.01	1.05	1.02	1.02	1.02	1.06	1.13	1.14	1.17
Other and unknown Hispanic	---	---	1.01	0.96	1.09	1.09	1.10	1.23	1.29	1.28	1.48	1.35
White, non-Hispanic (selected States)[2]	---	---	0.86	0.90	0.93	0.94	0.94	1.00	1.01	1.04	1.08	1.12
Black, non-Hispanic (selected States)[2]	---	---	2.46	2.66	2.93	2.97	2.97	2.99	2.99	2.98	3.02	3.05
Cigarette smoker[4]	---	---	---	---	1.73	1.73	1.74	1.77	1.81	1.85	1.85	1.83
Nonsmoker[4]	---	---	---	---	1.18	1.21	1.22	1.28	1.30	1.31	1.35	1.40

--- Data not available.

[1]Excludes live births with unknown birthweight. Percent based on live births with known birthweight.

[2]Trend data for Hispanics and non-Hispanics are affected by expansion of the reporting area for an Hispanic-origin item on the birth certificate and by immigration. These two factors affect numbers of events, composition of the Hispanic population, and maternal and infant health characteristics. The number of States in the reporting area increased from 22 in 1980, to 23 and the District of Columbia (DC) in 1983–87, 30 and DC in 1988, 47 and DC in 1989, 48 and DC in 1990, 49 and DC in 1991–92, and 50 and DC in 1993 and later years (see Appendix I, National Vital Statistics System).

[3]Includes mothers of all races.

[4]Percent based on live births with known smoking status of mother and known birthweight. Includes data for 43 States and the District of Columbia (DC) in 1989, 45 States and DC in 1990, 46 States and DC in 1991–93, and 46 States, DC, and New York City (NYC) in 1994–97. Excludes data for California, Indiana, New York (but includes NYC in 1994–97), and South Dakota (1989–97), Oklahoma (1989–90), and Louisiana and Nebraska (1989), which did not require the reporting of mother's tobacco use during pregnancy on the birth certificate (see Appendix I).

NOTES: The race groups, white, black, American Indian or Alaska Native, and Asian or Pacific Islander, include persons of Hispanic and non-Hispanic origin. Conversely, persons of Hispanic origin may be of any race. Data for additional years are available (see Appendix III).

SOURCES: Centers for Disease Control and Prevention, National Center for Health Statistics. Data computed by the Division of Health and Utilization Analysis from data compiled by the Division of Vital Statistics; Ventura SJ, Martin JA, Curtin SC, Mathews TJ. Births: Final data for 1997. National vital statistics reports; vol 48, no 18. Hyattsville, Maryland: 1999; Report of final natality statistics, for each data year 1970–96. Monthly vital statistics report. Hyattsville, Maryland.

Table 12. Low-birthweight live births among mothers 20 years of age and over, by mother's detailed race, Hispanic origin, and educational attainment: United States, 1989–97

[Data are based on the National Vital Statistics System]

Mother's education, race of mother, and Hispanic origin of mother	1989	1990	1991	1992	1993	1994	1995	1996	1997
Less than 12 years of education	Percent of live births weighing less than 2,500 grams[1]								
All races	9.0	8.6	8.7	8.4	8.6	8.5	8.4	8.3	8.4
White	7.3	7.0	7.1	6.9	7.1	7.1	7.1	7.1	7.2
Black	17.0	16.5	17.0	16.5	16.4	16.2	16.0	15.5	15.4
American Indian or Alaska Native	7.3	7.4	7.4	7.1	7.6	7.0	8.0	7.7	7.7
Asian or Pacific Islander	6.6	6.4	6.5	6.2	6.4	6.6	6.7	7.1	6.8
Chinese	5.4	5.2	5.0	4.4	4.6	4.6	5.3	5.0	5.1
Japanese	4.0	10.6	7.5	7.0	9.4	7.4	11.0	8.3	2.6
Filipino	6.9	7.2	7.4	6.8	6.2	8.2	7.5	8.0	7.8
Hawaiian and part Hawaiian	11.0	10.7	7.1	9.5	9.1	8.0	9.8	10.1	7.4
Other Asian or Pacific Islander	6.8	6.4	6.7	6.4	6.6	6.8	6.7	7.5	7.1
Hispanic origin (selected States)[2,3]	6.0	5.7	5.8	5.8	5.8	5.8	5.8	5.8	5.9
Mexican	5.3	5.2	5.3	5.3	5.4	5.4	5.4	5.4	5.6
Puerto Rican	11.3	10.3	11.2	10.4	10.3	10.7	10.5	10.4	10.6
Cuban	9.4	7.9	7.1	7.8	6.5	8.2	9.2	8.0	9.5
Central and South American	5.8	5.8	5.7	5.8	5.8	6.0	6.2	6.0	5.8
Other and unknown Hispanic	8.2	8.0	8.1	7.8	8.1	7.6	7.7	8.0	8.3
White, non-Hispanic (selected States)[2]	8.4	8.3	8.4	8.3	8.7	8.8	8.9	9.1	9.1
Black, non-Hispanic (selected States)[2]	17.6	16.7	17.2	16.7	16.7	16.6	16.2	15.8	15.6
12 years of education									
All races	7.1	7.1	7.3	7.2	7.4	7.5	7.6	7.7	7.7
White	5.7	5.8	5.9	5.9	6.1	6.3	6.4	6.6	6.6
Black	13.4	13.1	13.5	13.3	13.4	13.3	13.3	13.2	13.1
American Indian or Alaska Native	5.6	6.1	5.9	6.0	6.1	6.3	6.5	6.0	6.4
Asian or Pacific Islander	6.4	6.5	6.5	6.8	6.6	6.7	7.0	7.0	7.2
Chinese	5.1	4.9	5.5	5.7	4.9	5.3	5.7	4.9	5.2
Japanese	7.4	6.2	6.4	7.4	7.2	7.6	7.4	7.2	7.9
Filipino	6.8	7.6	6.9	7.4	6.5	7.5	7.7	7.8	8.2
Hawaiian and part Hawaiian	7.0	6.7	6.7	7.0	7.1	6.9	6.6	6.5	7.2
Other Asian or Pacific Islander	6.5	6.7	6.7	6.8	7.0	6.8	7.1	7.4	7.3
Hispanic origin (selected States)[2,3]	5.9	6.0	6.0	6.0	6.2	6.2	6.1	6.2	6.2
Mexican	5.2	5.5	5.4	5.5	5.7	5.8	5.6	5.8	5.7
Puerto Rican	8.8	8.3	8.4	8.3	8.5	8.1	8.7	8.8	8.7
Cuban	5.3	5.2	6.1	6.6	6.6	6.6	6.7	6.0	6.9
Central and South American	5.7	5.8	5.6	5.7	6.1	5.8	5.9	5.9	6.3
Other and unknown Hispanic	6.1	6.6	6.8	7.1	7.4	7.3	7.1	7.5	7.4
White, non-Hispanic (selected States)[2]	5.7	5.7	5.9	5.9	6.1	6.3	6.5	6.7	6.7
Black, non-Hispanic (selected States)[2]	13.6	13.2	13.6	13.4	13.5	13.4	13.4	13.3	13.2
13 years or more of education									
All races	5.5	5.4	5.6	5.6	5.8	5.9	6.0	6.2	6.4
White	4.6	4.6	4.7	4.8	5.0	5.1	5.3	5.5	5.7
Black	11.2	11.1	11.4	11.2	11.3	11.5	11.4	11.4	11.4
American Indian or Alaska Native	5.6	4.7	4.9	5.6	5.8	5.9	5.7	6.0	6.2
Asian or Pacific Islander	6.1	6.0	6.2	6.2	6.3	6.6	6.6	6.8	7.0
Chinese	4.5	4.4	4.9	4.7	4.9	4.6	5.1	5.0	4.9
Japanese	6.6	6.0	5.6	6.9	6.3	6.8	7.1	7.2	6.6
Filipino	7.2	7.0	7.1	7.3	6.9	7.5	7.6	7.8	8.1
Hawaiian and part Hawaiian	6.3	4.7	4.9	5.4	5.2	5.9	5.0	5.4	6.6
Other Asian or Pacific Islander	6.1	6.2	6.4	6.2	6.5	6.9	6.7	7.0	7.3
Hispanic origin (selected States)[2,3]	5.5	5.5	5.5	5.5	5.7	5.8	5.9	6.0	6.2
Mexican	5.1	5.2	5.0	5.1	5.5	5.5	5.6	5.6	5.8
Puerto Rican	7.4	7.4	7.5	7.5	7.4	7.3	7.9	7.8	8.2
Cuban	4.9	5.0	4.8	5.1	5.4	5.7	5.6	6.4	6.0
Central and South American	5.2	5.6	5.7	5.1	5.4	5.5	5.8	5.7	6.1
Other and unknown Hispanic	5.4	5.2	5.7	5.4	5.6	6.5	6.1	6.6	6.7
White, non-Hispanic (selected States)[2]	4.6	4.5	4.7	4.7	4.9	5.1	5.2	5.4	5.6
Black, non-Hispanic (selected States)[2]	11.2	11.1	11.4	11.2	11.4	11.5	11.5	11.4	11.5

[1]Excludes live births with unknown birthweight. Percent based on live births with known birthweight.
[2]Data shown only for States with an Hispanic-origin item and education of mother on their birth certificates. The number of States reporting both items increased from 45, the District of Columbia (DC), and New York City (NYC) in 1989, to 47, DC, and NYC in 1990–91, 49 and DC in 1992, and 50 and DC in 1993 and later years (see Appendix I, National Vital Statistics System).
[3]Includes mothers of all races.

NOTES: Includes data for 48 States, the District of Columbia (DC), and New York City (NYC) in 1989–91 and al' 50 States and DC starting in 1992. Excludes data for births to residents of upstate New York and Washington (1989–91), which did not require the reporting of education of mother on the birth certificate (see Appendix I). The race groups, white, black, American Indian or Alaska Native, and Asian or Pacific Islander, include persons of Hispanic and non-Hispanic origin. Conversely, persons of Hispanic origin may be of any race.

SOURCE: Centers for Disease Control and Prevention, National Center for Health Statistics. Data computed by the Division of Health and Utilization Analysis from data compiled by the Division of Vital Statistics.

[Data are based on the National Vital Statistics System]

Table 13 (page 1 of 2). Low-birthweight live births, according to detailed race of mother, Hispanic origin of mother, geographic division, and State: United States, average annual 1989–91, 1992–94, and 1995–97

Geographic division and State	All races			White, non-Hispanic			Black, non-Hispanic		
	1989–91	1992–94	1995–97	1989–91	1992–94	1995–97	1989–91	1992–94	1995–97
	Percent of live births weighing less than 2,500 grams								
United States[1]	7.04	7.19	7.41	5.65	5.90	6.34	13.50	13.39	13.15
New England[1]	5.97	6.19	6.59	5.16	5.38	5.86	12.21	12.06	11.78
Maine	5.14	5.38	5.97	5.19	5.43	6.01	*	*	*
New Hampshire[1]	4.97	5.12	5.38	4.93	5.00	5.26	*	*	*
Vermont	5.47	5.74	5.94	5.35	5.58	5.86	*	*	*
Massachusetts	5.88	6.16	6.57	5.13	5.36	5.89	11.30	11.68	11.22
Rhode Island	6.14	6.39	7.03	5.42	5.75	6.22	*11.51	*10.58	*11.06
Connecticut	6.80	6.88	7.21	5.20	5.42	5.92	13.77	12.97	12.67
Middle Atlantic	7.45	7.51	7.64	5.46	5.69	6.10	14.20	13.69	13.08
New York	7.71	7.64	7.70	5.40	5.60	5.98	13.94	13.23	12.40
New Jersey	7.21	7.46	7.69	5.28	5.62	6.08	13.89	13.93	13.71
Pennsylvania	7.17	7.31	7.49	5.63	5.85	6.24	15.06	14.54	14.09
East North Central	7.23	7.40	7.57	5.65	5.90	6.38	14.39	14.30	13.82
Ohio	7.21	7.44	7.62	5.96	6.21	6.57	13.81	13.81	13.57
Indiana	6.61	6.84	7.61	5.86	6.12	6.93	12.48	12.55	13.50
Illinois	7.68	7.89	7.92	5.56	5.82	6.34	14.69	14.92	14.34
Michigan	7.65	7.64	7.69	5.66	5.87	6.32	15.11	14.50	13.55
Wisconsin	5.92	6.14	6.23	4.92	5.17	5.40	14.18	13.83	13.25
West North Central	5.97	6.27	6.60	5.26	5.55	6.09	13.07	12.97	12.90
Minnesota	5.09	5.44	5.85	4.48	4.73	5.58	13.60	11.57	11.84
Iowa	5.50	5.78	6.23	5.28	5.50	5.95	*11.69	*12.85	*12.01
Missouri	7.18	7.47	7.61	5.92	6.22	6.56	13.38	13.51	13.47
North Dakota	5.11	5.27	5.73	4.98	5.14	5.66	*	*	*
South Dakota	5.27	5.51	5.65	5.08	5.32	5.62	*	*	*
Nebraska	5.56	5.86	6.54	5.04	5.40	6.25	*12.50	*12.30	*11.47
Kansas	6.19	6.50	6.76	5.57	5.98	6.28	12.37	12.28	12.88
South Atlantic	8.02	8.19	8.40	5.94	6.20	6.65	13.13	13.11	13.13
Delaware	7.67	7.60	8.55	5.63	5.83	6.82	13.76	13.13	13.74
Maryland	7.97	8.41	8.63	5.56	5.87	6.33	13.12	13.57	13.54
District of Columbia	15.45	14.35	13.70	*6.44	*5.05	*5.89	17.97	16.86	16.29
Virginia	7.18	7.40	7.69	5.58	5.76	6.18	12.44	12.50	12.59
West Virginia	6.86	7.30	8.05	6.61	7.10	7.86	*13.32	*12.23	*14.02
North Carolina	8.17	8.57	8.75	6.11	6.58	6.98	12.96	13.43	13.77
South Carolina	9.03	9.16	9.22	6.33	6.60	6.87	13.28	13.38	13.47
Georgia	8.53	8.63	8.70	6.07	6.20	6.58	12.93	12.97	12.94
Florida	7.51	7.56	7.86	5.88	6.12	6.60	12.66	12.29	12.27
East South Central	8.32	8.59	8.86	6.51	6.77	7.29	13.06	13.38	13.33
Kentucky	7.03	7.22	7.77	6.51	6.72	7.31	12.09	12.26	12.49
Tennessee	8.41	8.68	8.77	6.67	6.97	7.33	14.07	14.33	13.95
Alabama	8.46	8.72	9.18	6.28	6.57	7.24	12.64	12.88	13.24
Mississippi	9.56	9.95	9.93	6.53	6.76	7.23	12.87	13.38	13.10
West South Central[1]	7.39	7.45	7.65	5.95	6.14	6.59	13.30	13.21	13.13
Arkansas	8.22	8.18	8.35	6.58	6.79	7.07	13.59	12.93	13.12
Louisiana[1]	9.24	9.44	9.91	6.08	6.28	6.89	13.70	13.76	14.29
Oklahoma[1]	6.54	6.81	7.20	5.97	6.26	6.71	11.70	12.31	12.68
Texas	7.00	7.04	7.19	5.80	5.96	6.39	13.15	12.98	12.37
Mountain	6.76	6.97	7.26	6.33	6.59	6.96	14.16	14.20	14.04
Montana	5.76	6.08	6.18	5.71	5.96	5.90	*	*	*
Idaho	5.66	5.43	5.98	5.59	5.33	5.80	*	*	*
Wyoming	7.23	7.78	8.27	7.11	7.52	8.14	*	*	*
Colorado	7.99	8.48	8.70	7.28	7.86	8.22	15.20	15.76	15.44
New Mexico	7.14	7.29	7.61	6.71	7.15	7.52	*12.38	*11.49	*13.10
Arizona	6.38	6.63	6.78	6.08	6.33	6.65	12.82	13.12	13.11
Utah	5.81	5.81	6.50	5.63	5.69	6.29	*	*	*
Nevada	7.22	7.38	7.52	6.53	6.82	7.13	15.09	14.58	13.89
Pacific	5.81	5.92	6.02	5.06	5.22	5.42	12.85	12.51	11.89
Washington	5.33	5.26	5.56	4.95	4.91	5.21	11.84	11.12	10.70
Oregon	5.04	5.24	5.43	4.79	5.01	5.21	*11.83	*10.88	*10.92
California	5.90	6.03	6.11	5.13	5.36	5.55	12.99	12.68	12.02
Alaska	4.80	5.12	5.56	4.38	4.54	5.10	*9.17	*10.26	*12.64
Hawaii	6.99	7.07	7.18	5.51	5.45	4.97	*11.63	*11.56	*9.87

See footnotes at end of table.

[Data are based on the National Vital Statistics System]

Geographic division and State	Hispanic[2]			American Indian or Alaska Native[3]			Asian or Pacific Islander[3]		
	1989-91	1992-94	1995-97	1989-91	1992-94	1995-97	1989-91	1992-94	1995-97
	Percent of live births weighing less than 2,500 grams								
United States[4]	6.13	6.20	6.33	6.18	6.36	6.62	6.50	6.65	7.07
New England[4]	7.73	8.07	8.10	*7.62	*6.80	*9.16	6.68	6.78	7.09
Maine	*	*	*	*	*	*	*	*	*
New Hampshire[4]	- - -	- - -	*	*	*	*	*	*	*
Vermont	*	*	*	*	*	*	*	*	*
Massachusetts	7.30	7.74	7.91	*	*	*	6.36	6.39	6.70
Rhode Island	*6.87	*6.89	7.46	*	*	*	*8.21	*7.67	*7.70
Connecticut	8.74	8.96	8.64	*	*	*	*7.07	*7.68	*8.38
Middle Atlantic	8.01	7.79	7.70	*8.17	*8.41	*8.39	6.64	6.83	7.09
New York	8.18	7.83	7.64	*7.23	*8.12	*7.15	6.42	6.80	6.99
New Jersey	7.23	7.28	7.33	*	*9.30	*	6.81	6.61	7.29
Pennsylvania	8.78	8.97	9.23	*	*	*	7.38	7.36	7.20
East North Central	6.14	6.10	6.22	6.31	6.69	6.25	6.62	6.75	7.37
Ohio	7.88	7.39	7.26	*	*	*	*5.70	6.49	6.87
Indiana	6.04	6.48	6.79	*	*	*	*6.41	*5.63	*6.51
Illinois	5.94	5.94	6.01	*	*	*	7.18	7.28	8.01
Michigan	6.12	6.01	6.46	*6.95	*6.58	*6.10	6.35	6.68	7.03
Wisconsin	6.72	6.38	6.45	*5.28	*6.03	*4.95	*6.10	5.93	6.67
West North Central	6.12	5.87	6.22	6.01	6.36	6.26	6.35	6.75	6.89
Minnesota	*6.09	*5.70	6.46	*6.05	*6.83	*6.73	6.39	6.83	6.54
Iowa	*6.60	*6.05	*6.40	*	*	*	*6.54	*7.71	*8.30
Missouri	*5.37	*6.13	*6.36	*	*	*	*6.46	*7.05	*7.27
North Dakota	*	*	*	*6.19	*5.80	*5.52	*	*	*
South Dakota		*	*	5.95	6.39	*5.49	*	*	*
Nebraska	*6.38	*6.30	6.10	*5.10	*5.75	*6.12	*	*6.69	*7.24
Kansas	6.16	5.69	5.87	*	*	*	*5.99	*5.51	*6.35
South Atlantic	6.08	6.18	6.35	7.98	8.09	9.15	6.41	6.88	7.39
Delaware	*8.21	*6.68	*7.55	*	*	*	*	*	*
Maryland	5.80	6.21	6.08	*	*	*	6.30	6.55	7.05
District of Columbia	*6.79	*6.65	*7.10	*	*	*	*6.65	*7.59	*
Virginia	5.38	5.52	6.50	*	*	*	5.45	6.30	6.94
West Virginia	*	*	*	*	*	*	*	*	*
North Carolina	6.07	6.10	6.05	*8.41	*8.96	*9.98	*6.76	*7.31	7.54
South Carolina	*6.02	*5.47	*6.43	*	*	*	*7.14	*6.80	*7.56
Georgia	5.49	6.09	5.54	*	*	*	*6.72	6.50	7.66
Florida	6.18	6.27	6.50	*7.04	*5.82	*8.31	7.19	7.58	7.78
East South Central	*5.43	5.22	6.58	*6.44	*8.09	*7.57	*6.13	6.60	7.35
Kentucky	*	*5.49	*7.05	*	*	*	*	*5.04	*6.55
Tennessee	*5.40	*5.30	*6.59	*	*	*	*6.34	*6.90	*7.88
Alabama	*5.96	*5.09	*6.38	*	*	*	*5.73	*7.02	*7.48
Mississippi	*	*	*	*	*	*	*	*	*6.69
West South Central[4]	6.24	6.34	6.54	5.58	5.56	6.15	6.93	6.66	7.49
Arkansas	*5.21	*6.17	*5.97	*	*	*	*	*	*8.44
Louisiana[4]	- - -	*6.88	*5.97	*	*	*	*6.19	*5.82	*8.12
Oklahoma[4]	- - -	5.94	6.20	5.34	5.34	6.01	*6.56	*6.62	*6.85
Texas	6.25	6.34	6.55	*6.35	*6.35	*6.36	6.99	6.76	7.44
Mountain	7.07	7.15	7.24	6.11	6.22	6.54	7.58	7.75	8.41
Montana	*	*	*	*5.67	*6.08	*6.60	*	*	*
Idaho	*5.72	6.01	6.82	*	*	*	*	*	*
Wyoming	*7.56	*10.56	*8.39	*	*	*	*	*	*
Colorado	8.62	8.72	8.67	*8.83	*8.69	*8.47	*9.34	*9.15	*9.48
New Mexico	7.58	7.57	7.81	6.23	6.18	6.05	*	*7.11	*9.27
Arizona	6.21	6.46	6.51	5.99	6.05	6.41	*7.03	*7.63	*7.19
Utah	7.97	6.98	7.66	*5.09	*5.74	*6.94	*6.32	*6.38	7.55
Nevada	5.81	5.91	6.24	*5.40	*7.16	*6.84	*7.50	*7.58	*9.16
Pacific	5.24	5.42	5.51	5.89	6.00	6.00	6.36	6.45	6.78
Washington	5.14	5.05	5.31	6.14	5.52	6.30	6.05	5.74	5.93
Oregon	5.25	5.45	5.77	*5.08	*5.95	*5.77	*6.61	*6.20	6.07
California	5.22	5.42	5.50	6.38	6.66	6.24	6.14	6.27	6.67
Alaska	*3.55	*5.70	*6.28	5.28	5.30	5.35	*5.01	*6.63	*5.71
Hawaii	7.62	6.90	6.89	*	*	*	7.40	7.53	7.82

* Data for States with fewer than 5,000 live births for the 3-year period are considered unreliable. Data for States with fewer than 1,000 live births are considered highly unreliable and are not shown.

- - - Data not available.

[1]Percent low birthweight for white and black are substituted for non-Hispanic white and non-Hispanic black for those States and years in which Hispanic origin was not reported on the birth certificate: Louisiana 1989, Oklahoma 1989-90, and New Hampshire 1989-92.

[2]Persons of Hispanic origin may be of any race.   [3]Includes persons of Hispanic origin.

[4]Percent low birthweight for Hispanic origin excludes data from States not reporting Hispanic origin on the birth certificate for 1 or more years in any 3-year period.

SOURCE: Centers for Disease Control and Prevention, National Center for Health Statistics. Data computed by the Division of Health and Utilization Analysis from data compiled by the Division of Vital Statistics.

Table 14 (page 1 of 2). Very low-birthweight live births, according to detailed race of mother, Hispanic origin of mother, geographic division, and State: United States, average annual 1989–91, 1992–94, and 1995–97

[Data are based on the National Vital Statistics System]

Geographic division and State	All races			White, non-Hispanic			Black, non-Hispanic		
	1989–91	1992–94	1995–97	1989–91	1992–94	1995–97	1989–91	1992–94	1995–97
	Percent of live births weighing less than 1,500 grams								
United States[1]	1.28	1.32	1.38	0.94	0.98	1.08	2.95	2.98	3.02
New England[1]	1.12	1.12	1.24	0.90	0.89	1.02	2.91	2.98	3.03
Maine	0.85	0.92	1.10	0.87	0.92	1.10	*	*	*
New Hampshire[1]	0.93	0.83	0.93	0.91	0.80	0.90	*	*	*
Vermont	0.79	0.87	0.88	0.70	0.79	0.85	*	*	*
Massachusetts	1.10	1.12	1.22	0.92	0.92	1.01	2.56	2.75	2.90
Rhode Island	1.16	1.09	1.21	0.99	0.85	0.99	*2.73	*2.63	*2.18
Connecticut	1.37	1.33	1.49	0.91	0.91	1.09	3.47	3.37	3.35
Middle Atlantic	1.42	1.44	1.49	0.92	0.97	1.05	3.24	3.18	3.18
New York	1.44	1.47	1.50	0.86	0.95	0.98	3.13	3.11	3.03
New Jersey	1.41	1.47	1.56	0.97	1.01	1.10	3.12	3.29	3.49
Pennsylvania	1.38	1.36	1.42	0.96	0.98	1.09	3.61	3.23	3.25
East North Central	1.36	1.39	1.44	0.96	1.02	1.12	3.13	3.09	3.07
Ohio	1.32	1.35	1.43	1.01	1.04	1.15	2.98	2.96	3.06
Indiana	1.18	1.25	1.34	0.99	1.05	1.16	2.68	2.82	2.83
Illinois	1.46	1.53	1.54	0.95	1.04	1.16	3.10	3.16	3.11
Michigan	1.50	1.50	1.49	0.97	1.05	1.12	3.47	3.28	3.11
Wisconsin	1.08	1.08	1.18	0.85	0.86	0.96	3.03	2.84	3.01
West North Central	1.04	1.11	1.19	0.86	0.92	1.06	2.73	2.80	2.80
Minnesota	0.90	1.01	1.08	0.77	0.81	1.02	2.85	2.50	2.65
Iowa	0.91	0.98	1.20	0.85	0.90	1.12	*2.54	*2.85	*2.95
Missouri	1.26	1.31	1.31	0.93	1.00	1.04	2.81	2.80	2.81
North Dakota	0.84	0.95	1.00	0.82	0.89	0.97	*	*	*
South Dakota	0.90	0.87	1.01	0.86	0.79	0.94	*	*	*
Nebraska	0.95	0.98	1.20	0.85	0.92	1.17	*2.47	*2.41	*2.15
Kansas	1.09	1.19	1.24	0.95	1.03	1.09	2.51	3.14	3.11
South Atlantic	1.59	1.62	1.69	1.01	1.06	1.15	2.98	3.01	3.12
Delaware	1.63	1.49	1.77	1.04	0.96	1.29	3.43	3.22	3.30
Maryland	1.67	1.81	1.88	0.98	1.08	1.12	3.18	3.34	3.52
District of Columbia	3.79	3.35	3.51	*1.32	*0.61	*1.03	4.49	4.11	4.31
Virginia	1.41	1.46	1.52	0.96	1.00	1.07	2.89	2.90	2.97
West Virginia	1.15	1.18	1.36	1.07	1.14	1.32	*2.95	*2.02	*2.50
North Carolina	1.65	1.72	1.83	1.09	1.14	1.30	2.99	3.16	3.36
South Carolina	1.72	1.76	1.84	1.05	1.14	1.18	2.77	2.78	3.04
Georgia	1.67	1.72	1.74	1.00	1.06	1.10	2.85	2.93	2.99
Florida	1.43	1.45	1.49	0.99	1.03	1.11	2.79	2.77	2.79
East South Central	1.52	1.58	1.68	1.06	1.09	1.22	2.71	2.86	2.98
Kentucky	1.21	1.22	1.36	1.07	1.07	1.23	2.51	2.67	2.77
Tennessee	1.56	1.57	1.65	1.10	1.10	1.21	3.06	3.09	3.22
Alabama	1.61	1.70	1.87	1.06	1.10	1.28	2.66	2.85	3.09
Mississippi	1.70	1.87	1.87	0.94	1.08	1.13	2.52	2.72	2.72
West South Central[1]	1.26	1.32	1.37	0.92	0.98	1.08	2.70	2.83	2.88
Arkansas	1.33	1.43	1.57	0.98	1.11	1.24	2.46	2.49	2.75
Louisiana[1]	1.73	1.83	1.95	0.96	1.01	1.11	2.83	2.95	3.18
Oklahoma[1]	1.08	1.12	1.19	0.96	0.96	1.05	2.21	2.63	2.79
Texas	1.17	1.23	1.26	0.89	0.95	1.05	2.72	2.84	2.71
Mountain	1.01	1.02	1.11	0.93	0.94	1.04	2.73	2.66	2.69
Montana	0.87	0.82	1.03	0.82	0.80	0.97	*	*	*
Idaho	0.90	0.80	0.88	0.89	0.78	0.82	*	*	*
Wyoming	0.90	1.06	1.13	0.90	1.00	1.07	*	*	*
Colorado	1.08	1.18	1.27	0.94	1.05	1.18	2.73	2.95	2.79
New Mexico	0.94	1.04	1.06	0.96	1.09	1.08	*2.49	*1.91	*2.32
Arizona	1.08	1.06	1.13	1.01	0.98	1.07	2.88	2.72	2.69
Utah	0.86	0.85	1.01	0.83	0.82	0.95	*	*	*
Nevada	1.14	1.06	1.16	0.98	0.93	1.07	2.75	2.45	2.62
Pacific	0.99	1.02	1.05	0.83	0.86	0.90	2.71	2.77	2.59
Washington	0.85	0.83	0.94	0.76	0.78	0.87	2.73	2.22	2.29
Oregon	0.83	0.88	0.88	0.79	0.82	0.85	*1.95	*1.92	*2.04
California	1.02	1.06	1.09	0.86	0.89	0.92	2.73	2.82	2.62
Alaska	0.87	0.95	1.03	0.74	0.84	0.85	*2.12	*2.63	*2.88
Hawaii	1.03	1.00	1.04	0.94	0.74	0.83	*2.99	*2.92	*2.74

See footnotes at end of table.

Table 14 (page 2 of 2). Very low-birthweight live births, according to detailed race of mother, Hispanic origin of mother, geographic division, and State: United States, average annual 1989–91, 1992–94, and 1995–97

[Data are based on the National Vital Statistics System]

Geographic division and State	Hispanic[2]			American Indian or Alaska Native[3]			Asian or Pacific Islander[3]		
	1989–91	1992–94	1995–97	1989–91	1992–94	1995–97	1989–91	1992–94	1995–97
United States[4]	1.04	1.06	1.12	1.03	1.04	1.17	0.87	0.90	0.98
New England[4]	1.52	1.46	1.60	*1.71	*1.27	*1.67	0.83	0.90	1.06
Maine	*	*	*	*	*	*	*	*	*
New Hampshire[4]	- - -	- - -	*	*	*	*	*	*	*
Vermont	*	*	*	*	*	*	*	*	*
Massachusetts	1.47	1.45	1.53	*	*	*	0.77	0.78	0.86
Rhode Island	*1.25	*1.27	1.42	*	*	*	*0.83	*0.91	*1.17
Connecticut	1.70	1.54	1.79	*	*	*	*0.98	*1.22	*1.61
Middle Atlantic	1.43	1.40	1.45	*1.10	*1.25	*1.39	0.84	0.92	0.96
New York	1.47	1.37	1.43	*1.29	*1.14	*1.16	0.83	0.93	0.99
New Jersey	1.28	1.37	1.41	*	*1.30	*	0.83	0.80	0.92
Pennsylvania	1.57	1.76	1.68	*	*	*	0.89	1.09	0.88
East North Central	1.16	1.16	1.18	1.28	1.19	1.33	0.90	1.01	1.04
Ohio	1.46	1.56	1.32	*	*	*	*0.72	0.89	0.85
Indiana	1.10	1.36	1.33	*	*	*	*0.80	*0.88	*0.89
Illinois	1.14	1.12	1.12	*	*	*	0.93	1.15	1.14
Michigan	1.09	1.11	1.18	*1.56	*1.06	*1.60	0.86	0.97	0.94
Wisconsin	1.17	1.12	1.51	*1.03	*1.31	*0.73	*1.06	0.82	1.07
West North Central	1.08	0.94	1.16	1.06	1.16	1.43	0.90	0.92	0.89
Minnesota	*0.87	*1.04	1.27	*1.19	*1.19	*1.77	0.82	0.91	0.93
Iowa	*1.35	*1.15	*1.26	*	*	*	*1.02	*1.08	*1.26
Missouri	*1.08	*1.24	*1.29	*	*	*	*1.08	*0.90	*0.74
North Dakota	*	*	*	*0.94	*0.97	*1.00	*	*	*
South Dakota	*	*	*	1.09	1.32	*1.33	*	*	*
Nebraska	*1.00	*0.67	1.14	*0.78	*0.71	*0.77	*	*0.89	*0.83
Kansas	1.17	0.80	0.99	*	*	*	*0.55	*0.85	*0.78
South Atlantic	1.08	1.12	1.13	1.43	1.58	2.00	0.99	0.93	1.10
Delaware	*1.72	*1.26	*1.44	*	*	*	*	*	*
Maryland	1.05	1.06	1.09	*	*	*	1.01	0.91	1.16
District of Columbia	*1.25	*0.90	*1.53	*	*	*	*1.39	*0.88	*
Virginia	0.96	1.09	1.24	*	*	*	0.77	0.86	1.06
West Virginia	*	*	*	*	*	*	*	*	*
North Carolina	0.87	0.77	0.99	*1.60	*2.04	*2.65	*1.05	*0.91	1.09
South Carolina	*1.49	*1.01	*1.29	*	*	*	*0.85	*0.77	*1.12
Georgia	0.81	1.01	0.99	*	*	*	*0.98	0.99	1.22
Florida	1.11	1.18	1.15	*0.87	*0.81	*1.16	1.22	0.99	1.00
East South Central	*0.85	0.86	1.16	*1.01	*1.25	*1.54	*0.81	0.90	1.01
Kentucky	*	*0.73	*1.35	*	*	*	*	*0.42	*0.51
Tennessee	*0.76	*0.94	*0.99	*	*	*	*0.81	*0.99	*1.09
Alabama	*1.12	*0.91	*1.28	*	*	*	*0.55	*1.22	*1.39
Mississippi	*	*	*	*	*	*	*	*	*0.86
West South Central[4]	0.96	1.04	1.09	0.78	0.86	0.93	0.85	0.88	0.92
Arkansas	*0.72	*1.04	*1.14	*	*	*	*	*	*1.79
Louisiana[4]	- - -	*1.12	*0.92	*	*	*	*0.62	*0.65	*1.13
Oklahoma[4]	- - -	1.03	0.89	0.68	0.80	0.92	*1.08	*0.93	*0.57
Texas	0.96	1.04	1.10	*1.16	*1.06	*1.00	0.83	0.91	0.90
Mountain	1.01	1.05	1.12	0.97	0.90	0.98	1.00	1.00	1.09
Montana	*	*	*	*1.10	*0.66	*1.07	*	*	*
Idaho	*0.75	0.81	1.09	*	*	*	*	*	*
Wyoming	*0.92	*1.19	*1.49	*	*	*	*	*	*
Colorado	1.11	1.20	1.20	*1.45	*0.80	*0.86	*1.30	*1.17	*1.25
New Mexico	0.91	1.04	1.06	0.77	0.78	0.82	*	*0.80	*0.96
Arizona	1.02	1.05	1.11	0.99	0.90	0.98	*0.99	*0.95	*0.91
Utah	1.20	0.97	1.37	*0.87	*1.35	*1.46	*0.79	*0.73	*1.11
Nevada	0.93	0.84	0.94	*1.25	*1.68	*1.27	*0.93	*0.91	*1.13
Pacific	0.90	0.94	1.00	1.04	1.02	1.02	0.85	0.87	0.96
Washington	0.94	0.75	0.87	0.93	1.01	0.84	0.72	0.55	0.74
Oregon	1.04	1.03	0.88	*0.85	*1.39	*0.78	*0.71	*0.91	1.02
California	0.90	0.94	1.00	1.15	1.06	1.07	0.84	0.85	0.96
Alaska	*0.39	*0.58	*1.64	1.06	0.93	1.14	*0.80	*1.20	*0.86
Hawaii	1.21	1.02	0.92	*	*	*	0.96	1.02	1.04

* Data for States with fewer than 5,000 live births for the 3-year period are considered unreliable. Data for States with fewer than 1,000 live births are considered highly unreliable and are not shown.

- - - Data not available.

[1]Percent very low birthweight for white and black are substituted for non-Hispanic white and non-Hispanic black for those States and years in which Hispanic origin was not reported on the birth certificate: Louisiana 1989, Oklahoma 1989–90, and New Hampshire 1989–92.

[2]Persons of Hispanic origin may be of any race.   [3]Includes persons of Hispanic origin.

[4]Percent very low birthweight for Hispanic origin excludes data from States not reporting Hispanic origin on the birth certificate for 1 or more years in any 3-year period.

SOURCE: Centers for Disease Control and Prevention, National Center for Health Statistics. Data computed by the Division of Health and Utilization Analysis from data compiled by the Division of Vital Statistics.

Table 15. Legal abortion ratios, according to selected patient characteristics: United States, selected years 1973–96

[Data are based on reporting by State health departments and by hospitals and other medical facilities]

Characteristic	1973	1975	1980	1985	1989	1990	1991	1992	1993	1994	1995	1996
					Abortions per 100 live births[1]							
Total	19.6	27.2	35.9	35.4	34.6	34.5	33.9	33.5	33.4	32.1	31.1	31.4
Age												
Under 15 years	123.7	119.3	139.7	137.6	88.6	84.4	76.7	79.0	74.4	70.4	66.7	72.3
15–19 years	53.9	54.2	71.4	68.8	56.0	51.5	46.2	44.0	44.0	41.5	39.9	41.5
20–24 years	29.4	28.9	39.5	38.6	36.6	37.7	37.8	37.6	38.4	36.4	34.9	35.5
25–29 years	20.7	19.2	23.7	21.7	21.1	22.0	22.1	22.2	22.7	22.2	22.1	22.7
30–34 years	28.0	25.0	23.7	19.9	18.7	19.1	18.7	18.3	18.0	17.2	16.5	16.5
35–39 years	45.1	42.2	41.0	33.6	27.1	27.3	26.2	25.6	24.8	23.4	22.4	22.0
40 years and over	68.4	66.8	80.7	62.3	49.6	50.1	46.9	45.4	43.0	41.2	38.7	37.6
Race												
White[2]	32.6	27.7	33.2	27.7	25.2	25.8	24.6	23.6	23.1	21.7	20.4	20.2
Black[3]	42.0	47.6	54.3	47.2	49.6	52.1	50.2	51.8	55.2	53.8	53.4	55.5
Hispanic origin[4]												
Hispanic	- - -	- - -	- - -	- - -	- - -	- - -	30.0	30.7	28.9	27.8	26.5	27.6
Non-Hispanic	- - -	- - -	- - -	- - -	- - -	- - -	33.2	32.6	30.9	29.0	28.0	28.2
Marital status												
Married	7.6	9.6	10.5	8.0	8.1	8.9	8.9	8.4	8.4	7.9	7.6	8.0
Unmarried	139.8	161.0	147.6	117.4	92.1	87.9	81.5	79.0	78.9	68.9	65.0	65.0
Previous live births[5]												
0	43.7	38.4	45.7	45.1	36.8	35.8	34.8	32.7	32.4	30.9	28.6	28.7
1	23.5	22.0	20.2	21.6	21.2	23.0	23.2	22.9	23.1	22.3	22.1	22.3
2	36.8	36.8	29.5	29.9	28.9	31.7	31.9	31.9	32.2	30.9	30.9	31.1
3	46.9	47.7	29.8	18.2	26.5	30.2	31.0	30.8	31.5	30.8	31.0	31.5
4 or more[6]	44.7	43.5	24.3	21.5	22.3	27.1	22.6	25.5	23.4	23.3	24.1	24.9

- - - Data not available.

[1]For calculation of ratios according to each characteristic, abortions with the characteristic unknown have been distributed in proportion to abortions with the characteristic known.

[2]For 1989 and later years, white race includes women of Hispanic ethnicity.

[3]Before 1989 black race includes races other than white.

[4]Includes data for 20–22 States, the District of Columbia, and New York City in 1991–95, and 22 States and New York City in 1996. States with large Hispanic populations that are not included are California, Florida, and Illinois.

[5]For 1973–75 data indicate number of living children.

[6]For 1975 data refer to four previous live births, not four or more. For five or more previous live births, the ratio is 47.3.

NOTES: For each year since 1969 the Centers for Disease Control and Prevention has compiled total abortion data from 50 States, the District of Columbia (DC), and New York City (NYC). The number of States reporting each characteristic varies from year to year. For 1996, the number of areas included in the ratios for each characteristic was as follows: age, 45; race, 35; marital status, 34; previous live births, 39. Some data for 1995 have been revised and differ from the previous edition of Health, United States. Data for additional years are available (see Appendix III).

SOURCES: Centers for Disease Control and Prevention: Abortion Surveillance, 1973, 1975, 1979–80. Public Health Service, DHHS, Atlanta, Ga., May 1975, April 1977, May 1983; CDC Surveillance Summaries. Abortion Surveillance, United States, 1982–83, Vol. 36, No. 1SS, Public Health Service, DHHS, Atlanta, Ga., Feb. 1987; 1984 and 1985, Vol. 38, No. SS–2, Sept. 1989; 1986 and 1987, Vol. 39, No. SS–2, June 1990; 1988, Vol. 40, No. SS–2, July 1991; 1989, Vol. 41, No. SS–5, Sept. 1992; 1990, Vol. 42, No. SS–6, Dec. 1993; 1991, Vol. 44, No. SS–2, May 1995; 1992, Vol. 45, No. SS–3, May 1996; 1993 and 1994, Vol. 46, No. SS–4, Aug. 1997; 1995, Vol. 47, No. SS–2, July 1998; 1996, in press, 1999.

Table 16. Legal abortions, according to selected characteristics: United States, selected years 1973–96

[Data are based on reporting by State health departments and by hospitals and other facilities]

Characteristic	1973	1975	1980	1985	1989	1990	1991	1992	1993	1994	1995	1996
	Number of legal abortions reported in thousands											
Centers for Disease Control and Prevention	616	855	1,298	1,329	1,397	1,430	1,389	1,359	1,330	1,267	1,211	1,222
Alan Guttmacher Institute[1]	745	1,034	1,554	1,589	1,567	1,609	1,557	1,529	1,500	1,431	1,364	1,366
	Percent distribution[2]											
Total	100.0	100.0	100.0	100.0	100.0	100.0	100.0	100.0	100.0	100.0	100.0	100.0
Period of gestation[3]												
Under 9 weeks	36.1	44.6	51.7	50.3	49.8	51.6	52.3	52.1	52.3	53.7	54.0	54.6
Under 7 weeks	---	---	---	---	---	---	---	14.3	14.7	15.7	15.7	16.4
7 weeks	---	---	---	---	---	---	---	15.6	16.2	16.5	17.1	17.4
8 weeks	---	---	---	---	---	---	---	22.2	21.6	21.6	21.2	20.9
9–10 weeks	29.4	28.4	26.2	26.6	25.8	25.3	25.1	24.2	24.4	23.5	23.1	22.6
11–12 weeks	17.9	14.9	12.2	12.5	12.6	11.7	11.5	12.0	11.6	10.9	10.9	11.0
13–15 weeks	6.9	5.0	5.1	5.9	6.6	6.4	6.1	6.0	6.3	6.3	6.3	6.0
16–20 weeks	8.0	6.1	3.9	3.9	4.2	4.0	3.9	4.2	4.1	4.3	4.3	4.3
21 weeks and over	1.7	1.0	0.9	0.8	1.0	1.0	1.1	1.5	1.3	1.3	1.4	1.5
Type of procedure												
Curettage	88.4	90.9	95.5	97.5	98.8	98.8	98.9	98.9	99.0	99.1	98.9	98.8
Intrauterine instillation	10.4	6.2	3.1	1.7	0.9	0.8	0.7	0.7	0.6	0.5	0.5	0.4
Other[4]	1.2	2.8	1.4	0.8	0.3	0.4	0.4	0.4	0.4	0.4	0.6	0.8
Location of facility												
In State of residence	74.8	89.2	92.6	92.4	91.0	91.8	91.6	92.0	91.4	91.5	91.7	91.9
Out of State of residence	25.2	10.8	7.4	7.6	9.0	8.2	8.4	8.0	8.6	8.5	8.3	8.1
Previous induced abortions												
0	---	81.9	67.6	60.1	58.1	57.1	56.1	55.1	54.9	54.8	55.1	54.7
1	---	14.9	23.5	25.7	26.5	26.9	27.2	27.4	27.3	27.2	26.9	26.9
2	---	2.5	6.6	9.8	9.9	10.1	10.6	11.0	11.0	11.1	10.9	11.2
3 or more	---	0.7	2.3	4.4	5.5	5.9	6.1	6.5	6.7	7.0	7.1	7.2

- - - Data not available.

[1] No survey was conducted in 1983, 1986, 1989, 1990, 1993, or 1994; data for these years are estimated.

[2] Excludes cases for which selected characteristic is unknown.

[3] Percentages for under 7, 7, and 8 weeks may not add to percentage under 9 weeks because some States do not report abortions for detailed gestational age subgroups under 9 weeks.

[4] Includes hysterotomy and hysterectomy.

NOTES: For a discussion of the differences in reported legal abortions between the Centers for Disease Control and Prevention and the Alan Guttmacher Institute, see Appendix I. For each year since 1969 the Centers for Disease Control and Prevention has compiled total abortion data from 50 States, the District of Columbia (DC), and New York City (NYC). The number of States reporting each characteristic varies from year to year. For 1996, the number of areas included in the percentages for each characteristic was as follows: gestational age, 38 States, DC, and NYC; detailed gestational age under 9 weeks, 36 States and NYC; type of procedure, 39 States, DC, and NYC; residence, 43 States, DC, and NYC; previous induced abortions, 37 States and NYC. Some data for 1993–95 have been revised and differ from the previous edition of *Health, United States*. Data for additional years are available (see Appendix III).

SOURCES: Centers for Disease Control and Prevention: Abortion Surveillance, 1973, 1975, 1979–80. Public Health Service, DHHS, Atlanta, Ga., May 1975, April 1977, May 1983; CDC Surveillance Summaries. Abortion Surveillance, United States, 1982–83, Vol. 36, No. 1SS, Public Health Service, DHHS, Atlanta, Ga., Feb. 1987; 1984 and 1985, Vol. 38, No. SS–2, Sept. 1989; 1986 and 1987, Vol. 39, No. SS–2, June 1990; 1988, Vol. 40, No. SS–2, July 1991; 1989, Vol. 41, No. SS–5, Sept. 1992; 1990, Vol. 42, No. SS–6, Dec. 1993; 1991, Vol. 44, No. SS–2, May 1995; 1992, Vol. 45, No. SS–3, May 1996; 1993 and 1994, Vol. 46, No. SS–4, Aug. 1997; 1995, Vol. 47, No. SS–2, July 1998; 1996, in press, 1999; Henshaw, S. K.: Abortion incidence and services in the United States, 1995–1996. Fam. Plann. Perspect. 30(6), Nov.–Dec. 1998.

Table 17. Methods of contraception for women 15–44 years of age, according to race and age: United States, 1982, 1988, and 1995

[Data are based on household interviews of samples of women in the childbearing ages]

Method of contraception and age	All races			White			Black		
	1982	1988	1995	1982	1988	1995	1982	1988	1995
	Number of women in thousands								
15–44 years	54,099	57,900	60,201	45,367	47,076	47,981	6,985	7,679	8,460
15–19 years	9,521	9,179	8,961	7,815	7,313	6,838	1,416	1,409	1,454
20–24 years	10,629	9,413	9,041	8,855	7,401	7,015	1,472	1,364	1,386
25–34 years	19,644	21,726	20,758	16,485	17,682	16,609	2,479	2,865	2,861
35–44 years	14,305	17,582	21,440	12,212	14,681	17,519	1,618	2,041	2,758
All methods	Percent of women using contraception								
15–44 years	55.7	60.3	64.2	56.7	61.8	65.5	52.0	56.7	61.5
15–19 years	24.2	32.1	29.8	23.4	32.2	30.0	30.0	35.1	34.5
20–24 years	55.8	59.0	63.5	56.6	60.2	63.3	52.5	61.1	66.9
25–34 years	66.7	66.3	71.1	67.7	67.7	72.6	64.0	63.8	66.4
35–44 years	61.6	68.3	72.3	63.1	70.2	73.4	52.3	58.9	68.0
Female sterilization	Percent of contracepting women								
15–44 years	23.2	27.5	27.7	22.1	26.1	25.7	30.0	38.1	39.9
15–19 years	–	*1.5	*0.3	–	*1.6	–	–	*1.6	–
20–24 years	4.5	4.6	4.0	*3.8	3.9	3.5	9.8	9.1	7.2
25–34 years	22.1	25.0	23.8	20.2	23.2	21.3	33.5	39.9	40.3
35–44 years	43.5	47.6	45.0	41.9	44.7	41.7	56.8	70.5	66.3
Male sterilization									
15–44 years	10.9	11.7	10.9	12.2	13.6	12.7	*1.4	*0.9	1.7
15–19 years	*0.4	*0.2	–	*0.5	*0.3	–	–	–	–
20–24 years	*3.6	*1.8	*1.1	*4.2	*2.3	*1.3	*0.5	–	*0.2
25–34 years	10.1	10.2	7.8	11.3	11.7	8.9	*1.4	*1.1	*1.5
35–44 years	19.9	20.8	19.4	21.6	23.7	22.1	*3.1	*1.5	3.1
Birth control pill									
15–44 years	28.0	30.7	26.9	26.7	29.8	28.0	38.0	38.0	23.8
15–19 years	63.9	58.8	43.8	62.1	55.9	47.5	70.8	74.2	33.2
20–24 years	55.1	68.2	52.1	53.5	67.9	55.4	65.0	70.3	41.5
25–34 years	25.7	32.6	33.3	24.8	32.4	35.0	33.7	35.7	26.6
35–44 years	3.7	4.3	8.7	3.7	4.5	8.9	*5.1	*4.2	9.6
Intrauterine device									
15–44 years	7.1	2.0	0.8	6.9	1.8	0.8	9.1	3.1	*0.8
15–19 years	*1.3	–	–	*0.5	–	–	*4.9	–	–
20–24 years	4.2	*0.3	*0.3	*3.5	*0.3	*0.4	*6.2	*0.9	*0.2
25–34 years	9.7	2.1	0.8	9.4	1.7	0.7	13.0	*4.1	*1.5
35–44 years	6.9	3.1	1.1	7.0	3.0	1.2	*6.5	*4.3	*0.6
Diaphragm									
15–44 years	8.1	5.7	1.9	8.8	6.2	2.1	3.5	1.9	*0.8
15–19 years	*6.0	*1.0	*0.1	*7.1	*1.3	*0.2	*1.8	–	–
20–24 years	10.2	3.7	*0.6	11.3	4.1	*0.6	*2.8	*1.6	*0.7
25–34 years	10.3	7.3	1.7	11.3	8.0	1.8	*3.0	*1.7	*1.0
35–44 years	4.0	6.0	2.8	3.8	6.2	3.2	*6.0	*3.3	*0.9
Condom									
15–44 years	12.0	14.6	20.4	12.7	14.9	19.7	6.2	10.3	20.5
15–19 years	20.8	32.8	36.7	22.6	34.2	36.8	*12.6	22.7	37.8
20–24 years	10.7	14.5	26.4	11.4	15.8	23.8	*6.4	9.6	33.8
25–34 years	11.4	13.7	21.1	12.0	14.0	20.6	5.3	9.4	17.7
35–44 years	11.3	11.2	14.7	12.0	11.3	14.6	*4.5	7.0	12.2

– Quantity zero.
* Relative standard error greater than 30 percent.

NOTES: Method of contraception used in the month of interview. If multiple methods were reported, only the most effective method is shown in the table. Data for additional years are available (see Appendix III).

SOURCE: Centers for Disease Control and Prevention, National Center for Health Statistics, Division of Vital Statistics. Data from the National Survey of Family Growth.

Table 18. Breastfeeding by mothers 15–44 years of age by year of baby's birth, according to selected characteristics of mother: United States, average annual 1972–74 to 1993–94

[Data are based on household interviews of samples of women in the childbearing ages]

Selected characteristics of mother	1972–74	1975–77	1978–80	1981–83	1984–86	1987–89	1990–92	1993–94
	Percent of babies breastfed							
Total	30.1	36.7	47.5	58.1	54.5	52.3	54.2	58.1
Race and Hispanic origin[1]								
White, non-Hispanic	32.5	38.9	53.2	64.3	59.7	58.3	59.1	61.2
Black, non-Hispanic	12.5	16.8	19.6	26.0	22.9	21.0	22.9	27.5
Hispanic	33.1	42.9	46.3	52.8	58.9	51.3	58.8	67.4
Education[2]								
No high school diploma or GED[3] . . .	14.0	19.4	27.6	31.4	36.8	30.0	38.6	43.0
High school diploma or GED[3]	25.0	33.6	40.2	54.3	46.7	46.6	46.0	51.2
Some college, no bachelor's degree.	35.2	43.5	63.2	66.7	66.1	57.8	60.7	65.9
Bachelor's degree or higher.	65.5	66.9	71.3	83.2	75.3	79.2	80.8	80.6
Geographic region								
Northeast.	29.9	34.7	49.3	68.2	55.3	49.9	54.0	56.7
Midwest.	22.3	30.9	34.4	46.0	50.9	50.4	51.6	49.7
South	30.6	33.1	49.5	57.9	45.3	42.5	43.6	49.7
West.	47.1	54.5	66.6	69.9	70.9	69.1	70.5	79.3
Age at baby's birth								
Under 20 years	17.0	22.1	31.4	31.0	30.6	26.2	35.2	45.3
20–24 years.	28.7	33.5	44.7	50.8	50.2	46.7	44.7	50.9
25–29 years.	38.7	45.9	53.6	62.2	59.8	57.1	56.5	55.9
30–44 years.	43.1	47.5	55.2	73.1	65.9	65.3	67.5	71.1
	Percent of breastfed babies who were breastfed 3 months or more[4]							
Total	62.3	66.2	64.7	68.3	63.2	61.5	61.0	56.2
Race and Hispanic origin[1]								
White, non-Hispanic	62.1	66.7	67.6	68.1	62.5	62.3	62.6	56.8
Black, non-Hispanic	47.8	60.7	58.5	61.1	56.8	46.9	56.7	45.4
Hispanic	64.7	62.7	46.3	65.6	66.4	64.3	58.2	55.5
Education[2]								
No high school diploma or GED[3] . . .	54.4	54.7	53.7	50.5	59.8	57.3	55.5	44.5
High school diploma or GED[3]	53.7	62.5	59.4	59.6	58.0	58.3	58.2	49.7
Some college, no bachelor's degree.	69.5	77.2	63.8	73.3	63.4	60.7	53.8	60.2
Bachelor's degree or higher.	69.2	65.3	79.8	80.9	72.2	68.1	73.8	68.1
Geographic region								
Northeast.	64.6	68.2	71.2	75.0	64.8	59.7	72.7	58.7
Midwest.	44.4	54.3	53.1	64.4	60.4	58.6	63.1	56.7
South	72.6	74.1	67.6	65.0	60.3	55.2	50.8	50.9
West.	69.0	70.6	66.8	69.6	66.9	69.9	60.4	59.0
Age at baby's birth								
Under 20 years	50.0	61.0	48.2	49.1	62.5	56.3	31.9	22.6
20–24 years.	57.7	59.4	60.0	63.7	51.9	51.6	54.0	50.6
25–29 years.	68.3	71.5	65.1	70.8	65.6	58.3	59.7	63.7
30–44 years.	79.4	72.8	81.5	72.8	73.2	73.5	71.8	62.3

[1]Persons of Hispanic origin may be of any race.

[2]For women 22–44 years of age. Education is as of year of interview. See NOTES below.

[3]General equivalency diploma.

[4]For mothers interviewed in the first 3 months of 1995, only babies age 3 months and over are included so they would be eligible for breastfeeding for 3 months or more.

NOTES: Data on breastfeeding during 1972–83 are based on responses to questions in the National Survey of Family Growth (NSFG) Cycle 4, conducted in 1988. Data for 1984–94 are based on the NSFG Cycle 5, conducted in 1995. Data are based on all births to mothers 15–44 years of age at interview, including those births that occurred when the mothers were younger than 15 years of age.

SOURCE: Centers for Disease Control and Prevention, National Center for Health Statistics, Division of Vital Statistics. Data from the National Survey of Family Growth, Cycle 4 1988, Cycle 5 1995.

Table 19. Infant, neonatal, and postneonatal mortality rates, according to detailed race of mother and Hispanic origin of mother: United States, selected birth cohorts 1983–96

[Data are based on National Linked Birth/Infant Death Data Sets]

Race of mother and Hispanic origin of mother	Birth cohort								
	1983	1987	1990	1991	1995[1]	1996[1]	1983–85	1986–88	1989–91
	Infant deaths per 1,000 live births								
All mothers	10.9	9.8	8.9	8.6	7.6	7.3	10.6	9.8	9.0
White	9.3	8.2	7.3	7.1	6.3	6.1	9.0	8.2	7.4
Black	19.2	17.8	16.9	16.6	14.6	14.1	18.7	17.9	17.1
American Indian or Alaska Native	15.2	13.0	13.1	11.3	9.0	10.0	13.9	13.2	12.6
Asian or Pacific Islander	8.3	7.3	6.6	5.8	5.3	5.2	8.3	7.3	6.6
Chinese	9.5	6.2	4.3	4.6	3.8	3.2	7.4	5.8	5.1
Japanese	*	*6.6	*5.5	*4.2	*5.3	*4.2	6.0	6.9	5.3
Filipino	8.4	6.6	6.0	5.1	5.6	5.8	8.2	6.9	6.4
Hawaiian and part Hawaiian	*	*	*	*	*	*	11.3	11.1	9.0
Other Asian or Pacific Islander	8.1	7.6	7.4	6.3	5.5	5.7	8.6	7.6	7.0
Hispanic origin[2,3]	9.5	8.2	7.5	7.1	6.3	6.1	9.2	8.3	7.6
Mexican	9.1	8.0	7.2	6.9	6.0	5.8	8.8	7.9	7.2
Puerto Rican	12.9	9.9	9.9	9.7	8.9	8.6	12.3	11.1	10.4
Cuban	*7.5	7.1	7.2	5.2	5.3	5.1	8.0	7.3	6.2
Central and South American	8.5	7.8	6.8	5.9	5.5	5.0	8.2	7.6	6.6
Other and unknown Hispanic	10.6	8.7	8.0	8.2	7.4	7.7	9.9	9.0	8.2
White, non-Hispanic[3]	9.2	8.1	7.2	7.0	6.3	6.0	8.9	8.1	7.3
Black, non-Hispanic[3]	19.1	17.4	16.9	16.6	14.7	14.2	18.5	17.9	17.2
	Neonatal deaths per 1,000 live births								
All mothers	7.1	6.2	5.7	5.4	4.9	4.8	6.9	6.3	5.7
White	6.1	5.2	4.6	4.4	4.1	4.0	5.9	5.2	4.7
Black	12.5	11.8	11.1	10.7	9.6	9.4	12.2	11.7	11.1
American Indian or Alaska Native	7.5	6.2	6.1	5.5	4.0	4.7	6.7	5.9	5.9
Asian or Pacific Islander	5.2	4.5	3.9	3.6	3.4	3.3	5.2	4.5	3.9
Chinese	5.5	3.7	2.3	2.3	2.3	1.9	4.3	3.3	2.7
Japanese	*	*4.0	*3.5	*3.2	*3.3	*2.2	3.4	4.4	3.0
Filipino	5.6	4.1	3.5	3.4	3.4	4.1	5.3	4.5	4.0
Hawaiian and part Hawaiian	*	*	*	*	*	*	7.4	7.1	4.8
Other Asian or Pacific Islander	5.0	4.6	4.4	4.1	3.7	3.7	5.5	4.7	4.2
Hispanic origin[2,3]	6.2	5.3	4.8	4.5	4.1	4.0	6.0	5.3	4.8
Mexican	5.9	5.1	4.5	4.3	3.9	3.8	5.7	5.0	4.5
Puerto Rican	8.7	6.7	6.9	6.1	6.1	5.6	8.3	7.2	7.0
Cuban	*5.0	5.3	5.3	4.0	3.6	3.6	5.9	5.3	4.6
Central and South American	5.8	5.0	4.4	4.0	3.7	3.4	5.7	5.0	4.4
Other and unknown Hispanic	6.4	5.6	5.0	5.1	4.8	5.3	6.2	5.8	5.2
White, non-Hispanic[3]	6.0	5.0	4.5	4.3	4.0	3.9	5.8	5.1	4.6
Black, non-Hispanic[3]	12.1	11.3	11.0	10.7	9.6	9.4	11.8	11.4	11.1
	Postneonatal deaths per 1,000 live births								
All mothers	3.8	3.5	3.2	3.2	2.6	2.5	3.7	3.5	3.3
White	3.2	3.0	2.7	2.6	2.2	2.1	3.1	3.0	2.7
Black	6.7	6.1	5.9	5.9	5.0	4.8	6.4	6.2	6.0
American Indian or Alaska Native	7.7	6.8	7.0	5.8	5.1	5.3	7.2	7.3	6.7
Asian or Pacific Islander	3.1	2.8	2.7	2.2	1.9	1.9	3.1	2.8	2.6
Chinese	*	*2.5	2.0	2.3	1.5	1.2	3.1	2.5	2.4
Japanese	*	*	*	*	*	*	2.6	2.5	2.2
Filipino	*2.8	2.5	2.5	1.8	2.2	1.8	2.9	2.4	2.3
Hawaiian and part Hawaiian	*	*	*	*	*	*	*	*4.0	*4.1
Other Asian or Pacific Islander	3.0	2.9	3.0	2.3	1.9	2.0	3.1	2.9	2.8
Hispanic origin[2,3]	3.3	2.9	2.7	2.6	2.1	2.1	3.2	3.0	2.7
Mexican	3.2	2.9	2.7	2.6	2.1	2.1	3.2	2.9	2.7
Puerto Rican	4.2	3.2	3.0	3.5	2.8	3.0	4.0	3.9	3.4
Cuban	*	*	*	*	*	*	2.2	2.0	1.6
Central and South American	2.6	2.8	2.4	1.9	1.9	1.6	2.5	2.6	2.2
Other and unknown Hispanic	4.1	3.2	3.0	3.1	2.6	2.5	3.7	3.2	3.0
White, non-Hispanic[3]	3.2	3.0	2.7	2.7	2.2	2.1	3.1	3.0	2.7
Black, non-Hispanic[3]	7.0	6.2	5.9	5.9	5.0	4.8	6.7	6.4	6.1

* Infant and neonatal mortality rates for groups with fewer than 10,000 births are considered unreliable. Postneonatal mortality rates for groups with fewer than 20,000 births are considered unreliable. Infant and neonatal mortality rates for groups with fewer than 7,500 births are considered highly unreliable and are not shown. Postneonatal mortality rates for groups with fewer than 15,000 births are considered highly unreliable and are not shown.

[1]Rates based on a period file using weighted data. Data for 1995 and 1996 not strictly comparable with unweighted birth cohort data for earlier years (see Appendix I, National Vital Statistics System). The 1995 and 1996 weighted mortality rates shown in this table are less than 1 percent to 5 percent higher than unweighted rates for 1995 and 1996.

[2]Persons of Hispanic origin may be of any race.

[3]Data shown only for States with an Hispanic-origin item on their birth certificates. The number of States reporting the item increased from 23 and the District of Columbia (DC) in 1983–87, to 30 and DC in 1988, 47 and DC in 1989, 48 and DC in 1990, 49 and DC in 1991, and 50 and DC in 1995–96 (see Appendix I).

NOTES: The race groups, white, black, American Indian or Alaska Native, and Asian or Pacific Islander, include persons of Hispanic and non-Hispanic origin. National linked files do not exist for 1992–94 birth cohorts. Data for additional years are available (see Appendix III).

SOURCE: Centers for Disease Control and Prevention, National Center for Health Statistics. Data computed by the Division of Health and Utilization Analysis from data compiled by the Division of Vital Statistics for the National Linked Birth/Infant Death Data Sets.

Table 20. Infant mortality rates for mothers 20 years of age and over, according to educational attainment, detailed race of mother, and Hispanic origin of mother: United States, selected birth cohorts 1983–96

[Data are based on National Linked Birth/Infant Death Data Sets]

Education of mother, race of mother, and Hispanic origin of mother	1983	1987	1990	1991	1995[1]	1996[1]	1983–85	1986–88	1989–91
Less than 12 years of education				Infant deaths per 1,000 live births					
All mothers	15.0	13.6	10.8	10.5	8.9	8.5	14.6	13.8	11.1
White	12.5	11.5	9.0	8.8	7.6	7.1	12.4	11.4	9.2
Black	23.4	20.7	19.5	19.6	17.0	16.6	21.8	21.1	20.3
American Indian or Alaska Native	*	*	*14.3	*12.9	*	*	15.2	16.8	13.8
Asian or Pacific Islander[2]	*9.7	*7.3	6.6	6.3	5.7	6.4	9.5	8.2	6.9
Hispanic origin[3,4]	10.9	9.1	7.3	6.9	6.0	5.6	10.6	9.9	7.5
Mexican	8.7	8.1	7.0	6.6	5.8	5.4	9.5	8.3	7.1
Puerto Rican	*15.3	*10.7	10.1	10.3	10.6	9.1	14.1	12.8	11.7
Cuban	*	*	*	*	*	*	*	*	*
Central and South American	*	*9.2	7.0	5.8	5.1	4.7	8.6	9.2	6.8
Other and unknown Hispanic	*	*	9.9	9.9	*7.3	*7.9	10.1	10.6	10.0
White, non-Hispanic[4]	12.8	12.1	10.9	10.8	9.9	9.5	12.6	11.8	11.0
Black, non-Hispanic[4]	24.7	20.8	19.7	19.9	17.3	16.9	22.6	21.6	20.6
12 years of education									
All mothers	10.2	9.5	8.8	8.6	7.8	7.6	10.0	9.6	8.9
White	8.7	7.8	7.1	6.9	6.4	6.3	8.5	8.0	7.2
Black	17.8	17.0	16.0	16.2	14.7	13.8	17.7	17.1	16.4
American Indian or Alaska Native	*15.5	11.3	13.4	11.0	7.9	9.3	13.4	11.6	12.3
Asian or Pacific Islander[2]	10.0	7.6	7.5	6.6	5.5	5.9	9.3	7.9	7.5
Hispanic origin[3,4]	8.4	8.2	7.0	6.5	5.9	5.9	9.1	8.3	6.8
Mexican	*6.9	*8.3	6.8	6.4	5.7	5.6	7.8	8.2	6.5
Puerto Rican	*9.5	9.2	8.5	8.3	6.5	7.7	10.8	10.1	8.6
Cuban	*	*	*	*	*	*	*8.6	*6.6	7.6
Central and South American	*	7.9	6.5	5.5	6.1	5.3	8.7	7.4	6.3
Other and unknown Hispanic	8.8	7.1	7.4	6.3	6.5	7.6	8.8	7.7	7.0
White, non-Hispanic[4]	8.7	7.9	7.1	7.0	6.5	6.4	8.3	7.9	7.3
Black, non-Hispanic[4]	17.8	17.3	16.1	16.3	14.8	13.9	17.9	17.4	16.5
13 years or more of education									
All mothers	8.1	7.1	6.4	6.1	5.4	5.3	7.8	7.2	6.4
White	7.2	6.1	5.4	5.2	4.7	4.5	6.9	6.2	5.5
Black	15.3	14.6	13.7	13.1	11.9	11.7	15.3	14.9	13.7
American Indian or Alaska Native	*	*	*	*	*5.9	*7.1	10.4	8.4	8.1
Asian or Pacific Islander[2]	6.6	6.0	5.1	4.5	4.4	4.0	6.7	5.9	5.1
Hispanic origin[3,4]	9.0	6.6	5.7	5.5	5.0	5.1	7.4	7.0	5.8
Mexican	*	*	5.5	5.7	5.2	5.1	7.6	6.4	5.7
Puerto Rican	*	*	7.3	6.6	6.3	6.9	8.1	6.9	7.8
Cuban	*	*	*	*	*	*	*5.5	5.9	4.2
Central and South American	*	*	5.6	4.8	3.7	4.0	7.2	7.6	5.4
Other and unknown Hispanic	*	*	5.4	5.8	5.2	5.9	7.9	7.5	5.6
White, non-Hispanic[4]	7.0	6.0	5.4	5.2	4.6	4.5	6.8	6.1	5.4
Black, non-Hispanic[4]	14.8	14.5	13.7	13.2	12.0	11.7	14.7	14.9	13.8

* Infant mortality rates for groups with fewer than 10,000 births are considered unreliable. Infant mortality rates for groups with fewer than 7,500 births are considered highly unreliable and are not shown.

[1]Rates based on a period file using weighted data. Data for 1995 and 1996 not strictly comparable with unweighted birth cohort data for earlier years (see Appendix I, National Vital Statistics System). The 1995 and 1996 weighted mortality rates shown in this table are less than 1 percent to 4 percent higher than unweighted rates for 1995 and 1996.

[2]The States not reporting maternal education on the birth certificate accounted for 49–51 percent of the Asian or Pacific Islander births in the United States in 1983–87, 59 percent in 1988, and 12 percent in 1989–91. Starting in 1992 maternal education was reported by all 50 States and DC.

[3]Persons of Hispanic origin may be of any race.

[4]Data shown only for States with an Hispanic-origin item and education of mother on their birth certificates. The number of States reporting both items increased from 21 and the District of Columbia (DC) in 1983–87, to 26 and DC in 1988, 45 and DC in 1989, 47 and DC in 1990–91, and 50 and DC in 1995–96 (see Appendix I, National Vital Statistics System). The Hispanic-reporting States that did not report maternal education on the birth certificate during 1983–88 together accounted for 28–85 percent of the births in each Hispanic subgroup (except Cuban, 11–16 percent and Puerto Rican, 6–7 percent in 1983–87); and in 1989–91 accounted for 27–39 percent of Central and South American and Puerto Rican births and 2–9 percent of births in other Hispanic subgroups.

NOTES: Data for all mothers and by race based on data for 47 States and the District of Columbia (DC) in 1983–87, 46 States and DC in 1988, 48 States and DC in 1989–91, and 50 and DC in 1995–96. Excludes data for California and Texas (1983–88), Washington (1983–91), and New York (1988–91), which did not require the reporting of maternal education (see Appendix I). The race groups, white, black, American Indian or Alaska Native, and Asian or Pacific Islander, include persons of Hispanic and non-Hispanic origin. Persons of Hispanic origin may be of any race. National linked files do not exist for 1992–94 birth cohorts. Data for additional years are available (see Appendix III).

SOURCE: Centers for Disease Control and Prevention, National Center for Health Statistics. Data computed by the Division of Health and Utilization Analysis from data compiled by the Division of Vital Statistics for the National Linked Birth/Infant Death Data Sets.

Table 21. Infant mortality rates according to birthweight: United States, selected birth cohorts 1983–96

[Data are based on National Linked Birth/Infant Death Data Sets]

Birthweight	1983	1985	1986	1987	1988	1989	1990	1991	1995[1]	1996[1]
	Birth cohort									
	Infant deaths per 1,000 live births[2]									
All birthweights	10.9	10.4	10.1	9.8	9.6	9.5	8.9	8.6	7.6	7.3
Less than 2,500 grams	95.9	93.9	89.9	86.5	84.2	83.1	78.1	74.3	65.3	63.6
Less than 1,500 grams	400.6	387.7	371.8	358.0	348.7	343.1	317.6	305.4	270.7	261.5
Less than 500 grams	890.3	895.9	889.9	890.4	878.4	905.6	898.2	889.9	904.9	890.1
500–999 grams	584.2	559.2	537.4	507.9	502.0	480.4	440.1	422.6	351.0	336.9
1,000–1,499 grams	162.3	145.4	132.8	122.2	121.3	118.5	97.9	91.3	69.6	64.7
1,500–1,999 grams	58.4	54.0	51.9	48.8	48.9	46.0	43.8	40.4	33.5	30.6
2,000–2,499 grams	22.5	20.9	20.7	19.5	18.7	17.9	17.8	17.0	13.7	13.6
2,500 grams or more	4.7	4.3	4.3	4.1	4.0	4.0	3.7	3.6	3.0	2.8
2,500–2,999 grams	8.8	7.9	7.9	7.5	7.6	7.4	6.7	6.7	5.5	5.1
3,000–3,499 grams	4.4	4.3	4.1	4.0	3.9	3.8	3.7	3.5	2.9	2.7
3,500–3,999 grams	3.2	3.0	2.9	2.8	2.8	2.8	2.6	2.5	2.0	1.9
4,000 grams or more	3.3	3.2	3.0	3.0	2.9	2.6	2.4	2.4	2.0	1.8
4,000–4,499 grams	2.9	2.9	2.5	2.6	2.4	2.3	2.2	2.2	1.8	1.7
4,500–4,999 grams	3.9	3.8	3.6	3.4	3.4	3.1	2.5	3.0	2.2	2.1
5,000 grams or more[3]	14.4	14.7	16.3	15.8	20.7	9.6	9.8	8.2	8.5	6.2

[1]Rates based on a period file using weighted data; not stated birthweight imputed when period of gestation is known and proportionately distributed when period of gestation is unknown. Data for 1995 and 1996 not strictly comparable with unweighted and unimputed birth cohort data for earlier years (see Appendix I, National Vital Statistics System). The 1995 and 1996 weighted mortality rates with imputed birthweight shown in this table are less than 1 percent to 5 percent higher than unweighted rates with unimputed birthweight for 1995 and 1996.

[2]For calculation of birthweight-specific infant mortality rates, unknown birthweight has been distributed in proportion to known birthweight separately for live births (denominator) and infant deaths (numerator).

[3]In 1989 a birthweight-gestational age consistency check instituted for the natality file resulted in a decrease in the number of deaths to infants coded with birthweights of 5,000 grams or more and a discontinuity in the mortality trend for infants weighing 5,000 grams or more at birth. Starting with 1989 the rates are believed to be more accurate.

NOTES: National linked files do not exist for 1992–94 birth cohorts. Data for additional years are available (see Appendix III).

SOURCE: Centers for Disease Control and Prevention, National Center for Health Statistics. Data computed by the Division of Health and Utilization Analysis from data compiled by the Division of Vital Statistics for the National Linked Birth/Infant Death Data Sets.

Table 22. Infant mortality rates, fetal mortality rates, and perinatal mortality rates, according to race: United States, selected years 1950–97

[Data are based on the National Vital Statistics System]

Race and year	Infant[1]	Neonatal[1] Under 28 days	Neonatal[1] Under 7 days	Postneonatal[1]	Fetal mortality rate[2]	Late fetal mortality rate[3]	Perinatal mortality rate[4]
All races		Deaths per 1,000 live births					
1950[5]	29.2	20.5	17.8	8.7	18.4	14.9	32.5
1960[5]	26.0	18.7	16.7	7.3	15.8	12.1	28.6
1970	20.0	15.1	13.6	4.9	14.0	9.5	23.0
1980	12.6	8.5	7.1	4.1	9.1	6.2	13.2
1985	10.6	7.0	5.8	3.7	7.8	4.9	10.7
1989	9.8	6.2	5.1	3.6	7.5	4.5	9.6
1990	9.2	5.8	4.8	3.4	7.5	4.3	9.1
1991	8.9	5.6	4.6	3.4	7.3	4.1	8.7
1992	8.5	5.4	4.4	3.1	7.4	4.1	8.5
1993	8.4	5.3	4.3	3.1	7.1	3.8	8.1
1994	8.0	5.1	4.2	2.9	7.0	3.7	7.9
1995	7.6	4.9	4.0	2.7	7.0	3.6	7.6
1996	7.3	4.8	3.8	2.5	6.9	3.6	7.4
1997	7.2	4.8	3.8	2.5	6.8	3.5	7.3
Race of child:[6] White							
1950[5]	26.8	19.4	17.1	7.4	16.6	13.3	30.1
1960[5]	22.9	17.2	15.6	5.7	13.9	10.8	26.2
1970	17.8	13.8	12.5	4.0	12.3	8.6	21.0
1980	11.0	7.5	6.2	3.5	8.1	5.7	11.9
Race of mother:[7] White							
1980	10.9	7.4	6.1	3.5	8.1	5.7	11.8
1985	9.2	6.0	5.0	3.2	6.9	4.5	9.5
1989	8.1	5.1	4.2	2.9	6.4	4.0	8.2
1990	7.6	4.8	3.9	2.8	6.4	3.8	7.7
1991	7.3	4.5	3.7	2.8	6.2	3.7	7.4
1992	6.9	4.3	3.5	2.6	6.2	3.7	7.2
1993	6.8	4.3	3.5	2.5	6.1	3.4	6.9
1994	6.6	4.2	3.4	2.4	6.0	3.3	6.7
1995	6.3	4.1	3.3	2.2	5.9	3.3	6.5
1996	6.1	4.0	3.2	2.1	5.9	3.3	6.4
1997	6.0	4.0	3.2	2.0	5.8	3.2	6.3
Race of child:[6] Black							
1950[5]	43.9	27.8	23.0	16.1	32.1	- - -	- - -
1960[5]	44.3	27.8	23.7	16.5	- - -	- - -	- - -
1970	32.6	22.8	20.3	9.9	23.2	- - -	34.5
1980	21.4	14.1	11.9	7.3	14.4	8.9	20.7
Race of mother:[7] Black							
1980	22.2	14.6	12.3	7.6	14.7	9.1	21.3
1985	19.0	12.6	10.8	6.4	12.8	7.2	17.9
1989	18.6	11.9	10.1	6.7	13.1	6.8	16.8
1990	18.0	11.6	9.7	6.4	13.3	6.7	16.4
1991	17.6	11.2	9.4	6.3	12.8	6.4	15.7
1992	16.8	10.8	9.0	6.0	13.3	6.4	15.4
1993	16.5	10.7	9.0	5.8	12.8	5.8	14.7
1994	15.8	10.2	8.6	5.6	12.5	5.8	14.3
1995	15.1	9.8	8.2	5.3	12.7	5.7	13.8
1996	14.7	9.6	7.8	5.1	12.5	5.5	13.3
1997	14.2	9.4	7.8	4.8	12.5	5.5	13.2

- - - Data not available.

[1] Infant (under 1 year of age), neonatal (under 28 days), early neonatal (under 7 days), and postneonatal (28–365 days).
[2] Number of fetal deaths of 20 weeks or more gestation per 1,000 live births plus fetal deaths.
[3] Number of fetal deaths of 28 weeks or more gestation per 1,000 live births plus late fetal deaths.
[4] Number of late fetal deaths plus infant deaths within 7 days of birth per 1,000 live births plus late fetal deaths.
[5] Includes births and deaths of persons who were not residents of the 50 States and the District of Columbia.
[6] Infant deaths are tabulated by race of decedent; live births and fetal deaths are tabulated by race of child (see Appendix II, Race).
[7] Infant deaths are tabulated by race of decedent; fetal deaths and live births are tabulated by race of mother (see Appendix II, Race).

NOTES: Infant mortality rates in this table are based on infant deaths from the mortality file (numerator) and live births from the natality file (denominator). Inconsistencies in reporting race for the same infant between the birth and death certificate can result in underestimated infant mortality rates for races other than white or black. Infant mortality rates for minority population groups are available from the national linked files of live births and infant deaths and are presented in tables 19–21. Data for additional years are available (see Appendix III).

SOURCES: Centers for Disease Control and Prevention, National Center for Health Statistics: *Vital statistics of the United States, vol II, mortality, part A,* for data years 1950–93. Public Health Service. Washington. U.S. Government Printing Office; for 1994–97, unpublished data; Hoyert DL, Kochanek KD, Murphy SL. Deaths: Final data for 1997. National vital statistics reports; vol 48. Hyattsville, Maryland: 1999; and data computed by the Division of Health and Utilization Analysis from data compiled by the Division of Vital Statistics.

Table 23. Infant mortality rates, according to race, geographic division, and State: United States, average annual 1985–87, 1990–92, and 1995–97

[Data are based on the National Vital Statistics System]

Geographic division and State	All races 1985–87	All races 1990–92	All races 1995–97	White[1] 1985–87	White[1] 1990–92	White[1] 1995–97	Black[1] 1985–87	Black[1] 1990–92	Black[1] 1995–97
	Infant[2] deaths per 1,000 live births								
United States	10.4	8.9	7.4	8.8	7.3	6.1	18.9	17.5	14.7
New England	8.6	6.9	5.7	7.9	6.3	5.3	20.0	14.2	10.8
Maine	8.7	6.2	5.3	8.7	6.1	5.3	*	*	*
New Hampshire	8.7	6.4	4.9	8.6	6.3	4.9	*	*	*
Vermont	9.0	6.5	6.4	8.9	6.5	6.4	*	*	*
Massachusetts	8.3	6.7	5.1	7.4	6.2	4.8	19.6	12.5	8.9
Rhode Island	8.7	7.8	6.5	8.3	7.4	6.4	*14.5	*14.9	*9.3
Connecticut	9.2	7.6	6.9	7.8	6.3	6.0	21.3	16.5	13.9
Middle Atlantic	10.5	9.1	7.2	8.7	7.1	5.8	18.9	18.1	13.8
New York	10.7	9.3	7.1	9.0	7.3	5.9	17.5	17.2	12.4
New Jersey	9.9	8.7	6.6	7.9	6.3	5.2	19.3	18.5	13.9
Pennsylvania	10.5	9.2	7.7	8.7	7.3	6.2	22.3	20.1	17.4
East North Central	10.8	9.8	8.3	8.9	7.7	6.6	21.0	20.2	17.4
Ohio	10.1	9.6	8.1	8.9	7.9	6.7	17.5	18.4	16.4
Indiana	10.8	9.4	8.4	9.6	8.2	7.4	21.2	19.0	17.2
Illinois	11.8	10.5	8.8	9.1	7.6	6.7	22.2	21.2	18.0
Michigan	11.2	10.4	8.2	8.8	7.4	6.1	22.9	21.8	17.5
Wisconsin	9.0	7.9	7.0	8.2	7.1	6.1	17.9	15.5	17.1
West North Central	9.5	8.4	7.1	8.7	7.3	6.3	18.6	19.0	16.2
Minnesota	8.9	7.3	6.2	8.5	6.5	5.4	20.8	21.0	16.2
Iowa	9.0	8.1	7.1	8.8	7.8	6.8	*18.0	*18.3	*20.7
Missouri	10.4	9.4	7.5	9.0	7.5	6.2	18.3	18.6	15.3
North Dakota	8.6	8.0	6.2	8.2	7.5	5.9	*	*	*
South Dakota	11.0	9.6	7.6	8.9	8.0	5.9	*	*	*
Nebraska	9.4	7.7	7.9	8.7	6.9	7.5	*20.0	*18.9	*14.7
Kansas	9.2	8.7	7.6	8.5	7.7	6.7	18.4	19.8	19.3
South Atlantic	11.8	10.2	8.4	9.1	7.4	6.2	19.0	17.2	14.5
Delaware	12.7	10.2	7.6	10.1	7.6	5.9	21.4	18.8	13.4
Maryland	11.7	9.5	8.7	8.9	6.6	5.6	18.7	16.1	15.3
District of Columbia	20.4	20.4	14.8	11.0	10.9	5.8	23.7	24.0	18.1
Virginia	10.9	9.9	7.8	8.7	7.2	5.9	18.6	18.5	14.4
West Virginia	10.3	9.1	8.3	9.8	8.9	7.9	*23.3	*14.9	*19.6
North Carolina	11.7	10.5	9.2	9.2	7.8	6.9	18.2	16.7	15.6
South Carolina	13.4	11.1	9.2	9.7	7.8	6.3	19.4	16.6	14.6
Georgia	12.6	11.4	9.1	9.7	7.9	6.3	18.5	17.5	14.6
Florida	10.9	9.1	7.4	8.6	7.1	5.8	18.8	16.1	12.9
East South Central	11.8	10.2	9.1	9.4	7.8	7.1	18.5	16.5	15.0
Kentucky	10.3	8.6	7.5	9.7	8.0	7.1	16.1	14.2	11.8
Tennessee	11.4	9.9	8.8	8.9	7.4	6.7	19.8	18.0	16.6
Alabama	12.7	10.9	9.9	9.6	8.0	7.6	18.8	16.5	14.8
Mississippi	13.3	11.8	10.7	9.3	7.9	7.4	17.9	15.9	14.7
West South Central	10.1	8.5	7.2	8.7	7.2	6.2	16.6	14.7	12.8
Arkansas	10.8	9.9	8.9	9.4	8.3	7.6	15.3	15.5	14.1
Louisiana	11.9	10.4	9.5	8.4	7.4	6.4	17.4	14.6	14.0
Oklahoma	10.3	9.2	8.1	9.7	8.6	7.4	17.8	16.2	15.9
Texas	9.5	7.8	6.4	8.6	6.9	5.8	16.1	14.5	11.4
Mountain	9.5	8.1	6.7	9.1	7.6	6.4	18.5	18.3	15.1
Montana	10.0	7.9	7.0	9.1	7.0	6.6	*	*	*
Idaho	10.7	8.7	6.8	10.6	8.7	6.7	*	*	*
Wyoming	10.8	8.5	6.6	10.7	8.4	6.2	*	*	*
Colorado	9.3	8.3	6.7	8.9	7.7	6.4	19.3	17.4	15.9
New Mexico	9.4	8.2	6.2	9.0	7.8	5.9	*23.6	*23.4	*11.5
Arizona	9.5	8.6	7.4	8.9	7.9	7.0	18.1	19.2	17.2
Utah	9.0	6.5	5.7	9.0	6.4	5.7	*	*	*
Nevada	9.1	8.1	6.1	8.6	7.3	5.7	*17.0	17.4	12.5
Pacific	9.3	7.5	6.0	8.7	6.9	5.6	18.6	16.8	14.1
Washington	10.1	7.4	5.8	9.8	7.0	5.5	17.6	16.9	15.8
Oregon	9.9	7.5	5.8	9.7	7.2	5.7	*22.5	*21.5	*17.0
California	9.2	7.5	6.1	8.5	6.9	5.6	18.6	16.8	13.8
Alaska	10.7	9.3	7.5	8.9	7.7	6.2	*17.4	*13.2	*16.6
Hawaii	9.0	6.8	6.0	6.2	4.4	3.6	*20.8	*18.7	*13.9

* Data for States with fewer than 5,000 live births for the 3-year period are considered unreliable. Data for States with fewer than 1,000 live births are considered highly unreliable and are not shown.

[1]Deaths are tabulated by race of decedent; live births are tabulated by race of mother.

[2]Under 1 year of age.

NOTES: Infant mortality rates in this table are based on infant deaths from the mortality file (numerator) and live births from the natality file (denominator). Inconsistencies in reporting race for the same infant between the birth and death certificate can result in underestimated infant mortality rates for races other than white or black. Infant mortality rates for minority population groups are available from the national linked files of live births and infant deaths, tables 19–21.

SOURCE: Centers for Disease Control and Prevention, National Center for Health Statistics. Data computed by the Division of Health and Utilization Analysis from data compiled by the Division of Vital Statistics.

Table 24. Neonatal mortality rates, according to race, geographic division, and State: United States, average annual 1985–87, 1990–92, and 1995–97

[Data are based on the National Vital Statistics System]

Geographic division and State	All races 1985–87	All races 1990–92	All races 1995–97	White[1] 1985–87	White[1] 1990–92	White[1] 1995–97	Black[1] 1985–87	Black[1] 1990–92	Black[1] 1995–97
	Neonatal[2] deaths per 1,000 live births								
United States	6.7	5.6	4.8	5.7	4.6	4.0	12.4	11.2	9.6
New England	6.1	4.8	4.2	5.6	4.3	4.0	14.8	10.2	7.7
Maine	5.7	4.2	3.7	5.7	4.2	3.7	*	*	*
New Hampshire	5.9	3.7	3.5	5.9	3.7	3.5	*	*	*
Vermont	6.0	3.8	4.4	6.0	3.9	4.4	*	*	*
Massachusetts	5.8	4.7	3.8	5.3	4.3	3.6	14.0	8.9	6.0
Rhode Island	6.2	5.6	5.0	5.8	5.2	4.9	*11.6	*11.5	*7.5
Connecticut	6.9	5.5	5.1	5.8	4.6	4.5	16.4	11.8	10.4
Middle Atlantic	7.2	6.1	5.0	6.1	4.9	4.2	12.4	11.8	9.2
New York	7.3	6.3	5.0	6.3	5.1	4.2	11.4	11.2	8.2
New Jersey	6.7	5.8	4.6	5.5	4.4	3.8	12.4	11.7	9.1
Pennsylvania	7.2	6.1	5.4	6.0	4.9	4.3	15.0	13.2	11.9
East North Central	7.1	6.3	5.5	5.9	4.9	4.4	14.0	12.8	11.2
Ohio	6.4	6.0	5.4	5.7	5.0	4.5	11.0	11.5	10.8
Indiana	7.1	5.9	5.5	6.3	5.1	4.9	14.6	12.7	11.2
Illinois	8.0	6.9	5.9	6.3	5.2	4.6	14.4	13.2	11.4
Michigan	7.6	6.8	5.5	5.8	4.7	4.1	16.6	14.7	11.6
Wisconsin	5.5	4.7	4.6	4.9	4.3	4.0	11.7	8.0	10.2
West North Central	5.8	5.0	4.5	5.4	4.4	4.0	11.2	11.2	10.2
Minnesota	5.4	4.4	3.8	5.2	4.1	3.4	12.4	12.2	9.3
Iowa	5.7	4.6	4.7	5.5	4.4	4.5	*10.3	*11.2	*12.1
Missouri	6.5	5.7	4.7	5.7	4.6	3.9	11.1	11.1	9.8
North Dakota	4.8	5.0	3.8	4.7	5.0	3.9	*	*	*
South Dakota	5.8	5.3	4.0	5.3	4.8	3.4	*	*	*
Nebraska	5.9	4.3	5.5	5.5	3.9	5.2	*11.5	*10.2	*10.6
Kansas	5.6	5.2	5.0	5.2	4.6	4.4	11.3	11.4	12.4
South Atlantic	7.9	6.8	5.7	6.1	4.8	4.1	12.9	11.6	10.1
Delaware	9.2	6.9	5.0	7.5	5.4	3.6	15.0	12.0	9.6
Maryland	8.1	6.3	6.1	6.0	4.3	3.7	13.4	10.9	11.1
District of Columbia	15.5	14.4	10.7	8.0	8.1	4.3	18.1	16.8	13.1
Virginia	7.4	6.6	5.4	5.8	4.6	4.0	13.0	13.2	10.4
West Virginia	6.9	5.6	5.5	6.6	5.5	5.2	*15.9	*8.9	*13.9
North Carolina	7.8	7.1	6.3	6.1	5.1	4.7	12.4	11.7	10.9
South Carolina	9.1	7.3	6.4	6.6	5.1	4.2	13.3	10.9	10.4
Georgia	8.5	7.5	6.1	6.6	5.0	4.1	12.3	11.8	10.1
Florida	7.1	6.0	4.7	5.6	4.7	3.7	12.1	10.2	8.4
East South Central	7.7	6.4	5.7	6.1	4.7	4.4	12.1	10.8	9.6
Kentucky	6.6	4.9	4.6	6.2	4.5	4.4	10.8	8.5	7.5
Tennessee	7.4	6.2	5.3	5.6	4.5	3.9	13.3	11.7	10.1
Alabama	8.5	7.2	6.5	6.6	5.3	4.8	12.2	11.0	10.0
Mississippi	8.3	7.4	6.6	5.8	4.6	4.5	11.3	10.4	9.1
West South Central	6.3	5.1	4.3	5.5	4.3	3.7	10.3	8.7	7.8
Arkansas	6.2	5.4	5.4	5.6	4.5	4.5	8.3	8.7	8.5
Louisiana	7.7	6.3	6.1	5.6	4.6	4.1	11.1	8.8	9.1
Oklahoma	6.2	5.1	4.8	5.9	4.7	4.5	11.2	9.0	9.4
Texas	6.0	4.7	3.8	5.4	4.1	3.4	10.0	8.7	6.6
Mountain	5.5	4.5	4.2	5.3	4.3	4.1	11.7	10.3	9.0
Montana	5.1	3.6	4.0	4.7	3.4	3.9	*	*	*
Idaho	6.4	5.0	4.1	6.3	4.9	4.1	*	*	*
Wyoming	6.1	3.7	3.6	6.2	3.6	3.4	*	*	*
Colorado	5.6	4.7	4.4	5.3	4.3	4.2	11.8	10.7	10.2
New Mexico	5.6	4.7	3.8	5.4	4.7	3.8	*14.4	*11.7	*8.1
Arizona	5.8	5.1	4.8	5.5	4.7	4.7	12.7	11.9	10.5
Utah	4.9	3.5	3.6	4.9	3.5	3.6	*	*	*
Nevada	4.9	4.0	3.4	4.6	3.6	3.1	*10.3	8.3	6.5
Pacific	5.7	4.5	3.8	5.3	4.2	3.6	11.3	10.1	8.5
Washington	5.6	3.9	3.5	5.4	3.7	3.4	10.8	10.7	8.6
Oregon	5.2	4.0	3.4	5.1	3.9	3.3	*11.5	*11.3	*7.4
California	5.7	4.6	3.9	5.3	4.3	3.7	11.4	10.1	8.5
Alaska	5.6	4.2	3.9	4.9	3.7	3.4	*8.7	*5.6	*7.6
Hawaii	5.9	4.2	3.9	3.9	3.0	2.4	*13.2	*10.1	*10.3

* Data for States with fewer than 5,000 live births for the 3-year period are considered unreliable. Data for States with fewer than 1,000 live births are considered highly unreliable and are not shown.

[1]Deaths are tabulated by race of decedent; live births are tabulated by race of mother.

[2]Infants under 28 days of age.

NOTES: Infant mortality rates in this table are based on infant deaths from the mortality file (numerator) and live births from the natality file (denominator). Inconsistencies in reporting race for the same infant between the birth and death certificate can result in underestimated infant mortality rates for races other than white or black. Infant mortality rates for minority population groups are available from the national linked files of live births and infant deaths, tables 19–21.

SOURCE: Centers for Disease Control and Prevention, National Center for Health Statistics. Data computed by the Division of Health and Utilization Analysis from data compiled by the Division of Vital Statistics.

Table 25. Postneonatal mortality rates, according to race, geographic division, and State: United States, average annual 1985–87, 1990–92, and 1995–97

[Data are based on the National Vital Statistics System]

Geographic division and State	All races 1985–87	All races 1990–92	All races 1995–97	White[1] 1985–87	White[1] 1990–92	White[1] 1995–97	Black[1] 1985–87	Black[1] 1990–92	Black[1] 1995–97
	Postneonatal[2] deaths per 1,000 live births								
United States	3.6	3.3	2.6	3.1	2.7	2.1	6.5	6.3	5.0
New England	2.5	2.1	1.5	2.3	2.0	1.4	5.2	4.1	3.1
Maine	3.0	2.0	1.6	3.0	2.0	1.*	*	*	*
New Hampshire	2.8	2.7	.	2.8	2.6	1.4	*	*	*
Vermont	3.0	2.6	2.0	2.9	2.7	2.0	*	*	*
Massachusetts	2.4	2.0	1.4	2.2	1.8	1.2	5.7	3.6	2.9
Rhode Island	2.5	2.2	1.4	2.4	2.2	1.4	*3.0	*3.4	*1.8
Connecticut	2.3	2.2	1.8	2.0	1.8	1.5	4.9	4.7	3.6
Middle Atlantic	3.3	3.0	2.2	2.6	2.2	1.7	6.5	6.3	4.6
New York	3.4	3.0	2.2	2.7	2.2	1.7	6.0	5.9	4.2
New Jersey	3.2	2.8	2.0	2.4	1.9	1.4	6.9	6.8	4.8
Pennsylvania	3.3	3.1	2.4	2.7	2.5	1.9	7.4	6.9	5.5
East North Central	3.7	3.6	2.8	3.1	2.8	2.1	7.0	7.3	6.2
Ohio	3.6	3.6	2.7	3.2	2.9	2.2	6.5	7.0	5.6
Indiana	3.6	3.5	2.9	3.3	3.1	2.5	6.6	6.3	6.0
Illinois	3.9	3.6	2.9	2.8	2.4	2.1	7.8	8.0	6.6
Michigan	3.5	3.6	2.7	3.0	2.7	2.0	6.3	7.1	5.9
Wisconsin	3.5	3.2	2.5	3.3	2.7	2.0	6.2	7.5	6.9
West North Central	3.7	3.4	2.6	3.3	2.9	2.2	7.4	6.6	6.0
Minnesota	3.5	2.9	2.4	3.3	2.4	2.0	*8.4	*8.8	*6.8
Iowa	3.4	3.4	2.4	3.2	3.3	2.3	*7.7	*7.1	*8.6
Missouri	3.8	3.7	2.8	3.3	2.9	2.3	7.2	7.4	5.5
North Dakota	3.8	2.9	2.4	3.5	2.4	2.0	*	*	*
South Dakota	5.2	4.3	3.6	3.7	3.2	2.6	*	*	*
Nebraska	3.6	3.5	2.4	3.2	3.0	2.3	*8.5	*8.7	*4.1
Kansas	3.7	3.5	2.6	3.3	3.1	2.3	*7.1	*8.4	*6.9
South Atlantic	3.8	3.4	2.7	3.0	2.6	2.1	6.1	5.6	4.4
Delaware	3.4	3.3	2.7	2.6	2.2	2.3	*6.4	*6.8	*3.9
Maryland	3.6	3.2	2.6	2.9	2.3	1.9	5.3	5.2	4.2
District of Columbia	4.9	6.1	4.1	*3.0	*2.8	*1.5	5.6	7.2	5.0
Virginia	3.5	3.2	2.3	2.9	2.6	1.9	5.6	5.3	4.0
West Virginia	3.4	3.4	2.8	3.2	3.4	2.7	*7.4	*	*
North Carolina	3.9	3.4	2.9	3.1	2.7	2.2	5.8	5.0	4.8
South Carolina	4.2	3.8	2.8	3.1	2.7	2.0	6.1	5.7	4.2
Georgia	4.1	3.9	3.0	3.0	2.8	2.2	6.3	5.8	4.4
Florida	3.8	3.2	2.7	2.9	2.4	2.2	6.7	5.9	4.5
East South Central	4.1	3.8	3.4	3.3	3.1	2.7	6.4	5.8	5.5
Kentucky	3.6	3.7	2.8	3.5	3.5	2.7	5.2	5.7	4.3
Tennessee	4.0	3.8	3.5	3.3	3.0	2.7	6.5	6.3	6.4
Alabama	4.2	3.7	3.5	3.0	2.7	2.8	6.5	5.5	4.9
Mississippi	4.9	4.5	4.1	3.5	3.4	2.9	6.6	5.6	5.6
West South Central	3.8	3.5	2.9	3.2	2.9	2.5	6.3	6.0	5.0
Arkansas	4.5	4.5	3.6	3.8	3.8	3.1	7.0	6.8	5.6
Louisiana	4.1	4.0	3.4	2.8	2.8	2.3	6.3	5.8	4.9
Oklahoma	4.1	4.1	3.3	3.8	3.8	2.9	6.6	7.2	6.5
Texas	3.5	3.1	2.6	3.2	2.7	2.4	6.1	5.8	4.8
Mountain	4.0	3.6	2.5	3.8	3.3	2.3	6.7	8.0	6.2
Montana	4.9	4.2	3.0	4.4	3.6	2.7	*	*	*
Idaho	4.3	3.7	2.7	4.3	3.7	2.6	*	*	*
Wyoming	4.7	4.8	3.0	4.5	4.8	2.8	*	*	*
Colorado	3.7	3.6	2.3	3.6	3.4	2.2	*7.5	*6.7	*5.8
New Mexico	3.8	3.5	2.4	3.6	3.1	2.1	*	*	*
Arizona	3.7	3.5	2.6	3.4	3.2	2.3	*5.4	*7.3	*6.8
Utah	4.1	3.0	2.2	4.1	3.0	2.1	*	*	*
Nevada	4.1	4.1	2.8	4.0	3.7	2.6	*6.7	*9.1	*6.0
Pacific	3.7	3.0	2.2	3.4	2.8	2.0	7.3	6.7	5.5
Washington	4.5	3.4	2.3	4.3	3.3	2.1	*6.9	*6.1	*7.1
Oregon	4.7	3.5	2.5	4.6	3.4	2.3	*	*10.2	*9.6
California	3.5	2.9	2.2	3.2	2.7	2.0	7.2	6.7	5.3
Alaska	5.1	5.1	3.6	4.0	4.0	2.8	*	*	*
Hawaii	3.2	2.6	2.1	2.3	1.3	1.3	*	*	*

* Data for States with fewer than 10,000 live births for the 3-year period are considered unreliable. Data for States with fewer than 2,500 live births are considered highly unreliable and are not shown.
[1] Deaths are tabulated by race of decedent; live births are tabulated by race of mother.
[2] Infants 28–365 days of age.
NOTES: Infant mortality rates in this table are based on infant deaths from the mortality file (numerator) and live births from the natality file (denominator).
Inconsistencies in reporting race for the same infant between the birth and death certificate can result in underestimated infant mortality rates for races other than white or black. Infant mortality rates for minority population groups are available from the national linked files of live births and infant deaths, tables 19–21.
SOURCE: Centers for Disease Control and Prevention, National Center for Health Statistics. Data computed by the Division of Health and Utilization Analysis from data compiled by the Division of Vital Statistics.

Table 26. Infant mortality rates, feto-infant mortality rates, and postneonatal mortality rates, and average annual percent change: Selected countries, 1990 and 1995

[Data are based on reporting by countries]

Country[4]	Infant mortality rate[1]			Feto-infant mortality rate[2]			Postneonatal mortality rate[3]		
	1990[5]	1995[6]	Average annual percent change	1990[7]	1995[8]	Average annual percent change	1990[9]	1995[10]	Average annual percent change
Finland	5.64	3.93	−7.0	8.76	6.89	−4.7	1.91	1.24	−10.2
Singapore	6.67	4.01	−9.7	10.65	6.87	−8.4	2.01	1.91	−1.0
Sweden	5.96	4.13	−7.1	9.50	7.48	−4.7	2.46	1.27	−12.4
Norway	7.02	4.13	−10.1	11.55	7.68	−7.8	3.10	1.41	−14.6
Japan	4.60	4.26	−1.5	8.38	7.36	−2.6	1.99	2.05	0.6
Hong Kong	6.13	4.57	−5.7	10.23	8.42	−3.8	2.33	2.00	−3.0
France	7.33	4.86	−7.9	13.75	9.29	−6.3	3.79	1.96	−12.4
Switzerland	6.83	5.05	−5.9	11.42	9.10	−4.4	3.05	1.63	−11.8
Denmark	7.39	5.07	−7.3	12.03	9.59	−4.4	2.84	1.30	−14.5
Germany	7.05	5.30	−5.5	9.77	9.70	−0.1	3.32	2.12	−8.6
Austria	7.84	5.42	−7.1	11.39	8.61	−5.4	3.41	2.06	−9.6
Netherlands	7.06	5.46	−5.0	12.74	11.19	−2.6	2.42	1.62	−7.7
Spain	7.60	5.49	−6.3	11.58	8.91	−5.1	2.62	1.96	−5.6
Australia	8.17	5.66	−7.1	12.06	9.51	−4.6	3.31	1.92	−10.3
Belgium	7.94	6.05	−5.3	13.18	10.78	−3.9	3.87	4.03	1.4
Italy	8.01	6.12	−5.2	13.29	11.59	−3.4	1.82	1.68	−2.0
England and Wales	7.88	6.14	−4.9	12.44	10.27	−3.8	3.32	1.98	−9.8
Canada	6.84	6.14	−2.1	10.74	12.17	2.5	2.22	1.95	−2.6
Scotland	7.73	6.24	−4.2	12.92	11.09	−3.0	3.35	2.23	−7.8
Ireland	8.20	6.37	−4.9	14.25	12.78	−2.2	3.57	1.69	−13.9
New Zealand	8.31	6.68	−4.3	12.37	10.23	−6.1	4.24	3.53	−5.9
Israel	9.84	6.86	−7.0	13.96	11.11	−4.5	3.46	2.33	−7.6
Northern Ireland	7.47	7.08	−1.1	11.45	11.64	0.3	3.48	1.89	−14.2
Portugal	10.99	7.51	−7.3	17.84	12.92	−6.2	3.99	2.77	−7.0
United States	9.22	7.59	−3.8	13.21	11.20	−3.2	3.38	2.67	−4.6
Czech Republic	10.80	7.70	−6.5	14.10	10.79	−4.4	3.08	2.76	−2.2
Greece	9.32	8.15	−2.6	16.39	13.75	−3.5	2.81	2.36	−3.4
Cuba	10.74	9.40	−2.6	22.94	20.01	−2.3	3.91	3.36	−2.5
Hungary	14.82	10.66	−6.4	20.27	14.12	−7.0	3.99	3.36	−3.4
Kuwait	17.33	10.93	−5.6	25.39	18.18	−3.6	5.22	3.34	−6.2
Slovakia	13.46	10.99	−3.3	18.02	14.85	−3.2	4.24	3.13	−4.9
Chile	16.82	11.10	−8.0	22.81	15.59	−7.3	7.90	5.04	−8.6
Puerto Rico	14.77	11.47	−6.1	24.46	21.51	−3.2	2.36	2.83	4.6
Costa Rica	15.26	13.25	−2.8	23.97	21.82	−4.6	6.14	4.72	−5.1
Poland	16.01	13.60	−3.2	21.49	19.30	−1.8	4.43	3.53	−4.4
Bulgaria	14.77	14.80	0.0	20.74	21.03	0.3	7.06	7.03	−0.1
Russian Federation	17.64	18.21	0.6	26.53	25.47	−0.8	6.67	7.19	1.5
Romania	30.09	21.24	−6.7	36.92	27.29	−5.9	18.24	11.98	−8.1

0.0 Quantity more than zero but less than 0.05.
[1]Number of deaths of infants under 1 year per 1,000 live births.
[2]Number of late fetal deaths plus infant deaths under 1 year per 1,000 live births plus late fetal deaths.
[3]Number of postneonatal deaths per 1,000 live births.
[4]Refers to countries, territories, cities, or geographic areas.
[5]Data for Kuwait are for 1987. Data for Slovakia are for 1989.
[6]Data for Puerto Rico are for 1994.
[7]Data for Kuwait are for 1986. Data for France, Czech Republic, Cuba, Slovakia, and Poland are for 1989.
[8]Data for Costa Rica are for 1992. Data for New Zealand are for 1993. Data for Italy and Puerto Rico are for 1994.
[9]Data for Kuwait are for 1987. Data for Belgium, Cuba, and Slovakia are for 1989.
[10]Data for Belgium are for 1992. Data for New Zealand are for 1993. Data for Finland, Northern Ireland, Italy, Kuwait, and Puerto Rico are for 1994.

NOTES: Rankings are from lowest to highest infant mortality rates based on the latest data available for countries or geographic areas with at least 1 million population and with "complete" counts of live births and infant deaths as indicated in the United Nations Demographic Yearbook, 1996 edition. Some of the international variation in infant mortality rates (IMR) is due to differences among countries in distinguishing between fetal and infant deaths. The feto-infant mortality rate (FIMR) is an alternative measure of pregnancy outcome that reduces the effect of international differences in distinguishing between fetal and infant deaths. The United States ranks 25th on the IMR, 21st on the FIMR, and 23rd on the postneonatal mortality rate.

SOURCES: World Health Organization: World Health Statistics Annuals. Vols. 1990–1996. Geneva; United Nations: Demographic Yearbook 1991 and 1996. New York; Centers for Disease Control and Prevention, National Center for Health Statistics. Vital statistics of the United States, 1990 and 1995, vol II, mortality, part A. Washington: Public Health Service. 1994 and unpublished.

[Data are based on reporting by countries]

Country[1]	At birth		At 65 years	
	1990[2]	1995[3]	1990[2]	1995[3]
Male	Life expectancy in years			
Japan	76.2	76.4	16.5	16.5
Sweden	74.8	76.2	15.5	16.0
Israel	74.6	75.3	15.6	15.8
Canada	74.0	75.2	15.5	16.1
Switzerland	74.0	75.1	15.3	16.1
Greece	74.6	75.1	15.8	16.2
Australia	73.3	75.0	14.7	15.6
Norway	73.4	74.9	14.6	15.2
Netherlands	73.9	74.6	14.4	14.7
Italy	73.6	74.4	15.0	15.5
England and Wales	73.2	74.3	14.3	14.7
France	73.4	74.2	16.1	16.6
Spain	73.4	74.2	15.5	16.0
Austria	72.6	73.5	14.7	15.2
Singapore	72.3	73.4	14.4	14.9
Germany	72.0	73.3	14.1	14.7
New Zealand	71.9	73.3	14.3	15.0
Northern Ireland	71.8	73.1	13.2	14.1
Belgium	72.3	73.0	14.0	14.5
Cuba	72.9	73.0	15.9	15.7
Costa Rica	72.1	73.0	14.0	15.2
Finland	71.0	72.8	13.8	14.5
Denmark	72.2	72.8	14.0	14.1
Ireland	72.0	72.5	13.2	13.4
United States	71.8	72.5	15.1	15.6
Scotland	71.2	72.2	13.2	13.8
Chile	69.4	71.6	14.0	14.6
Portugal	70.1	71.2	13.8	14.3
Czech Republic	67.6	69.7	11.7	12.7
Puerto Rico	69.1	69.6	14.9	16.3
Slovakia	68.3	68.2	13.0	12.7
Poland	66.5	67.6	12.5	12.9
Bulgaria	68.2	67.1	12.8	12.6
Romania	66.6	65.5	13.3	12.8
Hungary	65.1	65.3	12.1	12.1
Russian Federation[4]	63.8	58.3	11.9	11.0
Female				
Japan	82.5	82.9	20.6	20.9
France	81.8	82.6	20.7	21.4
Switzerland	81.0	81.9	19.7	20.5
Sweden	80.8	81.6	19.4	19.8
Spain	80.5	81.5	19.2	19.9
Canada	80.8	81.2	19.9	20.1
Australia	79.6	80.9	18.7	19.5
Italy	80.4	80.8	19.0	19.4
Norway	79.9	80.7	18.7	19.3
Netherlands	80.3	80.4	19.2	19.1
Greece	79.8	80.3	18.3	18.5
Finland	79.0	80.3	17.9	18.7
Austria	79.2	80.1	18.2	18.8
Germany	78.6	79.8	17.8	18.6
Belgium	79.1	79.8	18.4	18.9
England and Wales	78.9	79.6	18.2	18.5
Israel	78.1	79.3	17.3	17.8
Singapore	77.5	79.0	17.2	18.1
United States	78.8	78.9	18.9	18.9
New Zealand	78.1	78.9	18.1	18.6

See footnotes at end of table.

Table 27 (page 2 of 2). **Life expectancy at birth and at 65 years of age, according to sex: Selected countries, 1990 and 1995**

[Data are based on reporting by countries]

	At birth		At 65 years	
Country[1]	1990[2]	1995[3]	1990[2]	1995[3]
Female—Con.	Life expectancy in years			
Puerto Rico	77.2	78.9	17.5	19.4
Portugal	77.3	78.6	17.0	17.7
Northern Ireland	77.5	78.5	17.1	17.7
Ireland	77.7	78.1	17.0	17.0
Denmark	77.9	77.9	18.0	17.6
Chile	76.5	77.9	17.6	17.9
Costa Rica	76.9	77.8	16.8	17.6
Scotland	77.0	77.6	16.9	17.1
Cuba	76.8	76.9	17.8	17.6
Czech Republic	75.5	76.7	15.3	16.2
Poland	75.6	76.4	16.2	16.5
Slovakia	76.5	76.3	16.6	16.3
Bulgaria	74.9	74.9	15.3	15.5
Hungary	73.8	74.6	15.4	15.8
Romania	73.1	73.4	15.2	15.3
Russian Federation[4]	74.3	71.6	15.7	15.0

[1]Refers to countries, territories, cities, or geographic areas.
[2]Data for Slovakia are for 1987. Data for Costa Rica are for 1988. Data for Australia, Belgium, and Puerto Rico are for 1989.
[3]Data for Australia, Bulgaria, Chile, Costa Rica, France, Norway, Spain, and Switzerland are for 1994. Data for Ireland, Italy, and New Zealand are for 1993. Data for Puerto Rico are for 1992.
[4]Data for 1990 from Goskomstat 1997 (Demographic Yearbook of Russia, 1996).

NOTES: Rankings are from highest to lowest life expectancy based on the latest available data for countries or geographic areas with at least 1 million population. This table is based on official mortality data from the countries concerned, as submitted to the United Nations Demographic Yearbook or the World Health Statistics Annual.

SOURCES: World Health Organization: World Health Statistics Annuals. Vols. 1990–1996. Geneva; United Nations: Demographic Yearbook 1991 and 1996. New York; Centers for Disease Control and Prevention, National Center for Health Statistics. Vital statistics of the United States, 1990 and 1995, vol II, mortality, part A. Washington: Public Health Service. 1994 and unpublished.

Table 28. Life expectancy at birth, at 65 years of age, and at 75 years of age, according to race and sex: United States, selected years 1900–97

[Data are based on the National Vital Statistics System]

Specified age and year	All races			White			Black		
	Both sexes	Male	Female	Both sexes	Male	Female	Both sexes	Male	Female
At birth				Remaining life expectancy in years					
1900[1,2]	47.3	46.3	48.3	47.6	46.6	48.7	[3]33.0	[3]32.5	[3]33.5
1950[2]	68.2	65.6	71.1	69.1	66.5	72.2	60.7	58.9	62.7
1960[2]	69.7	66.6	73.1	70.6	67.4	74.1	63.2	60.7	65.9
1970	70.8	67.1	74.7	71.7	68.0	75.6	64.1	60.0	68.3
1980	73.7	70.0	77.4	74.4	70.7	78.1	68.1	63.8	72.5
1985	74.7	71.1	78.2	75.3	71.8	78.7	69.3	65.0	73.4
1986	74.7	71.2	78.2	75.4	71.9	78.8	69.1	64.8	73.4
1987	74.9	71.4	78.3	75.6	72.1	78.9	69.1	64.7	73.4
1988	74.9	71.4	78.3	75.6	72.2	78.9	68.9	64.4	73.2
1989	75.1	71.7	78.5	75.9	72.5	79.2	68.8	64.3	73.3
1990	75.4	71.8	78.8	76.1	72.7	79.4	69.1	64.5	73.6
1991	75.5	72.0	78.9	76.3	72.9	79.6	69.3	64.6	73.8
1992	75.8	72.3	79.1	76.5	73.2	79.8	69.6	65.0	73.9
1993	75.5	72.2	78.8	76.3	73.1	79.5	69.2	64.6	73.7
1994	75.7	72.4	79.0	76.5	73.3	79.6	69.5	64.9	73.9
1995	75.8	72.5	78.9	76.5	73.4	79.6	69.6	65.2	73.9
1996	76.1	73.1	79.1	76.8	73.9	79.7	70.2	66.1	74.2
1997	76.5	73.6	79.4	77.1	74.3	79.9	71.1	67.2	74.7
At 65 years									
1900–1902[1,2]	11.9	11.5	12.2	- - -	11.5	12.2	- - -	10.4	11.4
1950[2]	13.9	12.8	15.0	- - -	12.8	15.1	13.9	12.9	14.9
1960[2]	14.3	12.8	15.8	14.4	12.9	15.9	13.9	12.7	15.1
1970	15.2	13.1	17.0	15.2	13.1	17.1	14.2	12.5	15.7
1980	16.4	14.1	18.3	16.5	14.2	18.4	15.1	13.0	16.8
1985	16.7	14.5	18.5	16.8	14.5	18.7	15.2	13.0	16.9
1986	16.8	14.6	18.6	16.9	14.7	18.7	15.2	13.0	17.0
1987	16.9	14.7	18.7	17.0	14.8	18.8	15.2	13.0	17.0
1988	16.9	14.7	18.6	17.0	14.8	18.7	15.1	12.9	16.9
1989	17.1	15.0	18.8	17.2	15.1	18.9	15.2	13.0	16.9
1990	17.2	15.1	18.9	17.3	15.2	19.1	15.4	13.2	17.2
1991	17.4	15.3	19.1	17.5	15.4	19.2	15.5	13.4	17.2
1992	17.5	15.4	19.2	17.6	15.5	19.3	15.7	13.5	17.4
1993	17.3	15.3	18.9	17.4	15.4	19.0	15.5	13.4	17.1
1994	17.4	15.5	19.0	17.5	15.6	19.1	15.7	13.6	17.2
1995	17.4	15.6	18.9	17.6	15.7	19.1	15.6	13.6	17.1
1996	17.5	15.7	19.0	17.6	15.8	19.1	15.8	13.9	17.2
1997	17.7	15.9	19.2	17.8	16.0	19.3	16.1	14.2	17.6
At 75 years									
1980	10.4	8.8	11.5	10.4	8.8	11.5	9.7	8.3	10.7
1985	10.6	9.0	11.7	10.6	9.0	11.7	10.1	8.7	11.1
1986	10.7	9.1	11.7	10.7	9.1	11.8	10.1	8.6	11.1
1987	10.7	9.1	11.8	10.7	9.1	11.8	10.1	8.6	11.1
1988	10.6	9.1	11.7	10.7	9.1	11.7	10.0	8.5	11.0
1989	10.9	9.3	11.9	10.9	9.3	11.9	10.1	8.6	11.0
1990	10.9	9.4	12.0	11.0	9.4	12.0	10.2	8.6	11.2
1991	11.1	9.5	12.1	11.1	9.5	12.1	10.2	8.7	11.2
1992	11.2	9.6	12.2	11.2	9.6	12.2	10.4	8.9	11.4
1993	10.9	9.5	11.9	11.0	9.5	12.0	10.2	8.7	11.1
1994	11.0	9.6	12.0	11.1	9.6	12.0	10.3	8.9	11.2
1995	11.0	9.7	11.9	11.1	9.7	12.0	10.2	8.8	11.1
1996	11.1	9.8	12.0	11.1	9.8	12.0	10.3	9.0	11.2
1997	11.2	9.9	12.1	11.2	9.9	12.1	10.7	9.3	11.5

- - - Data not available.

[1]Death registration area only. The death registration area increased from 10 States and the District of Columbia in 1900 to the coterminous United States in 1933.
[2]Includes deaths of persons who were not residents of the 50 States and the District of Columbia.
[3]Figure is for the all other population.

NOTES: Beginning in 1997 life table methodology was revised to construct complete life tables by single years of age that extend to age 100. Previously abridged life tables were constructed for five-year age groups ending with the age group 85 years and over. Data for additional years are available (see Appendix III).

SOURCES: U.S. Bureau of the Census: U.S. Life Tables 1890, 1901, 1910, and 1901–1910, by Glover JW. Washington. U.S. Government Printing Office, 1921; Centers for Disease Control and Prevention, National Center for Health Statistics: Vital Statistics Rates in the United States, 1940–1960, by Grove RD and Hetzel AM. DHEW Pub. No. (PHS) 1677. Public Health Service. Washington. U.S. Government Printing Office, 1968; Hoyert DL, Kochanek KD, Murphy SL. Deaths: Final data for 1997. National vital statistics reports; vol 48. Hyattsville, Maryland: 1999; unpublished data from the Division of Vital Statistics; data for 1960 and earlier years for the black population were computed by the Office of Research and Methodology from data compiled by the Division of Vital Statistics.

Table 29 (page 1 of 2). Age-adjusted death rates, according to detailed race, Hispanic origin, geographic division, and State: United States, average annual 1984–86, 1989–91, and 1995–97

[Data are based on the National Vital Statistics System]

Geographic division and State	All persons 1984–86	All persons 1989–91	All persons 1995–97	White 1995–97	Black 1995–97	American Indian or Alaska Native 1995–97	Asian or Pacific Islander 1995–97	Hispanic 1995–97	White, non-Hispanic 1995–97
				Deaths per 100,000 resident population[1]					
United States	547.7	522.0	491.4	466.7	736.5	462.9	278.7	365.6	469.0
New England	514.4	473.0	444.6	438.5	626.5	*	237.1	316.2	433.9
Maine	530.2	490.3	470.0	472.0	*	*	*	*	460.6
New Hampshire	519.8	473.7	448.5	449.7	*	*	225.4	179.7	437.6
Vermont	528.5	480.5	456.5	457.2	*	*	*	*	458.0
Massachusetts	518.7	475.0	439.7	434.9	599.8	*	264.4	317.2	432.7
Rhode Island	517.3	478.8	448.0	441.4	682.9	*	255.5	256.7	435.1
Connecticut	497.3	461.4	441.8	425.6	659.5	*	173.2	347.9	420.8
Middle Atlantic	566.2	537.2	491.3	466.2	698.6	*	240.9	389.1	457.7
New York	573.0	549.7	488.1	466.8	639.9	*	257.2	412.7	448.2
New Jersey	553.6	522.3	481.2	450.8	751.6	*	188.4	296.2	452.7
Pennsylvania	562.5	525.8	500.5	473.7	801.4	*	263.6	490.3	471.0
East North Central	553.0	525.3	496.7	466.9	769.7	*	229.6	305.2	465.7
Ohio	561.6	528.1	505.9	484.5	718.8	*	198.8	364.7	481.3
Indiana	551.2	524.1	509.7	491.9	761.6	*	218.4	278.1	493.5
Illinois	559.5	541.5	506.9	463.2	828.3	*	222.0	294.7	463.2
Michigan	569.6	534.3	494.5	456.4	753.0	*	260.8	342.4	452.7
Wisconsin	488.5	463.9	441.2	428.2	724.4	*	287.3	225.1	429.5
West North Central	497.1	471.9	458.3	442.6	753.4	*	301.0	348.4	440.0
Minnesota	462.6	431.2	412.8	404.4	675.7	813.1	335.0	449.1	401.1
Iowa	472.7	448.9	430.7	427.2	704.6	*	301.2	335.0	427.0
Missouri	549.7	527.8	521.5	496.1	778.5	*	307.9	357.5	496.1
North Dakota	449.6	435.9	419.1	404.9	*	960.3	*	*	394.1
South Dakota	497.2	459.4	444.9	411.9	*	1,126.1	*	*	412.0
Nebraska	484.1	464.1	442.9	431.7	776.5	905.8	237.8	315.4	427.9
Kansas	494.0	467.6	459.6	447.2	722.7	*	254.8	316.3	439.8
South Atlantic	565.0	540.0	514.4	466.4	753.0	*	219.7	329.9	471.7
Delaware	573.9	549.4	518.9	481.2	748.5	*	154.5	336.4	480.5
Maryland	577.6	544.9	519.0	454.1	747.8	*	223.6	93.7	462.0
District of Columbia	765.8	824.5	774.4	401.5	1,003.6	*	210.0	88.6	438.6
Virginia	564.2	528.6	499.1	459.2	720.2	*	227.0	186.7	462.1
West Virginia	593.6	576.5	551.0	547.9	717.3	*	*	199.3	549.2
North Carolina	576.9	556.7	533.0	480.3	759.7	602.6	247.3	168.8	481.2
South Carolina	618.6	596.4	573.8	504.8	785.6	*	239.2	190.5	506.0
Georgia	614.9	592.6	560.3	502.4	764.2	*	263.3	216.1	502.7
Florida	521.2	497.9	478.3	450.0	715.0	*	188.0	362.0	458.9
East South Central	598.3	584.0	571.5	531.2	782.9	*	248.5	312.4	531.3
Kentucky	592.6	571.0	548.6	537.7	741.3	*	274.6	433.7	537.4
Tennessee	583.7	566.9	564.6	527.2	821.7	*	281.0	340.4	527.1
Alabama	604.5	593.7	576.3	526.7	764.7	*	138.0	279.6	527.3
Mississippi	625.3	621.3	611.7	539.0	784.6	*	288.6	186.5	539.5
West South Central	564.6	548.6	521.5	496.4	735.7	*	227.8	411.6	532.3
Arkansas	575.7	564.7	561.1	531.1	788.3	*	331.8	177.1	532.4
Louisiana	623.7	621.1	589.8	519.1	783.0	*	254.1	249.0	525.0
Oklahoma	550.4	534.1	540.4	537.4	707.0	*	279.4	- - -	- - -
Texas	549.4	530.1	495.7	478.6	702.3	*	217.8	415.9	487.2
Mountain	502.4	479.1	459.2	452.4	596.6	626.7	286.2	428.7	447.3
Montana	513.7	484.1	460.8	446.8	*	814.9	*	335.0	445.0
Idaho	488.7	456.8	433.3	432.3	*	582.6	336.1	305.1	433.9
Wyoming	507.5	484.7	467.5	462.5	*	866.5	*	431.5	461.0
Colorado	478.9	456.1	428.7	426.2	572.5	371.9	240.9	430.8	421.2
New Mexico	518.5	497.3	473.8	465.8	462.1	600.7	297.2	473.6	447.6
Arizona	511.9	488.4	476.5	464.6	631.0	686.3	250.3	436.2	458.0
Utah	465.8	426.8	406.6	405.0	625.7	462.4	348.2	394.0	402.1
Nevada	586.6	569.3	543.8	543.8	653.5	428.1	335.5	260.0	551.1

See footnotes at end of table.

Table 29 (page 2 of 2). Age-adjusted death rates, according to detailed race, Hispanic origin, geographic division, and State: United States, average annual 1984–86, 1989–91, and 1995–97

[Data are based on the National Vital Statistics System]

Geographic division and State	All persons			White	Black	American Indian or Alaska Native	Asian or Pacific Islander	Hispanic	White, non-Hispanic
	1984–86	1989–91	1995–97	1995–97	1995–97	1995–97	1995–97	1995–97	1995–97
	Deaths per 100,000 resident population[1]								
Pacific	516.6	491.9	446.7	448.2	681.8	*	307.0	335.4	459.1
Washington	496.9	463.7	436.8	435.1	618.6	565.1	290.7	289.8	435.6
Oregon	510.9	479.9	461.6	460.1	668.6	*	306.1	280.3	461.5
California	523.4	500.7	449.0	451.0	691.5	*	285.7	337.4	467.3
Alaska	561.8	525.6	475.6	440.1	468.7	727.8	335.4	282.9	442.0
Hawaii	418.6	405.5	385.1	368.4	307.1	*	396.2	336.5	374.4

* Data for States with population under 10,000 in the middle year of a 3-year period or fewer than 50 deaths for the 3-year period are considered unreliable and are not shown. Data for American Indians or Alaska Natives in States with more than 10 percent misclassification of American Indian or Alaska Native deaths on death certificates or without information on misclassification are also not shown. (Support Services International, Inc. Methodology for adjusting IHS mortality data for miscoding race-ethnicity of American Indians and Alaska Natives on State death certificates. Report submitted to Indian Health Service. 1996.) Division death rates for American Indians or Alaska Natives are not shown when any State within the division does not meet reliability criteria.

- - - Data not available.

[1] Average annual death rate. Denominators are population estimates for the middle year of each 3-year period, multiplied by 3.

NOTES: The race groups, white, black, American Indian or Alaska Native, and Asian or Pacific Islander, include persons of Hispanic and non-Hispanic origin. Conversely, persons of Hispanic origin may be of any race. Consistency of race identification between the death certificate (source of data for numerator of death rates) and data from the Census Bureau (denominator) is high for individual white and black persons; however, persons identified as American Indian, Asian, or Hispanic origin in data from the Census Bureau are sometimes misreported as white or non-Hispanic on the death certificate, causing death rates to be underestimated by 22–30 percent for American Indians, about 12 percent for Asians, and about 7 percent for persons of Hispanic origin. (Sorlie PD, Rogot E, and Johnson NJ: Validity of demographic characteristics on the death certificate, *Epidemiology* 3(2):181–184, 1992.) See Appendix II for age-adjustment procedure. Data for additional years are available (see Appendix III).

SOURCES: Centers for Disease Control and Prevention, National Center for Health Statistics. Rates computed by the Division of Health and Utilization Analysis from mortality data compiled by the Division of Vital Statistics and from State population estimates prepared by the U.S. Bureau of the Census: 1985 estimate from 0792I intercensal series; 1990 from April 1, 1990 MARS Census File; 1993–94 from vintage 1994 postcensal series; 1995 from vintage 1996 postcensal series; 1996 from vintage 1997 postcensal series.

Table 30 (page 1 of 4). Age-adjusted death rates for selected causes of death, according to sex, detailed race, and Hispanic origin: United States, selected years 1950–97

[Data are based on the National Vital Statistics System]

Sex, race, Hispanic origin, and cause of death	1950[1]	1960[1]	1970	1980	1985	1990	1994	1995	1996	1997
All persons	Deaths per 100,000 resident population									
All causes	841.5	760.9	714.3	585.8	548.9	520.2	507.4	503.9	491.6	479.1
Natural causes	766.6	695.2	636.9	519.7	493.0	465.1	454.4	451.7	440.6	429.2
Diseases of heart	307.2	286.2	253.6	202.0	181.4	152.0	140.4	138.3	134.5	130.5
Ischemic heart disease	---	---	---	149.8	126.1	102.6	91.4	89.5	86.7	82.9
Cerebrovascular diseases	88.8	79.7	66.3	40.8	32.5	27.7	26.5	26.7	26.4	25.9
Malignant neoplasms	125.4	125.8	129.8	132.8	134.4	135.0	131.5	129.9	127.9	125.6
Respiratory system	12.8	19.2	28.4	36.4	39.1	41.4	40.1	39.7	39.3	38.7
Colorectal	---	17.7	16.8	15.5	14.9	13.6	12.8	12.7	12.2	12.0
Prostate[2]	13.4	13.1	13.3	14.4	14.7	16.7	16.0	15.4	14.9	13.9
Breast[3]	22.2	22.3	23.1	22.7	23.3	23.1	21.3	21.0	20.2	19.4
Chronic obstructive pulmonary diseases	4.4	8.2	13.2	15.9	18.8	19.7	21.0	20.8	21.0	21.1
Pneumonia and influenza	26.2	28.0	22.1	12.9	13.5	14.0	13.0	12.9	12.8	12.9
Chronic liver disease and cirrhosis	8.5	10.5	14.7	12.2	9.7	8.6	7.9	7.6	7.5	7.4
Diabetes mellitus	14.3	13.6	14.1	10.1	9.7	11.7	12.9	13.3	13.6	13.5
Human immunodeficiency virus infection	---	---	---	---	---	9.8	15.4	15.6	11.1	5.8
External causes	73.9	65.7	77.4	66.1	55.9	55.1	53.0	52.2	50.9	49.9
Unintentional injuries	57.5	49.9	53.7	42.3	34.8	32.5	30.3	30.5	30.4	30.1
Motor vehicle-related injuries	23.3	22.5	27.4	22.9	18.8	18.5	16.1	16.3	16.2	15.9
Suicide	11.0	10.6	11.8	11.4	11.5	11.5	11.2	11.2	10.8	10.6
Homicide and legal intervention	5.4	5.2	9.1	10.8	8.3	10.2	10.3	9.4	8.5	8.0
Male										
All causes	1,001.6	949.3	931.6	777.2	723.0	680.2	654.6	646.3	623.7	602.8
Natural causes	---	---	---	675.5	637.9	595.8	573.6	567.0	547.2	528.0
Diseases of heart	383.8	375.5	348.5	280.4	250.1	206.7	188.5	184.9	178.8	173.1
Ischemic heart disease	---	---	---	214.8	179.6	144.0	127.0	123.9	119.3	114.2
Cerebrovascular diseases	91.9	85.4	73.2	44.9	35.5	30.2	29.0	28.9	28.5	27.9
Malignant neoplasms	130.8	143.0	157.4	165.5	166.1	166.3	159.6	156.8	153.8	150.4
Respiratory system	21.3	34.8	50.6	59.7	60.7	61.0	56.5	55.3	54.2	52.8
Colorectal	---	18.6	18.7	18.3	17.9	16.8	15.6	15.3	14.8	14.6
Prostate	13.4	13.1	13.3	14.4	14.7	16.7	16.0	15.4	14.9	13.9
Chronic obstructive pulmonary diseases	6.0	13.7	23.4	26.1	28.1	27.2	26.9	26.3	25.9	26.1
Pneumonia and influenza	30.6	35.0	28.8	17.4	18.4	18.5	16.7	16.5	16.2	16.2
Chronic liver disease and cirrhosis	11.4	14.5	20.2	17.1	13.7	12.2	11.3	11.0	10.7	10.5
Diabetes mellitus	11.4	12.0	13.5	10.2	10.0	12.3	13.9	14.4	14.9	14.8
Human immunodeficiency virus infection	---	---	---	---	---	17.7	26.4	26.2	18.1	9.1
External causes	---	---	---	101.7	85.2	84.4	81.0	79.3	76.5	74.8
Unintentional injuries	83.7	73.9	80.7	64.0	51.8	47.7	44.0	44.1	43.3	42.9
Motor vehicle-related injuries	36.4	34.5	41.1	34.3	27.3	26.3	22.5	22.7	22.3	21.7
Suicide	17.3	16.6	17.3	18.0	18.8	19.0	18.7	18.6	18.0	17.4
Homicide and legal intervention	8.4	7.9	14.9	17.4	12.8	16.3	16.4	14.7	13.3	12.5
Female										
All causes	688.4	590.6	532.5	432.6	410.3	390.6	385.2	385.2	381.0	375.7
Natural causes	---	---	---	400.1	382.2	363.5	359.2	359.1	354.8	349.8
Diseases of heart	233.9	205.7	175.2	140.3	127.4	108.9	101.6	100.4	98.2	95.4
Ischemic heart disease	---	---	---	98.8	84.2	70.2	63.1	61.9	60.4	57.6
Cerebrovascular diseases	86.0	74.7	60.8	37.6	30.0	25.7	24.5	24.8	24.6	24.2
Malignant neoplasms	120.8	111.2	108.8	109.2	111.7	112.7	111.1	110.4	108.8	107.3
Respiratory system	4.6	5.2	10.1	18.3	22.5	26.2	27.3	27.5	27.5	27.5
Colorectal	---	16.9	16.9	13.4	12.6	11.3	10.6	10.6	10.2	10.0
Breast	22.2	22.3	23.1	22.7	23.3	23.1	21.3	21.0	20.2	19.4
Chronic obstructive pulmonary diseases	2.9	3.5	5.4	8.9	12.5	14.7	17.1	17.1	17.6	17.7
Pneumonia and influenza	22.0	21.8	16.7	9.8	10.1	11.0	10.4	10.4	10.4	10.5
Chronic liver disease and cirrhosis	5.8	6.9	9.8	7.9	6.1	5.3	4.8	4.6	4.5	4.5
Diabetes mellitus	17.1	15.0	14.4	10.0	9.4	11.1	12.1	12.4	12.5	12.4
Human immunodeficiency virus infection	---	---	---	---	---	2.1	4.8	5.2	4.2	2.6
External causes	---	---	---	32.5	28.1	27.0	26.1	26.1	26.2	25.9
Unintentional injuries	31.7	26.8	28.2	21.8	18.7	17.9	17.2	17.5	17.9	17.8
Motor vehicle-related injuries	10.7	11.0	14.4	11.8	10.5	10.7	9.9	10.0	10.2	10.2
Suicide	4.9	5.0	6.8	5.4	4.9	4.5	4.2	4.1	4.0	4.1
Homicide and legal intervention	2.5	2.6	3.7	4.5	3.9	4.2	4.0	4.0	3.6	3.3

See footnotes at end of table.

Table 30 (page 2 of 4). Age-adjusted death rates for selected causes of death, according to sex, detailed race, and Hispanic origin: United States, selected years 1950–97

[Data are based on the National Vital Statistics System]

Sex, race, Hispanic origin, and cause of death	1950[1]	1960[1]	1970	1980	1985	1990	1994	1995	1996	1997
White				Deaths per 100,000 resident population						
All causes	800.4	727.0	679.6	559.4	524.9	492.8	479.8	476.9	466.8	456.5
Natural causes	---	---	---	497.7	471.9	442.0	431.4	428.5	419.2	409.7
Diseases of heart	300.5	281.5	249.1	197.6	176.6	146.9	135.4	133.1	129.8	125.9
Ischemic heart disease	---	---	---	150.6	126.6	102.5	91.1	89.0	86.4	82.5
Cerebrovascular diseases	83.2	74.2	61.8	38.0	30.1	25.5	24.5	24.7	24.5	24.0
Malignant neoplasms	124.7	124.2	127.8	129.6	131.2	131.5	128.6	127.0	125.2	122.9
Respiratory system	13.0	19.1	28.0	35.6	38.4	40.6	39.7	39.3	38.9	38.4
Colorectal	---	17.9	16.9	15.4	14.7	13.3	12.5	12.3	11.8	11.6
Prostate[2]	13.1	12.4	12.3	13.2	13.4	15.3	14.6	14.0	13.5	12.6
Breast[3]	22.5	22.4	23.4	22.8	23.4	22.9	20.9	20.5	19.8	18.9
Chronic obstructive pulmonary diseases	4.3	8.2	13.4	16.3	19.2	20.1	21.6	21.3	21.5	21.7
Pneumonia and influenza	22.9	24.6	19.8	12.2	12.9	13.4	12.5	12.4	12.2	12.4
Chronic liver disease and cirrhosis	8.6	10.3	13.4	11.0	8.9	8.0	7.5	7.4	7.3	7.3
Diabetes mellitus	13.9	12.8	12.9	9.1	8.6	10.4	11.5	11.7	12.0	11.9
Human immunodeficiency virus infection	---	---	---	---	---	8.0	11.2	11.1	7.2	3.3
External causes	---	---	---	61.9	53.0	50.8	48.5	48.4	47.5	46.8
Unintentional injuries	55.7	47.6	51.0	41.5	34.2	31.8	29.5	29.9	29.9	29.6
Motor vehicle-related injuries	23.1	22.3	26.9	23.4	19.1	18.6	16.2	16.4	16.3	15.9
Suicide	11.6	11.1	12.4	12.1	12.3	12.2	11.9	11.9	11.6	11.3
Homicide and legal intervention	2.6	2.7	4.7	6.9	5.4	5.9	5.8	5.5	4.9	4.7
Black										
All causes	1,236.7	1,073.3	1,044.0	842.5	793.6	789.2	772.1	765.7	738.3	705.3
Natural causes	---	---	---	740.2	713.5	701.3	686.5	685.8	662.3	632.7
Diseases of heart	379.6	334.5	307.6	255.7	240.6	213.5	198.8	198.8	191.5	185.7
Ischemic heart disease	---	---	---	150.5	130.9	113.2	103.8	103.4	99.4	96.3
Cerebrovascular diseases	150.9	140.3	114.5	68.5	55.8	48.4	45.4	45.0	44.2	42.5
Malignant neoplasms	129.1	142.3	156.7	172.1	176.6	182.0	173.8	171.6	167.8	165.2
Respiratory system	10.4	20.3	33.5	46.5	50.3	54.0	50.6	49.9	48.9	47.9
Colorectal	---	15.2	16.6	16.9	17.9	17.9	17.2	17.3	16.8	16.8
Prostate[2]	16.9	22.2	25.4	29.1	31.2	35.3	35.3	34.0	33.8	31.4
Breast[3]	19.3	21.3	21.5	23.3	25.5	27.5	26.9	27.5	26.5	26.7
Chronic obstructive pulmonary diseases	---	---	---	12.5	15.3	16.9	17.7	17.6	17.8	17.4
Pneumonia and influenza	57.0	56.4	40.4	19.2	18.8	19.8	17.5	17.8	17.8	17.2
Chronic liver disease and cirrhosis	7.2	11.7	24.8	21.6	16.3	13.7	10.7	9.9	9.2	8.7
Diabetes mellitus	17.2	22.0	26.5	20.3	20.1	24.8	27.4	28.5	28.8	28.9
Human immunodeficiency virus infection	---	---	---	---	---	25.7	49.4	51.8	41.4	24.9
External causes	---	---	---	101.2	80.1	87.8	85.6	79.8	76.0	72.6
Unintentional injuries	70.9	66.4	74.4	51.2	42.3	39.7	38.1	37.4	36.7	36.1
Motor vehicle-related injuries	24.7	23.4	30.6	19.7	17.4	18.4	16.6	16.6	16.7	16.8
Suicide	4.2	4.7	6.1	6.4	6.4	7.0	7.1	6.9	6.6	6.3
Homicide and legal intervention	30.5	27.4	46.1	40.6	29.2	39.5	38.2	33.4	30.6	28.1
American Indian or Alaska Native										
All causes	---	---	---	564.1	468.2	445.1	460.7	468.5	456.7	465.3
Natural causes	---	---	---	436.5	375.1	360.3	374.9	385.4	374.5	381.1
Diseases of heart	---	---	---	131.2	119.6	107.1	104.9	104.5	100.8	102.6
Ischemic heart disease	---	---	---	87.4	77.3	66.6	65.8	65.4	63.8	64.2
Cerebrovascular diseases	---	---	---	26.6	22.5	19.3	20.2	21.6	21.1	19.9
Malignant neoplasms	---	---	---	70.6	72.0	75.0	78.1	80.8	84.9	86.6
Respiratory system	---	---	---	15.0	18.8	20.5	23.7	23.7	24.4	25.3
Colorectal	---	---	---	5.6	6.3	6.4	7.5	7.6	8.5	9.1
Prostate[2]	---	---	---	9.6	8.9	7.7	9.2	8.8	9.8	8.6
Breast[3]	---	---	---	8.1	8.0	10.0	10.4	10.4	12.7	9.4
Chronic obstructive pulmonary diseases	---	---	---	7.5	9.8	12.8	13.3	13.8	12.6	15.3
Pneumonia and influenza	---	---	---	19.4	14.9	15.2	14.8	14.2	14.0	13.4
Chronic liver disease and cirrhosis	---	---	---	38.6	23.6	19.8	21.4	24.3	20.7	20.6
Diabetes mellitus	---	---	---	20.0	18.7	20.8	25.9	27.3	27.8	30.4
Human immunodeficiency virus infection	---	---	---	---	---	1.8	5.4	7.0	4.2	2.4
External causes	---	---	---	127.6	93.1	84.8	85.8	83.0	82.1	84.3
Unintentional injuries	---	---	---	95.1	66.2	59.0	58.3	56.7	57.6	58.5
Motor vehicle-related injuries	---	---	---	54.4	36.3	33.2	31.4	33.1	34.0	32.3
Suicide	---	---	---	12.8	12.1	12.4	14.0	12.2	13.0	12.9
Homicide and legal intervention	---	---	---	16.0	12.2	11.1	11.9	11.9	10.1	11.0

See footnotes at end of table.

Table 30 (page 3 of 4). Age-adjusted death rates for selected causes of death, according to sex, detailed race, and Hispanic origin: United States, selected years 1950–97

[Data are based on the National Vital Statistics System]

Sex, race, Hispanic origin, and cause of death	1950[1]	1960[1]	1970	1980	1985	1990	1994	1995	1996	1997
Asian or Pacific Islander				Deaths per 100,000 resident population						
All causes	---	---	---	315.6	305.7	297.6	299.2	298.9	277.4	274.8
Natural causes	---	---	---	280.7	274.4	266.7	269.5	269.2	250.3	247.0
Diseases of heart	---	---	---	93.9	88.6	78.5	79.7	78.9	71.7	69.8
Ischemic heart disease	---	---	---	67.5	58.8	49.7	50.5	49.3	44.8	43.5
Cerebrovascular diseases	---	---	---	29.0	25.5	25.0	25.4	25.8	23.9	24.4
Malignant neoplasms	---	---	---	77.2	80.2	79.8	81.8	81.1	76.3	75.4
Respiratory system	---	---	---	18.1	17.2	18.3	18.5	18.5	17.4	17.4
Colorectal	---	---	---	9.3	9.6	8.3	8.4	8.2	7.7	7.6
Prostate[2]	---	---	---	4.0	5.9	6.9	6.4	7.4	5.8	5.3
Breast[3]	---	---	---	9.2	9.6	10.0	10.5	11.0	8.9	9.2
Chronic obstructive pulmonary diseases	---	---	---	5.9	8.4	8.7	8.5	9.0	8.6	8.6
Pneumonia and influenza	---	---	---	9.1	9.1	10.4	10.5	10.8	9.9	10.1
Chronic liver disease and cirrhosis	---	---	---	4.5	4.2	3.7	3.2	2.7	2.6	2.4
Diabetes mellitus	---	---	---	6.9	6.1	7.4	8.0	9.2	8.8	9.3
Human immunodeficiency virus infection	---	---	---	---	---	2.1	3.5	3.1	2.2	0.9
External causes	---	---	---	34.9	31.4	30.9	29.7	29.7	27.1	27.7
Unintentional injuries	---	---	---	21.7	20.1	19.3	17.2	17.1	16.1	16.7
Motor vehicle-related injuries	---	---	---	12.6	12.0	12.5	10.3	10.8	9.5	9.7
Suicide	---	---	---	6.7	6.4	6.0	6.6	6.6	6.0	6.2
Homicide and legal intervention	---	---	---	5.6	4.2	5.2	5.4	5.4	4.6	4.3
Hispanic[4]										
All causes	---	---	---	---	397.4	400.2	383.8	386.8	365.9	350.3
Natural causes	---	---	---	---	342.7	342.4	330.3	334.0	316.9	304.5
Diseases of heart	---	---	---	---	116.0	102.8	91.9	92.1	88.6	86.8
Ischemic heart disease	---	---	---	---	77.8	68.0	59.9	60.1	58.2	56.8
Cerebrovascular diseases	---	---	---	---	23.8	21.0	19.5	20.3	19.5	19.4
Malignant neoplasms	---	---	---	---	75.8	82.4	79.5	79.7	77.8	76.4
Respiratory system	---	---	---	---	14.3	16.9	15.5	15.6	15.4	15.2
Colorectal	---	---	---	---	7.5	8.2	7.9	7.6	7.3	7.5
Prostate[2]	---	---	---	---	8.5	9.5	11.0	10.9	9.9	8.6
Breast[3]	---	---	---	---	11.8	14.1	12.6	12.7	12.8	12.6
Chronic obstructive pulmonary diseases	---	---	---	---	8.2	8.7	9.0	9.4	8.9	8.7
Pneumonia and influenza	---	---	---	---	12.0	11.5	9.8	9.9	9.7	10.0
Chronic liver disease and cirrhosis	---	---	---	---	16.3	14.2	13.7	12.9	12.6	12.0
Diabetes mellitus	---	---	---	---	12.8	15.7	18.0	19.3	18.8	18.7
Human immunodeficiency virus infection	---	---	---	---	---	15.5	23.6	23.9	16.3	8.2
External causes	---	---	---	---	54.7	57.8	53.6	52.9	49.0	45.8
Unintentional injuries	---	---	---	---	31.8	32.2	29.2	29.8	29.0	27.7
Motor vehicle-related injuries	---	---	---	---	16.9	19.3	16.6	16.6	16.1	15.2
Suicide	---	---	---	---	6.1	7.3	7.2	7.2	6.7	6.1
Homicide and legal intervention	---	---	---	---	15.7	17.7	16.1	15.0	12.4	11.1

See footnotes at end of table.

Table 30 (page 4 of 4). Age-adjusted death rates for selected causes of death, according to sex, detailed race, and Hispanic origin: United States, selected years 1950–97

[Data are based on the National Vital Statistics System]

Sex, race, Hispanic origin, and cause of death	1950[1]	1960[1]	1970	1980	1985	1990	1994	1995	1996	1997
White, non-Hispanic[4]					Deaths per 100,000 resident population					
All causes	---	---	---	---	510.7	493.1	478.1	475.2	466.7	458.5
Natural causes	---	---	---	---	460.7	444.2	431.7	428.8	420.7	412.6
Diseases of heart	---	---	---	---	173.0	148.2	136.4	134.1	131.0	127.5
Ischemic heart disease	---	---	---	---	125.4	103.7	91.9	89.8	87.4	83.6
Cerebrovascular diseases	---	---	---	---	29.2	25.7	24.4	24.6	24.4	24.0
Malignant neoplasms	---	---	---	---	128.3	134.2	130.7	129.2	127.6	125.3
Respiratory system	---	---	---	---	38.0	41.9	40.9	40.5	40.2	39.8
Colorectal	---	---	---	---	14.4	13.6	12.7	12.5	12.1	11.8
Prostate[2]	---	---	---	---	13.0	15.6	14.7	14.1	13.6	12.7
Breast[3]	---	---	---	---	23.3	23.5	21.3	20.9	20.1	19.2
Chronic obstructive pulmonary diseases	---	---	---	---	19.7	20.7	22.1	21.8	22.1	22.4
Pneumonia and influenza	---	---	---	---	13.2	13.3	12.4	12.3	12.2	12.4
Chronic liver disease and cirrhosis	---	---	---	---	8.5	7.5	6.9	6.8	6.7	6.7
Diabetes mellitus	---	---	---	---	8.0	10.1	11.0	11.2	11.5	11.3
Human immunodeficiency virus infection	---	---	---	---	---	7.0	9.6	9.4	6.0	2.6
External causes	---	---	---	---	50.0	48.9	46.4	46.4	46.0	45.9
Unintentional injuries	---	---	---	---	31.9	31.3	28.9	29.3	29.3	29.4
Motor vehicle-related injuries	---	---	---	---	17.8	18.4	15.8	16.0	16.0	15.8
Suicide	---	---	---	---	12.7	12.7	12.2	12.2	12.0	11.8
Homicide and legal intervention	---	---	---	---	4.5	4.2	4.1	3.8	3.5	3.5

- - - Data not available.

[1] Includes deaths of persons who were not residents of the 50 States and the District of Columbia.
[2] Male only.
[3] Female only.
[4] Excludes data from States lacking an Hispanic-origin item on their death certificates. See Appendix I, National Vital Statistics System.

NOTES: For data years shown, code numbers for cause of death are based on the current revision of *International Classification of Diseases*. See Appendix II, tables IV, V. Categories for coding human immunodeficiency virus infection deaths were introduced in the United States in 1987. Consistency of race identification between the death certificate (source of data for numerator of death rates) and data from the Census Bureau (denominator) is high for individual white and black persons; however, persons identified as American Indian, Asian, or Hispanic origin in data from the Census Bureau are sometimes misreported as white or non-Hispanic on the death certificate, causing death rates to be underestimated by 22–30 percent for American Indians, about 12 percent for Asians, and about 7 percent for persons of Hispanic origin. (Sorlie PD, Rogot E, and Johnson NJ: Validity of demographic characteristics on the death certificate, *Epidemiology* 3(2):181–184, 1992.) See Appendix II for age-adjustment procedure. Data for additional years are available (see Appendix III).

SOURCES: Centers for Disease Control and Prevention, National Center for Health Statistics: Grove, RD, Hetzel, AM. *Vital statistics rates in the United States, 1940–1960*. Washington: U.S. Government Printing Office. 1968; *Vital statistics of the United States, vol II, mortality, part A*, for data years 1960–93. Public Health Service. Washington. U.S. Government Printing Office; for 1994–97, unpublished data; data computed by Division of Health and Utilization Analysis from numerator data compiled by Division of Vital Statistics and denominator data from table 1 and unpublished Hispanic population estimates prepared by the Housing and Household Economic Statistics Division, U.S. Bureau of the Census.

Table 31 (page 1 of 5). Years of potential life lost before age 75 for selected causes of death, according to sex, detailed race, and Hispanic origin: United States, selected years 1980–97

[Data are based on the National Vital Statistics System]

Sex, race, Hispanic origin, and cause of death	Crude			Age adjusted[1]				
	1980	1990	1997	1980	1990	1995	1996	1997
All persons	Years lost before age 75 per 100,000 population under 75 years of age							
All causes	10,267.6	8,997.0	7,873.3	9,813.5	8,518.3	8,128.2	7,748.0	7,398.4
Diseases of heart	2,065.3	1,517.6	1,368.9	1,877.5	1,363.0	1,259.2	1,222.6	1,190.2
Ischemic heart disease	1,454.3	942.1	786.4	1,307.4	834.8	727.9	704.9	670.2
Cerebrovascular diseases	332.9	246.2	238.5	302.9	221.1	211.5	210.2	207.1
Malignant neoplasms	1,932.4	1,863.4	1,734.6	1,815.2	1,713.9	1,587.7	1,554.2	1,523.5
Respiratory system	521.1	538.0	479.9	479.5	486.3	432.7	424.1	410.6
Colorectal	175.8	153.4	143.0	158.5	137.3	128.3	123.5	123.3
Prostate[2]	78.8	89.5	69.7	67.2	76.6	66.6	64.6	59.7
Breast[3]	408.5	416.5	368.1	393.0	381.9	340.0	324.3	314.3
Chronic obstructive pulmonary diseases	164.5	182.5	187.0	141.4	156.9	161.4	161.1	158.9
Pneumonia and influenza	156.4	139.9	123.8	149.1	128.5	115.3	114.5	112.6
Chronic liver disease and cirrhosis	254.1	178.4	161.7	259.1	168.8	149.7	145.7	141.7
Diabetes mellitus	124.6	147.0	172.0	115.1	133.0	149.9	153.5	149.9
Human immunodeficiency virus infection	- - -	391.2	225.3	- - -	366.2	570.3	401.9	208.7
Unintentional injuries	1,688.7	1,221.2	1,060.7	1,688.3	1,263.0	1,155.5	1,136.5	1,115.2
Motor vehicle-related injuries	1,017.6	752.4	608.6	1,010.8	788.8	687.9	680.8	661.1
Suicide	401.6	404.8	371.5	402.8	405.9	405.6	387.8	378.0
Homicide and legal intervention	459.5	452.3	335.7	460.9	466.4	436.4	394.7	368.9
White male								
All causes	12,454.3	10,629.4	9,116.7	11,877.4	10,064.6	9,546.4	8,980.1	8,533.2
Diseases of heart	2,907.1	2,058.7	1,826.4	2,681.9	1,856.8	1,678.9	1,623.5	1,576.7
Ischemic heart disease	2,241.0	1,416.9	1,162.9	2,060.2	1,269.3	1,085.7	1,044.7	990.1
Cerebrovascular diseases	309.0	222.9	219.8	280.2	198.6	195.7	194.4	189.8
Malignant neoplasms	2,087.1	1,970.9	1,806.5	1,939.8	1,793.9	1,653.5	1,620.7	1,576.4
Respiratory system	744.8	700.1	591.9	680.6	627.7	537.8	525.5	503.6
Colorectal	194.2	174.7	160.3	176.2	155.7	144.8	138.8	137.5
Prostate	72.6	85.0	64.0	59.1	68.3	58.1	56.3	51.5
Chronic obstructive pulmonary diseases	219.3	208.9	201.4	187.1	177.2	169.4	167.5	169.3
Pneumonia and influenza	156.0	143.3	129.5	147.4	130.5	117.9	115.1	116.1
Chronic liver disease and cirrhosis	306.4	233.5	231.8	307.9	219.1	208.8	205.1	200.8
Diabetes mellitus	114.7	141.0	166.5	107.4	127.5	145.7	153.0	143.4
Human immunodeficiency virus infection	- - -	589.3	220.1	- - -	544.3	707.8	448.0	200.7
Unintentional injuries	2,553.8	1,766.9	1,486.9	2,523.6	1,821.5	1,638.4	1,591.5	1,561.2
Motor vehicle-related injuries	1,579.9	1,085.4	824.6	1,549.8	1,134.9	957.0	933.1	897.1
Suicide	663.0	694.0	636.6	656.4	692.2	703.8	665.7	644.7
Homicide and legal intervention	455.2	384.7	290.5	452.6	391.6	372.5	327.7	314.5
Black male								
All causes	21,081.4	20,744.8	16,621.0	22,338.5	21,250.2	20,272.8	18,994.6	17,373.4
Diseases of heart	3,383.9	2,769.2	2,576.9	4,179.5	3,338.2	3,151.1	2,969.9	2,918.1
Ischemic heart disease	1,805.9	1,249.8	1,128.4	2,283.2	1,561.4	1,411.1	1,326.2	1,308.8
Cerebrovascular diseases	714.1	546.4	515.8	870.2	655.6	601.0	583.0	578.8
Malignant neoplasms	2,495.1	2,444.5	2,178.4	3,070.6	3,021.7	2,654.4	2,576.8	2,517.0
Respiratory system	911.8	899.8	727.8	1,160.8	1,150.8	941.0	918.1	865.6
Colorectal	176.1	188.6	196.9	215.9	234.0	223.7	225.6	229.1
Prostate	136.9	143.7	127.4	159.1	177.6	166.5	160.2	154.6
Chronic obstructive pulmonary diseases	223.3	241.4	226.4	258.7	278.7	275.3	266.7	250.8
Pneumonia and influenza	467.1	399.2	276.2	492.6	416.8	321.2	328.4	291.7
Chronic liver disease and cirrhosis	610.1	390.5	239.5	791.8	461.4	320.5	293.5	265.3
Diabetes mellitus	199.8	263.0	336.0	245.5	317.8	373.8	357.4	380.2
Human immunodeficiency virus infection	- - -	1,622.4	1,300.2	- - -	1,625.8	2,928.0	2,270.3	1,288.0
Unintentional injuries	2,934.4	2,308.7	1,929.9	2,931.3	2,265.6	2,042.6	1,983.7	1,925.4
Motor vehicle-related injuries	1,289.2	1,163.1	982.7	1,281.2	1,143.1	1,007.9	997.1	987.6
Suicide	415.7	482.3	436.8	428.1	478.0	489.3	465.6	443.1
Homicide and legal intervention	2,872.4	3,197.7	2,216.1	2,939.9	3,096.6	2,663.5	2,448.4	2,251.2

See footnotes at end of table.

Table 31 (page 2 of 5). Years of potential life lost before age 75 for selected causes of death, according to sex, detailed race, and Hispanic origin: United States, selected years 1980–97

[Data are based on the National Vital Statistics System]

Sex, race, Hispanic origin, and cause of death	Crude			Age adjusted[1]				
	1980	1990	1997	1980	1990	1995	1996	1997
American Indian or Alaska Native male[4]	Years lost before age 75 per 100,000 population under 75 years of age							
All causes	16,368.1	11,879.5	11,278.4	16,915.2	12,125.2	12,349.1	11,607.8	11,907.9
Diseases of heart	1,667.6	1,287.0	1,328.9	2,299.7	1,660.5	1,592.9	1,564.5	1,616.5
Ischemic heart disease	1,024.5	712.6	809.3	1,511.6	985.1	1,016.3	965.7	1,007.5
Cerebrovascular diseases	190.2	160.3	165.2	256.4	194.1	270.1	234.2	196.2
Malignant neoplasms	661.4	725.2	1,042.4	912.9	948.4	1,053.0	1,030.9	1,261.7
Respiratory system	174.5	206.2	280.6	256.6	293.1	325.1	358.1	366.9
Colorectal	44.9	53.1	113.0	64.6	68.9	97.4	103.6	135.5
Prostate	34.2	22.5	25.5	53.1	33.5	43.0	58.3	36.4
Chronic obstructive pulmonary diseases	78.2	100.3	166.8	106.2	128.2	134.3	99.1	200.1
Pneumonia and influenza	343.1	230.2	239.1	370.1	227.5	240.0	274.9	249.0
Chronic liver disease and cirrhosis	943.9	445.9	539.3	1,259.9	530.2	735.9	555.6	586.7
Diabetes mellitus	183.1	191.6	284.8	255.3	256.1	324.7	360.0	358.1
Human immunodeficiency virus infection	- - -	130.2	145.1	- - -	130.3	429.3	264.8	139.7
Unintentional injuries	5,731.6	3,600.0	3,125.9	5,509.9	3,508.2	3,289.7	3,130.9	3,107.1
Motor vehicle-related injuries	3,329.6	2,095.9	1,802.3	3,146.2	2,047.2	1,936.6	1,925.0	1,786.1
Suicide	984.6	968.2	917.1	921.0	945.1	880.4	867.0	913.0
Homicide and legal intervention	1,029.4	778.2	743.7	1,003.6	754.5	823.3	677.3	731.5
Asian or Pacific Islander male[5]								
All causes	6,131.1	5,414.5	4,853.1	6,342.7	5,638.0	5,310.0	5,101.5	4,944.2
Diseases of heart	1,027.0	740.6	795.9	1,237.1	877.9	852.2	873.7	855.5
Ischemic heart disease	697.6	413.4	441.7	863.6	507.1	487.2	493.2	485.7
Cerebrovascular diseases	201.0	176.2	211.1	238.4	208.1	234.7	219.3	224.9
Malignant neoplasms	969.1	965.7	997.0	1,160.1	1,132.1	1,072.9	1,031.3	1,062.2
Respiratory system	239.3	192.8	213.5	304.7	245.4	231.4	227.6	236.6
Colorectal	84.1	85.6	96.7	104.8	103.7	109.2	89.1	103.0
Prostate	10.3	18.6	14.1	12.9	25.0	20.1	21.9	16.7
Chronic obstructive pulmonary diseases	67.1	61.6	68.1	76.8	77.7	75.1	88.3	75.7
Pneumonia and influenza	94.1	72.2	74.2	93.9	79.4	73.3	75.5	78.9
Chronic liver disease and cirrhosis	94.7	84.8	60.1	112.1	95.7	64.4	61.8	59.9
Diabetes mellitus	63.6	60.2	77.4	76.6	74.1	82.2	98.5	85.9
Human immunodeficiency virus infection	- - -	145.8	60.5	- - -	134.5	202.4	133.0	54.7
Unintentional injuries	1,196.8	986.7	747.9	1,143.8	957.1	797.1	788.6	755.2
Motor vehicle-related injuries	732.6	657.3	418.7	699.8	634.9	505.4	477.7	425.7
Suicide	320.0	336.5	319.5	308.9	320.5	361.0	324.6	324.1
Homicide and legal intervention	317.1	347.5	285.4	304.4	330.7	371.5	323.8	291.9
Hispanic male[6]								
All causes	- - -	10,217.2	7,677.6	- - -	10,469.6	9,989.4	8,861.4	8,054.4
Diseases of heart	- - -	897.3	806.6	- - -	1,301.8	1,155.8	1,124.6	1,079.4
Ischemic heart disease	- - -	483.5	412.6	- - -	759.4	650.8	631.2	596.6
Cerebrovascular diseases	- - -	168.7	178.5	- - -	228.9	232.4	233.5	228.9
Malignant neoplasms	- - -	810.1	796.5	- - -	1,131.3	1,104.4	1,042.3	1,041.3
Respiratory system	- - -	169.2	141.8	- - -	267.8	235.0	224.2	210.5
Colorectal	- - -	64.1	69.4	- - -	98.7	98.5	91.8	98.8
Prostate	- - -	22.0	22.5	- - -	37.8	46.9	44.4	35.9
Chronic obstructive pulmonary diseases	- - -	54.6	55.4	- - -	74.8	79.0	72.2	73.2
Pneumonia and influenza	- - -	139.4	107.9	- - -	152.5	129.1	119.0	118.0
Chronic liver disease and cirrhosis	- - -	340.2	281.1	- - -	454.0	395.8	377.9	350.7
Diabetes mellitus	- - -	107.2	141.6	- - -	160.0	206.8	204.0	200.9
Human immunodeficiency virus infection	- - -	964.3	434.6	- - -	972.6	1,330.6	869.6	434.1
Unintentional injuries	- - -	2,120.1	1,600.7	- - -	1,972.7	1,757.9	1,632.1	1,551.3
Motor vehicle-related injuries	- - -	1,305.0	900.2	- - -	1,202.0	1,002.9	922.9	872.0
Suicide	- - -	450.2	390.1	- - -	434.3	464.3	413.3	383.7
Homicide and legal intervention	- - -	1,466.4	877.3	- - -	1,330.1	1,182.4	949.7	841.0

See footnotes at end of table.

[Data are based on the National Vital Statistics System]

Sex, race, Hispanic origin, and cause of death	Crude			Age adjusted[1]				
	1980	1990	1997	1980	1990	1995	1996	1997
White, non-Hispanic male[6]	Years lost before age 75 per 100,000 population under 75 years of age							
All causes	- - -	10,530.0	9,197.1	- - -	9,803.6	9,226.3	8,744.4	8,407.2
Diseases of heart	- - -	2,175.5	1,962.2	- - -	1,877.0	1,697.9	1,643.2	1,607.4
Ischemic heart disease	- - -	1,515.2	1,265.6	- - -	1,294.4	1,107.3	1,065.8	1,018.1
Cerebrovascular diseases	- - -	228.8	223.2	- - -	195.0	188.5	185.9	183.9
Malignant neoplasms	- - -	2,102.1	1,943.4	- - -	1,835.5	1,679.9	1,651.4	1,610.1
Respiratory system	- - -	760.4	655.8	- - -	649.2	554.8	544.1	524.7
Colorectal	- - -	187.9	172.6	- - -	159.8	147.5	141.5	139.8
Prostate	- - -	92.8	69.8	- - -	70.4	58.6	56.8	52.4
Chronic obstructive pulmonary diseases	- - -	227.2	222.0	- - -	183.2	173.2	172.0	175.8
Pneumonia and influenza	- - -	141.3	130.6	- - -	125.3	113.6	110.9	113.3
Chronic liver disease and cirrhosis	- - -	219.1	219.3	- - -	198.2	187.3	183.8	181.6
Diabetes mellitus	- - -	144.7	168.1	- - -	125.9	140.0	147.5	137.8
Human immunodeficiency virus infection	- - -	531.4	181.6	- - -	485.9	618.2	384.0	164.1
Unintentional injuries	- - -	1,689.9	1,444.2	- - -	1,769.3	1,581.6	1,549.9	1,540.1
Motor vehicle-related injuries	- - -	1,041.9	799.8	- - -	1,111.0	928.0	914.2	889.4
Suicide	- - -	719.4	665.5	- - -	720.9	723.2	692.1	676.5
Homicide and legal intervention	- - -	239.2	191.4	- - -	242.3	219.0	200.3	204.4
White female								
All causes	6,655.6	5,740.0	5,373.7	6,185.7	5,225.3	5,005.0	4,899.9	4,821.5
Diseases of heart	1,142.1	864.1	784.8	915.3	689.3	648.9	637.1	626.2
Ischemic heart disease	758.1	521.1	434.3	584.8	399.6	356.1	352.2	332.0
Cerebrovascular diseases	275.0	200.1	189.8	231.4	165.4	156.8	157.3	153.2
Malignant neoplasms	1,774.6	1,760.8	1,668.5	1,595.5	1,528.7	1,425.7	1,403.1	1,379.3
Respiratory system	305.8	391.8	388.2	267.5	326.9	316.0	312.3	305.4
Colorectal	165.1	133.2	122.1	137.5	109.5	101.2	96.8	97.6
Breast	418.8	420.7	361.3	390.0	373.0	324.1	308.5	298.9
Chronic obstructive pulmonary diseases	117.4	164.6	182.4	94.8	128.9	143.4	142.0	140.1
Pneumonia and influenza	103.6	92.3	90.5	97.0	81.8	78.8	79.8	79.0
Chronic liver disease and cirrhosis	145.2	95.5	92.0	138.7	84.6	75.9	77.1	76.3
Diabetes mellitus	108.0	121.8	136.6	91.4	101.0	110.3	110.9	111.1
Human immunodeficiency virus infection	- - -	43.4	40.2	- - -	41.8	98.1	73.2	38.5
Unintentional injuries	793.0	610.1	576.8	816.8	654.1	629.2	634.9	627.6
Motor vehicle-related injuries	525.0	426.7	379.9	539.1	464.8	429.5	434.7	428.0
Suicide	193.0	166.1	156.5	196.1	165.3	154.0	153.6	155.3
Homicide and legal intervention	132.0	117.2	92.9	136.1	123.5	124.0	111.1	101.2
Black female								
All causes	11,795.1	10,966.0	9,560.3	11,863.1	10,662.7	10,179.7	10,012.6	9,475.2
Diseases of heart	2,020.0	1,665.2	1,535.1	2,189.5	1,756.0	1,627.8	1,636.2	1,534.8
Ischemic heart disease	987.7	711.9	634.2	1,078.5	762.1	680.9	682.3	636.6
Cerebrovascular diseases	600.9	458.3	426.7	656.7	481.2	417.3	422.9	419.4
Malignant neoplasms	1,855.8	1,893.9	1,839.9	2,085.5	2,041.9	1,911.8	1,845.0	1,837.9
Respiratory system	279.5	344.9	341.4	322.0	382.4	347.6	337.5	345.2
Colorectal	162.6	164.4	153.3	179.2	178.3	165.8	160.8	153.2
Breast	382.8	465.4	479.4	448.6	505.6	495.9	484.0	472.7
Chronic obstructive pulmonary diseases	109.0	149.0	172.7	116.3	157.4	172.8	187.4	172.2
Pneumonia and influenza	252.3	214.2	180.5	245.2	206.1	184.0	177.2	177.9
Chronic liver disease and cirrhosis	323.8	193.2	115.8	378.0	203.4	130.0	119.8	113.2
Diabetes mellitus	248.3	279.1	314.6	271.6	299.0	318.0	329.5	318.3
Human immunodeficiency virus infection	- - -	427.1	517.8	- - -	402.5	913.5	757.5	492.1
Unintentional injuries	898.9	767.7	735.7	876.0	748.3	730.1	751.9	734.6
Motor vehicle-related injuries	362.9	381.2	394.5	354.7	376.7	370.2	396.9	400.4
Suicide	88.3	90.0	73.6	91.2	89.0	77.5	74.7	74.5
Homicide and legal intervention	605.3	619.7	417.7	593.1	596.5	505.6	470.5	422.2

See footnotes at end of table.

[Data are based on the National Vital Statistics System]

Sex, race, Hispanic origin, and cause of death	Crude			Age adjusted[1]				
	1980	1990	1997	1980	1990	1995	1996	1997
American Indian or Alaska Native female[4]	Years lost before age 75 per 100,000 population under 75 years of age							
All causes	9,077.4	6,086.8	6,368.4	9,126.7	6,192.2	6,788.9	6,797.2	6,563.6
Diseases of heart	714.8	647.0	684.4	870.8	753.2	781.6	738.7	754.3
Ischemic heart disease	323.4	299.7	323.3	442.1	381.1	408.3	376.3	365.1
Cerebrovascular diseases	158.3	167.1	200.4	204.2	191.7	199.2	194.6	218.5
Malignant neoplasms	775.0	860.2	942.9	980.9	1,012.8	978.0	1,105.9	1,035.1
Respiratory system	67.2	138.6	150.3	94.9	177.3	170.1	178.1	177.4
Colorectal	45.8	56.2	78.2	63.9	68.3	92.3	85.7	87.0
Breast	125.9	150.1	140.9	173.5	178.3	179.5	210.0	154.7
Chronic obstructive pulmonary diseases	*	80.1	106.6	*	94.2	126.1	110.1	119.1
Pneumonia and influenza	216.4	152.9	118.1	210.9	154.4	144.7	141.1	128.1
Chronic liver disease and cirrhosis	681.0	381.8	408.2	842.4	415.9	427.7	428.0	423.1
Diabetes mellitus	190.5	186.6	269.2	260.4	233.0	318.5	317.8	306.4
Human immunodeficiency virus infection	- - -	*	*	- - -	*	96.8	*	*
Unintentional injuries	2,170.7	1,185.9	1,327.1	2,056.6	1,155.4	1,337.2	1,350.9	1,302.8
Motor vehicle-related injuries	1,486.8	778.5	846.9	1,412.6	772.9	955.5	924.6	844.2
Suicide	211.6	153.9	160.1	212.9	152.8	176.3	243.1	164.0
Homicide and legal intervention	342.9	226.8	227.5	345.9	219.8	238.7	211.8	223.4
Asian or Pacific Islander female[5]								
All causes	3,893.8	3,264.7	3,060.5	3,918.3	3,308.2	3,159.5	2,949.8	2,992.2
Diseases of heart	378.1	318.1	326.1	420.4	343.0	358.9	318.8	322.5
Ischemic heart disease	167.1	148.3	145.8	200.5	164.1	157.6	139.0	143.8
Cerebrovascular diseases	192.2	175.3	173.1	215.6	190.0	157.3	158.6	168.0
Malignant neoplasms	870.0	847.0	896.4	949.9	893.7	959.1	886.9	863.2
Respiratory system	98.1	110.7	125.2	113.1	121.6	129.8	106.4	121.0
Colorectal	79.7	69.7	76.3	89.9	75.7	70.0	77.5	72.5
Breast	175.7	173.1	181.7	190.0	182.0	211.1	164.1	170.4
Chronic obstructive pulmonary diseases	22.1	47.4	43.3	23.2	50.4	41.5	52.8	42.2
Pneumonia and influenza	49.6	59.6	47.3	52.3	60.7	46.6	45.8	47.4
Chronic liver disease and cirrhosis	34.0	30.3	20.2	39.6	32.2	25.1	18.8	19.1
Diabetes mellitus	53.1	44.5	60.6	62.6	50.2	64.7	61.4	60.7
Human immunodeficiency virus infection	- - -	*	*	- - -	*	23.3	18.2	*
Unintentional injuries	486.4	419.6	396.9	481.7	424.0	398.0	349.5	412.5
Motor vehicle-related injuries	338.1	325.0	279.4	333.1	328.3	297.2	246.4	293.7
Suicide	159.2	114.7	116.5	151.0	111.3	132.2	116.5	118.6
Homicide and legal intervention	131.0	117.9	93.0	124.8	113.0	113.0	97.4	94.8
Hispanic female[6]								
All causes	- - -	4,753.5	4,137.4	- - -	4,662.3	4,378.8	4,211.1	4,114.5
Diseases of heart	- - -	442.2	391.4	- - -	556.9	485.5	458.9	466.2
Ischemic heart disease	- - -	219.8	190.2	- - -	297.0	249.6	241.9	242.3
Cerebrovascular diseases	- - -	151.9	135.8	- - -	182.8	165.6	155.1	155.8
Malignant neoplasms	- - -	828.7	810.4	- - -	1,014.7	937.1	942.3	936.4
Respiratory system	- - -	66.3	72.6	- - -	88.9	82.1	85.3	90.4
Colorectal	- - -	54.4	52.7	- - -	70.9	67.2	64.8	63.7
Breast	- - -	201.4	189.3	- - -	254.2	217.8	220.2	221.7
Chronic obstructive pulmonary diseases	- - -	50.6	51.1	- - -	61.6	64.2	58.0	58.4
Pneumonia and influenza	- - -	93.0	80.0	- - -	87.7	71.2	74.8	79.3
Chronic liver disease and cirrhosis	- - -	93.1	81.8	- - -	115.7	90.2	95.5	95.2
Diabetes mellitus	- - -	103.4	133.8	- - -	137.0	168.8	164.2	167.9
Human immunodeficiency virus infection	- - -	152.9	114.6	- - -	146.0	309.8	224.2	114.4
Unintentional injuries	- - -	556.5	516.0	- - -	526.1	501.7	520.7	505.9
Motor vehicle-related injuries	- - -	382.4	349.4	- - -	368.1	349.7	355.6	348.6
Suicide	- - -	89.8	64.6	- - -	88.4	75.9	84.8	66.7
Homicide and legal intervention	- - -	227.5	146.6	- - -	214.0	197.1	158.8	142.5

See footnotes at end of table.

[Data are based on the National Vital Statistics System]

Sex, race, Hispanic origin, and cause of death	Crude			Age adjusted[1]				
	1980	1990	1997	1980	1990	1995	1996	1997
White, non-Hispanic female[6]	Years lost before age 75 per 100,000 population under 75 years of age							
All causes	- - -	5,788.3	5,474.7	- - -	5,189.9	4,968.7	4,874.5	4,814.2
Diseases of heart	- - -	902.4	832.5	- - -	691.9	654.2	643.8	636.7
Ischemic heart disease	- - -	549.4	464.6	- - -	402.7	360.4	356.9	337.8
Cerebrovascular diseases	- - -	205.5	195.2	- - -	163.4	153.7	155.6	151.2
Malignant neoplasms	- - -	1,861.9	1,772.5	- - -	1,563.0	1,453.5	1,429.5	1,404.2
Respiratory system	- - -	428.1	429.9	- - -	343.6	333.1	328.9	321.8
Colorectal	- - -	142.6	130.9	- - -	112.6	103.3	98.6	99.9
Breast	- - -	444.4	381.9	- - -	381.3	330.9	313.4	303.0
Chronic obstructive pulmonary diseases	- - -	176.9	199.4	- - -	132.5	147.7	147.0	145.2
Pneumonia and influenza	- - -	90.2	90.6	- - -	78.1	77.7	78.0	76.6
Chronic liver disease and cirrhosis	- - -	95.6	91.9	- - -	82.0	74.0	74.9	73.5
Diabetes mellitus	- - -	123.2	134.6	- - -	98.9	105.1	105.7	105.4
Human immunodeficiency virus infection	- - -	29.1	28.6	- - -	28.2	69.4	51.2	27.6
Unintentional injuries	- - -	607.4	577.8	- - -	661.1	636.4	637.3	639.6
Motor vehicle-related injuries	- - -	425.1	379.2	- - -	470.9	433.2	436.7	436.0
Suicide	- - -	172.6	168.2	- - -	170.9	160.7	159.8	165.8
Homicide and legal intervention	- - -	102.3	83.3	- - -	108.3	105.9	99.5	92.0

- - - Data not available.

* Based on fewer than 20 deaths.

[1]See Appendix II for age-adjustment procedure.

[2]Male only.

[3]Female only.

[4]Interpretation of trends should take into account that population estimates for American Indians increased by 45 percent between 1980 and 1990, partly due to better enumeration techniques in the 1990 decennial census and to the increased tendency for people to identify themselves as American Indian in 1990.

[5]Interpretation of trends should take into account that the Asian population in the United States more than doubled between 1980 and 1990, primarily due to immigration.

[6]Excludes data from States lacking an Hispanic-origin item on their death certificates. See Appendix I, National Vital Statistics System.

NOTES: For data years shown, the code numbers for cause of death are based on the *International Classification of Diseases, Ninth Revision*, described in Appendix II, table V. Categories for coding human immunodeficiency virus infection were introduced in the United States in 1987. Years of potential life lost (YPLL) before age 75 provides a measure of the impact of mortality on the population under 75 years of age. These data are presented as YPLL–75 because the average life expectancy in the United States is over 75 years. YPLL–65 was calculated in *Health, United States, 1995* and earlier editions. See Appendix II, YPLL, for method of calculation. The race groups, white, black, Asian or Pacific Islander, and American Indian or Alaska Native, include persons of Hispanic and non-Hispanic origin. Conversely, persons of Hispanic origin may be of any race. Consistency of race identification between the death certificate (source of data for numerator of death rates) and data from the Census Bureau (denominator) is high for individual white and black persons; however, persons identified as American Indian, Asian, or Hispanic origin in data from the Census Bureau are sometimes misreported as white or non-Hispanic on the death certificate, causing death rates to be underestimated by 22–30 percent for American Indians, about 12 percent for Asians, and about 7 percent for persons of Hispanic origin. (Sorlie PD, Rogot E, and Johnson NJ: Validity of demographic characteristics on the death certificate, *Epidemiology* 3(2):181–184, 1992.) YPLL rates for minority groups may also be underestimated. Data for additional years are available (see Appendix III).

SOURCES: Centers for Disease Control and Prevention, National Center for Health Statistics. *Vital statistics of the United States, vol II, mortality, part A*, for data years 1950–93. Public Health Service. Washington. U.S. Government Printing Office; for 1994–97, unpublished data; data computed by the Division of Health and Utilization Analysis from numerator data compiled by the Division of Vital Statistics and denominator data from unrounded national population estimates for race groups from table 1 and unpublished Hispanic population estimates prepared by the Housing and Household Economic Statistics Division, U.S. Bureau of the Census.

[Data are based on the National Vital Statistics System]

Sex, race, Hispanic origin, and rank order	1980		1997	
	Cause of death	Deaths	Cause of death	Deaths
All persons				
...	All causes	1,989,841	All causes	2,314,245
1............	Diseases of heart	761,085	Diseases of heart	726,974
2............	Malignant neoplasms	416,509	Malignant neoplasms	539,577
3............	Cerebrovascular diseases	170,225	Cerebrovascular diseases	159,791
4............	Unintentional injuries	105,718	Chronic obstructive pulmonary diseases	109,029
5............	Chronic obstructive pulmonary diseases	56,050	Unintentional injuries	95,644
6............	Pneumonia and influenza	54,619	Pneumonia and influenza	86,449
7............	Diabetes mellitus	34,851	Diabetes mellitus	62,636
8............	Chronic liver disease and cirrhosis	30,583	Suicide	30,535
9............	Atherosclerosis	29,449	Nephritis, nephrotic syndrome, and nephrosis	25,331
10............	Suicide	26,869	Chronic liver disease and cirrhosis	25,175
Male				
...	All causes	1,075,078	All causes	1,154,039
1............	Diseases of heart	405,661	Diseases of heart	356,598
2............	Malignant neoplasms	225,948	Malignant neoplasms	281,110
3............	Unintentional injuries	74,180	Cerebrovascular diseases	62,564
4............	Cerebrovascular diseases	69,973	Unintentional injuries	61,963
5............	Chronic obstructive pulmonary diseases	38,625	Chronic obstructive pulmonary diseases	55,984
6............	Pneumonia and influenza	27,574	Pneumonia and influenza	39,284
7............	Suicide	20,505	Diabetes mellitus	28,187
8............	Chronic liver disease and cirrhosis	19,768	Suicide	24,492
9............	Homicide and legal intervention	19,088	Chronic liver disease and cirrhosis	16,260
10............	Diabetes mellitus	14,325	Homicide and legal intervention	15,449
Female				
...	All causes	914,763	All causes	1,160,206
1............	Diseases of heart	355,424	Diseases of heart	370,376
2............	Malignant neoplasms	190,561	Malignant neoplasms	258,467
3............	Cerebrovascular diseases	100,252	Cerebrovascular diseases	97,227
4............	Unintentional injuries	31,538	Chronic obstructive pulmonary diseases	53,045
5............	Pneumonia and influenza	27,045	Pneumonia and influenza	47,165
6............	Diabetes mellitus	20,526	Diabetes mellitus	34,449
7............	Atherosclerosis	17,848	Unintentional injuries	33,681
8............	Chronic obstructive pulmonary diseases	17,425	Alzheimer's disease	15,437
9............	Chronic liver disease and cirrhosis	10,815	Nephritis, nephrotic syndrome, and nephrosis	13,191
10............	Certain conditions originating in the perinatal period	9,815	Septicemia	12,741
White				
...	All causes	1,738,607	All causes	1,996,393
1............	Diseases of heart	683,347	Diseases of heart	639,225
2............	Malignant neoplasms	368,162	Malignant neoplasms	468,521
3............	Cerebrovascular diseases	148,734	Cerebrovascular diseases	138,324
4............	Unintentional injuries	90,122	Chronic obstructive pulmonary diseases	100,770
5............	Chronic obstructive pulmonary diseases	52,375	Unintentional injuries	79,922
6............	Pneumonia and influenza	48,369	Pneumonia and influenza	76,875
7............	Diabetes mellitus	28,868	Diabetes mellitus	49,850
8............	Atherosclerosis	27,069	Suicide	27,513
9............	Chronic liver disease and cirrhosis	25,240	Chronic liver disease and cirrhosis	21,683
10............	Suicide	24,829	Alzheimer's disease	21,192
Black				
...	All causes	233,135	All causes	276,520
1............	Diseases of heart	72,956	Diseases of heart	77,174
2............	Malignant neoplasms	45,037	Malignant neoplasms	61,333
3............	Cerebrovascular diseases	20,135	Cerebrovascular diseases	18,131
4............	Unintentional injuries	13,480	Unintentional injuries	12,665
5............	Homicide and legal intervention	10,283	Diabetes mellitus	11,130
6............	Certain conditions originating in the perinatal period	6,961	Homicide and legal intervention	9,253
7............	Pneumonia and influenza	5,648	Human immunodeficiency virus infection	8,525
8............	Diabetes mellitus	5,544	Pneumonia and influenza	7,920
9............	Chronic liver disease and cirrhosis	4,790	Chronic obstructive pulmonary diseases	6,908
10............	Nephritis, nephrotic syndrome, and nephrosis	3,416	Certain conditions originating in the perinatal period	4,714

See footnotes at end of table.

[Data are based on the National Vital Statistics System]

Sex, race, Hispanic origin, and rank order	1980		1997	
	Cause of death	Deaths	Cause of death	Deaths
American Indian or Alaska Native				
. . .	All causes	6,923	All causes	10,576
1.	Diseases of heart	1,494	Diseases of heart	2,383
2.	Unintentional injuries	1,290	Malignant neoplasms	1,817
3.	Malignant neoplasms	770	Unintentional injuries	1,330
4.	Chronic liver disease and cirrhosis	410	Diabetes mellitus	645
5.	Cerebrovascular diseases	322	Cerebrovascular diseases	497
6.	Pneumonia and influenza	257	Chronic liver disease and cirrhosis	426
7.	Homicide and legal intervention	219	Pneumonia and influenza	354
8.	Diabetes mellitus	210	Chronic obstructive pulmonary diseases	349
9.	Certain conditions originating in the perinatal period	199	Suicide	290
10.	Suicide	181	Homicide and legal intervention	251
Asian or Pacific Islander				
. . .	All causes	11,071	All causes	30,756
1.	Diseases of heart	3,265	Diseases of heart	8,192
2.	Malignant neoplasms	2,522	Malignant neoplasms	7,906
3.	Cerebrovascular diseases	1,028	Cerebrovascular diseases	2,839
4.	Unintentional injuries	810	Unintentional injuries	1,727
5.	Pneumonia and influenza	342	Pneumonia and influenza	1,300
6.	Suicide	249	Diabetes mellitus	1,011
7.	Certain conditions originating in the perinatal period	246	Chronic obstructive pulmonary diseases	1,002
8.	Diabetes mellitus	227	Suicide	629
9.	Homicide and legal intervention	211	Homicide and legal intervention	429
10.	Chronic obstructive pulmonary diseases	207	Congenital anomalies	309
Hispanic				
. . .		- - -	All causes	95,460
1.		- - -	Diseases of heart	23,824
2.		- - -	Malignant neoplasms	18,635
3.		- - -	Unintentional injuries	7,932
4.		- - -	Cerebrovascular diseases	5,306
5.		- - -	Diabetes mellitus	4,538
6.		- - -	Homicide and legal intervention	3,248
7.		- - -	Pneumonia and influenza	3,119
8.		- - -	Chronic liver disease and cirrhosis	2,793
9.		- - -	Chronic obstructive pulmonary diseases	2,477
10.		- - -	Human immunodeficiency virus infection	2,300
White male				
. . .	All causes	933,878	All causes	986,884
1.	Diseases of heart	364,679	Diseases of heart	313,316
2.	Malignant neoplasms	198,188	Malignant neoplasms	243,192
3.	Unintentional injuries	62,963	Cerebrovascular diseases	53,158
4.	Cerebrovascular diseases	60,095	Unintentional injuries	51,396
5.	Chronic obstructive pulmonary diseases	35,977	Chronic obstructive pulmonary diseases	51,184
6.	Pneumonia and influenza	23,810	Pneumonia and influenza	34,386
7.	Suicide	18,901	Diabetes mellitus	22,968
8.	Chronic liver disease and cirrhosis	16,407	Suicide	22,042
9.	Diabetes mellitus	12,125	Chronic liver disease and cirrhosis	14,045
10.	Atherosclerosis	10,543	Nephritis, nephrotic syndrome, and nephrosis	10,002
Black male				
. . .	All causes	130,138	All causes	144,110
1.	Diseases of heart	37,877	Diseases of heart	37,212
2.	Malignant neoplasms	25,861	Malignant neoplasms	32,719
3.	Unintentional injuries	9,701	Unintentional injuries	8,582
4.	Cerebrovascular diseases	9,194	Cerebrovascular diseases	7,794
5.	Homicide and legal intervention	8,385	Homicide and legal intervention	7,601
6.	Certain conditions originating in the perinatal period	3,869	Human immunodeficiency virus infection	6,078
7.	Pneumonia and influenza	3,386	Diabetes mellitus	4,440
8.	Chronic liver disease and cirrhosis	3,020	Pneumonia and influenza	3,978
9.	Chronic obstructive pulmonary diseases	2,429	Chronic obstructive pulmonary diseases	3,966
10.	Diabetes mellitus	2,010	Certain conditions originating in the perinatal period	2,624

See footnotes at end of table.

Table 32 (page 3 of 4). Leading causes of death and numbers of deaths, according to sex, detailed race, and Hispanic origin: United States, 1980 and 1997

[Data are based on the National Vital Statistics System]

Sex, race, Hispanic origin, and rank order	1980 Cause of death	Deaths	1997 Cause of death	Deaths
American Indian or Alaska Native male				
...	All causes	4,193	All causes	5,985
1.	Unintentional injuries	946	Diseases of heart	1,347
2.	Diseases of heart	917	Malignant neoplasms	977
3.	Malignant neoplasms	408	Unintentional injuries	927
4.	Chronic liver disease and cirrhosis	239	Diabetes mellitus	291
5.	Homicide and legal intervention	164	Chronic liver disease and cirrhosis	244
6.	Cerebrovascular diseases	163	Suicide	241
7.	Pneumonia and influenza	148	Cerebrovascular diseases	213
8.	Suicide	147	Chronic obstructive pulmonary diseases	206
9.	Certain conditions originating in the perinatal period	107	Homicide and legal intervention	189
10.	Diabetes mellitus	86	Pneumonia and influenza	186
Asian or Pacific Islander male				
...	All causes	6,809	All causes	17,060
1.	Diseases of heart	2,174	Diseases of heart	4,723
2.	Malignant neoplasms	1,485	Malignant neoplasms	4,222
3.	Unintentional injuries	556	Cerebrovascular diseases	1,399
4.	Cerebrovascular diseases	521	Unintentional injuries	1,058
5.	Pneumonia and influenza	227	Pneumonia and influenza	734
6.	Suicide	159	Chronic obstructive pulmonary diseases	628
7.	Chronic obstructive pulmonary diseases	158	Diabetes mellitus	488
8.	Homicide and legal intervention	151	Suicide	445
9.	Certain conditions originating in the perinatal period	128	Homicide and legal intervention	316
10.	Diabetes mellitus	103	Certain conditions originating in the perinatal period	177
Hispanic male				
...		---	All causes	54,348
1.		---	Diseases of heart	12,654
2.		---	Malignant neoplasms	9,865
3.		---	Unintentional injuries	5,978
4.		---	Homicide and legal intervention	2,800
5.		---	Cerebrovascular diseases	2,510
6.		---	Diabetes mellitus	2,083
7.		---	Chronic liver disease and cirrhosis	2,003
8.		---	Human immunodeficiency virus infection	1,856
9.		---	Pneumonia and influenza	1,608
10.		---	Suicide	1,479
White female				
...	All causes	804,729	All causes	1,009,509
1.	Diseases of heart	318,668	Diseases of heart	325,909
2.	Malignant neoplasms	169,974	Malignant neoplasms	225,329
3.	Cerebrovascular diseases	88,639	Cerebrovascular diseases	85,166
4.	Unintentional injuries	27,159	Chronic obstructive pulmonary diseases	49,586
5.	Pneumonia and influenza	24,559	Pneumonia and influenza	42,489
6.	Diabetes mellitus	16,743	Unintentional injuries	28,526
7.	Atherosclerosis	16,526	Diabetes mellitus	26,882
8.	Chronic obstructive pulmonary diseases	16,398	Alzheimer's disease	14,613
9.	Chronic liver disease and cirrhosis	8,833	Nephritis, nephrotic syndrome, and nephrosis	10,676
10.	Certain conditions originating in the perinatal period	6,512	Septicemia	10,199
Black female				
...	All causes	102,997	All causes	132,410
1.	Diseases of heart	35,079	Diseases of heart	39,962
2.	Malignant neoplasms	19,176	Malignant neoplasms	28,614
3.	Cerebrovascular diseases	10,941	Cerebrovascular diseases	10,337
4.	Unintentional injuries	3,779	Diabetes mellitus	6,690
5.	Diabetes mellitus	3,534	Unintentional injuries	4,083
6.	Certain conditions originating in the perinatal period	3,092	Pneumonia and influenza	3,942
7.	Pneumonia and influenza	2,262	Chronic obstructive pulmonary diseases	2,942
8.	Homicide and legal intervention	1,898	Human immunodeficiency virus infection	2,447
9.	Chronic liver disease and cirrhosis	1,770	Septicemia	2,370
10.	Nephritis, nephrotic syndrome, and nephrosis	1,722	Nephritis, nephrotic syndrome, and nephrosis	2,295

See footnotes at end of table.

Table 32 (page 4 of 4). Leading causes of death and numbers of deaths, according to sex, detailed race, and Hispanic origin: United States, 1980 and 1997

[Data are based on the National Vital Statistics System]

Sex, race, Hispanic origin, and rank order	1980 Cause of death	1980 Deaths	1997 Cause of death	1997 Deaths
American Indian or Alaska Native female				
...	All causes	2,730	All causes	4,591
1	Diseases of heart	577	Diseases of heart	1,036
2	Malignant neoplasms	362	Malignant neoplasms	840
3	Unintentional injuries	344	Unintentional injuries	403
4	Chronic liver disease and cirrhosis	171	Diabetes mellitus	354
5	Cerebrovascular diseases	159	Cerebrovascular diseases	284
6	Diabetes mellitus	124	Chronic liver disease and cirrhosis	182
7	Pneumonia and influenza	109	Pneumonia and influenza	168
8	Certain conditions originating in the perinatal period	92	Chronic obstructive pulmonary diseases	143
9	Nephritis, nephrotic syndrome, and nephrosis	56	Nephritis, nephrotic syndrome, and nephrosis	68
10	Homicide and legal intervention	55	Homicide and legal intervention	62
Asian or Pacific Islander female				
...	All causes	4,262	All causes	13,696
1	Diseases of heart	1,091	Malignant neoplasms	3,684
2	Malignant neoplasms	1,037	Diseases of heart	3,469
3	Cerebrovascular diseases	507	Cerebrovascular diseases	1,440
4	Unintentional injuries	254	Unintentional injuries	669
5	Diabetes mellitus	124	Pneumonia and influenza	566
6	Certain conditions originating in the perinatal period	118	Diabetes mellitus	523
7	Pneumonia and influenza	115	Chronic obstructive pulmonary diseases	374
8	Congenital anomalies	104	Suicide	184
9	Suicide	90	Nephritis, nephrotic syndrome, and nephrosis	152
10	Homicide and legal intervention	60	Congenital anomalies	149
Hispanic female				
...	- - -	- - -	All causes	41,112
1	- - -	- - -	Diseases of heart	11,170
2	- - -	- - -	Malignant neoplasms	8,770
3	- - -	- - -	Cerebrovascular diseases	2,796
4	- - -	- - -	Diabetes mellitus	2,455
5	- - -	- - -	Unintentional injuries	1,954
6	- - -	- - -	Pneumonia and influenza	1,511
7	- - -	- - -	Chronic obstructive pulmonary diseases	1,120
8	- - -	- - -	Certain conditions originating in the perinatal period	831
9	- - -	- - -	Chronic liver disease and cirrhosis	790
10	- - -	- - -	Congenital anomalies	759

. . . Category not applicable.
- - - Data not available.

NOTES: For data years shown, the code numbers for cause of death are based on the *International Classification of Diseases, 9th Revision*, described in Appendix II, table V. Categories for the coding and classification of human immunodeficiency virus infection were introduced in the United States beginning with mortality data for 1987.

SOURCES: Centers for Disease Control and Prevention, National Center for Health Statistics. *Vital statistics of the United States, vol II, mortality, part A*, 1980. Washington: Public Health Service. 1985; Hoyert DL, Kochanek KD, Murphy SL. Deaths: Final data for 1997. National vital statistics reports; vol 48. Hyattsville, Maryland: 1999; and data computed by the Division of Health and Utilization Analysis from data compiled by the Division of Vital Statistics.

Table 33 (page 1 of 2). Leading causes of death and numbers of deaths, according to age: United States, 1980 and 1997

[Data are based on the National Vital Statistics System]

Age and rank order	1980 Cause of death	Deaths	1997 Cause of death	Deaths
Under 1 year				
. . .	All causes	45,526	All causes	28,045
1.	Congenital anomalies	9,220	Congenital anomalies	6,178
2.	Sudden infant death syndrome	5,510	Disorders relating to short gestation and unspecified low birthweight	3,925
3.	Respiratory distress syndrome	4,989	Sudden infant death syndrome	2,991
4.	Disorders relating to short gestation and unspecified low birthweight	3,648	Respiratory distress syndrome	1,301
5.	Newborn affected by maternal complications of pregnancy	1,572	Newborn affected by maternal complications of pregnancy	1,244
6.	Intrauterine hypoxia and birth asphyxia	1,497	Newborn affected by complications of placenta, cord, and membranes	960
7.	Unintentional injuries	1,166	Infections specific to the perinatal period	777
8.	Birth trauma	1,058	Unintentional injuries	765
9.	Pneumonia and influenza	1,012	Intrauterine hypoxia and birth asphyxia	452
10.	Newborn affected by complications of placenta, cord, and membranes	985	Pneumonia and influenza	421
1–4 years				
. . .	All causes	8,187	All causes	5,501
1.	Unintentional injuries	3,313	Unintentional injuries	2,005
2.	Congenital anomalies	1,026	Congenital anomalies	589
3.	Malignant neoplasms	573	Malignant neoplasms	438
4.	Diseases of heart	338	Homicide and legal intervention	375
5.	Homicide and legal intervention	319	Diseases of heart	212
6.	Pneumonia and influenza	267	Pneumonia and influenza	180
7.	Meningitis	223	Certain conditions originating in the perinatal period	75
8.	Meningococcal infection	110	Septicemia	73
9.	Certain conditions originating in the perinatal period	84	Benign neoplasms	65
10.	Septicemia	71	Cerebrovascular diseases	56
5–14 years				
. . .	All causes	10,689	All causes	8,061
1.	Unintentional injuries	5,224	Unintentional injuries	3,371
2.	Malignant neoplasms	1,497	Malignant neoplasms	1,030
3.	Congenital anomalies	561	Homicide and legal intervention	457
4.	Homicide and legal intervention	415	Congenital anomalies	447
5.	Diseases of heart	330	Diseases of heart	313
6.	Pneumonia and influenza	194	Suicide	307
7.	Suicide	142	Pneumonia and influenza	141
8.	Benign neoplasms	104	Chronic obstructive pulmonary diseases	129
9.	Cerebrovascular diseases	95	Human immunodeficiency virus infection	102
10.	Chronic obstructive pulmonary diseases	85	Benign neoplasms	76
10.	. . .		Cerebrovascular diseases	76
15–24 years				
. . .	All causes	49,027	All causes	31,544
1.	Unintentional injuries	26,206	Unintentional injuries	13,367
2.	Homicide and legal intervention	6,647	Homicide and legal intervention	6,146
3.	Suicide	5,239	Suicide	4,186
4.	Malignant neoplasms	2,683	Malignant neoplasms	1,645
5.	Diseases of heart	1,223	Diseases of heart	1,098
6.	Congenital anomalies	600	Congenital anomalies	420
7.	Cerebrovascular diseases	418	Human immunodeficiency virus infection	276
8.	Pneumonia and influenza	348	Pneumonia and influenza	220
9.	Chronic obstructive pulmonary diseases	141	Chronic obstructive pulmonary diseases	201
10.	Anemias	133	Cerebrovascular diseases	188

See footnotes at end of table.

Table 33 (page 2 of 2). Leading causes of death and numbers of deaths, according to age: United States, 1980 and 1997

[Data are based on the National Vital Statistics System]

Age and rank order	1980		1997	
	Cause of death	Deaths	Cause of death	Deaths
25–44 years				
...	All causes	108,658	All causes	134,946
1.............	Unintentional injuries	26,722	Unintentional injuries	27,129
2.............	Malignant neoplasms	17,551	Malignant neoplasms	21,706
3.............	Diseases of heart	14,513	Diseases of heart	16,513
4.............	Homicide and legal intervention	11,136	Suicide	12,402
5.............	Suicide	9,855	Human immunodeficiency virus infection	11,066
6.............	Chronic liver disease and cirrhosis	4,782	Homicide and legal intervention	8,752
7.............	Cerebrovascular diseases	3,154	Chronic liver disease and cirrhosis	4,024
8.............	Diabetes mellitus	1,472	Cerebrovascular diseases	3,465
9.............	Pneumonia and influenza	1,467	Diabetes mellitus	2,478
10............	Congenital anomalies	817	Pneumonia and influenza	1,928
45–64 years				
...	All causes	425,338	All causes	376,875
1.............	Diseases of heart	148,322	Malignant neoplasms	131,743
2.............	Malignant neoplasms	135,675	Diseases of heart	101,235
3.............	Cerebrovascular diseases	19,909	Unintentional injuries	17,521
4.............	Unintentional injuries	18,140	Cerebrovascular diseases	15,371
5.............	Chronic liver disease and cirrhosis	16,089	Chronic obstructive pulmonary diseases	12,947
6.............	Chronic obstructive pulmonary diseases	11,514	Diabetes mellitus	12,705
7.............	Diabetes mellitus	7,977	Chronic liver disease and cirrhosis	10,875
8.............	Suicide	7,079	Suicide	7,894
9.............	Pneumonia and influenza	5,804	Pneumonia and influenza	5,992
10............	Homicide and legal intervention	4,057	Human immunodeficiency virus infection	4,578
65 years and over				
...	All causes	1,341,848	All causes	1,728,872
1.............	Diseases of heart	595,406	Diseases of heart	606,913
2.............	Malignant neoplasms	258,389	Malignant neoplasms	382,913
3.............	Cerebrovascular diseases	146,417	Cerebrovascular diseases	140,366
4.............	Pneumonia and influenza	45,512	Chronic obstructive pulmonary diseases	94,411
5.............	Chronic obstructive pulmonary diseases	43,587	Pneumonia and influenza	77,561
6.............	Atherosclerosis	28,081	Diabetes mellitus	47,289
7.............	Diabetes mellitus	25,216	Unintentional injuries	31,386
8.............	Unintentional injuries	24,844	Alzheimer's disease	22,154
9.............	Nephritis, nephrotic syndrome, and nephrosis	12,968	Nephritis, nephrotic syndrome, and nephrosis	21,787
10............	Chronic liver disease and cirrhosis	9,519	Septicemia	18,079

... Category not applicable.

NOTES: For data years shown, the code numbers for cause of death are based on the *International Classification of Diseases, 9th Revision*, described in Appendix II, table V. Categories for the coding and classification of human immunodeficiency virus infection were introduced in the United States beginning with mortality data for 1987.

SOURCES: Centers for Disease Control and Prevention, National Center for Health Statistics. *Vital statistics of the United States, vol II, mortality, part A*, 1980. Washington: Public Health Service. 1985; Hoyert DL, Kochanek KD, Murphy SL. Deaths: Final data for 1997. National vital statistics reports; vol 48. Hyattsville, Maryland: 1999; and data computed by the Division of Health and Utilization Analysis from data compiled by the Division of Vital Statistics.

Table 34 (page 1 of 2). Age-adjusted death rates, according to race, sex, region, and urbanization: United States, average annual 1984–86, 1989–91, and 1994–96

[Data are based on the National Vital Statistics System]

Sex, region, and urbanization[1]	All races			White			Black		
	1984–86	1989–91	1994–96	1984–86	1989–91	1994–96	1984–86	1989–91	1994–96
Both sexes	Deaths per 100,000 resident population[2]								
All regions:									
Large core metropolitan	575.2	556.5	524.5	536.9	510.8	479.5	810.4	826.5	791.2
Large fringe metropolitan	511.5	474.1	454.2	504.0	464.6	444.6	710.5	691.7	668.6
Medium/small metropolitan	538.2	509.2	496.3	517.7	486.0	473.7	785.2	777.8	748.9
Urban nonmetropolitan	549.8	529.4	514.5	531.1	509.0	496.1	791.6	793.7	743.9
Rural	549.4	534.1	521.1	528.7	511.1	499.7	755.9	758.8	719.5
Northeast:									
Large core metropolitan	592.7	577.4	538.6	552.5	528.1	493.7	799.0	811.6	749.1
Large fringe metropolitan	515.2	472.4	451.4	509.2	464.7	445.3	694.6	670.8	631.4
Medium/small metropolitan	527.4	486.8	470.1	519.0	476.2	458.3	761.4	737.7	739.3
Urban nonmetropolitan	543.3	501.2	482.3	542.8	500.6	482.1	726.4	667.9	613.5
Rural	527.7	497.5	469.0	528.7	497.8	470.3	*	*	*
South:									
Large core metropolitan	587.5	577.7	551.0	522.8	500.5	471.5	834.7	857.8	844.9
Large fringe metropolitan	522.6	491.1	471.2	506.8	472.4	452.1	710.9	695.6	668.9
Medium/small metropolitan	559.4	534.7	523.2	522.6	494.6	485.6	797.5	792.2	757.4
Urban nonmetropolitan	594.4	579.4	566.5	560.0	542.4	534.0	799.9	803.7	757.3
Rural	595.7	583.8	572.7	566.8	553.5	546.2	757.8	759.1	724.9
Midwest:									
Large core metropolitan	600.9	582.4	561.6	544.9	512.1	488.4	824.8	841.3	819.8
Large fringe metropolitan	519.4	478.5	464.4	510.8	467.8	453.1	751.9	727.8	727.7
Medium/small metropolitan	522.1	490.4	479.6	510.0	475.3	463.1	752.8	748.2	750.5
Urban nonmetropolitan	503.8	484.4	470.6	501.5	481.1	467.7	718.3	721.0	644.5
Rural	503.4	488.0	476.0	493.6	475.4	463.0	704.1	782.8	564.0
West:									
Large core metropolitan	527.5	504.0	468.5	523.4	499.9	466.1	757.8	768.1	719.3
Large fringe metropolitan	475.9	445.2	420.4	479.9	448.0	422.1	661.2	661.8	654.5
Medium/small metropolitan	508.5	487.1	470.5	510.1	488.8	472.9	714.5	710.9	638.2
Urban nonmetropolitan	515.3	493.8	472.7	508.7	486.4	467.4	654.1	660.3	498.0
Rural	502.6	468.6	443.4	502.1	465.2	442.5	*	*	*
Male									
All regions:									
Large core metropolitan	757.7	733.5	680.1	707.5	671.9	619.8	1,092.0	1,130.3	1,065.0
Large fringe metropolitan	664.1	607.8	568.8	655.4	595.6	556.5	918.7	899.6	850.8
Medium/small metropolitan	709.8	663.5	633.8	685.5	633.7	604.6	1,029.6	1,035.8	981.6
Urban nonmetropolitan	729.7	695.0	658.3	707.8	669.7	635.3	1,042.4	1,054.4	973.8
Rural	730.3	704.7	669.2	704.7	675.2	641.4	1,005.9	1,016.6	953.0
Northeast:									
Large core metropolitan	784.9	767.6	700.7	730.3	699.5	640.5	1,095.2	1,127.6	1,015.5
Large fringe metropolitan	671.2	607.9	569.6	663.8	597.8	562.2	910.3	881.3	809.0
Medium/small metropolitan	697.0	635.0	600.8	686.6	621.3	585.6	996.3	982.0	960.5
Urban nonmetropolitan	712.7	652.1	609.5	713.1	652.2	609.9	868.0	808.6	735.7
Rural	696.7	651.2	585.1	699.0	651.3	585.5	*	*	*
South:									
Large core metropolitan	778.7	772.0	723.0	693.6	668.2	617.6	1,124.5	1,179.1	1,145.6
Large fringe metropolitan	683.6	636.4	595.3	664.4	611.9	570.5	926.3	915.0	861.2
Medium/small metropolitan	742.2	702.4	674.7	697.4	649.6	625.5	1,053.6	1,066.2	1,004.9
Urban nonmetropolitan	800.1	772.2	736.6	760.2	725.6	695.1	1,064.3	1,082.9	1,004.8
Rural	799.1	778.8	743.9	764.2	740.2	708.1	1,011.1	1,021.8	966.1
Midwest:									
Large core metropolitan	798.5	769.5	732.6	725.8	674.0	632.9	1,107.7	1,147.9	1,112.1
Large fringe metropolitan	674.9	611.2	577.4	664.9	598.2	563.7	957.4	929.9	907.9
Medium/small metropolitan	689.7	638.2	610.3	675.5	619.2	589.5	974.4	979.6	963.9
Urban nonmetropolitan	667.9	635.4	600.4	665.7	632.1	597.6	880.0	874.5	792.4
Rural	666.2	639.7	607.8	653.9	624.4	592.6	891.7	945.5	639.8
West:									
Large core metropolitan	684.5	652.2	599.6	679.9	646.9	595.2	994.0	1,011.4	926.8
Large fringe metropolitan	607.8	561.4	519.3	613.8	565.4	520.6	810.0	812.3	790.3
Medium/small metropolitan	657.4	620.9	587.7	661.6	624.4	590.0	881.1	874.2	770.5
Urban nonmetropolitan	661.0	624.5	585.3	653.2	615.4	578.6	782.9	763.5	555.8
Rural	646.2	596.0	553.3	646.4	590.4	552.6	*	*	*

See footnotes at end of table.

Table 34 (page 2 of 2). Age-adjusted death rates, according to race, sex, region, and urbanization: United States, average annual 1984–86, 1989–91, and 1994–96

[Data are based on the National Vital Statistics System]

Sex, region, and urbanization[1]	All races			White			Black		
	1984–86	1989–91	1994–96	1984–86	1989–91	1994–96	1984–86	1989–91	1994–96
Female	Deaths per 100,000 resident population[2]								
All regions:									
Large core metropolitan........	432.6	413.5	395.3	403.7	379.9	361.7	599.4	598.2	582.0
Large fringe metropolitan.......	391.1	367.3	359.6	384.9	360.2	352.2	544.3	526.3	520.8
Medium/small metropolitan......	402.6	385.4	382.4	385.3	367.6	365.0	597.9	580.6	567.8
Urban nonmetropolitan.........	402.6	393.3	392.2	386.4	376.6	377.3	598.1	594.9	565.9
Rural	391.6	385.4	387.9	374.8	367.4	371.5	550.4	551.1	528.4
Northeast:									
Large core metropolitan........	446.7	428.3	408.6	417.1	392.6	374.6	589.3	585.4	554.7
Large fringe metropolitan.......	395.3	367.0	355.9	390.5	361.4	350.9	527.6	507.3	491.5
Medium/small metropolitan......	398.9	372.8	365.0	392.3	365.1	356.3	575.4	545.3	556.4
Urban nonmetropolitan.........	408.0	379.9	375.8	407.2	379.2	375.8	592.0	532.7	476.7
Rural	383.7	366.8	366.2	383.5	367.0	368.1	*	*	*
South:									
Large core metropolitan........	436.5	420.2	408.3	386.9	362.9	348.6	617.0	616.0	616.3
Large fringe metropolitan.......	392.5	372.4	366.9	379.1	358.2	352.3	539.7	523.9	515.9
Medium/small metropolitan......	414.5	399.7	398.3	383.1	368.9	369.0	605.6	587.8	570.5
Urban nonmetropolitan.........	428.4	423.7	425.0	397.2	392.8	397.9	600.1	596.6	571.2
Rural	421.7	417.3	422.3	397.2	392.6	402.3	550.8	549.2	529.8
Midwest:									
Large core metropolitan........	451.7	438.3	426.0	410.7	389.0	375.2	610.0	611.5	598.0
Large fringe metropolitan.......	398.8	375.2	374.1	391.5	366.8	365.0	586.8	565.3	578.9
Medium/small metropolitan......	394.0	375.7	375.4	383.8	364.0	362.6	578.4	567.5	578.7
Urban nonmetropolitan.........	371.5	361.9	361.8	369.1	358.9	358.9	575.5	585.1	511.8
Rural	360.7	355.1	356.5	353.4	345.2	345.8	*	*	*
West:									
Large core metropolitan........	398.8	377.2	353.4	395.2	373.3	350.9	564.9	565.2	542.3
Large fringe metropolitan.......	368.9	348.9	335.8	371.5	351.0	337.5	525.6	519.5	525.3
Medium/small metropolitan......	380.7	370.5	365.0	381.3	371.3	367.2	551.3	552.7	506.3
Urban nonmetropolitan.........	384.3	376.0	367.3	379.8	370.8	363.6	521.7	566.7	433.1
Rural	364.6	345.9	334.9	363.6	345.2	333.9	*	*	*

* Data for groups with population under 5,000 in the middle year of a 3-year period are considered unreliable and are not shown.
[1] Urbanization categories for county of residence of decedent are based on a modification of the 1993 classification of counties by the Department of Agriculture. See Appendix II, Urbanization.
[2] Average annual death rate.

NOTES: Denominators for rates are population estimates for the middle year of each 3-year period multiplied by 3. See Appendix II for age-adjustment procedure.

SOURCE: Centers for Disease Control and Prevention, National Center for Health Statistics. Data computed by the Division of Health and Utilization Analysis using the Compressed Mortality File. See Appendix I, National Vital Statistics System.

Table 35. Age-adjusted death rates for persons 25–64 years of age for selected causes of death, according to sex and educational attainment: Selected States, 1994–97

[Data are based on the National Vital Statistics System]

	Both sexes			Male			Female		
	Years of educational attainment[1]			Years of educational attainment[1]			Years of educational attainment[1]		
Cause of death and year	Less than 12	12	13 or more	Less than 12	12	13 or more	Less than 12	12	13 or more
All causes				Deaths per 100,000 population					
1994	571.0	486.1	243.4	762.6	679.2	309.9	379.8	327.6	173.3
1995	581.2	491.7	240.4	770.5	684.9	303.0	391.3	332.4	174.5
1996	556.0	472.4	230.4	733.0	642.6	287.2	379.4	328.9	171.4
1997	531.7	453.6	221.6	690.9	608.0	270.4	370.3	322.3	171.1
Chronic and non-communicable diseases									
1994	415.8	360.0	183.2	529.8	476.5	216.2	307.2	271.6	147.1
1995	420.4	362.9	181.7	531.6	479.3	212.2	314.2	274.4	147.9
1996	408.6	355.1	178.7	519.3	460.0	209.9	303.8	272.7	145.1
1997	395.9	348.9	177.2	497.3	447.9	207.0	299.1	269.7	145.4
Injury and adverse effects									
1994	98.7	75.3	32.1	153.2	121.6	46.0	40.3	32.6	18.1
1995	99.6	76.3	31.8	153.4	122.8	45.6	41.5	33.1	18.0
1996	94.8	74.9	32.1	143.0	118.6	45.7	42.1	33.6	18.5
1997	95.4	75.4	32.0	142.2	113.7	45.7	42.4	34.4	18.5
Communicable diseases									
1994	56.5	50.8	28.1	79.7	81.2	47.9	32.2	23.3	8.1
1995	61.3	52.5	27.0	85.5	82.9	45.3	35.7	24.8	8.6
1996	52.6	42.4	19.5	70.7	63.9	31.4	33.4	22.6	7.7
1997	40.4	29.2	12.4	51.4	41.4	17.6	28.7	18.2	7.2
HIV infection									
1994	36.3	36.3	21.0	54.2	62.3	38.9	17.2	12.4	2.9
1995	39.9	37.7	20.1	58.7	63.6	36.9	19.6	13.8	3.4
1996	31.8	27.5	12.7	44.9	44.8	23.1	17.5	11.2	2.4
1997	19.3	14.1	5.7	25.9	22.6	9.9	12.0	6.2	1.6
Other communicable diseases									
1994	20.2	14.5	7.1	25.5	18.8	8.9	15.0	10.9	5.2
1995	21.4	14.8	6.9	26.8	19.3	8.4	16.0	11.0	5.2
1996	20.8	14.9	6.8	25.8	19.1	8.3	16.0	11.4	5.3
1997	21.1	15.1	6.7	25.4	18.9	7.7	16.8	12.0	5.7

[1]Educational attainment for the numerator is based on the death certificate item "highest grade completed." Educational attainment for the denominator is based on answers to the Current Population Survey question "What is the highest level of school completed or highest degree received?" (Kominski R, Adams A. Educational Attainment in the United States: March 1993 and 1992, U.S. Bureau of the Census, Current Population Reports, P20–476, Washington, DC. 1994.)

NOTES: See Appendix II for age-adjustment procedure. Code numbers for cause of death are based on the *International Classification of Diseases, 9th Revision*. See Appendix II, table V. Based on data from 45 States and the District of Columbia (DC) in 1994–96 and 46 States and DC in 1997. See Appendix I. Death records with education not stated are not included in the calculation of age-adjusted death rates shown in this table. Percent not stated averages 3–9 percent of the deaths comprising the age-adjusted death rates for causes of death in this table. Misreporting of education on the death certificate tends to overstate the death rate for high school graduates (12 years of education) because there is a tendency for some people who did not graduate from high school to be reported as high school graduates on the death certificate; by extension, the death rate for the group with less than 12 years of education tends to be understated. Data for the elderly population are not shown because percent with education not stated is somewhat higher for this group and because of possible bias due to misreporting of education on the death certificate. (Sorlie PD, Johnson NJ: Validity of education information on the death certificate, *Epidemiology* 7(4):437–439, 1996.)

SOURCES: Centers for Disease Control and Prevention, National Center for Health Statistics. Rates computed by the Division of Health and Utilization Analysis from vital statistics data compiled by the Division of Vital Statistics; and from unpublished population estimates prepared by the Housing and Household Economic Statistics Division, U.S. Bureau of the Census.

Table 36 (page 1 of 4). Death rates for all causes, according to sex, detailed race, Hispanic origin, and age: United States, selected years 1950–97

[Data are based on the National Vital Statistics System]

Sex, race, Hispanic origin, and age	1950[1]	1960[1]	1970	1980	1985	1990	1995	1996	1997	1995–97[2]
All persons				Deaths per 100,000 resident population						
All ages, age adjusted	841.5	760.9	714.3	585.8	548.9	520.2	503.9	491.6	479.1	491.4
All ages, crude	963.8	954.7	945.3	878.3	876.9	863.8	880.0	872.5	864.7	872.3
Under 1 year	3,299.2	2,696.4	2,142.4	1,288.3	1,088.1	971.9	768.8	755.7	738.7	754.5
1–4 years	139.4	109.1	84.5	63.9	51.8	46.8	40.6	38.3	35.8	38.3
5–14 years	60.1	46.6	41.3	30.6	26.5	24.0	22.5	21.7	20.8	21.7
15–24 years	128.1	106.3	127.7	115.4	94.9	99.2	95.3	89.6	86.2	90.3
25–34 years	178.7	146.4	157.4	135.5	124.4	139.2	141.3	126.7	115.0	127.8
35–44 years	358.7	299.4	314.5	227.9	207.7	223.2	240.8	221.3	203.2	221.6
45–54 years	853.9	756.0	730.0	584.0	519.3	473.4	460.1	445.9	430.8	445.2
55–64 years	1,901.0	1,735.1	1,658.8	1,346.3	1,294.2	1,196.9	1,114.5	1,094.1	1,063.6	1,090.5
65–74 years	4,104.3	3,822.1	3,582.7	2,994.9	2,862.8	2,648.6	2,563.5	2,538.4	2,509.8	2,537.3
75–84 years	9,331.1	8,745.2	8,004.4	6,692.6	6,398.7	6,007.2	5,851.8	5,803.1	5,728.2	5,793.3
85 years and over	20,196.9	19,857.5	16,344.9	15,980.3	15,712.4	15,327.4	15,469.5	15,327.2	15,345.2	15,379.3
Male										
All ages, age adjusted	1,001.6	949.3	931.6	777.2	723.0	680.2	646.3	623.7	602.8	624.0
All ages, crude	1,106.1	1,104.5	1,090.3	976.9	948.6	918.4	914.1	896.4	880.8	897.0
Under 1 year	3,728.0	3,059.3	2,410.0	1,428.5	1,219.9	1,082.8	843.8	828.0	812.8	828.3
1–4 years	151.7	119.5	93.2	72.6	58.5	52.4	44.8	42.2	39.7	42.3
5–14 years	70.9	55.7	50.5	36.7	31.8	28.5	26.7	25.4	24.0	25.4
15–24 years	167.9	152.1	188.5	172.3	138.9	147.4	140.5	130.6	124.0	131.6
25–34 years	216.5	187.9	215.3	196.1	179.6	204.3	204.7	178.6	160.1	181.4
35–44 years	428.8	372.8	402.6	299.2	278.9	310.4	333.0	298.1	265.7	298.5
45–54 years	1,067.1	992.2	958.5	767.3	671.6	610.3	598.9	573.8	550.5	573.7
55–64 years	2,395.3	2,309.5	2,282.7	1,815.1	1,711.4	1,553.4	1,416.7	1,388.7	1,336.6	1,380.2
65–74 years	4,931.4	4,914.4	4,873.8	4,105.2	3,856.3	3,491.5	3,284.6	3,233.4	3,191.2	3,236.5
75–84 years	10,426.0	10,178.4	10,010.2	8,816.7	8,501.6	7,888.6	7,377.1	7,249.8	7,116.1	7,244.8
85 years and over	21,636.0	21,186.3	17,821.5	18,801.1	18,614.1	18,056.6	17,978.9	17,547.7	17,461.9	17,655.0
Female										
All ages, age adjusted	688.4	590.6	532.5	432.6	410.3	390.6	385.2	381.0	375.7	380.6
All ages, crude	823.5	809.2	807.8	785.3	809.1	812.0	847.3	849.7	849.2	848.8
Under 1 year	2,854.6	2,321.3	1,863.7	1,141.7	950.6	855.7	690.1	680.0	661.1	677.1
1–4 years	126.7	98.4	75.4	54.7	44.8	41.0	36.2	34.3	31.8	34.1
5–14 years	48.9	37.3	31.8	24.2	21.0	19.3	18.2	17.8	17.4	17.8
15–24 years	89.1	61.3	68.1	57.5	49.6	49.0	48.1	46.2	46.3	46.9
25–34 years	142.7	106.6	101.6	75.9	69.4	74.2	77.9	74.7	69.9	74.2
35–44 years	290.3	229.4	231.1	159.3	138.7	137.9	150.1	145.4	141.4	145.6
45–54 years	641.5	526.7	517.2	412.9	375.2	342.7	327.6	323.3	316.1	322.2
55–64 years	1,404.8	1,196.4	1,098.9	934.3	925.6	878.8	840.8	826.7	815.2	827.5
65–74 years	3,333.2	2,871.8	2,579.7	2,144.7	2,096.9	1,991.2	1,986.1	1,979.0	1,959.0	1,974.8
75–84 years	8,399.6	7,633.1	6,677.6	5,440.1	5,162.1	4,883.1	4,882.7	4,868.3	4,820.5	4,856.8
85 years and over	19,194.7	19,008.4	15,518.0	14,746.9	14,553.9	14,274.3	14,492.4	14,444.7	14,492.3	14,476.4
White male										
All ages, age adjusted	963.1	917.7	893.4	745.3	693.3	644.3	610.5	591.4	573.8	591.7
All ages, crude	1,089.5	1,098.5	1,086.7	983.3	963.6	930.9	932.1	918.1	906.3	918.7
Under 1 year	3,400.5	2,694.1	2,113.2	1,230.3	1,056.5	896.1	717.5	683.3	678.1	693.0
1–4 years	135.5	104.9	83.6	66.1	52.8	45.9	38.8	37.1	35.1	37.0
5–14 years	67.2	52.7	48.0	35.0	30.1	26.4	24.5	23.2	22.1	23.3
15–24 years	152.4	143.7	170.8	167.0	134.2	131.3	122.3	113.9	109.0	115.0
25–34 years	185.3	163.2	176.6	171.3	158.8	176.1	177.7	154.8	140.3	157.8
35–44 years	380.9	332.6	343.5	257.4	243.1	268.2	287.7	259.6	235.3	260.6
45–54 years	984.5	932.2	882.9	698.9	611.7	548.7	534.6	515.5	495.8	514.8
55–64 years	2,304.4	2,225.2	2,202.6	1,728.5	1,625.8	1,467.2	1,330.8	1,305.2	1,252.4	1,295.7
65–74 years	4,864.9	4,848.4	4,810.1	4,035.7	3,770.7	3,397.7	3,199.0	3,158.3	3,122.7	3,160.2
75–84 years	10,526.3	10,299.6	10,098.8	8,829.8	8,486.1	7,844.9	7,320.6	7,205.5	7,086.0	7,201.5
85 years and over	22,116.3	21,750.0	18,551.7	19,097.3	18,980.1	18,268.3	18,152.9	17,870.5	17,767.1	17,924.9

See footnotes at end of table.

Table 36 (page 2 of 4). Death rates for all causes, according to sex, detailed race, Hispanic origin, and age: United States, selected years 1950–97

[Data are based on the National Vital Statistics System]

Sex, race, Hispanic origin, and age	1950[1]	1960[1]	1970	1980	1985	1990	1995	1996	1997	1995–97[2]
Black male					Deaths per 100,000 resident population					
All ages, age adjusted	1,373.1	1,246.1	1,318.6	1,112.8	1,053.4	1,061.3	1,016.7	967.0	911.9	964.3
All ages, crude	1,260.3	1,181.7	1,186.6	1,034.1	989.3	1,008.0	980.7	939.9	893.9	937.8
Under 1 year	- - -	5,306.8	4,298.9	2,586.7	2,219.9	2,112.4	1,590.8	1,748.2	1,671.6	1,666.7
1–4 years	- - -	208.5	150.5	110.5	90.1	85.8	77.5	71.4	67.2	72.1
5–14 years	95.1	75.1	67.1	47.4	42.3	41.2	40.2	38.1	34.8	37.7
15–24 years	289.7	212.0	320.6	209.1	173.6	252.2	249.2	233.0	215.8	232.6
25–34 years	503.5	402.5	559.5	407.3	351.9	430.8	416.5	361.0	308.6	362.1
35–44 years	878.1	762.0	956.6	689.8	630.2	699.6	721.2	629.2	523.7	623.0
45–54 years	1,905.0	1,624.8	1,777.5	1,479.9	1,292.9	1,261.0	1,273.0	1,190.6	1,114.1	1,189.9
55–64 years	3,773.2	3,316.4	3,256.9	2,873.0	2,779.8	2,618.4	2,437.5	2,395.1	2,320.0	2,383.4
65–74 years	5,310.3	5,798.7	5,803.2	5,131.1	5,172.4	4,946.1	4,610.5	4,431.5	4,298.3	4,445.5
75–84 years	- - -	8,605.1	9,454.9	9,231.6	9,262.3	9,129.5	8,778.8	8,614.9	8,296.8	8,559.1
85 years and over	- - -	14,844.8	12,222.3	16,098.8	15,774.2	16,954.9	16,728.7	16,006.3	16,083.5	16,263.5
American Indian or Alaska Native male[3]										
All ages, age adjusted	- - -	- - -	- - -	732.5	602.6	573.1	580.4	555.9	584.1	573.4
All ages, crude	- - -	- - -	- - -	597.1	492.5	476.4	502.3	489.8	519.2	503.8
Under 1 year	- - -	- - -	- - -	1,598.1	1,080.0	1,056.6	689.3	874.4	903.0	820.5
1–4 years	- - -	- - -	- - -	82.7	105.3	77.4	81.2	72.9	51.6	68.7
5–14 years	- - -	- - -	- - -	43.7	39.2	33.4	30.3	37.8	28.7	32.3
15–24 years	- - -	- - -	- - -	311.1	214.4	219.8	202.3	174.7	180.3	185.5
25–34 years	- - -	- - -	- - -	360.6	275.0	256.1	284.2	260.0	245.4	263.0
35–44 years	- - -	- - -	- - -	556.8	363.5	365.4	420.5	370.0	389.3	392.9
45–54 years	- - -	- - -	- - -	871.3	687.9	619.9	668.1	580.2	673.4	640.6
55–64 years	- - -	- - -	- - -	1,547.5	1,319.1	1,211.3	1,369.5	1,348.0	1,409.6	1,376.1
65–74 years	- - -	- - -	- - -	2,968.4	2,692.3	2,461.7	2,605.2	2,640.7	2,847.2	2,698.8
75–84 years	- - -	- - -	- - -	5,607.0	5,572.7	5,389.2	4,780.0	4,633.8	4,796.3	4,736.8
85 years and over	- - -	- - -	- - -	12,635.2	8,900.0	11,243.9	7,404.3	7,686.7	7,888.1	7,676.6
Asian or Pacific Islander male[4]										
All ages, age adjusted	- - -	- - -	- - -	416.6	396.9	377.8	384.4	355.8	350.3	361.7
All ages, crude	- - -	- - -	- - -	375.3	344.6	334.3	354.9	350.7	351.7	352.4
Under 1 year	- - -	- - -	- - -	816.5	750.0	605.3	427.3	457.6	426.3	436.8
1–4 years	- - -	- - -	- - -	50.9	43.4	45.0	26.8	24.6	25.5	25.6
5–14 years	- - -	- - -	- - -	23.4	22.5	20.7	18.8	17.1	17.3	17.7
15–24 years	- - -	- - -	- - -	80.8	76.0	76.0	81.2	73.2	67.2	73.7
25–34 years	- - -	- - -	- - -	83.5	77.3	79.6	80.5	75.6	71.8	75.9
35–44 years	- - -	- - -	- - -	128.3	114.4	130.8	131.4	125.0	115.7	123.8
45–54 years	- - -	- - -	- - -	342.3	284.8	287.1	286.9	277.0	274.8	279.3
55–64 years	- - -	- - -	- - -	881.1	869.4	789.1	745.1	726.3	750.8	740.8
65–74 years	- - -	- - -	- - -	2,236.1	2,102.0	2,041.4	1,975.8	1,948.4	1,892.6	1,937.9
75–84 years	- - -	- - -	- - -	5,389.5	5,551.2	5,008.6	5,182.4	4,844.3	4,749.1	4,910.4
85 years and over	- - -	- - -	- - -	13,753.6	12,750.0	12,446.3	17,273.0	11,637.4	11,796.3	13,060.5
Hispanic male[5]										
All ages, age adjusted	- - -	- - -	- - -	- - -	524.8	531.2	515.0	474.8	447.7	477.6
All ages, crude	- - -	- - -	- - -	- - -	374.6	411.6	412.1	381.3	360.5	383.8
Under 1 year	- - -	- - -	- - -	- - -	1,041.8	921.8	687.2	686.2	654.3	675.6
1–4 years	- - -	- - -	- - -	- - -	53.8	53.8	39.7	37.3	34.1	37.0
5–14 years	- - -	- - -	- - -	- - -	23.0	26.0	25.3	23.5	18.7	22.4
15–24 years	- - -	- - -	- - -	- - -	147.5	159.3	168.7	140.3	129.1	145.0
25–34 years	- - -	- - -	- - -	- - -	202.0	234.0	215.7	175.0	154.5	181.1
35–44 years	- - -	- - -	- - -	- - -	290.3	341.8	343.3	279.7	235.7	283.5
45–54 years	- - -	- - -	- - -	- - -	495.4	533.9	533.3	493.7	456.1	492.4
55–64 years	- - -	- - -	- - -	- - -	1,129.2	1,123.7	1,058.7	1,032.0	957.8	1,014.6
65–74 years	- - -	- - -	- - -	- - -	2,488.9	2,368.2	2,322.2	2,245.4	2,251.7	2,272.1
75–84 years	- - -	- - -	- - -	- - -	5,724.6	5,369.1	5,199.0	4,966.4	4,750.3	4,959.3
85 years and over	- - -	- - -	- - -	- - -	11,856.1	12,272.1	12,242.7	10,617.7	10,487.1	11,039.5

See footnotes at end of table.

[Data are based on the National Vital Statistics System]

Sex, race, Hispanic origin, and age	1950[1]	1960[1]	1970	1980	1985	1990	1995	1996	1997	1995–97[2]
White, non-Hispanic male[5]					Deaths per 100,000 resident population					
All ages, age adjusted	---	---	---	---	669.7	643.1	605.7	589.5	575.3	590.1
All ages, crude	---	---	---	---	956.3	985.9	989.0	982.1	977.3	982.8
Under 1 year	---	---	---	---	1,002.5	865.4	695.7	654.6	662.4	671.0
1–4 years	---	---	---	---	48.8	43.8	37.5	36.2	34.8	36.2
5–14 years	---	---	---	---	28.9	25.7	23.6	22.5	22.4	22.9
15–24 years	---	---	---	---	125.0	123.4	110.6	105.6	102.7	106.3
25–34 years	---	---	---	---	151.2	165.3	166.4	147.2	134.8	149.7
35–44 years	---	---	---	---	231.8	257.1	275.9	252.3	231.4	253.0
45–54 years	---	---	---	---	587.6	544.5	526.1	509.0	494.0	509.3
55–64 years	---	---	---	---	1,550.8	1,479.7	1,337.0	1,308.7	1,264.7	1,302.9
65–74 years	---	---	---	---	3,648.0	3,434.5	3,221.9	3,181.1	3,154.6	3,185.9
75–84 years	---	---	---	---	8,364.2	7,920.4	7,368.2	7,274.5	7,154.7	7,263.1
85 years and over	---	---	---	---	18,637.2	18,505.4	18,157.7	18,110.1	18,066.9	18,110.3
White female										
All ages, age adjusted	645.0	555.0	501.7	411.1	391.0	369.9	364.9	361.9	358.0	361.6
All ages, crude	803.3	800.9	812.6	806.1	840.1	846.9	891.3	896.2	897.8	895.1
Under 1 year	2,566.8	2,007.7	1,614.6	962.5	799.3	690.0	571.6	558.0	546.0	558.5
1–4 years	112.2	85.2	66.1	49.3	40.0	36.1	31.2	28.5	28.0	29.2
5–14 years	45.1	34.7	29.9	22.9	19.5	17.9	16.6	16.4	15.6	16.2
15–24 years	71.5	54.9	61.6	55.5	48.1	45.9	44.3	42.7	43.8	43.6
25–34 years	112.8	85.0	84.1	65.4	59.4	61.5	64.3	62.7	60.0	62.3
35–44 years	235.8	191.1	193.3	138.2	121.9	117.4	125.8	121.6	120.9	122.7
45–54 years	546.4	458.8	462.9	372.7	341.7	309.3	294.4	290.5	285.0	289.9
55–64 years	1,293.8	1,078.9	1,014.9	876.2	869.1	822.7	788.4	779.5	766.3	778.0
65–74 years	3,242.8	2,779.3	2,470.7	2,066.6	2,027.1	1,923.5	1,924.5	1,919.8	1,900.5	1,915.0
75–84 years	8,481.5	7,696.6	6,698.7	5,401.7	5,111.6	4,839.1	4,831.1	4,826.5	4,786.3	4,814.3
85 years and over	19,679.5	19,477.7	15,980.2	14,979.6	14,745.4	14,400.6	14,639.1	14,642.9	14,681.4	14,654.8
Black female										
All ages, age adjusted	1,106.7	916.9	814.4	631.1	594.8	581.6	571.0	561.0	545.5	559.0
All ages, crude	1,002.0	905.0	829.2	733.3	734.2	747.9	759.0	753.5	742.8	751.7
Under 1 year	---	4,162.2	3,368.8	2,123.7	1,821.4	1,735.5	1,342.0	1,444.0	1,383.9	1,387.8
1–4 years	---	173.3	129.4	84.4	71.1	67.6	62.9	63.7	51.0	59.3
5–14 years	72.8	53.8	43.8	30.5	28.6	27.5	26.5	25.9	27.2	26.5
15–24 years	213.1	107.5	111.9	70.5	59.6	68.7	70.3	66.8	62.0	66.3
25–34 years	393.3	273.2	231.0	150.0	137.6	159.5	166.6	153.8	134.6	151.7
35–44 years	758.1	568.5	533.0	323.9	276.5	298.6	327.7	316.4	287.1	310.1
45–54 years	1,576.4	1,177.0	1,043.9	768.2	667.6	639.4	619.0	610.1	590.4	606.0
55–64 years	3,089.4	2,510.9	1,986.2	1,561.0	1,532.5	1,452.6	1,350.3	1,311.7	1,307.3	1,322.8
65–74 years	4,000.2	4,064.2	3,860.9	3,057.4	2,967.8	2,865.7	2,823.7	2,787.0	2,739.7	2,783.3
75–84 years	---	6,730.0	6,691.5	6,212.1	6,078.0	5,688.3	5,840.3	5,775.9	5,669.3	5,760.9
85 years and over	---	13,052.6	10,706.6	12,367.2	12,703.0	13,309.5	13,472.2	13,398.5	13,701.7	13,526.0
American Indian or Alaska Native female[3]										
All ages, age adjusted	---	---	---	414.1	353.3	335.1	368.0	367.7	359.9	365.1
All ages, crude	---	---	---	380.1	342.5	330.4	390.6	396.0	392.6	393.1
Under 1 year	---	---	---	1,352.6	910.5	688.7	756.5	718.2	646.1	707.3
1–4 years	---	---	---	87.5	54.8	37.8	60.0	67.1	66.8	64.6
5–14 years	---	---	---	33.5	23.0	25.5	22.5	23.7	22.2	22.8
15–24 years	---	---	---	90.3	72.8	69.0	64.8	62.5	57.5	61.5
25–34 years	---	---	---	178.5	121.5	102.3	115.5	108.9	116.3	113.6
35–44 years	---	---	---	286.0	185.6	156.4	194.2	196.3	195.6	195.4
45–54 years	---	---	---	491.4	415.5	380.9	386.9	435.4	387.4	403.3
55–64 years	---	---	---	837.1	851.9	805.9	917.6	862.2	866.9	881.8
65–74 years	---	---	---	1,765.5	1,630.3	1,679.4	1,894.3	1,878.8	1,920.5	1,898.0
75–84 years	---	---	---	3,612.9	3,200.0	3,073.2	3,591.1	3,657.1	3,531.6	3,592.5
85 years and over	---	---	---	8,567.4	7,740.0	8,201.1	6,521.3	6,193.5	5,773.6	6,139.6

See footnotes at end of table.

Table 36 (page 4 of 4). Death rates for all causes, according to sex, detailed race, Hispanic origin, and age: United States, selected years 1950–97

[Data are based on the National Vital Statistics System]

Sex, race, Hispanic origin, and age	1950[1]	1960[1]	1970	1980	1985	1990	1995	1996	1997	1995–97[2]
Asian or Pacific Islander female[4]					Deaths per 100,000 resident population					
All ages, age adjusted	---	---	---	224.6	228.5	228.9	231.4	214.4	214.7	219.3
All ages, crude	---	---	---	222.5	224.9	234.3	257.7	257.9	264.3	260.1
Under 1 year	---	---	---	755.8	622.0	518.2	359.9	347.4	343.7	350.2
1–4 years	---	---	---	35.4	36.8	32.0	23.8	25.6	24.7	24.7
5–14 years	---	---	---	21.5	19.1	13.0	14.7	11.4	13.8	13.3
15–24 years	---	---	---	32.3	30.7	28.8	33.5	30.6	33.4	32.5
25–34 years	---	---	---	45.4	36.5	37.5	38.1	35.4	32.4	35.2
35–44 years	---	---	---	89.7	77.8	69.9	68.6	68.7	74.1	70.5
45–54 years	---	---	---	214.1	184.9	182.7	191.2	173.8	166.6	176.6
55–64 years	---	---	---	440.8	468.0	483.4	475.6	417.7	423.4	437.9
65–74 years	---	---	---	1,027.7	1,130.8	1,089.2	1,061.5	1,090.8	1,117.3	1,090.8
75–84 years	---	---	---	2,833.6	2,873.9	3,127.9	3,278.9	3,118.8	3,052.1	3,141.8
85 years and over	---	---	---	7,923.3	9,808.3	10,254.0	11,256.4	8,599.1	8,414.1	9,197.3
Hispanic female[5]										
All ages, age adjusted	---	---	---	---	286.6	284.9	274.4	268.0	263.4	268.4
All ages, crude	---	---	---	---	251.9	285.4	290.8	289.8	288.0	289.5
Under 1 year	---	---	---	---	793.0	746.6	575.0	540.2	572.3	562.5
1–4 years	---	---	---	---	42.3	42.1	33.5	29.6	28.4	30.5
5–14 years	---	---	---	---	16.0	17.3	15.5	16.9	15.6	16.0
15–24 years	---	---	---	---	36.3	40.6	40.6	39.2	38.3	39.3
25–34 years	---	---	---	---	56.3	62.9	63.1	61.1	54.6	59.6
35–44 years	---	---	---	---	100.0	109.3	121.0	108.2	101.1	109.7
45–54 years	---	---	---	---	251.3	253.3	238.9	231.8	228.3	232.8
55–64 years	---	---	---	---	620.3	607.5	586.2	580.9	580.3	582.4
65–74 years	---	---	---	---	1,449.3	1,453.8	1,399.6	1,400.0	1,381.9	1,393.6
75–84 years	---	---	---	---	3,549.8	3,351.3	3,275.0	3,279.4	3,220.5	3,257.3
85 years and over	---	---	---	---	10,216.9	10,098.7	9,613.6	8,783.9	8,708.6	9,002.7
White, non-Hispanic female[5]										
All ages, age adjusted	---	---	---	---	385.3	372.2	366.4	364.1	360.9	363.8
All ages, crude	---	---	---	---	861.7	903.6	956.7	965.0	971.2	964.3
Under 1 year	---	---	---	---	762.8	655.3	550.2	541.1	519.6	536.9
1–4 years	---	---	---	---	36.6	34.0	30.0	27.8	27.3	28.4
5–14 years	---	---	---	---	19.0	17.6	16.4	15.9	15.3	15.9
15–24 years	---	---	---	---	47.9	46.0	44.0	42.4	44.1	43.5
25–34 years	---	---	---	---	59.0	60.6	62.8	61.7	60.0	61.5
35–44 years	---	---	---	---	122.8	116.8	124.0	121.1	121.7	122.3
45–54 years	---	---	---	---	335.7	312.1	296.1	292.0	287.3	291.7
55–64 years	---	---	---	---	853.3	834.5	797.2	787.6	775.7	786.7
65–74 years	---	---	---	---	1,997.8	1,940.2	1,940.3	1,937.1	1,920.3	1,932.6
75–84 years	---	---	---	---	5,058.5	4,887.3	4,860.2	4,868.1	4,831.1	4,852.9
85 years and over	---	---	---	---	14,561.4	14,533.1	14,724.6	14,826.1	14,864.0	14,806.2

- - - Data not available.

[1]Includes deaths of persons who were not residents of the 50 States and the District of Columbia.

[2]Average annual death rate.

[3]Interpretation of trends should take into account that population estimates for American Indians increased by 45 percent between 1980 and 1990, partly due to better enumeration techniques in the 1990 decennial census and to the increased tendency for people to identify themselves as American Indian in 1990.

[4]Interpretation of trends should take into account that the Asian population in the United States more than doubled between 1980 and 1990, primarily due to immigration.

[5]Excludes data from States lacking an Hispanic-origin item on their death certificates. See Appendix I, National Vital Statistics System.

NOTES: The race groups, white, black, Asian or Pacific Islander, and American Indian or Alaska Native, include persons of Hispanic and non-Hispanic origin. Conversely, persons of Hispanic origin may be of any race. Consistency of race identification between the death certificate (source of data for numerator of death rates) and data from the Census Bureau (denominator) is high for individual white and black persons; however, persons identified as American Indian, Asian, or Hispanic origin in data from the Census Bureau are sometimes misreported as white or non-Hispanic on the death certificate, causing death rates to be underestimated by 22–30 percent for American Indians, about 12 percent for Asians, and about 7 percent for persons of Hispanic origin. (Sorlie PD, Rogot E, and Johnson NJ: Validity of demographic characteristics on the death certificate, *Epidemiology* 3(2):181–184, 1992.) See Appendix II for age-adjustment procedure. Data for additional years are available (see Appendix III).

SOURCES: Centers for Disease Control and Prevention, National Center for Health Statistics. Grove RD and Hetzel AM. *Vital statistics rates in the United States, 1940–60.* Washington: Public Health Service, 1968; *Vital statistics of the United States, vol II, mortality, part A,* for data years 1950–93. Public Health Service. Washington. U.S. Government Printing Office; for 1994–97, unpublished data; data computed by the Division of Health and Utilization Analysis from numerator data compiled by the Division of Vital Statistics and denominator data from national population estimates for race groups from table 1 and unpublished Hispanic population estimates prepared by the Housing and Household Economic Statistics Division, U.S. Bureau of the Census.

Table 37 (page 1 of 3). Death rates for diseases of heart according to sex, detailed race, Hispanic origin, and age: United States, selected years 1950–97

[Data are based on the National Vital Statistics System]

Sex, race, Hispanic origin, and age	1950[1]	1960[1]	1970	1980	1985	1990	1994	1995	1996	1997	1995–97[2]
All persons				Deaths per 100,000 resident population							
All ages, age adjusted	307.2	286.2	253.6	202.0	181.4	152.0	140.4	138.3	134.5	130.5	134.4
All ages, crude	355.5	369.0	362.0	336.0	324.1	289.5	281.3	280.7	276.4	271.6	276.2
Under 1 year	3.5	6.6	13.1	22.8	25.0	20.1	17.7	17.1	16.6	16.4	16.7
1–4 years	1.3	1.3	1.7	2.6	2.2	1.9	1.8	1.6	1.4	1.4	1.5
5–14 years	2.1	1.3	0.8	0.9	1.0	0.9	0.9	0.8	0.9	0.8	0.8
15–24 years	6.8	4.0	3.0	2.9	2.8	2.5	2.8	2.9	2.7	3.0	2.9
25–34 years	19.4	15.6	11.4	8.3	8.3	7.6	8.5	8.5	8.3	8.3	8.4
35–44 years	86.4	74.6	66.7	44.6	38.1	31.4	31.8	32.0	30.5	30.1	30.8
45–54 years	308.6	271.8	238.4	180.2	153.8	120.5	112.6	111.0	108.2	104.9	108.0
55–64 years	808.1	737.9	652.3	494.1	443.0	367.3	329.9	322.9	315.2	302.4	313.4
65–74 years	1,839.8	1,740.5	1,558.2	1,218.6	1,089.8	894.3	817.4	799.9	776.2	753.7	776.7
75–84 years	4,310.1	4,089.4	3,683.8	2,993.1	2,693.1	2,295.7	2,093.0	2,064.7	2,010.2	1,943.6	2,005.2
85 years and over	9,150.6	9,317.8	7,891.3	7,777.1	7,384.1	6,739.9	6,494.9	6,484.1	6,314.5	6,198.9	6,329.4
Male											
All ages, age adjusted	383.8	375.5	348.5	280.4	250.1	206.7	188.5	184.9	178.8	173.1	178.9
All ages, crude	423.4	439.5	422.5	368.6	344.1	297.6	284.3	282.7	277.4	272.2	277.4
Under 1 year	4.0	7.8	15.1	25.5	27.8	21.9	18.6	17.5	17.4	18.0	17.6
1–4 years	1.4	1.4	1.9	2.8	2.2	1.9	1.8	1.7	1.4	1.5	1.5
5–14 years	2.0	1.4	0.9	1.0	0.9	0.9	0.9	0.8	0.9	0.9	0.9
15–24 years	6.8	4.2	3.7	3.7	3.5	3.1	3.4	3.6	3.3	3.6	3.5
25–34 years	22.9	20.1	15.2	11.4	11.6	10.3	11.0	11.4	11.0	10.8	11.1
35–44 years	118.4	112.7	103.2	68.7	58.6	48.1	46.6	47.2	44.2	43.7	45.0
45–54 years	440.5	420.4	376.4	282.6	237.8	183.0	170.6	168.6	161.8	157.7	162.6
55–64 years	1,104.5	1,066.9	987.2	746.8	659.1	537.3	478.1	465.4	453.8	434.6	451.1
65–74 years	2,292.3	2,291.3	2,170.3	1,728.0	1,535.8	1,250.0	1,133.1	1,102.3	1,065.0	1,031.1	1,066.2
75–84 years	4,825.0	4,742.4	4,534.8	3,834.3	3,496.9	2,968.2	2,655.1	2,615.0	2,529.4	2,443.6	2,527.4
85 years and over	9,659.8	9,788.9	8,426.2	8,752.7	8,251.8	7,418.4	7,123.0	7,039.6	6,834.0	6,658.5	6,838.3
Female											
All ages, age adjusted	233.9	205.7	175.2	140.3	127.4	108.9	101.6	100.4	98.2	95.4	98.0
All ages, crude	288.4	300.6	304.5	305.1	305.2	281.8	278.5	278.8	275.5	271.1	275.1
Under 1 year	2.9	5.4	10.9	20.0	22.0	18.3	16.7	16.7	15.7	14.7	15.7
1–4 years	1.2	1.1	1.6	2.5	2.2	1.9	1.8	1.5	1.4	1.2	1.4
5–14 years	2.2	1.2	0.8	0.9	1.0	0.8	0.8	0.7	0.8	0.7	0.7
15–24 years	6.7	3.7	2.3	2.1	2.1	1.8	2.1	2.2	2.0	2.4	2.2
25–34 years	16.2	11.3	7.7	5.3	5.0	5.0	6.0	5.6	5.6	5.8	5.6
35–44 years	55.1	38.2	32.2	21.4	18.3	15.1	17.2	17.1	16.8	16.5	16.8
45–54 years	177.2	127.5	109.9	84.5	74.4	61.0	57.1	56.0	56.9	54.3	55.7
55–64 years	510.0	429.4	351.6	272.1	252.1	215.7	195.8	193.9	189.3	182.1	188.4
65–74 years	1,419.3	1,261.3	1,082.7	828.6	746.1	616.8	566.3	557.8	543.8	529.4	543.8
75–84 years	3,872.0	3,582.7	3,120.8	2,497.0	2,220.4	1,893.8	1,741.3	1,715.2	1,674.7	1,616.6	1,668.2
85 years and over	8,796.1	9,016.8	7,591.8	7,350.5	7,037.6	6,478.1	6,252.7	6,267.8	6,108.0	6,013.7	6,127.5
White male											
All ages, age adjusted	381.1	375.4	347.6	277.5	246.2	202.0	183.8	179.7	174.5	168.7	174.2
All ages, crude	433.0	454.6	438.3	384.0	360.3	312.7	300.1	297.9	293.3	287.7	292.9
45–54 years	423.6	413.2	365.7	269.8	225.5	170.6	157.7	155.7	149.8	145.4	150.2
55–64 years	1,081.7	1,056.0	979.3	730.6	640.1	516.7	458.6	443.0	431.8	411.2	428.5
65–74 years	2,308.3	2,297.9	2,177.2	1,729.7	1,522.7	1,230.5	1,114.7	1,080.5	1,049.5	1,015.1	1,048.5
75–84 years	4,907.3	4,839.9	4,617.6	3,883.2	3,527.0	2,983.4	2,661.8	2,616.1	2,536.0	2,453.7	2,533.5
85 years and over	9,950.5	10,135.8	8,818.0	8,958.0	8,481.7	7,558.7	7,262.2	7,165.5	7,014.5	6,829.7	6,998.6
Black male											
All ages, age adjusted	415.5	381.2	375.9	327.3	310.8	275.9	254.0	255.9	242.6	236.2	244.7
All ages, crude	348.4	330.6	330.3	301.0	288.6	256.8	240.4	244.2	234.8	230.8	236.5
45–54 years	624.1	514.0	512.8	433.4	385.2	328.9	316.5	317.1	297.7	293.7	302.4
55–64 years	1,434.0	1,236.8	1,135.4	987.2	935.3	824.0	742.3	757.8	740.9	727.8	742.0
65–74 years	2,140.1	2,281.4	2,237.8	1,847.2	1,839.2	1,632.9	1,479.3	1,482.9	1,381.3	1,335.4	1,399.3
75–84 years	- - -	3,533.6	3,783.4	3,578.8	3,436.6	3,107.1	2,874.5	2,881.4	2,762.0	2,641.6	2,759.4
85 years and over	- - -	6,037.9	5,367.6	6,819.5	6,393.5	6,479.6	5,919.4	5,985.7	5,675.4	5,538.7	5,727.3

See footnotes at end of table.

Table 37 (page 2 of 3). Death rates for diseases of heart, according to sex, detailed race, Hispanic origin, and age: United States, selected years 1950–97

[Data are based on the National Vital Statistics System]

Sex, race, Hispanic origin, and age	1950[1]	1960[1]	1970	1980	1985	1990	1994	1995	1996	1997	1995–97[2]
American Indian or Alaska Native male[3]				Deaths per 100,000 resident population							
All ages, age adjusted	---	---	---	180.9	162.2	144.6	145.5	136.7	131.6	136.5	135.0
All ages, crude	---	---	---	130.6	117.9	108.0	116.7	110.4	110.7	116.8	112.7
45–54 years	---	---	---	238.1	209.1	173.8	181.2	151.4	157.5	171.8	160.5
55–64 years	---	---	---	496.3	438.3	411.0	414.2	403.2	404.9	427.2	412.0
65–74 years	---	---	---	1,009.4	984.6	839.1	937.5	918.5	778.0	828.1	840.9
75–84 years	---	---	---	2,062.2	2,118.2	1,788.8	1,628.4	1,534.9	1,546.5	1,513.8	1,531.3
85 years and over	---	---	---	4,413.7	2,766.7	3,860.3	3,072.1	2,308 7	2,660.1	2,764.2	2,593.9
Asian or Pacific Islander male[4]											
All ages, age adjusted	---	---	---	136.7	123.4	102.6	107.6	106.2	98.1	95.9	99.4
All ages, crude	---	---	---	119.8	103.5	88.7	96.9	96.9	97.3	97.4	97.2
45–54 years	---	---	---	112.0	81.1	70.4	80.4	73.4	75.4	72.1	73.6
55–64 years	---	---	---	306.7	291.2	226.1	229.1	214.3	220.7	218.3	217.9
65–74 years	---	---	---	852.4	753.5	623.5	623.5	605.8	581.2	585.1	590.4
75–84 years	---	---	---	2,010.9	2,025.6	1,642.2	1,576.3	1,680.5	1,534.8	1,432.1	1,541.0
85 years and over	---	---	---	5,923.0	4,937.5	4,617.8	6,158.3	6,372.3	4,338.0	4,392.5	4,850.5
Hispanic male[5]											
All ages, age adjusted	---	---	---	---	152.3	136.3	123.5	121.9	117.6	113.4	117.4
All ages, crude	---	---	---	---	92.1	91.0	87.4	87.5	85.8	83.9	85.7
45–54 years	---	---	---	---	128.0	116.4	102.1	103.0	98.7	96.2	99.1
55–64 years	---	---	---	---	398.8	363.0	308.3	306.0	310.0	276.9	297.2
65–74 years	---	---	---	---	972.6	829.9	769.4	750.0	725.7	737.2	737.5
75–84 years	---	---	---	---	2,160.8	1,971.3	1,770.0	1,734.5	1,688.6	1,628.7	1,680.9
85 years and over	---	---	---	---	4,791.2	4,711.9	4,726.9	4,699.7	4,078.6	3,844.6	4,172.2
White, non-Hispanic male[5]											
All ages, age adjusted	---	---	---	---	240.3	204.1	185.3	181.2	176.2	171.1	176.1
All ages, crude	---	---	---	---	362.8	336.5	324.2	322.0	318.9	315.0	318.6
45–54 years	---	---	---	---	219.9	172.8	160.1	157.5	152.1	148.5	152.6
55–64 years	---	---	---	---	610.6	521.3	464.2	448.0	435.1	418.1	433.5
65–74 years	---	---	---	---	1,471.3	1,243.4	1,123.6	1,088.3	1,056.4	1,025.1	1,056.6
75–84 years	---	---	---	---	3,514.1	3,007.7	2,674.1	2,635.6	2,559.8	2,477.3	2,555.5
85 years and over	---	---	---	---	8,539.3	7,663.4	7,260.9	7,166.3	7,109.2	6,954.2	7,073.5
White female											
All ages, age adjusted	223.6	197.1	167.8	134.6	121.7	103.1	96.1	94.9	92.9	90.4	92.7
All ages, crude	289.4	306.5	313.8	319.2	321.8	298.4	296.8	297.4	294.2	289.8	293.8
45–54 years	141.9	103.4	91.4	71.2	62.5	50.2	47.0	45.9	46.9	44.9	45.9
55–64 years	460.2	383.0	317.7	248.1	227.1	192.4	174.7	173.1	167.8	162.5	167.8
65–74 years	1,400.9	1,229.8	1,044.0	796.7	713.3	583.6	535.6	526.3	515.1	500.7	514.1
75–84 years	3,925.2	3,629.7	3,143.5	2,493.6	2,207.5	1,874.3	1,717.6	1,689.8	1,652.9	1,595.9	1,645.6
85 years and over	9,084.7	9,280.8	7,839.9	7,501.6	7,170.0	6,563.4	6,342.8	6,352.6	6,211.4	6,108.0	6,222.0
Black female											
All ages, age adjusted	349.5	292.6	251.7	201.1	188.3	168.1	158.0	156.3	153.4	147.6	152.4
All ages, crude	289.9	268.5	261.0	249.7	250.3	237.0	230.6	231.1	229.0	224.2	228.1
45–54 years	526.8	360.7	290.9	202.4	176.2	155.3	146.4	143.1	144.7	134.8	140.7
55–64 years	1,210.7	952.3	710.5	530.1	510.7	442.0	392.2	384.9	388.4	364.8	379.2
65–74 years	1,659.4	1,680.5	1,553.2	1,210.3	1,149.9	1,017.5	941.7	933.7	890.0	871.6	898.3
75–84 years	---	2,926.9	2,964.1	2,707.2	2,533.4	2,250.9	2,158.1	2,163.1	2,097.7	2,030.5	2,096.3
85 years and over	---	5,650.0	5,003.8	5,796.5	5,686.5	5,766.1	5,531.8	5,614.8	5,493.6	5,542.5	5,549.4

See footnotes at end of table.

Table 37 (page 3 of 3). Death rates for diseases of heart. according to sex, detailed race, Hispanic origin, and age: United States, selected years 1950–97

[Data are based on the National Vital Statistics System]

Sex, race, Hispanic origin, and age	1950[1]	1960[1]	1970	1980	1985	1990	1994	1995	1996	1997	1995–97[2]
American Indian or Alaska Native female[3]				Deaths per 100,000 resident population							
All ages, age adjusted	---	---	---	88.4	83.7	76.6	71.3	77.3	74.9	73.9	75.3
All ages, crude	---	---	---	80.3	84.3	77.5	82.1	87.0	86.7	88.6	87.4
45–54 years	---	---	---	65.2	59.2	62.0	48.7	69.2	61.1	59.7	63.2
55–64 years	---	---	---	193.5	230.8	197.0	196.8	210.2	192.5	172.8	191.5
65–74 years	---	---	---	577.2	472.7	492.8	429.9	503.3	512.8	473.8	496.5
75–84 years	---	---	---	1,364.3	1,258.8	1,050.3	1,055.6	1,045.6	1,030.0	1,115.2	1,064.5
85 years and over	---	---	---	2,893.3	3,180.0	2,868.7	2,490.9	2,209.8	2,108.8	2,019.5	2,106.8
Asian or Pacific Islander female[4]											
All ages, age adjusted	---	---	---	55.8	59.6	58.3	57.7	57.7	50.9	49.3	52.2
All ages, crude	---	---	---	57.0	60.3	62.0	66.7	68.2	66.8	66.9	67.3
45–54 years	---	---	---	28.6	23.8	17.5	22.1	21.6	17.2	18.8	19.1
55–64 years	---	---	---	92.9	103.0	99.0	93.3	93.0	82.3	80.5	85.0
65–74 years	---	---	---	313.3	341.0	323.9	295.7	294.9	282.0	272.8	282.8
75–84 years	---	---	---	1,053.2	1,056.5	1,130.9	1,110.7	1,063.0	1,009.8	944.0	1,001.5
85 years and over	---	---	---	3,211.0	4,208.3	4,161.2	4,376.5	4,717.9	3,394.7	3,326.2	3,701.8
Hispanic female[5]											
All ages, age adjusted	---	---	---	---	86.5	76.0	67.0	68.1	64.7	64.7	65.7
All ages, crude	---	---	---	---	75.0	79.4	75.6	78.9	77.0	78.3	78.1
45–54 years	---	---	---	---	46.6	43.5	31.8	32.0	31.3	31.5	31.6
55–64 years	---	---	---	---	184.8	153.2	134.3	137.3	125.1	129.5	130.5
65–74 years	---	---	---	---	534.0	460.4	399.3	402.4	387.6	391.9	393.9
75–84 years	---	---	---	---	1,456.5	1,259.7	1,163.5	1,150.1	1,152.8	1,102.4	1,134.2
85 years and over	---	---	---	---	4,523.4	4,440.3	3,783.1	4,243.9	3,673.8	3,748.7	3,870.3
White, non-Hispanic female[5]											
All ages, age adjusted	---	---	---	---	120.2	103.7	96.5	95.4	93.6	91.3	93.4
All ages, crude	---	---	---	---	334.2	320.0	320.6	321.4	318.9	315.6	318.6
45–54 years	---	---	---	---	61.3	50.2	47.5	46.6	47.5	45.7	46.6
55–64 years	---	---	---	---	219.6	193.6	175.5	173.6	169.0	163.9	168.8
65–74 years	---	---	---	---	700.4	584.7	537.2	529.1	518.0	504.0	517.1
75–84 years	---	---	---	---	2,201.4	1,890.2	1,728.0	1,697.8	1,663.5	1,609.4	1,656.2
85 years and over	---	---	---	---	7,164.7	6,615.2	6,354.2	6,384.5	6,285.4	6,176.4	6,280.0

--- Data not available.

[1]Includes deaths of persons who were not residents of the 50 States and the District of Columbia.

[2]Average annual death rate.

[3]Interpretation of trends should take into account that population estimates for American Indians increased by 45 percent between 1980 and 1990, partly due to better enumeration techniques in the 1990 decennial census and to the increased tendency for people to identify themselves as American Indian in 1990.

[4]Interpretation of trends should take into account that the Asian population in the United States more than doubled between 1980 and 1990, primarily due to immigration.

[5]Excludes data from States lacking an Hispanic-origin item on their death certificates. See Appendix I, National Vital Statistics System.

NOTES: For data years shown, the code numbers for cause of death are based on the then current *International Classification of Diseases*, which are described in Appendix II, tables IV and V. Age groups were selected to minimize the presentation of unstable age-specific death rates based on small numbers of deaths and for consistency among comparison groups. The race groups, white, black, Asian or Pacific Islander, and American Indian or Alaska Native, include persons of Hispanic and non-Hispanic origin. Conversely, persons of Hispanic origin may be of any race. Consistency of race identification between the death certificate (source of data for numerator of death rates) and data from the Census Bureau (denominator) is high for individual white and black persons; however, persons identified as American Indian, Asian, or Hispanic origin in data from the Census Bureau are sometimes misreported as white or non-Hispanic on the death certificate, causing death rates to be underestimated by 22–30 percent for American Indians, about 12 percent for Asians, and about 7 percent for persons of Hispanic origin. (Sorlie PD, Rogot E, and Johnson NJ: Validity of demographic characteristics on the death certificate, *Epidemiology* 3(2):181–184, 1992.) See Appendix II for age-adjustment procedure. Data for additional years are available (see Appendix III).

SOURCES: Centers for Disease Control and Prevention, National Center for Health Statistics. *Vital statistics of the United States, vol II, mortality, part A*, for data years 1950–93. Public Health Service. Washington. U.S. Government Printing Office; for 1994–97, unpublished data; data computed by the Division of Health and Utilization Analysis from numerator data compiled by the Division of Vital Statistics and denominator data from national population estimates for race groups from table 1 and unpublished Hispanic population estimates prepared by the Housing and Household Economic Statistics Division, U.S. Bureau of the Census.

Table 38 (page 1 of 3). Death rates for cerebrovascular diseases, according to sex, detailed race, Hispanic origin, and age: United States, selected years 1950–97

[Data are based on the National Vital Statistics System]

Sex, race, Hispanic origin, and age	1950[1]	1960[1]	1970	1980	1985	1990	1994	1995	1996	1997	1995–97[2]
All persons				Deaths per 100,000 resident population							
All ages, age adjusted	88.8	79.7	66.3	40.8	32.5	27.7	26.5	26.7	26.4	25.9	26.3
All ages, crude	104.0	108.0	101.9	75.1	64.3	57.9	58.9	60.1	60.3	59.7	60.0
Under 1 year	5.1	4.1	5.0	4.4	3.7	3.8	5.1	5.8	6.2	7.0	6.3
1–4 years	0.9	0.8	1.0	0.5	0.3	0.3	0.3	0.4	0.3	0.4	0.3
5–14 years	0.5	0.7	0.7	0.3	- - -	0.2	0.2	0.2	0.2	0.2	0.2
15–24 years	1.6	1.8	1.6	1.0	.5	0.6	0.5	0.5	0.5	0.5	0.5
25–34 years	4.2	4.7	4.5	2.6	2.2	2.2	1.9	1.8	1.8	1.7	1.8
35–44 years	18.7	14.7	15.6	8.5	7.2	6.5	6.5	6.5	6.3	6.3	6.4
45–54 years	70.4	49.2	41.6	25.2	21.3	18.7	17.9	17.6	17.9	16.9	17.5
55–64 years	194.2	147.3	115.8	65.2	54.8	48.0	45.6	46.1	45.3	44.4	45.2
65–74 years	554.7	469.2	384.1	219.5	172.8	144.4	135.7	137.2	135.5	134.8	135.9
75–84 years	1,499.6	1,491.3	1,254.2	788.6	601.5	499.3	480.2	481.4	477.0	462.0	473.3
85 years and over	2,990.1	3,680.5	3,014.3	2,288.9	1,865.1	1,633.9	1,604.1	1,636.5	1,612.7	1,584.6	1,610.7
Male											
All ages, age adjusted	91.9	85.4	73.2	44.9	35.5	30.2	29.0	28.9	28.5	27.9	28.4
All ages, crude	102.5	104.5	94.5	63.6	52.5	46.8	47.4	48.0	48.1	47.8	48.0
Under 1 year	6.4	5.0	5.8	5.0	4.6	4.4	5.8	6.3	6.5	7.6	6.8
1–4 years	1.1	0.9	1.2	0.4	0.4	0.3	0.4	0.4	0.3	0.5	0.4
5–14 years	0.5	0.7	0.8	0.3	0.2	0.2	0.2	0.2	0.2	0.2	0.2
15–24 years	1.8	1.9	1.8	1.1	0.7	0.7	0.5	0.5	0.5	0.6	0.5
25–34 years	4.2	4.5	4.4	2.6	2.2	2.1	1.8	1.9	1.7	1.7	1.8
35–44 years	17.5	14.6	15.7	8.7	7.4	6.8	7.1	7.1	6.7	6.5	6.7
45–54 years	67.9	52.2	44.4	27.3	23.2	20.5	20.1	19.8	20.0	19.2	19.6
55–64 years	205.2	163.8	138.7	74.7	63.5	54.4	52.5	53.4	52.5	51.4	52.4
65–74 years	589.6	530.7	449.5	259.2	201.4	166.8	156.0	155.9	154.7	153.1	154.6
75–84 years	1,543.6	1,555.9	1,361.6	868.3	661.2	552.7	524.6	517.1	508.7	488.7	504.5
85 years and over	3,048.6	3,643.1	2,895.2	2,199.2	1,730.1	1,533.2	1,521.8	1,537.7	1,512.7	1,500.7	1,516.4
Female											
All ages, age adjusted	86.0	74.7	60.8	37.6	30.0	25.7	24.5	24.8	24.6	24.2	24.5
All ages, crude	105.6	111.4	109.0	86.1	75.5	68.6	69.8	71.7	71.9	71.2	71.6
Under 1 year	3.7	3.2	4.0	3.8	2.7	3.1	4.3	5.2	5.9	6.3	5.8
1–4 years	0.7	0.7	0.7	0.5	0.3	0.3	*	0.3	0.3	0.3	0.3
5–14 years	0.4	0.6	0.6	0.3	0.3	0.2	0.2	0.2	0.2	0.2	0.2
15–24 years	1.5	1.6	1.4	0.8	0.8	0.6	0.5	0.4	0.4	0.5	0.4
25–34 years	4.3	4.9	4.7	2.6	2.1	2.2	2.1	1.7	1.8	1.7	1.7
35–44 years	19.9	14.8	15.6	8.4	6.9	6.1	5.9	6.0	5.9	6.2	6.0
45–54 years	72.9	46.3	39.0	23.3	19.4	17.0	15.8	15.5	15.9	14.8	15.4
55–64 years	183.1	131.8	95.3	56.9	47.2	42.2	39.3	39.4	38.8	37.9	38.7
65–74 years	522.1	415.7	333.3	189.0	150.7	126.9	119.5	122.2	120.1	120.1	120.8
75–84 years	1,462.2	1,441.1	1,183.1	741.6	566.3	467.4	452.4	458.7	456.5	444.4	453.1
85 years and over	2,949.4	3,704.4	3,081.0	2,328.2	1,918.9	1,672.7	1,635.9	1,675.0	1,652.4	1,618.4	1,648.1
White male											
All ages, age adjusted	87.0	80.3	68.8	41.9	33.0	27.7	26.6	26.5	26.3	25.7	26.1
All ages, crude	100.5	102.7	93.5	63.3	52.7	47.0	48.1	48.6	49.1	48.8	48.8
45–54 years	53.7	40.9	35.6	21.7	18.1	15.4	15.2	14.8	15.2	14.6	14.9
55–64 years	182.2	139.0	119.9	64.2	54.6	45.8	44.1	44.7	43.4	42.3	43.4
65–74 years	569.7	501.0	420.0	240.4	186.4	153.2	143.6	143.5	142.0	141.8	142.4
75–84 years	1,556.3	1,564.8	1,361.6	854.8	650.0	540.7	511.0	503.1	500.1	480.3	494.2
85 years and over	3,127.1	3,734.8	3,018.1	2,236.9	1,765.6	1,549.8	1,539.8	1,550.0	1,537.7	1,530.6	1,539.2
Black male											
All ages, age adjusted	146.2	141.2	122.5	77.5	62.7	56.1	52.4	52.2	50.9	48.6	50.5
All ages, crude	122.0	122.9	108.8	73.1	59.2	53.1	50.5	51.0	50.1	48.3	49.8
45–54 years	211.9	166.1	136.1	82.1	71.1	68.4	64.7	64.1	62.1	59.8	61.9
55–64 years	522.8	439.9	343.4	189.8	160.7	141.8	134.2	134.1	137.5	135.5	135.7
65–74 years	783.6	899.2	780.1	472.8	379.7	327.2	293.2	291.5	292.2	274.3	285.9
75–84 years	- - -	1,475.2	1,445.7	1,067.6	814.4	723.7	702.0	700.2	653.0	600.5	650.3
85 years and over	- - -	2,700.0	1,963.1	1,873.2	1,429.0	1,430.5	1,319.8	1,393.9	1,329.5	1,281.6	1,333.5

See footnotes at end of table.

[Data are based on the National Vital Statistics System]

Sex, race, Hispanic origin, and age	1950[1]	1960[1]	1970	1980	1985	1990	1994	1995	1996	1997	1995–97[2]
American Indian or Alaska Native male[3]				Deaths per 100,000 resident population							
All ages, age adjusted	---	---	---	30.7	24.9	20.5	22.0	23.5	21.4	20.1	21.6
All ages, crude	---	---	---	23.2	18.5	16.0	18.7	20.1	18.7	18.5	19.1
45–54 years	---	---	---	*	*	*	*	28.4	19.9	*	20.8
55–64 years	---	---	---	72.0	*	39.8	43.3	45.7	42.9	49.4	46.0
65–74 years	---	---	---	170.5	200.0	120.3	141.3	153.1	139.1	112.5	134.7
75–84 years	---	---	---	535.1	372.7	325.9	333.2	290.1	319.4	324.0	311.9
85 years and over	---	---	---	1,384.7	733.3	949.8	845.9	748.8	550.4	707.9	667.0
Asian or Pacific Islander male[4]											
All ages, age adjusted	---	---	---	32.3	28.0	26.9	30.1	31.2	26.9	28.3	28.6
All ages, crude	---	---	---	28.7	24.0	23.4	27.2	28.6	27.0	28.8	28.2
45–54 years	---	---	---	17.0	13.9	15.6	20.3	17.3	19.5	18.3	18.4
55–64 years	---	---	---	59.9	48.8	51.8	49.8	62.1	55.6	58.0	58.5
65–74 years	---	---	---	197.9	155.6	167.9	166.9	162.3	161.4	160.9	161.5
75–84 years	---	---	---	619.5	583.7	485.7	564.9	571.8	430.0	524.0	506.2
85 years and over	---	---	---	1,399.0	1,387.5	1,196.6	1,702.9	1,808.5	1,348.7	1,219.4	1,409.3
Hispanic male[5]											
All ages, age adjusted	---	---	---	---	27.7	22.7	23.3	23.1	22.3	22.1	22.4
All ages, crude	---	---	---	---	17.2	15.6	16.9	17.1	16.8	16.7	16.8
45–54 years	---	---	---	---	23.6	20.0	21.9	20.5	23.1	20.4	21.3
55–64 years	---	---	---	---	63.9	49.4	48.4	46.1	50.7	52.7	49.9
65–74 years	---	---	---	---	163.5	126.4	133.5	132.2	114.8	134.9	127.3
75–84 years	---	---	---	---	396.7	356.6	343.3	349.9	348.6	304.2	333.0
85 years and over	---	---	---	---	1,152.1	866.3	980.0	996.3	866.3	787.8	875.1
White, non-Hispanic male[5]											
All ages, age adjusted	---	---	---	---	31.6	27.9	26.4	26.3	26.1	25.6	26.0
All ages, crude	---	---	---	---	52.2	50.7	51.7	52.3	53.0	53.1	52.8
45–54 years	---	---	---	---	16.0	14.9	14.5	14.1	14.2	13.9	14.1
55–64 years	---	---	---	---	50.5	45.2	43.4	43.9	42.0	41.1	42.3
65–74 years	---	---	---	---	178.5	154.8	143.2	143.1	142.0	141.1	142.1
75–84 years	---	---	---	---	637.0	548.8	514.7	507.4	505.1	486.0	499.2
85 years and over	---	---	---	---	1,735.1	1,583.6	1,544.5	1,552.4	1,560.6	1,562.9	1,558.8
White female											
All ages, age adjusted	79.7	68.7	56.2	35.2	27.9	23.8	22.8	23.1	22.9	22.5	22.9
All ages, crude	103.3	110.1	109.8	88.8	78.4	71.8	73.9	76.0	76.3	75.7	76.0
45–54 years	55.0	33.8	30.5	18.7	15.5	13.5	12.3	12.7	12.8	11.6	12.4
55–64 years	156.9	103.0	78.1	48.7	40.0	35.8	33.7	33.6	33.3	31.8	32.9
65–74 years	498.1	383.3	303.2	172.8	137.9	116.3	109.7	112.6	110.2	111.4	111.4
75–84 years	1,471.3	1,444.7	1,176.8	730.3	552.9	457.6	442.8	449.5	446.7	437.5	444.5
85 years and over	3,017.9	3,795.7	3,167.6	2,367.8	1,944.9	1,691.4	1,656.7	1,690.0	1,679.3	1,645.8	1,671.3
Black female											
All ages, age adjusted	155.6	139.5	107.9	61.7	50.6	42.7	40.1	39.6	39.2	37.9	38.9
All ages, crude	128.3	127.7	112.2	77.9	68.6	60.7	59.3	60.4	59.7	58.0	59.4
45–54 years	248.9	166.2	119.4	61.9	50.8	44.1	43.1	36.4	38.6	38.6	37.9
55–64 years	567.7	452.0	272.4	138.7	113.6	97.0	84.8	85.5	82.9	84.0	84.1
65–74 years	754.4	830.5	673.5	362.2	285.6	236.8	217.9	221.2	216.4	204.8	214.1
75–84 years	---	1,413.1	1,338.3	918.6	753.8	596.0	582.2	583.2	586.5	540.0	569.7
85 years and over	---	2,578.9	2,210.5	1,896.3	1,657.1	1,496.5	1,447.9	1,568.8	1,443.6	1,433.1	1,480.4

See footnotes at end of table.

Table 38 (page 3 of 3). Death rates for cerebrovascular diseases, according to sex, detailed race, Hispanic origin, and age: United States, selected years 1950–97

[Data are based on the National Vital Statistics System]

Sex, race, Hispanic origin, and age	1950[1]	1960[1]	1970	1980	1985	1990	1994	1995	1996	1997	1995–97[2]
American Indian or Alaska Native female[3]					Deaths per 100,000 resident population						
All ages, age adjusted	---	---	---	23.3	20.6	18.5	18.8	19.9	20.6	19.9	20.1
All ages, crude	---	---	---	22.1	21.8	19.3	21.9	23.8	25.5	24.3	24.6
45–54 years	---	---	---	*	*	*	*	*	24.6	*	18.4
55–64 years	---	---	---	*	40.4	40.7	44.4	43.5	29.7	49.4	40.9
65–74 years	---	---	---	128.3	121.2	100.5	121.6	112.3	127.7	109.0	116.3
75–84 years	---	---	---	404.2	317.6	282.0	296.9	321.7	354.9	319.7	332.1
85 years and over	---	---	---	1,123.6	1,000.0	776.2	654.9	697.3	700.0	570.0	651.9
Asian or Pacific Islander female[4]											
All ages, age adjusted	---	---	---	25.9	23.6	23.4	21.8	21.6	21.5	21.4	21.5
All ages, crude	---	---	---	26.5	23.3	24.3	24.9	24.9	27.5	27.8	26.8
45–54 years	---	---	---	20.3	15.1	19.7	14.8	16.2	16.2	14.2	15.5
55–64 years	---	---	---	44.5	49.0	42.5	35.4	39.1	36.3	40.7	38.7
65–74 years	---	---	---	136.1	130.8	124.0	111.7	103.3	111.2	109.3	108.0
75–84 years	---	---	---	449.6	387.0	396.6	394.3	405.2	409.2	409.8	408.2
85 years and over	---	---	---	1,545.2	1,383.3	1,395.0	1,452.4	1,432.5	1,243.3	1,097.8	1,234.3
Hispanic female[5]											
All ages, age adjusted	---	---	---	---	20.6	19.5	16.5	18.1	17.1	17.0	17.4
All ages, crude	---	---	---	---	18.3	20.2	18.2	20.1	19.6	19.6	19.8
45–54 years	---	---	---	---	15.8	15.2	14.2	15.1	15.3	12.7	14.3
55–64 years	---	---	---	---	35.8	38.8	32.3	35.7	35.2	32.4	34.4
65–74 years	---	---	---	---	108.6	102.9	84.7	98.2	90.3	96.8	95.1
75–84 years	---	---	---	---	339.8	309.5	274.2	287.4	284.3	286.3	286.0
85 years and over	---	---	---	---	1,191.5	1,060.4	825.7	932.4	837.8	774.5	842.8
White, non-Hispanic female[5]											
All ages, age adjusted	---	---	---	---	27.2	23.9	22.8	23.1	23.0	22.6	22.9
All ages, crude	---	---	---	---	81.0	77.4	80.0	82.2	82.9	82.6	82.5
45–54 years	---	---	---	---	14.3	13.2	12.0	12.4	12.4	11.3	12.0
55–64 years	---	---	---	---	37.8	35.7	33.5	33.0	32.7	31.5	32.4
65–74 years	---	---	---	---	133.5	117.1	110.1	112.4	110.7	111.5	111.5
75–84 years	---	---	---	---	551.6	463.1	447.3	452.9	450.4	442.0	448.3
85 years and over	---	---	---	---	1,926.2	1,720.4	1,666.4	1,704.8	1,707.4	1,675.3	1,695.5

- - - Data not available.
* Based on fewer than 20 deaths.
[1]Includes deaths of persons who were not residents of the 50 States and the District of Columbia.
[2]Average annual death rate.
[3]Interpretation of trends should take into account that population estimates for American Indians increased by 45 percent between 1980 and 1990, partly due to better enumeration techniques in the 1990 decennial census and to the increased tendency for people to identify themselves as American Indian in 1990.
[4]Interpretation of trends should take into account that the Asian population in the United States more than doubled between 1980 and 1990, primarily due to immigration.
[5]Excludes data from States lacking an Hispanic-origin item on their death certificates. See Appendix I, National Vital Statistics System.

NOTES: For data years shown, the code numbers for cause of death are based on the then current *International Classification of Diseases*, which are described in Appendix II, tables IV and V. Age groups were selected to minimize the presentation of unstable age-specific death rates based on small numbers of deaths and for consistency among comparison groups. The race groups, white, black, Asian or Pacific Islander, and American Indian or Alaska Native, include persons of Hispanic and non-Hispanic origin. Conversely, persons of Hispanic origin may be of any race. Consistency of race identification between the death certificate (source of data for numerator of death rates) and data from the Census Bureau (denominator) is high for individual white and black persons; however, persons identified as American Indian, Asian, or Hispanic origin in data from the Census Bureau are sometimes misreported as white or non-Hispanic on the death certificate, causing death rates to be underestimated by 22–30 percent for American Indians, about 12 percent for Asians, and about 7 percent for persons of Hispanic origin. (Sorlie PD, Rogot E, and Johnson NJ: Validity of demographic characteristics on the death certificate, *Epidemiology* 3(2):181–184, 1992.) See Appendix II for age-adjustment procedure. Data for additional years are available (see Appendix III).

SOURCES: Centers for Disease Control and Prevention, National Center for Health Statistics. Grove RD and Hetzel AM. *Vital statistics rates in the United States, 1940–60*. Washington: Public Health Service, 1968; *Vital statistics of the United States, vol II, mortality, part A*, for data years 1950–93. Public Health Service. Washington. U.S. Government Printing Office; for 1994–97, unpublished data; data computed by the Division of Health and Utilization Analysis from numerator data compiled by the Division of Vital Statistics and denominator data from national population estimates for race groups from table 1 and unpublished Hispanic population estimates prepared by the Housing and Household Economic Statistics Division, U.S. Bureau of the Census.

Table 39 (page 1 of 4). Death rates for malignant neoplasms, according to sex, detailed race, Hispanic origin, and age: United States, selected years 1950–97

[Data are based on the National Vital Statistics System]

Sex, race, Hispanic origin, and age	1950[1]	1960[1]	1970	1980	1985	1990	1994	1995	1996	1997	1995–97[2]
All persons				Deaths per 100,000 resident population							
All ages, age adjusted	125.4	125.8	129.8	132.8	134.4	135.0	131.5	129.9	127.9	125.6	127.8
All ages, crude	139.8	149.2	162.8	183.9	194.0	203.2	205.2	204.9	203.4	201.6	203.3
Under 1 year	8.7	7.2	4.7	3.2	3.1	2.3	1.5	1.8	2.3	2.4	2.2
1–4 years	11.7	10.9	7.5	4.5	3.8	3.5	3.3	3.1	2.7	2.9	2.9
5–14 years	6.7	6.8	6.0	4.3	3.5	3.1	2.8	2.7	2.7	2.7	2.7
15–24 years	8.6	8.3	8.3	6.3	5.4	4.9	4.8	4.6	4.5	4.5	4.5
25–34 years	20.0	19.5	16.5	13.7	13.2	12.6	12.2	11.9	12.0	11.6	11.9
35–44 years	62.7	59.7	59.5	48.6	45.9	43.3	40.4	40.3	39.3	38.9	39.5
45–54 years	175.1	177.0	182.5	180.0	170.1	158.9	145.9	142.2	137.9	135.1	138.3
55–64 years	390.7	396.8	423.0	436.1	454.6	449.6	424.6	416.0	406.5	395.7	405.9
65–74 years	698.8	713.9	751.2	817.9	845.5	872.3	875.4	868.2	861.6	847.3	859.1
75–84 years	1,153.3	1,127.4	1,169.2	1,232.3	1,271.8	1,348.5	1,367.4	1,364.8	1,351.5	1,335.2	1,350.3
85 years and over	1,451.0	1,450.0	1,320.7	1,594.6	1,615.4	1,752.9	1,789.0	1,823.8	1,798.3	1,805.0	1,808.8
Male											
All ages, age adjusted	130.8	143.0	157.4	165.5	166.1	166.3	159.6	156.8	153.8	150.4	153.6
All ages, crude	142.9	162.5	182.1	205.3	213.4	221.3	220.7	219.5	217.2	214.6	217.0
Under 1 year	9.7	7.7	4.4	3.7	3.0	2.4	1.4	1.8	2.2	2.3	2.1
1–4 years	12.5	12.4	8.3	5.2	4.3	3.7	3.5	3.6	3.1	3.1	3.3
5–14 years	7.4	7.6	6.7	4.9	3.9	3.5	3.1	3.0	3.0	2.8	2.9
15–24 years	9.7	10.2	10.4	7.8	6.4	5.7	5.8	5.5	5.1	5.2	5.3
25–34 years	17.7	18.8	16.3	13.4	13.2	12.6	12.1	11.7	11.5	11.5	11.5
35–44 years	45.6	48.9	53.0	44.0	42.4	38.5	36.7	36.5	35.6	34.5	35.5
45–54 years	156.2	170.8	183.5	188.7	175.2	162.5	148.8	143.7	140.7	138.0	140.7
55–64 years	413.1	459.9	511.8	520.8	536.9	532.9	495.3	480.5	469.1	453.4	467.5
65–74 years	791.5	890.5	1,006.8	1,093.2	1,105.2	1,122.2	1,102.5	1,089.9	1,080.9	1,058.4	1,076.4
75–84 years	1,332.6	1,389.4	1,588.3	1,790.5	1,839.7	1,914.4	1,862.6	1,842.3	1,802.7	1,770.2	1,804.3
85 years and over	1,668.3	1,741.2	1,720.8	2,369.5	2,451.8	2,739.9	2,805.8	2,837.3	2,733.1	2,712.5	2,759.1
Female											
All ages, age adjusted	120.8	111.2	108.8	109.2	111.7	112.7	111.1	110.4	108.8	107.3	108.8
All ages, crude	136.8	136.4	144.4	163.6	175.7	186.0	190.5	191.0	190.2	189.2	190.1
Under 1 year	7.6	6.8	5.0	2.7	3.2	2.2	1.6	1.8	2.4	2.5	2.2
1–4 years	10.8	9.3	6.7	3.7	3.4	3.2	3.0	2.6	2.3	2.6	2.5
5–14 years	6.0	6.0	5.2	3.6	3.1	2.8	2.4	2.4	2.4	2.5	2.4
15–24 years	7.6	6.5	6.2	4.8	4.3	4.1	3.9	3.6	3.8	3.7	3.7
25–34 years	22.2	20.1	16.7	14.0	13.2	12.6	12.3	12.2	12.6	11.7	12.2
35–44 years	79.3	70.0	65.6	53.1	49.2	48.1	44.1	44.0	42.9	43.1	43.4
45–54 years	194.0	183.0	181.5	171.8	165.3	155.5	143.1	140.7	135.2	132.3	136.0
55–64 years	368.2	337.7	343.2	361.7	381.8	375.2	360.7	357.5	349.6	343.2	350.0
65–74 years	612.3	560.2	557.9	607.1	645.3	677.4	694.7	690.7	685.2	676.8	684.3
75–84 years	1,000.7	924.1	891.9	903.1	937.8	1,010.3	1,057.5	1,061.5	1,060.0	1,050.6	1,057.3
85 years and over	1,299.7	1,263.9	1,096.7	1,255.7	1,281.4	1,372.1	1,397.1	1,429.1	1,426.8	1,439.2	1,431.8
White male											
All ages, age adjusted	130.9	141.6	154.3	160.5	160.4	160.3	154.4	151.8	149.2	145.9	148.9
All ages, crude	147.2	166.1	185.1	208.7	218.1	227.7	228.9	228.1	225.8	223.3	225.7
25–34 years	17.7	18.8	16.2	13.6	13.1	12.3	11.8	11.3	11.3	11.2	11.3
35–44 years	44.5	46.3	50.1	41.1	39.8	35.8	34.5	34.2	33.5	32.3	33.3
45–54 years	150.8	164.1	172.0	175.4	162.0	149.9	138.0	134.3	131.8	129.0	131.6
55–64 years	409.4	450.9	498.1	497.4	512.0	508.2	474.7	460.0	448.9	432.4	446.9
65–74 years	798.7	887.3	997.0	1,070.7	1,076.5	1,090.7	1,074.6	1,064.6	1,057.3	1,038.7	1,053.6
75–84 years	1,367.6	1,413.7	1,592.7	1,779.7	1,817.1	1,883.2	1,831.2	1,810.9	1,771.0	1,746.1	1,775.3
85 years and over	1,732.7	1,791.4	1,772.2	2,375.6	2,449.1	2,715.1	2,780.3	2,805.2	2,723.9	2,695.5	2,740.1
Black male											
All ages, age adjusted	126.1	158.5	198.0	229.9	239.9	248.1	232.6	226.8	221.9	214.8	221.1
All ages, crude	106.6	136.7	171.6	205.5	214.9	221.9	212.1	209.1	207.3	203.0	206.5
25–34 years	18.0	18.4	18.8	14.1	14.9	15.7	15.5	15.2	14.0	14.5	14.6
35–44 years	55.7	72.9	81.3	73.8	69.9	64.3	57.2	57.5	55.0	54.3	55.6
45–54 years	211.7	244.7	311.2	333.0	315.9	302.6	269.5	250.7	242.7	235.3	242.7
55–64 years	490.8	579.7	689.2	812.5	851.3	859.2	772.7	755.3	741.2	723.3	739.8
65–74 years	636.4	938.5	1,168.9	1,417.2	1,532.8	1,613.9	1,547.8	1,509.6	1,473.2	1,412.4	1,464.7
75–84 years	---	1,053.3	1,624.8	2,029.6	2,229.6	2,478.3	2,456.3	2,426.8	2,421.8	2,298.4	2,381.1
85 years and over	---	1,155.2	1,387.0	2,393.9	2,629.0	3,238.3	3,274.6	3,338.2	3,209.7	3,306.2	3,284.0

See footnotes at end of table.

Table 39 (page 2 of 4). **Death rates for malignant neoplasms, according to sex, detailed race, Hispanic origin, and age: United States, selected years 1950–97**

[Data are based on the National Vital Statistics System]

Sex, race, Hispanic origin, and age	1950[1]	1960[1]	1970	1980	1985	1990	1994	1995	1996	1997	1995–97[2]
American Indian or Alaska Native male[3]				Deaths per 100,000 resident population							
All ages, age adjusted	---	---	---	82.1	87.1	83.5	91.3	94.0	94.0	104.0	97.4
All ages, crude	---	---	---	58.1	62.8	61.4	70.7	74.2	75.9	84.7	78.3
25–34 years	---	---	---	*	*	*	*	*	*	*	6.8
35–44 years	---	---	---	*	28.8	22.8	18.9	16.0	18.4	25.0	19.9
45–54 years	*---	---	---	86.9	89.4	86.9	79.8	88.0	76.0	109.3	91.4
55–64 years	---	---	---	213.4	276.6	246.2	287.8	300.3	325.5	336.2	321.0
65–74 years	---	---	---	613.0	584.6	530.6	728.3	670.4	680.1	761.6	704.5
75–84 years	---	---	---	936.4	963.6	1,038.4	892.8	1,111.9	1,036.6	1,041.1	1,061.6
85 years and over	---	---	---	1,471.2	1,133.3	1,654.4	1,135.4	1,081.5	1,284.2	1,011.3	1,124.0
Asian or Pacific Islander male[4]											
All ages, age adjusted	---	---	---	96.4	101.0	99.6	100.9	98.3	93.8	91.7	94.3
All ages, crude	---	---	---	81.9	82.6	82.7	88.1	87.1	87.1	87.0	87.1
25–34 years	---	---	---	6.3	10.0	9.2	9.9	8.8	7.8	9.4	8.7
35–44 years	---	---	---	29.4	25.7	27.7	27.8	27.4	27.4	26.1	27.0
45–54 years	---	---	---	108.2	98.0	92.6	95.4	86.6	85.7	89.0	87.1
55–64 years	---	---	---	298.5	315.0	274.6	270.3	255.4	247.5	261.6	254.9
65–74 years	---	---	---	581.2	631.3	687.2	659.5	640.6	663.6	596.2	632.9
75–84 years	---	---	---	1,147.6	1,251.2	1,229.9	1,288.8	1,278.9	1,199.8	1,160.3	1,209.0
85 years and over	---	---	---	1,798.7	1,800.0	1,837.0	2,385.5	2,712.8	1,668.4	1,674.0	1,922.8
Hispanic male[5]											
All ages, age adjusted	---	---	---	---	92.1	99.8	97.4	98.6	93.1	91.4	94.2
All ages, crude	---	---	---	---	56.1	65.5	67.4	68.9	65.8	65.4	66.6
25–34 years	---	---	---	---	9.7	8.0	9.3	9.2	8.0	8.8	8.7
35–44 years	---	---	---	---	23.0	22.5	22.5	25.4	22.0	22.5	23.3
45–54 years	---	---	---	---	83.4	96.6	85.5	85.8	81.6	87.3	84.9
55–64 years	---	---	---	---	259.0	294.0	269.9	276.8	262.2	256.0	264.7
65–74 years	---	---	---	---	599.1	655.5	663.9	667.1	647.9	627.2	646.9
75–84 years	---	---	---	---	1,216.6	1,233.4	1,241.4	1,272.1	1,178.3	1,123.5	1,187.1
85 years and over	---	---	---	---	1,700.7	2,019.4	1,962.5	1,858.7	1,637.8	1,658.8	1,709.4
White, non-Hispanic male[5]											
All ages, age adjusted	---	---	---	---	156.0	163.3	156.8	154.0	151.7	148.6	151.4
All ages, crude	---	---	---	---	217.4	246.2	248.1	247.1	246.2	244.7	246.0
25–34 years	---	---	---	---	13.5	12.8	12.1	11.4	11.8	11.5	11.6
35–44 years	---	---	---	---	39.1	36.8	35.4	34.7	34.4	33.1	34.1
45–54 years	---	---	---	---	159.9	153.9	141.0	137.0	134.9	131.9	134.5
55–64 years	---	---	---	---	496.4	520.6	486.4	469.9	458.6	443.3	457.1
65–74 years	---	---	---	---	1,044.2	1,109.0	1,091.2	1,081.1	1,073.6	1,057.8	1,070.9
75–84 years	---	---	---	---	1,766.1	1,906.6	1,846.0	1,825.6	1,791.6	1,765.7	1,793.6
85 years and over	---	---	---	---	2,327.6	2,744.4	2,776.3	2,814.6	2,764.3	2,738.3	2,771.4
White female											
All ages, age adjusted	119.4	109.5	107.6	107.7	110.5	111.2	109.9	108.9	107.6	106.0	107.5
All ages, crude	139.9	139.8	149.4	170.3	184.4	196.1	201.9	202.4	201.8	200.4	201.6
25–34 years	20.9	18.8	16.3	13.5	12.7	11.9	11.8	11.5	12.1	11.2	11.6
35–44 years	74.5	66.6	62.4	50.9	47.3	46.2	41.8	42.0	40.5	40.6	41.0
45–54 years	185.8	175.7	177.3	166.4	161.6	150.9	139.4	136.1	131.0	128.4	131.8
55–64 years	362.5	329.0	338.6	355.5	376.3	368.5	356.5	352.6	347.3	339.6	346.4
65–74 years	616.5	562.1	554.7	605.2	644.9	675.1	694.3	689.6	684.6	674.6	683.0
75–84 years	1,026.6	939.3	903.5	905.4	938.2	1,011.8	1,056.5	1,060.2	1,059.9	1,049.7	1,056.5
85 years and over	1,348.3	1,304.9	1,126.6	1,266.8	1,285.4	1,372.3	1,395.6	1,428.2	1,430.1	1,435.8	1,431.4

See footnotes at end of table.

Table 39 (page 3 of 4). Death rates for malignant neoplasms, according to sex, detailed race, Hispanic origin, and age: United States, selected years 1950–97

[Data are based on the National Vital Statistics System]

Sex, race, Hispanic origin, and age	1950[1]	1960[1]	1970	1980	1985	1990	1994	1995	1996	1997	1995–97[2]
Black female					Deaths per 100,000 resident population						
All ages, age adjusted	131.9	127.8	123.5	129.7	131.8	137.2	133.7	134.1	130.7	131.2	132.0
All ages, crude	111.8	113.8	117.3	136.5	145.2	156.1	157.6	159.1	157.9	160.5	159.2
25–34 years	34.3	31.0	20.9	18.3	17.2	18.7	16.3	16.8	16.4	16.2	16.5
35–44 years	119.8	102.4	94.6	73.5	69.0	67.4	64.6	62.2	62.8	62.9	62.6
45–54 years	277.0	254.8	228.6	230.2	212.4	209.9	192.0	192.7	182.8	180.6	185.2
55–64 years	484.6	442.7	404.8	450.4	474.9	482.4	445.8	443.6	422.2	426.4	430.6
65–74 years	477.3	541.6	615.8	662.4	704.2	773.2	794.5	799.6	790.6	789.7	793.3
75–84 years	- - -	696.3	763.3	923.9	986.3	1,059.9	1,139.3	1,154.1	1,150.9	1,166.5	1,157.2
85 years and over	- - -	728.9	791.5	1,159.9	1,284.2	1,431.3	1,469.2	1,490.3	1,507.2	1,602.3	1,534.3
American Indian or Alaska Native female[3]											
All ages, age adjusted	- - -	- - -	- - -	62.1	60.5	69.6	68.0	70.7	78.6	72.8	74.0
All ages, crude	- - -	- - -	- - -	50.4	52.5	62.1	65.8	69.9	77.1	71.8	73.0
25–34 years	- - -	- - -	- - -	*	*	*	*	11.1	*	11.0	9.8
35–44 years	- - -	- - -	- - -	36.9	23.4	31.0	24.1	33.5	38.5	36.8	36.3
45–54 years	- - -	- - -	- - -	96.9	90.1	104.5	86.4	85.2	111.2	88.3	94.9
55–64 years	- - -	- - -	- - -	198.4	192.3	213.3	224.9	223.2	249.2	245.5	239.5
65–74 years	- - -	- - -	- - -	350.8	378.8	438.9	440.7	427.7	487.3	467.5	461.0
75–84 years	- - -	- - -	- - -	446.4	505.9	554.3	618.5	723.9	721.4	613.4	684.8
85 years and over	- - -	- - -	- - -	786.5	700.0	843.7	708.6	736.6	638.0	561.9	640.0
Asian or Pacific Islander female[4]											
All ages, age adjusted	- - -	- - -	- - -	59.8	62.8	63.6	67.3	68.4	63.2	63.0	64.7
All ages, crude	- - -	- - -	- - -	54.1	57.5	60.5	69.7	71.5	69.7	71.1	70.8
25–34 years	- - -	- - -	- - -	9.5	9.9	7.3	10.1	10.6	9.6	7.0	9.0
35–44 years	- - -	- - -	- - -	38.7	33.1	29.8	30.1	28.6	29.9	31.5	30.0
45–54 years	- - -	- - -	- - -	99.8	91.3	93.9	90.2	98.0	88.7	81.1	88.9
55–64 years	- - -	- - -	- - -	174.7	195.5	196.2	198.4	211.4	179.6	176.7	188.6
65–74 years	- - -	- - -	- - -	301.9	330.8	346.2	352.2	351.2	347.8	376.4	358.8
75–84 years	- - -	- - -	- - -	522.1	589.1	641.4	769.7	722.6	703.6	662.1	694.1
85 years and over	- - -	- - -	- - -	800.0	908.3	971.7	1,214.4	1,307.7	917.8	1,014.0	1,053.6
Hispanic female[5]											
All ages, age adjusted	- - -	- - -	- - -	- - -	64.1	70.0	67.1	66.1	66.7	65.4	66.1
All ages, crude	- - -	- - -	- - -	- - -	49.8	60.7	60.7	60.5	62.1	61.4	61.4
25–34 years	- - -	- - -	- - -	- - -	9.7	9.7	10.3	9.2	10.3	10.3	9.9
35–44 years	- - -	- - -	- - -	- - -	30.9	34.8	33.4	31.2	30.0	30.5	30.6
45–54 years	- - -	- - -	- - -	- - -	90.1	100.5	95.2	89.7	85.3	84.7	86.5
55–64 years	- - -	- - -	- - -	- - -	199.4	205.4	200.0	197.6	202.4	201.6	200.6
65–74 years	- - -	- - -	- - -	- - -	356.3	404.8	384.5	382.3	405.3	388.2	392.0
75–84 years	- - -	- - -	- - -	- - -	599.7	663.0	628.4	659.6	637.8	622.4	639.3
85 years and over	- - -	- - -	- - -	- - -	906.1	1,022.7	912.9	938.2	913.9	888.6	911.9

See footnotes at end of table.

Table 39 (page 4 of 4). Death rates for malignant neoplasms, according to sex, detailed race, Hispanic origin, and age: United States, selected years 1950–97

[Data are based on the National Vital Statistics System]

Sex, race, Hispanic origin, and age	1950[1]	1960[1]	1970	1980	1985	1990	1994	1995	1996	1997	1995–97[2]
White, non-Hispanic female[5]					Deaths per 100,000 resident population						
All ages, age adjusted	- - -	- - -	- - -	- - -	108.9	113.6	111.7	111.1	109.8	108.1	109.6
All ages, crude	- - -	- - -	- - -	- - -	187.1	210.6	217.5	218.4	218.3	217.3	218.0
25–34 years	- - -	- - -	- - -	- - -	12.2	11.9	11.8	11.7	12.2	11.2	11.7
35–44 years	- - -	- - -	- - -	- - -	47.2	47.0	42.1	42.7	41.2	41.4	41.8
45–54 years	- - -	- - -	- - -	- - -	158.8	154.9	141.7	139.3	133.9	131.2	134.7
55–64 years	- - -	- - -	- - -	- - -	372.7	379.5	366.1	362.7	356.6	348.5	355.8
65–74 years	- - -	- - -	- - -	- - -	638.3	688.5	706.8	703.1	697.9	688.7	696.6
75–84 years	- - -	- - -	- - -	- - -	917.7	1,027.2	1,069.6	1,070.5	1,075.3	1,063.9	1,069.8
85 years and over	- - -	- - -	- - -	- - -	1,241.6	1,385.7	1,397.7	1,438.4	1,448.8	1,452.5	1,446.7

- - - Data not available.

* Based on fewer than 20 deaths.

[1]Includes deaths of persons who were not residents of the 50 States and the District of Columbia.

[2]Average annual death rate.

[3]Interpretation of trends should take into account that population estimates for American Indians increased by 45 percent between 1980 and 1990, partly due to better enumeration techniques in the 1990 decennial census and to the increased tendency for people to identify themselves as American Indian in 1990.

[4]Interpretation of trends should take into account that the Asian population in the United States more than doubled between 1980 and 1990, primarily due to immigration.

[5]Excludes data from States lacking an Hispanic-origin item on their death certificates. See Appendix I, National Vital Statistics System.

NOTES: For data years shown, the code numbers for cause of death are based on the then current *International Classification of Diseases*, which are described in Appendix II, tables IV and V. Age groups were selected to minimize the presentation of unstable age-specific death rates based on small numbers of deaths and for consistency among comparison groups. The race groups, white, black, Asian or Pacific Islander, and American Indian or Alaska Native, include persons of Hispanic and non-Hispanic origin. Conversely, persons of Hispanic origin may be of any race. Consistency of race identification between the death certificate (source of data for numerator of death rates) and data from the Census Bureau (denominator) is high for individual white and black persons; however, persons identified as American Indian, Asian, or Hispanic origin in data from the Census Bureau are sometimes misreported as white or non-Hispanic on the death certificate, causing death rates to be underestimated by 22–30 percent for American Indians, about 12 percent for Asians, and about 7 percent for persons of Hispanic origin. (Sorlie PD, Rogot E, and Johnson NJ: Validity of demographic characteristics on the death certificate, *Epidemiology* 3(2):181–184, 1992.) See Appendix II for age-adjustment procedure. Data for additional years are available (see Appendix III).

SOURCES: Centers for Disease Control and Prevention, National Center for Health Statistics. Grove RD and Hetzel AM. *Vital statistics rates in the United States, 1940–60*. Washington: Public Health Service, 1968; *Vital statistics of the United States, vol II, mortality, part A*, for data years 1950–93. Public Health Service. Washington. U.S. Government Printing Office; for 1994–97, unpublished data; data computed by the Division of Health and Utilization Analysis from numerator data compiled by the Division of Vital Statistics and denominator data from national population estimates for race groups from table 1 and unpublished Hispanic population estimates prepared by the Housing and Household Economic Statistics Division, U.S. Bureau of the Census.

Table 40 (page 1 of 3). Death rates for malignant neoplasms of respiratory system, according to sex, detailed race, Hispanic origin, and age: United States, selected years 1950–97

[Data are based on the National Vital Statistics System]

Sex, race, Hispanic origin, and age	1950[1]	1960[1]	1970	1980	1985	1990	1994	1995	1996	1997	1995–97[2]
All persons	Deaths per 100,000 resident population										
All ages, age adjusted	12.8	19.2	28.4	36.4	39.1	41.4	40.1	39.7	39.3	38.7	39.2
All ages, crude	14.1	22.2	34.2	47.9	53.5	58.9	59.4	59.5	59.3	59.2	59.3
Under 25 years	0.1	0.1	0.1	0.1	0.1	0.1	0.1	0.1	0.0	0.0	0.0
25–34 years	0.9	1.1	1.0	0.8	0.8	0.8	0.7	0.7	0.8	0.7	0.7
35–44 years	5.1	7.3	11.6	9.6	8.2	7.2	6.5	6.4	6.5	6.5	6.5
45–54 years	22.9	32.0	46.2	56.5	53.1	48.8	40.9	39.8	38.5	36.2	38.1
55–64 years	55.2	81.5	116.2	144.3	159.8	166.5	153.5	148.2	144.3	139.7	144.0
65–74 years	69.3	117.2	174.6	243.1	270.3	298.1	305.9	306.1	305.2	304.4	305.2
75–84 years	69.3	102.9	175.1	251.4	292.4	344.1	367.4	372.7	375.1	379.1	375.7
85 years and over	64.0	79.1	113.5	184.5	205.0	252.9	278.7	294.0	290.9	308.2	297.9
Male											
All ages, age adjusted	21.3	34.8	50.6	59.7	60.7	61.0	56.5	55.3	54.2	52.8	54.0
All ages, crude	23.1	38.5	57.0	71.9	75.6	78.3	75.4	74.6	73.6	72.7	73.6
Under 25 years	0.2	0.1	0.1	0.1	0.1	0.1	0.1	0.1	0.0	0.1	0.1
25–34 years	1.3	1.7	1.5	1.0	0.9	1.0	0.8	0.8	0.9	0.8	0.8
35–44 years	8.1	11.4	17.0	12.6	10.6	9.1	8.0	7.6	7.8	7.5	7.6
45–54 years	39.3	54.7	72.1	79.8	71.0	63.0	51.9	49.9	48.5	45.2	47.8
55–64 years	94.2	150.2	202.3	223.8	233.6	232.6	206.8	196.1	190.7	182.7	189.7
65–74 years	116.3	221.7	340.7	422.0	432.5	447.3	434.5	432.4	424.6	418.8	425.3
75–84 years	105.1	188.5	354.2	511.5	558.9	594.4	576.7	573.4	566.9	562.9	567.6
85 years and over	95.4	132.2	215.3	386.3	457.3	538.0	556.1	567.6	543.2	568.8	559.9
Female											
All ages, age adjusted	4.6	5.2	10.1	18.3	22.5	26.2	27.3	27.5	27.5	27.5	27.5
All ages, crude	5.2	6.2	12.6	25.2	32.6	40.4	44.2	45.1	45.6	46.3	45.6
Under 25 years	0.1	0.1	0.1	0.1	0.1	0.0	*	0.0	*	*	0.0
25–34 years	0.6	0.6	0.6	0.6	0.7	0.6	0.6	0.7	0.7	0.6	0.6
35–44 years	2.3	3.4	6.5	6.8	5.8	5.4	4.9	5.1	5.3	5.6	5.4
45–54 years	6.7	10.1	22.2	34.8	36.2	35.3	30.4	30.1	29.0	27.5	28.8
55–64 years	15.4	17.0	38.9	74.5	94.5	107.6	105.3	104.8	102.2	100.7	102.6
65–74 years	26.7	26.2	45.6	106.1	145.3	181.7	203.6	205.0	209.0	212.0	208.7
75–84 years	38.8	36.5	56.5	98.0	135.7	194.5	236.4	245.1	251.1	258.9	251.8
85 years and over	42.0	45.2	56.5	96.3	104.2	142.8	171.8	187.5	190.6	203.2	193.9
White male											
All ages, age adjusted	21.6	34.6	49.9	58.0	58.7	59.0	54.8	53.7	52.6	51.4	52.5
All ages, crude	24.1	39.6	58.3	73.4	77.6	81.0	78.5	77.8	76.8	76.0	76.9
45–54 years	39.1	53.0	67.6	74.3	65.5	57.9	47.4	46.0	45.0	41.7	44.2
55–64 years	95.9	149.8	199.3	215.0	223.3	222.5	199.4	188.2	182.4	175.2	181.9
65–74 years	119.4	225.1	344.8	418.4	425.2	438.2	427.0	426.1	419.1	414.2	419.8
75–84 years	109.1	191.9	360.7	516.1	561.7	593.6	571.8	569.2	562.7	559.1	563.6
85 years and over	102.7	133.9	221.8	391.5	463.8	540.4	552.3	565.3	547.5	573.6	562.2
Black male											
All ages, age adjusted	16.9	36.6	60.8	82.0	87.7	91.0	82.8	80.5	78.5	75.4	78.1
All ages, crude	14.3	31.1	51.2	70.8	75.5	77.8	72.5	71.2	70.1	68.3	69.9
45–54 years	41.1	75.0	123.5	142.8	133.1	125.0	104.2	96.4	92.5	86.3	91.5
55–64 years	78.8	161.8	250.3	340.3	373.2	377.5	322.2	315.0	310.8	292.2	305.9
65–74 years	65.2	184.6	322.2	499.4	565.9	613.4	581.1	573.9	550.0	534.5	552.6
75–84 years	- - -	126.3	290.6	499.6	579.0	669.9	708.1	695.3	692.3	693.3	693.6
85 years and over	- - -	110.3	154.4	337.7	409.7	535.7	623.2	607.3	566.3	588.8	587.2
American Indian or Alaska Native male[3]											
All ages, age adjusted	- - -	- - -	- - -	23.2	28.4	29.7	31.1	32.7	34.5	35.5	34.3
All ages, crude	- - -	- - -	- - -	15.7	19.6	21.1	23.0	25.1	26.4	27.9	26.5
45–54 years	- - -	- - -	- - -	*	*	26.6	22.6	28.4	26.2	33.8	29.6
55–64 years	- - -	- - -	- - -	80.0	95.7	106.8	119.8	114.3	142.9	129.5	129.0
65–74 years	- - -	- - -	- - -	221.2	234.6	206.7	290.8	258.7	273.1	283.7	272.0
75–84 years	- - -	- - -	- - -	*	281.8	371.4	220.1	368.6	325.0	361.2	351.4
85 years and over	- - -	- - -	- - -	*	*	*	*	*	*	*	216.2

See footnotes at end of table.

[Data are based on the National Vital Statistics System]

Sex, race, Hispanic origin, and age	1950[1]	1960[1]	1970	1980	1985	1990	1994	1995	1996	1997	1995–97[2]
Asian or Pacific Islander male[4]				Deaths per 100,000 resident population							
All ages, age adjusted	---	---	---	27.6	26.9	26.8	28.0	25.8	25.8	25.2	25.5
All ages, crude	---	---	---	22.9	21.3	21.7	23.9	22.4	23.4	23.3	23.0
45–54 years	---	---	---	34.0	23.8	19.3	23.6	20.2	17.3	18.3	18.6
55–64 years	---	---	---	98.0	101.2	79.7	76.4	69.6	71.8	74.6	72.1
65–74 years	---	---	---	179.9	188.9	222.6	218.8	197.0	213.4	202.4	204.4
75–84 years	---	---	---	308.1	297.7	319.7	369.3	341.7	350.8	311.9	334.0
85 years and over	---	---	---	*	375.0	438.2	535.8	607.6	352.2	375.9	423.1
Hispanic male[5]											
All ages, age adjusted	---	---	---	---	24.0	27.7	24.8	25.2	23.9	23.1	24.0
All ages, crude	---	---	---	---	13.9	17.4	16.5	16.9	16.1	15.9	16.3
45–54 years	---	---	---	---	18.3	23.4	21.1	19.8	20.7	18.8	19.7
55–64 years	---	---	---	---	73.8	88.0	73.0	75.2	72.3	66.5	71.2
65–74 years	---	---	---	---	181.3	210.7	187.6	196.9	189.6	187.4	191.2
75–84 years	---	---	---	---	306.6	328.8	323.6	324.5	297.0	290.7	303.1
85 years and over	---	---	---	---	418.8	458.1	410.8	385.4	302.6	369.8	351.2
White, non-Hispanic male[5]											
All ages, age adjusted	---	---	---	---	57.2	60.5	56.3	55.0	54.0	53.0	54.0
All ages, crude	---	---	---	---	77.5	88.1	85.7	85.0	84.5	84.3	84.6
45–54 years	---	---	---	---	65.4	60.4	49.1	47.7	46.6	43.5	45.9
55–64 years	---	---	---	---	218.3	229.8	206.9	194.7	188.8	182.8	188.7
65–74 years	---	---	---	---	413.7	447.5	437.0	435.1	429.0	425.9	430.0
75–84 years	---	---	---	---	538.4	602.5	577.5	575.2	571.0	568.6	571.5
85 years and over	---	-	---	---	433.2	544.3	547.8	565.3	556.1	581.2	567.8
White female											
All ages, age adjusted	4.6	5.1	10.1	18.2	22.7	26.5	27.7	27.9	28.0	28.0	28.0
All ages, crude	5.4	6.4	13.1	26.5	34.8	43.4	47.9	48.9	49.6	50.2	49.6
45–54 years	6.5	9.8	22.1	33.9	36.2	35.2	30.5	30.1	23.1	27.4	28.8
55–64 years	15.5	16.7	39.3	74.2	94.7	108.0	107.1	106.8	105.1	102.9	104.9
65–74 years	27.2	26.5	45.4	108.1	149.0	185.3	207.9	208.7	213.9	216.8	213.1
75–84 years	40.0	36.5	56.8	99.3	138.7	199.0	241.2	250.8	256.3	264.2	257.2
85 years and over	44.0	45.2	57.4	96.8	103.2	143.2	173.2	188.4	193.1	205.2	195.7
Black female											
All ages, age adjusted	4.1	5.5	10.9	19.5	22.8	27.5	27.7	27.8	27.6	28.3	27.9
All ages, crude	3.4	4.9	10.1	19.3	23.5	29.2	30.8	31.3	31.6	32.9	31.9
45–54 years	8.8	12.8	25.3	46.4	41.5	43.4	36.0	36.6	34.9	34.9	35.4
55–64 years	15.3	20.7	36.4	83.8	107.8	122.8	111.6	110.0	103.2	105.3	106.2
65–74 years	16.4	20.7	49.3	91.7	120.6	169.9	196.4	202.0	203.0	206.6	203.9
75–84 years	---	33.1	52.6	81.1	105.6	153.8	198.2	195.3	213.6	225.1	211.5
85 years and over	---	44.7	47.6	90.5	117.3	138.1	157.3	171.4	167.0	190.9	176.6
American Indian or Alaska Native female[3]											
All ages, age adjusted	---	---	---	8.1	11.1	13.5	17.7	16.4	16.0	16.9	16.5
All ages, crude	---	---	---	6.4	9.2	11.3	16.5	15.5	15.4	16.0	15.7
45–54 years	---	---	---	*	*	22.9	23.0	*	*	*	13.9
55–64 years	---	---	---	*	38.5	53.7	66.6	49.3	62.3	70.0	60.7
65–74 years	---	---	---	*	100.0	80.9	123.7	136.1	102.1	136.3	124.8
75–84 years	---	---	---	*	*	111.8	181.4	193.0	196.7	152.4	180.2
85 years and over	---	---	---	*	*	*	*	*	*	*	74.1

See footnotes at end of table.

Table 40 (page 3 of 3). Death rates for malignant neoplasms of respiratory system, according to sex, detailed race, Hispanic origin, and age: United States, selected years 1950–97

[Data are based on the National Vital Statistics System]

Sex, race, Hispanic origin, and age	1950[1]	1960[1]	1970	1980	1985	1990	1994	1995	1996	1997	1995–97[2]
Asian or Pacific Islander female[4]				Deaths per 100,000 resident population							
All ages, age adjusted	---	---	---	9.5	9.2	11.3	11.2	13.0	10.9	11.5	11.7
All ages, crude	---	---	---	8.4	8.2	10.6	11.4	13.6	12.2	13.0	12.9
45–54 years	---	---	---	13.5	12.8	11.6	11.2	12.1	11.2	10.0	11.0
55–64 years	---	---	---	25.4	26.0	39.5	36.3	39.1	30.1	32.5	33.8
65–74 years	---	---	---	62.4	63.2	71.6	72.7	87.8	76.9	80.4	81.6
75–84 years	---	---	---	117.7	100.0	139.4	147.7	165.0	150.4	150.7	154.8
85 years and over	---	---	---	*	*	172.9	174.9	291.1	185.5	173.5	207.5
Hispanic female[5]											
All ages, age adjusted	---	---	---	---	6.7	8.7	8.5	8.2	8.6	8.9	8.6
All ages, crude	---	---	---	---	5.2	7.5	7.7	7.5	8.1	8.3	8.0
45–54 years	---	---	---	---	6.8	9.0	9.2	7.3	6.3	7.4	7.0
55–64 years	---	---	---	---	18.7	26.0	26.9	25.1	27.2	28.2	26.9
65–74 years	---	---	---	---	51.4	68.1	62.5	57.8	67.6	68.2	64.7
75–84 years	---	---	---	---	79.1	95.8	88.9	106.7	102.0	103.0	103.9
85 years and over	---	---	---	---	121.4	125.1	138.8	120.5	125.8	118.9	121.7
White, non-Hispanic female[5]											
All ages, age adjusted	---	---	---	---	23.2	27.5	28.8	29.1	29.2	29.2	29.2
All ages, crude	---	---	---	---	36.5	47.2	52.5	53.7	54.6	55.5	54.6
45–54 years	---	---	---	---	37.5	37.2	32.1	32.0	30.9	29.0	30.6
55–64 years	---	---	---	---	95.5	113.7	112.5	112.7	110.6	108.4	110.6
65–74 years	---	---	---	---	152.7	190.5	214.6	215.9	221.5	225.0	220.8
75–84 years	---	---	---	---	141.8	203.5	246.8	255.2	262.1	270.3	262.6
85 years and over	---	---	---	---	104.5	143.9	172.1	189.6	195.8	208.0	198.0

- - - Data not available.

* Based on fewer than 20 deaths.

0.0 Quantity more than zero but less than 0.05.

[1]Includes deaths of persons who were not residents of the 50 States and the District of Columbia.

[2]Average annual death rate.

[3]Interpretation of trends should take into account that population estimates for American Indians increased by 45 percent between 1980 and 1990, partly due to better enumeration techniques in the 1990 decennial census and to the increased tendency for people to identify themselves as American Indian in 1990.

[4]Interpretation of trends should take into account that the Asian population in the United States more than doubled between 1980 and 1990, primarily due to immigration.

[5]Excludes data from States lacking an Hispanic-origin item on their death certificates. See Appendix I, National Vital Statistics System.

NOTES: For data years shown, the code numbers for cause of death are based on the then current International Classification of Diseases, which are described in Appendix II, tables IV and V. Age groups were selected to minimize the presentation of unstable age-specific death rates based on small numbers of deaths and for consistency among comparison groups. The race groups, white, black, Asian or Pacific Islander, and American Indian or Alaska Native, include persons of Hispanic and non-Hispanic origin. Conversely, persons of Hispanic origin may be of any race. Consistency of race identification between the death certificate (source of data for numerator of death rates) and data from the Census Bureau (denominator) is high for individual white and black persons; however, persons identified as American Indian, Asian, or Hispanic origin in data from the Census Bureau are sometimes misreported as white or non-Hispanic on the death certificate, causing death rates to be underestimated by 22–30 percent for American Indians, about 12 percent for Asians, and about 7 percent for persons of Hispanic origin. (Sorlie PD, Rogot E, and Johnson NJ: Validity of demographic characteristics on the death certificate, Epidemiology 3(2):181–184, 1992.) See Appendix II for age-adjustment procedure. Data for additional years are available (see Appendix III).

SOURCES: Centers for Disease Control and Prevention, National Center for Health Statistics. Grove RD and Hetzel AM. Vital statistics rates in the United States, 1940–60. Washington: Public Health Service, 1968; Vital statistics of the United States, vol II, mortality, part A, for data years 1950–93. Public Health Service. Washington. U.S. Government Printing Office; for 1994–97, unpublished data; data computed by the Division of Health and Utilization Analysis from numerator data compiled by the Division of Vital Statistics and denominator data from national population estimates for race groups from table 1 and unpublished Hispanic population estimates prepared by the Housing and Household Economic Statistics Division, U.S. Bureau of the Census.

Table 41 (page 1 of 2). Death rates for malignant neoplasm of breast for females, according to detailed race, Hispanic origin, and age: United States, selected years 1950–97

[Data are based on the National Vital Statistics System]

Race, Hispanic origin, and age	1950[1]	1960[1]	1970	1980	1985	1990	1994	1995	1996	1997	1995–97[2]
All persons					Deaths per 100,000 resident population						
All ages, age adjusted	22.2	22.3	23.1	22.7	23.3	23.1	21.3	21.0	20.2	19.4	20.2
All ages, crude	24.7	26.1	28.4	30.6	32.8	34.0	32.7	32.6	31.8	30.7	31.7
Under 25 years	*	*	*	*	0.0	*	*	*	0.0	*	0.0
25–34 years	3.8	3.8	3.9	3.3	3.0	2.9	2.7	2.7	2.7	2.6	2.7
35–44 years	20.8	20.2	20.4	17.9	17.5	17.8	15.2	15.0	14.2	14.0	14.4
45–54 years	46.9	51.4	52.6	48.1	47.1	45.4	41.6	41.4	38.8	37.8	39.3
55–64 years	70.4	70.8	77.6	80.5	84.2	78.6	69.8	69.8	67.4	64.4	67.2
65–74 years	94.0	90.0	93.8	101.1	107.8	111.7	105.6	103.3	99.1	94.1	98.9
75–84 years	139.8	129.9	127.4	126.4	136.2	146.3	145.9	142.0	139.8	132.2	137.9
85 years and over	195.5	191.9	157.1	169.3	178.5	196.8	197.5	203.7	204.9	198.5	202.3
White											
All ages, age adjusted	22.5	22.4	23.4	22.8	23.4	22.9	20.9	20.5	19.8	18.9	19.7
All ages, crude	25.7	27.2	29.9	32.3	34.7	35.9	34.4	34.1	33.3	31.9	33.1
35–44 years	20.8	19.7	20.2	17.3	16.8	17.1	14.2	14.1	12.9	12.9	13.3
45–54 years	47.1	51.2	53.0	48.1	46.8	44.3	40.2	39.2	36.9	36.1	37.4
55–64 years	70.9	71.8	79.3	81.3	84.7	78.5	69.1	68.7	67.2	62.8	66.2
65–74 years	96.3	91.6	95.9	103.7	109.9	113.3	106.5	103.9	99.8	93.6	99.2
75–84 years	143.6	132.8	129.6	128.4	138.8	148.2	147.1	143.0	140.6	132.3	138.6
85 years and over	204.2	199.7	161.9	171.7	180.9	198.0	197.8	205.9	207.1	199.9	204.3
Black											
All ages, age adjusted	19.3	21.3	21.5	23.3	25.5	27.5	26.9	27.5	26.5	26.7	26.9
All ages, crude	16.4	18.7	19.7	22.9	25.9	29.0	29.6	30.2	29.9	30.4	30.2
35–44 years	21.0	24.8	24.4	24.1	26.1	25.8	24.6	23.1	24.6	23.1	23.6
45–54 years	46.5	54.4	52.0	52.7	55.5	60.5	58.3	62.6	59.1	56.4	59.3
55–64 years	64.3	63.2	64.7	79.9	90.4	93.1	87.5	88.8	82.9	88.1	86.6
65–74 years	67.0	72.3	77.3	84.3	100.7	112.2	116.0	117.3	109.9	117.7	115.0
75–84 years	---	87.5	101.8	114.1	117.6	140.5	150.7	151.6	152.9	154.0	152.8
85 years and over	---	92.1	112.1	149.9	159.4	201.5	209.9	198.6	206.9	211.2	205.7
American Indian or Alaska Native[3]											
All ages, age adjusted	---	---	---	8.1	8.0	10.0	10.4	10.4	12.7	9.4	10.8
All ages, crude	---	---	---	6.1	6.9	8.6	9.6	9.8	12.1	9.0	10.3
35–44 years	---	---	---	*	*	*	*	*	*	*	7.5
45–54 years	---	---	---	*	*	23.9	22.1	24.0	28.0	19.6	23.8
55–64 years	---	---	---	*	*	*	29.6	39.1	43.9	32.9	38.6
65–74 years	---	---	---	*	*	*	60.8	45.4	66.0	48.2	53.2
75–84 years	---	---	---	*	*	*	*	*	*	*	55.3
85 years and over	---	---	---	*	*	*	*	*	*	*	80.0
Asian or Pacific Islander[4]											
All ages, age adjusted	---	---	---	9.2	9.6	10.0	10.5	11.0	8.9	9.2	9.7
All ages, crude	---	---	---	8.2	8.6	9.3	10.7	11.1	9.6	9.9	10.2
35–44 years	---	---	---	10.4	7.2	8.4	8.5	8.3	8.8	8.2	8.4
45–54 years	---	---	---	23.4	21.9	26.4	26.4	30.2	22.0	23.2	25.0
55–64 years	---	---	---	35.7	39.5	33.8	33.5	39.4	23.0	33.1	31.7
65–74 years	---	---	---	*	32.5	38.5	35.5	37.4	40.2	34.1	37.2
75–84 years	---	---	---	*	50.0	48.0	63.3	44.9	51.0	40.6	45.4
85 years and over	---	---	---	*	*	*	111.7	*	*	68.8	61.8
Hispanic[5]											
All ages, age adjusted	---	---	---	---	11.8	14.1	12.6	12.7	12.8	12.6	12.7
All ages, crude	---	---	---	---	8.8	11.5	10.7	10.9	11.4	11.2	11.2
35–44 years	---	---	---	---	10.4	11.7	11.6	9.7	11.0	9.9	10.2
45–54 years	---	---	---	---	26.4	32.8	28.0	27.7	27.4	26.7	27.3
55–64 years	---	---	---	---	43.5	45.8	43.0	43.8	39.7	45.4	43.0
65–74 years	---	---	---	---	40.9	64.8	51.2	55.7	56.5	52.9	55.0
75–84 years	---	---	---	---	64.5	67.2	72.8	75.5	85.6	71.6	77.5
85 years and over	---	---	---	---	85.7	102.8	76.2	105.4	104.5	101.9	103.8

See footnotes at end of table.

Table 41 (page 2 of 2). Death rates for malignant neoplasm of breast for females, according to detailed race, Hispanic origin, and age: United States, selected years 1950–97

[Data are based on the National Vital Statistics System]

Race, Hispanic origin, and age	1950[1]	1960[1]	1970	1980	1985	1990	1994	1995	1996	1997	1995–97[2]
White, non-Hispanic[5]					Deaths per 100,000 resident population						
All ages, age adjusted	- - -	- - -	- - -	- - -	23.3	23.5	21.3	20.9	20.1	19.2	20.1
All ages, crude	- - -	- - -	- - -	- - -	35.6	38.5	37.0	36.8	35.9	34.4	35.7
35–44 years	- - -	- - -	- - -	- - -	16.9	17.5	14.3	14.4	12.9	13.1	13.4
45–54 years	- - -	- - -	- - -	- - -	46.8	45.2	40.8	39.9	37.5	36.7	38.0
55–64 years . . . . , . .	- - -	- - -	- - -	- - -	85.1	80.6	70.5	70.2	69.0	63.8	67.6
65–74 years	- - -	- - -	- - -	- - -	108.6	115.7	109.0	106.2	102.0	95.7	101.3
75–84 years	- - -	- - -	- - -	- - -	139.4	151.4	149.2	145.2	142.6	134.4	140.6
85 years and over	- - -	- - -	- - -	- - -	175.6	201.5	200.0	208.3	211.7	203.3	207.7

* Based on fewer than 20 deaths.
0.0 Quantity more than zero but less than 0.05.
- - - Data not available.
[1]Includes deaths of persons who were not residents of the 50 States and the District of Columbia.
[2]Average annual death rate.
[3]Interpretation of trends should take into account that population estimates for American Indians increased by 45 percent between 1980 and 1990, partly due to better enumeration techniques in the 1990 decennial census and to the increased tendency for people to identify themselves as American Indian in 1990.
[4]Interpretation of trends should take into account that the Asian population in the United States more than doubled between 1980 and 1990, primarily due to immigration.
[5]Excludes data from States lacking an Hispanic-origin item on their death certificates. See Appendix I, National Vital Statistics System.

NOTES: For data years shown, the code numbers for cause of death are based on the then current *International Classification of Diseases*, which are described in Appendix II, tables IV and V. Age groups were selected to minimize the presentation of unstable age-specific death rates based on small numbers of deaths and for consistency among comparison groups. The race groups, white, black, Asian or Pacific Islander, and American Indian or Alaska Native, include persons of Hispanic and non-Hispanic origin. Conversely, persons of Hispanic origin may be of any race. Consistency of race identification between the death certificate (source of data for numerator of death rates) and data from the Census Bureau (denominator) is high for individual white and black persons; however, persons identified as American Indian, Asian, or Hispanic origin in data from the Census Bureau are sometimes misreported as white or non-Hispanic on the death certificate, causing death rates to be underestimated by 22–30 percent for American Indians, about 12 percent for Asians, and about 7 percent for persons of Hispanic origin. (Sorlie PD, Rogot E, and Johnson NJ: Validity of demographic characteristics on the death certificate, *Epidemiology* 3(2):181–184, 1992.) See Appendix II for age-adjustment procedure. Data for additional years are available (see Appendix III).

SOURCES: Centers for Disease Control and Prevention, National Center for Health Statistics. *Vital statistics of the United States, vol II, mortality, part A*, for data years 1950–93. Public Health Service. Washington. U.S. Government Printing Office; for 1994–97, unpublished data; data computed by the Division of Health and Utilization Analysis from numerator data compiled by the Division of Vital Statistics and denominator data from national population estimates for race groups from table 1 and unpublished Hispanic population estimates prepared by the Housing and Household Economic Statistics Division, U.S. Bureau of the Census.

Table 42 (page 1 of 3). Death rates for chronic obstructive pulmonary diseases, according to sex, detailed race, Hispanic origin, and age: United States, selected years 1980–97

[Data are based on the National Vital Statistics System]

Sex, race, Hispanic origin, and age	1980	1985	1990	1991	1992	1993	1994	1995	1996	1997	1995–97[1]
All persons					Deaths per 100,000 resident population						
All ages, age adjusted	15.9	18.8	19.7	20.1	19.9	21.4	21.0	20.8	21.0	21.1	21.0
All ages, crude	24.7	31.4	34.9	35.9	36.0	39.2	39.0	39.2	40.0	40.7	40.0
Under 1 year	1.6	1.4	1.4	1.5	1.1	1.4	1.4	1.1	1.0	1.3	1.1
1–4 years	0.4	0.3	0.4	0.3	0.4	0.3	0.3	0.2	0.3	0.3	0.3
5–14 years	0.2	0.3	0.3	0.3	0.3	0.4	0.3	0.4	0.4	0.3	0.4
15–24 years	·0.3	0.5	0.5	0.6	0.5	0.6	0.6	0.7	0.7	0.5	0.6
25–34 years	0.5	0.6	0.7	0.8	0.7	0.7	0.9	0.9	0.9	0.9	0.9
35–44 years	1.6	1.6	1.6	1.7	1.8	1.8	1.8	2.0	2.0	2.0	2.0
45–54 years	9.8	10.2	9.1	9.1	8.3	8.7	9.0	8.9	8.7	8.4	8.6
55–64 years	42.7	47.9	48.9	49.7	48.3	51.0	49.2	47.3	47.0	46.3	46.9
65–74 years	129.1	149.2	152.5	156.3	155.5	167.8	163.8	160.6	161.6	165.3	162.5
75–84 years	224.4	289.5	321.1	327.0	326.5	357.3	351.9	351.8	358.3	359.6	356.6
85 years and over	274.0	365.4	433.3	446.9	460.9	493.9	509.7	527.8	540.9	561.9	543.9
Male											
All ages, age adjusted	26.1	28.1	27.2	27.0	26.4	27.8	26.9	26.3	25.9	26.1	26.1
All ages, crude	35.1	40.3	40.8	41.1	40.5	43.2	42.3	42.0	42.0	42.7	42.2
Under 1 year	1.9	2.0	1.6	1.6	1.7	1.5	1.7	1.4	1.3	1.6	1.5
1–4 years	0.5	*	0.5	0.4	0.4	0.4	0.3	0.2	0.4	0.3	0.3
5–14 years	0.2	0.3	0.4	0.4	0.3	0.4	0.4	0.5	0.5	0.4	0.5
15–24 years	0.4	0.4	0.5	0.6	0.6	0.7	0.8	0.7	0.7	0.7	0.7
25–34 years	0.6	0.6	0.7	0.8	0.7	0.6	0.9	0.9	0.8	1.0	0.9
35–44 years	1.7	1.6	1.7	1.8	1.8	1.8	1.8	1.7	1.9	1.9	1.8
45–54 years	12.1	11.3	9.4	9.3	8.7	9.5	9.3	9.0	8.9	8.8	8.9
55–64 years	59.9	60.8	58.6	57.5	56.3	58.1	55.9	52.9	52.2	50.5	51.8
65–74 years	210.0	218.9	204.0	202.4	199.7	208.4	202.0	196.9	192.6	201.3	196.9
75–84 years	437.4	505.2	500.0	495.4	478.6	512.1	490.4	482.5	478.8	469.6	476.8
85 years and over	583.4	758.1	815.1	830.8	830.9	883.1	874.9	896.2	878.6	902.8	892.6
Female											
All ages, age adjusted	8.9	12.5	14.7	15.5	15.5	17.1	17.1	17.1	17.6	17.7	17.5
All ages, crude	15.0	23.0	29.2	31.1	31.8	35.4	35.9	36.4	38.0	38.8	37.8
Under 1 year	1.3	*	1.2	1.4	*	1.2	1.1	*	*	*	0.8
1–4 years	*	*	*	*	0.4	*	*	*	*	*	0.2
5–14 years	0.3	0.4	0.3	0.3	0.3	0.3	0.2	0.2	0.4	0.3	0.3
15–24 years	0.3	0.5	0.5	0.5	0.5	0.4	0.5	0.6	0.6	0.4	0.5
25–34 years	0.5	0.6	0.7	0.7	0.6	0.8	0.9	0.9	0.9	0.8	0.9
35–44 years	1.5	1.5	1.5	1.7	1.7	1.8	1.7	2.2	2.1	2.1	2.1
45–54 years	7.7	9.2	8.8	8.9	7.9	8.0	8.7	8.8	8.4	8.1	8.4
55–64 years	27.6	36.6	40.3	42.7	41.0	44.6	43.1	42.2	42.4	42.6	42.4
65–74 years	67.1	95.5	112.3	120.2	120.7	135.6	133.4	131.5	136.7	136.1	134.7
75–84 years	98.7	162.7	214.2	225.1	233.4	261.5	265.2	268.8	280.4	287.6	279.1
85 years and over	138.7	208.6	286.0	298.6	317.6	344.6	368.8	384.3	406.7	424.5	405.6
White male											
All ages, age adjusted	26.7	28.7	27.4	27.4	26.8	28.2	27.3	26.6	26.3	26.5	26.5
All ages, crude	37.9	43.7	44.3	44.9	44.4	47.3	46.4	46.1	46.1	47.0	46.4
35–44 years	1.2	1.3	1.3	1.4	1.5	1.3	1.4	1.4	1.5	1.5	1.5
45–54 years	11.4	10.5	8.6	8.4	8.3	9.0	8.7	8.3	8.5	8.3	8.3
55–64 years	60.0	60.6	58.7	57.8	56.6	58.5	56.7	53.2	52.3	51.0	52.2
65–74 years	218.4	225.2	208.1	206.7	204.6	213.3	206.9	201.6	198.4	207.5	202.5
75–84 years	459.8	525.5	513.5	511.8	494.1	525.2	504.2	496.3	491.1	481.4	489.4
85 years and over	611.2	798.1	847.0	867.4	862.5	917.6	907.7	924.0	917.5	940.1	927.4
Black male											
All ages, age adjusted	20.9	24.8	26.5	25.9	24.8	26.6	25.7	25.4	24.8	24.5	24.9
All ages, crude	19.3	23.4	25.2	24.5	23.8	25.7	24.9	24.9	24.7	24.6	24.7
35–44 years	5.8	5.3	5.3	5.5	4.7	5.4	4.9	4.3	5.2	4.8	4.8
45–54 years	19.7	19.5	18.8	19.8	15.1	16.9	16.6	17.3	15.4	14.9	15.8
55–64 years	66.6	69.6	67.4	66.7	64.8	65.9	61.0	62.0	63.2	56.6	60.5
65–74 years	142.0	178.2	184.5	183.2	175.1	184.9	181.7	175.1	161.6	170.7	169.1
75–84 years	229.8	321.8	390.9	357.8	354.5	407.1	374.1	366.5	380.7	374.9	374.1
85 years and over	271.6	374.2	498.0	482.6	559.8	560.6	561.7	613.6	579.5	586.5	592.8

See footnotes at end of table.

Table 42 (page 2 of 3). Death rates for chronic obstructive pulmonary diseases, according to sex, detailed race, Hispanic origin, and age: United States, selected years 1980–97

[Data are based on the National Vital Statistics System]

Sex, race, Hispanic origin, and age	1980	1985	1990	1991	1992	1993	1994	1995	1996	1997	1995–97[1]
American Indian or Alaska Native male[2]				Deaths per 100,000 resident population							
All ages, age adjusted	11.2	14.1	18.5	15.5	14.7	17.3	16.5	16.4	13.7	20.3	16.9
All ages, crude	8.4	10.5	13.8	11.8	11.3	13.4	13.4	13.4	11.9	17.9	14.4
35–44 years	*	*	*	*	*	*	*	*	*	*	*
45–54 years	*	*	*	*	*	*	*	*	*	*	7.5
55–64 years	*	46.8	*	38.6	39.8	42.4	33.3	39.2	*	54.0	40.2
65–74 years	*	*	135.7	132.4	102.9	138.9	130.4	129.3	115.9	127.8	124.3
75–84 years	*	272.7	363.8	221.4	276.8	313.9	301.8	253.8	229.7	339.9	276.2
85 years and over	*	*	*	*	*	*	*	*	421.9	488.8	432.3
Asian or Pacific Islander male[3]											
All ages, age adjusted	9.8	12.0	13.1	12.2	11.6	13.5	12.8	13.5	13.0	12.7	13.0
All ages, crude	8.7	10.1	11.3	10.8	10.3	11.9	11.5	12.3	12.7	12.9	12.7
35–44 years	*	*	*	*	*	*	*	*	*	*	1.2
45–54 years	*	*	*	*	*	*	*	*	*	*	3.0
55–64 years	*	24.4	22.1	15.5	19.6	19.8	15.7	16.4	19.2	16.6	17.4
65–74 years	70.6	72.7	91.4	86.9	94.6	94.1	85.5	91.7	89.9	86.2	89.2
75–84 years	155.7	246.5	258.6	250.8	206.1	278.2	264.2	263.6	294.8	276.3	278.8
85 years and over	472.4	462.5	615.2	561.5	483.8	645.7	660.6	847.8	421.7	568.2	581.8
Hispanic male[4]											
All ages, age adjusted	---	11.8	12.2	12.8	11.3	12.4	12.4	12.7	11.4	11.5	11.9
All ages, crude	---	7.2	8.4	9.0	8.1	9.0	9.0	9.4	8.7	9.0	9.0
35–44 years	---	*	*	*	2.1	1.3	1.3	1.1	1.1	1.5	1.2
45–54 years	---	5.9	4.1	4.7	4.5	3.1	4.6	3.9	4.0	3.5	3.8
55–64 years	---	21.5	17.2	21.9	16.5	21.1	18.2	18.8	18.8	17.6	18.4
65–74 years	---	67.5	81.0	82.9	76.7	77.1	80.3	78.8	68.4	77.2	74.8
75–84 years	---	261.8	252.4	255.1	223.9	244.4	253.5	273.8	240.3	220.2	243.3
85 years and over	---	462.5	613.9	566.7	483.5	666.5	616.2	634.5	579.5	634.3	615.5
White, non-Hispanic male[4]											
All ages, age adjusted	---	29.1	28.2	27.7	27.2	28.5	27.8	27.1	26.9	27.3	27.1
All ages, crude	---	45.3	48.5	48.4	48.2	51.5	50.7	50.4	50.9	52.2	51.2
35–44 years	---	1.3	1.4	1.4	1.4	1.3	1.4	1.4	1.5	1.5	1.4
45–54 years	---	10.7	9.0	8.5	8.3	9.2	8.9	8.5	8.7	8.6	8.6
55–64 years	---	61.6	61.3	59.2	58.5	60.1	58.8	55.2	54.1	53.3	54.2
65–74 years	---	229.9	213.4	209.5	208.4	217.6	211.5	206.5	204.0	214.2	208.2
75–84 years	---	528.7	523.7	514.1	498.2	529.8	510.3	501.9	499.5	491.0	497.3
85 years and over	---	782.4	860.6	876.1	873.1	909.1	908.6	924.5	928.0	951.1	934.9
White female											
All ages, age adjusted	9.2	12.9	15.2	16.1	16.1	17.8	17.8	17.8	18.3	18.5	18.2
All ages, crude	16.4	25.5	32.8	35.0	35.8	40.0	40.6	41.2	43.0	44.1	42.8
35–44 years	1.3	1.3	1.2	1.3	1.3	1.4	1.3	1.7	1.7	1.7	1.7
45–54 years	7.6	9.1	8.3	8.4	7.5	7.6	8.3	8.4	8.0	7.8	8.1
55–64 years	28.7	37.8	41.9	44.7	43.2	47.0	45.2	44.3	44.6	44.8	44.5
65–74 years	71.0	101.1	118.8	127.0	127.7	143.8	141.8	139.8	145.3	145.3	143.5
75–84 years	104.0	171.0	226.3	238.3	246.9	276.1	280.1	282.8	296.4	304.2	294.6
85 years and over	144.2	217.6	298.4	311.6	330.7	361.2	384.9	402.0	423.6	445.0	423.9
Black female											
All ages, age adjusted	6.3	8.8	10.7	11.3	11.2	12.2	12.4	12.5	13.1	12.7	12.8
All ages, crude	6.8	10.0	12.6	13.4	13.7	14.9	15.4	15.8	17.0	16.5	16.4
35–44 years	3.4	2.8	3.8	4.1	4.3	5.3	5.1	5.4	5.0	5.0	5.1
45–54 years	9.3	11.2	14.0	15.0	13.3	12.6	13.5	12.9	13.2	12.2	12.8
55–64 years	20.8	30.6	33.4	34.0	32.1	35.2	35.8	34.7	34.8	35.8	35.1
65–74 years	32.7	48.3	64.7	70.4	73.5	78.3	79.2	78.3	84.3	81.4	81.4
75–84 years	41.1	76.6	96.0	96.0	105.6	120.2	122.1	136.6	137.6	136.9	137.0
85 years and over	63.2	94.0	133.0	142.3	169.0	163.5	195.0	191.4	236.5	220.9	216.6

See footnotes at end of table.

[Data are based on the National Vital Statistics System]

Sex, race, Hispanic origin, and age	1980	1985	1990	1991	1992	1993	1994	1995	1996	1997	1995–97[1]
American Indian or Alaska Native female[2]					Deaths per 100,000 resident population						
All ages, age adjusted	4.5	6.5	8.9	9.4	9.3	13.3	11.1	12.0	11.8	11.4	11.7
All ages, crude	3.8	5.9	8.7	9.6	9.3	12.9	11.5	12.5	13.4	12.2	12.7
35–44 years	*	*	*	*	*	*	*	*	*	*	*
45–54 years	*	*	*	*	*	*	*	*	*	*	7.9
55–64 years	*	*	*	*	*	38.1	34.0	40.6	32.6	35.7	36.2
65–74 years	*	*	56.4	71.4	62.3	114.6	73.8	77.8	78.7	88.1	81.6
75–84 years	*	*	116.7	150.0	128.9	172.2	189.7	168.9	192.9	137.5	166.0
85 years and over	*	*	*	*	*	*	*	*	265.8	171.0	207.4
Asian or Pacific Islander female[3]											
All ages, age adjusted	2.5	5.4	5.2	5.5	4.5	5.0	5.3	5.8	5.3	5.6	5.5
All ages, crude	2.6	5.1	5.2	5.7	4.9	5.4	5.8	6.5	6.5	7.2	6.7
35–44 years	*	*	*	*	*	*	*	*	*	*	1.4
45–54 years	*	*	*	*	*	*	*	3.6	*	*	3.0
55–64 years	*	13.5	15.2	12.1	9.2	7.8	9.4	10.0	11.1	9.2	10.1
65–74 years	*	35.0	26.5	38.4	29.6	31.0	29.4	29.8	32.7	32.2	31.6
75–84 years	*	76.1	80.6	86.3	79.7	102.4	105.5	120.1	81.1	117.7	106.0
85 years and over	*	208.3	232.5	226.3	190.7	191.8	238.0	272.6	240.9	242.3	249.4
Hispanic female[4]											
All ages, age adjusted	- - -	5.7	6.4	6.4	5.9	6.9	6.7	7.1	7.2	6.7	7.0
All ages, crude	- - -	4.8	6.3	6.7	6.3	7.3	7.3	7.9	8.3	7.8	8.0
35–44 years	- - -	*	*	*	1.3	1.2	1.3	1.5	1.3	1.1	1.3
45–54 years	- - -	*	4.9	4.7	4.2	3.6	4.1	4.6	4.1	4.4	4.4
55–64 years	- - -	13.8	14.4	12.7	10.8	12.2	12.1	12.5	13.0	11.7	12.4
65–74 years	- - -	35.0	36.6	37.4	34.5	44.8	41.2	41.4	40.9	38.6	40.3
75–84 years	- - -	99.1	101.1	106.3	109.2	123.0	114.5	116.7	134.1	119.3	123.4
85 years and over	- - -	175.0	269.0	293.9	250.2	290.5	308.4	367.2	342.8	322.6	342.7
White, non-Hispanic female[4]											
All ages, age adjusted	- - -	13.6	15.7	16.4	16.4	18.2	18.3	18.3	18.9	19.1	18.8
All ages, crude	- - -	27.7	35.7	37.6	38.7	43.3	44.4	45.0	47.2	48.6	46.9
35–44 years	- - -	1.2	1.2	1.3	1.3	1.4	1.3	1.7	1.7	1.8	1.7
45–54 years	- - -	9.6	8.5	8.5	7.5	7.7	8.5	8.6	8.2	8.1	8.3
55–64 years	- - -	39.8	43.7	46.3	44.8	49.0	47.3	46.6	46.8	47.3	46.9
65–74 years	- - -	107.6	122.8	129.6	130.8	147.0	146.2	144.0	150.4	151.2	148.5
75–84 years	- - -	179.4	231.9	240.4	250.1	280.1	285.6	288.4	302.5	310.9	300.8
85 years and over	- - -	221.4	302.1	310.6	330.9	358.7	383.6	401.2	426.8	447.9	425.7

* Based on fewer than 20 deaths.

- - - Data not available.

[1]Average annual death rate.

[2]Interpretation of trends should take into account that population estimates for American Indians increased by 45 percent between 1980 and 1990, partly due to better enumeration techniques in the 1990 decennial census and to the increased tendency for people to identify themselves as American Indian in 1990.

[3]Interpretation of trends should take into account that the Asian population in the United States more than doubled between 1980 and 1990, primarily due to immigration.

[4]Excludes data from States lacking an Hispanic-origin item on their death certificates. See Appendix I, National Vital Statistics System.

NOTES: For data years shown, the code numbers for cause of death are based on the then current *International Classification of Diseases*, which are described in Appendix II, tables IV and V. Age groups were selected to minimize the presentation of unstable age-specific death rates based on small numbers of deaths and for consistency among comparison groups. The race groups, white, black, Asian or Pacific Islander, and American Indian or Alaska Native, include persons of Hispanic and non-Hispanic origin. Conversely, persons of Hispanic origin may be of any race. Consistency of race identification between the death certificate (source of data for numerator of death rates) and data from the Census Bureau (denominator) is high for individual white and black persons; however, persons identified as American Indian, Asian, or Hispanic origin in data from the Census Bureau are sometimes misreported as white or non-Hispanic on the death certificate, causing death rates to be underestimated by 22–30 percent for American Indians, about 12 percent for Asians, and about 7 percent for persons of Hispanic origin. (Sorlie PD, Rogot E, and Johnson NJ: Validity of demographic characteristics on the death certificate, *Epidemiology* 3(2):181–184, 1992.) See Appendix II for age-adjustment procedure. Data for additional years are available (see Appendix III).

SOURCES: Centers for Disease Control and Prevention, National Center for Health Statistics. *Vital statistics of the United States, vol II, mortality, part A*, for data years 1980–93. Public Health Service. Washington. U.S. Government Printing Office; for 1994–97, unpublished data; data computed by the Division of Health and Utilization Analysis from numerator data compiled by the Division of Vital Statistics and denominator data from national population estimates for race groups from table 1 and unpublished Hispanic population estimates prepared by the Housing and Household Economic Statistics Division, U.S. Bureau of the Census.

Table 43 (page 1 of 2). Death rates for human immunodeficiency virus (HIV) infection, according to sex, detailed race, Hispanic origin, and age: United States, selected years 1987–97

[Data are based on the National Vital Statistics System]

Sex, race, Hispanic origin, and age	1987	1989	1990	1991	1992	1993	1994	1995	1996	1997	1995–97[1]
All persons					Deaths per 100,000 resident population						
All ages, age adjusted	5.5	8.7	9.8	11.3	12.6	13.8	15.4	15.6	11.1	5.8	10.8
All ages, crude	5.6	8.9	10.1	11.7	13.2	14.5	16.2	16.4	11.7	6.2	11.4
Under 1 year	2.3	3.1	2.7	2.3	2.5	2.2	2.5	1.5	1.1	*	1.0
1–4 years	0.7	0.8	0.8	1.0	1.0	1.3	1.3	1.3	0.9	0.4	0.9
5–14 years	0.1	0.2	0.2	0.3	0.3	0.4	0.5	0.5	0.5	0.3	0.4
15–24 years	1.3	1.6	1.5	1.7	1.6	1.7	1.8	1.7	1.1	0.8	1.2
25–34 years	11.7	17.9	19.7	22.1	24.6	27.0	29.3	29.1	19.9	10.1	19.8
35–44 years	14.0	23.5	27.4	31.2	35.6	39.1	44.1	44.4	31.4	16.1	30.5
45–54 years	8.0	13.3	15.2	18.4	20.3	22.6	25.6	26.3	19.3	10.4	18.5
55–64 years	3.5	5.4	6.2	7.4	8.5	8.8	10.4	11.0	8.4	4.9	8.1
65–74 years	1.3	1.8	2.0	2.4	2.8	2.9	3.1	3.6	2.7	1.8	2.7
75–84 years	0.8	0.7	0.7	0.9	0.8	0.8	0.9	0.7	0.8	0.6	0.7
85 years and over	*	*	*	*	*	*	*	*	*	*	0.3
Male											
All ages, age adjusted	10.0	15.8	17.7	20.1	22.3	24.1	26.4	26.2	18.1	9.1	17.8
All ages, crude	10.2	16.4	18.5	21.2	23.6	25.5	28.0	28.0	19.5	9.8	19.0
Under 1 year	2.2	2.7	2.4	2.1	2.3	2.1	2.1	1.7	1.1	*	1.1
1–4 years	0.7	0.7	0.8	1.0	1.1	1.3	1.2	1.2	0.9	0.3	0.8
5–14 years	0.2	0.2	0.3	0.3	0.4	0.4	0.5	0.5	0.5	0.3	0.4
15–24 years	2.2	2.6	2.2	2.4	2.3	2.3	2.3	2.1	1.3	0.8	1.4
25–34 years	20.7	31.5	34.5	38.3	42.2	46.0	48.5	47.1	31.4	15.1	31.3
35–44 years	26.3	43.6	50.2	56.9	63.5	68.5	76.2	75.9	51.8	25.5	50.8
45–54 years	15.5	25.6	29.1	34.4	38.1	41.7	46.3	46.9	33.6	17.4	32.2
55–64 years	6.8	10.5	12.0	14.0	15.9	16.5	19.1	19.9	14.9	8.5	14.4
65–74 years	2.4	3.3	3.7	4.5	5.3	5.4	5.8	6.4	5.1	3.4	5.0
75–84 years	1.2	1.2	1.1	1.5	1.6	1.4	1.4	1.3	1.5	1.0	1.3
85 years and over	*	*	*	*	*	*	*	*	*	*	*
Female											
All ages, age adjusted	1.1	1.8	2.1	2.7	3.2	3.8	4.8	5.2	4.2	2.6	4.0
All ages, crude	1.1	1.8	2.2	2.7	3.2	3.9	4.9	5.3	4.3	2.7	4.1
Under 1 year	2.5	3.5	3.0	2.4	2.7	2.4	2.9	1.2	*	*	0.9
1–4 years	0.7	0.8	0.8	1.1	1.0	1.3	1.3	1.5	1.0	0.4	0.9
5–14 years	*	0.1	0.2	0.2	0.2	0.4	0.5	0.5	0.4	0.2	0.4
15–24 years	0.3	0.6	0.7	0.9	0.9	1.1	1.3	1.4	1.0	0.7	1.0
25–34 years	2.8	4.4	4.9	6.0	6.9	8.0	10.1	11.1	8.5	5.1	8.3
35–44 years	2.1	3.9	5.2	6.1	8.2	10.2	12.5	13.4	11.3	6.8	10.4
45–54 years	0.8	1.6	1.9	3.1	3.4	4.4	5.8	6.7	5.7	3.8	5.3
55–64 years	0.5	0.8	1.1	1.5	1.9	1.9	2.6	2.9	2.5	1.6	2.3
65–74 years	0.5	0.7	0.8	0.8	0.9	1.0	1.0	1.4	0.8	0.5	0.9
75–84 years	0.5	0.4	0.4	0.5	0.4	0.4	0.6	0.3	0.3	0.4	0.0
85 years and over	*	*	*	*	*	*	*	*	*	*	*
All ages, age adjusted											
White male	8.4	13.2	15.0	16.7	18.1	19.0	20.1	19.6	12.5	5.6	12.5
Black male	25.4	40.3	44.2	52.9	61.8	70.0	81.7	84.3	66.4	38.5	62.7
American Indian or Alaska Native male	*	2.9	3.3	6.5	4.9	8.3	9.3	11.3	6.9	3.6	7.2
Asian or Pacific Islander male	2.2	3.6	4.0	4.0	4.3	5.1	6.6	5.8	4.1	1.6	3.8
Hispanic male[2]	17.8	27.0	27.2	30.1	33.0	33.6	39.3	39.0	26.0	13.1	25.5
White, non-Hispanic male[2]	6.4	12.2	13.4	14.8	15.9	16.7	17.7	17.1	10.7	4.6	10.7
White female	0.6	0.9	1.1	1.3	1.6	1.9	2.3	2.5	1.8	1.0	1.8
Black female	4.7	8.1	9.9	12.0	14.3	17.3	21.8	24.0	20.2	13.3	19.1
American Indian or Alaska Native female	*	*	*	*	*	*	*	2.7	*	*	1.8
Asian or Pacific Islander female	*	*	*	*	0.5	0.7	0.7	0.6	0.5	*	0.4
Hispanic female[2]	2.1	4.0	3.7	4.8	5.6	6.5	7.7	8.5	6.2	3.3	5.9
White, non-Hispanic female[2]	0.2	0.6	0.7	0.9	1.0	1.2	1.6	1.8	1.3	0.7	1.2

See footnotes at end of table.

Table 43 (page 2 of 2). Death rates for human immunodeficiency virus (HIV) infection, according to sex, detailed race, Hispanic origin, and age: United States, selected years 1987–97

[Data are based on the National Vital Statistics System]

Sex, race, Hispanic origin, and age	1987	1989	1990	1991	1992	1993	1994	1995	1996	1997	1995–97[1]
Age 25–44 years	Deaths per 100,000 resident population										
All races	12.7	20.5	23.2	26.5	29.9	32.9	36.7	36.9	25.9	13.2	25.3
White male	19.2	30.8	35.0	39.3	42.8	45.5	48.4	46.9	29.6	13.2	29.9
Black male	60.2	94.1	102.0	117.9	137.4	155.3	178.0	182.0	139.1	76.7	132.2
American Indian or Alaska Native male	*	7.4	7.7	13.9	13.4	20.9	23.6	31.3	18.4	10.7	19.9
Asian or Pacific Islander male	4.1	7.5	8.1	9.0	9.4	10.8	13.8	12.8	8.1	3.6	8.1
Hispanic male[2]	36.8	58.2	59.3	63.9	68.9	71.0	78.0	78.9	50.5	24.9	50.5
White, non-Hispanic male[2]	14.3	28.2	31.6	34.9	38.1	40.2	43.4	41.5	25.8	11.0	26.1
White female	1.2	1.9	2.3	3.0	3.6	4.4	5.5	6.0	4.4	2.4	4.3
Black female	11.6	20.1	23.6	27.2	34.4	40.4	49.8	54.5	46.6	29.3	43.4
American Indian or Alaska Native female	*	*	*	*	*	*	*	*	*	*	3.7
Asian or Pacific Islander female	*	*	*	*	*	1.2	1.5	1.2	*	*	0.9
Hispanic female[2]	4.9	9.3	8.9	10.1	12.5	14.2	17.3	18.0	12.8	6.7	12.4
White, non-Hispanic female[2]	0.3	1.3	1.5	1.9	2.3	2.9	3.9	4.2	3.1	1.7	3.0
Age 45–64 years											
All races	5.8	9.7	11.1	13.4	15.2	16.8	19.3	20.1	15.0	8.3	14.3
White male	9.9	16.4	18.6	21.2	23.4	24.7	26.4	26.3	17.4	8.0	17.1
Black male	27.3	46.1	53.0	71.4	86.4	101.2	127.1	136.6	114.1	71.8	106.7
American Indian or Alaska Native male	*	*	*	*	*	*	*	*	*	*	5.8
Asian or Pacific Islander male	*	6.1	6.5	5.3	7.1	9.2	10.6	9.5	8.2	2.4	6.5
Hispanic male[2]	25.8	37.0	37.9	45.0	52.5	52.2	69.2	67.1	48.8	24.7	45.9
White, non-Hispanic male[2]	8.0	15.3	16.9	18.8	20.3	21.5	22.6	22.6	14.3	6.4	14.3
White female	0.5	0.7	0.9	1.2	1.5	1.8	2.1	2.4	1.9	1.1	1.8
Black female	2.6	5.6	7.5	12.2	12.9	16.5	24.1	27.2	24.4	17.6	23.0
American Indian or Alaska Native female	*	*	*	*	*	*	*	*	*	*	*
Asian or Pacific Islander female	*	*	*	*	*	*	*	*	*	*	*
Hispanic female[2]	*	3.5	3.1	6.2	6.8	8.2	9.9	12.4	9.7	5.3	9.0
White, non-Hispanic female[2]	0.3	0.5	0.7	0.8	1.0	1.1	1.4	1.5	1.2	0.7	1.1

* Based on fewer than 20 deaths.
[1] Average annual death rate.
[2] Data shown only for States with an Hispanic-origin item on their death certificates. See Appendix I, National Vital Statistics System.

NOTES: Categories for the coding and classification of human immunodeficiency virus infection were introduced in the United States beginning with mortality data for 1987. Age groups were selected to minimize the presentation of unstable age-specific death rates based on small numbers of deaths and for consistency among comparison groups. The race groups, white, black, Asian or Pacific Islander, and American Indian or Alaska Native, include persons of Hispanic and non-Hispanic origin. Conversely, persons of Hispanic origin may be of any race. Consistency of race identification between the death certificate (source of data for numerator of death rates) and data from the Census Bureau (denominator) is high for individual white and black persons; however, persons identified as American Indian, Asian, or Hispanic origin in data from the Census Bureau are sometimes misreported as white or non-Hispanic on the death certificate, causing death rates to be underestimated by 22–30 percent for American Indians, about 12 percent for Asians, and about 7 percent for persons of Hispanic origin. (Sorlie PD, Rogot E, and Johnson NJ: Validity of demographic characteristics on the death certificate, *Epidemiology* 3(2):181–184, 1992.) See Appendix II for age-adjustment procedure. Data for additional years are available (see Appendix III).

SOURCES: Centers for Disease Control and Prevention, National Center for Health Statistics. *Vital statistics of the United States, vol II, mortality, part A*, for data years 1987–93. Public Health Service. Washington. U.S. Government Printing Office; for 1994–97, unpublished data; data computed by the Division of Health and Utilization Analysis from numerator data compiled by the Division of Vital Statistics and denominator data from national population estimates for race groups from table 1 and unpublished Hispanic population estimates prepared by the Housing and Household Economic Statistics Division, U.S. Bureau of the Census.

Table 44. Maternal mortality for complications of pregnancy, childbirth, and the puerperium, according to race, Hispanic origin, and age: United States, selected years 1950–97

[Data are based on the National Vital Statistics System]

Race, Hispanic origin, and age	1950[1]	1960[1]	1970	1980	1985	1990	1994	1995	1996	1997
	Number of deaths									
All persons	2,960	1,579	803	334	295	343	328	277	294	327
White	1,873	936	445	193	156	177	193	129	159	179
Black	1,041	624	342	127	124	153	118	133	121	125
American Indian or Alaska Native	---	---	---	3	7	4	–	1	6	2
Asian or Pacific Islander	---	---	---	11	8	9	17	14	8	21
Hispanic[2]	---	---	---	---	29	47	64	43	39	57
White, non-Hispanic[2]	---	---	---	---	60	125	127	84	114	121
All persons	Deaths per 100,000 live births									
All ages, age adjusted	73.7	32.1	21.5	9.4	7.6	7.6	7.9	6.3	6.4	7.6
All ages, crude	83.3	37.1	21.5	9.2	7.8	8.2	8.3	7.1	7.6	8.4
Under 20 years	70.7	22.7	18.9	7.6	6.9	7.5	6.9	3.9	*	5.7
20–24 years	47.6	20.7	13.0	5.8	5.4	6.1	7.6	5.7	5.0	6.6
25–29 years	63.5	29.8	17.0	7.7	6.4	6.0	7.1	6.0	6.6	7.9
30–34 years	107.7	50.3	31.6	13.6	8.9	9.5	6.5	7.3	7.6	8.3
35 years and over[3]	222.0	104.3	81.9	36.3	25.0	20.7	18.3	15.9	19.0	16.1
White										
All ages, age adjusted	53.1	22.4	14.4	6.7	4.9	5.1	5.8	3.6	4.1	5.2
All ages, crude	61.1	26.0	14.3	6.6	5.1	5.4	6.2	4.2	5.1	5.8
Under 20 years	44.9	14.8	13.8	5.8	*	*	6.2	*	*	*
20–24 years	35.7	15.3	8.4	4.2	3.3	3.9	4.7	3.5	*	4.2
25–29 years	45.0	20.3	11.1	5.4	4.6	4.8	6.1	4.0	4.0	5.4
30–34 years	75.9	34.3	18.7	9.3	5.1	5.0	5.0	4.0	5.0	5.4
35 years and over[3]	174.1	73.9	59.3	25.5	17.5	12.6	12.0	9.1	14.9	11.5
Black										
All ages, age adjusted	---	92.0	65.5	24.9	22.1	21.7	18.1	20.9	19.9	20.1
All ages, crude	---	103.6	60.9	22.4	21.3	22.4	18.5	22.1	20.3	20.8
Under 20 years	---	54.8	32.3	13.1	*	*	*	*	*	*
20–24 years	---	56.9	41.9	13.9	14.6	14.7	18.2	15.3	15.1	15.3
25–29 years	---	92.8	65.2	22.4	19.4	14.9	*	21.0	25.5	24.3
30–34 years	---	150.6	117.8	44.0	38.0	44.2	*	31.2	28.6	32.9
35 years and over[3]	---	299.5	207.5	100.6	77.2	79.7	64.5	61.4	49.9	40.4
Hispanic[2,4]										
All ages, age adjusted	---	---	---	---	7.1	7.4	9.1	5.4	4.8	7.6
All ages, crude	---	---	---	---	7.8	7.9	9.6	6.3	5.6	8.0
White, non-Hispanic[2]										
All ages, age adjusted	---	---	---	---	4.0	4.4	4.9	3.3	3.9	4.4
All ages, crude	---	---	---	---	4.3	4.8	5.2	3.5	4.8	5.2

- - - Data not available.
– Quantity zero.
* Based on fewer than 20 deaths.
[1]Includes deaths of persons who were not residents of the 50 States and the District of Columbia.
[2]Hispanic and White, non-Hispanic data exclude data from States lacking an Hispanic-origin item on their death and birth certificates. See Appendix I, National Vital Statistics System.
[3]Rates computed by relating deaths of women 35 years and over to live births to women 35–49 years.
[4]Age-specific maternal mortality rates are not calculated because rates based on fewer than 20 deaths are unreliable.

NOTES: For data years shown, the code numbers for cause of death are based on the then current *International Classification of Diseases*, described in Appendix II, tables IV and V. The race groups, white, black, Asian or Pacific Islander, and American Indian or Alaska Native, include persons of Hispanic and non-Hispanic origin. Conversely, persons of Hispanic origin may be of any race. For 1950 and 1960, rates are based on live births by race of child; for all other years, rates are based on live births by race of mother. See Appendix II, Race. Rates are not calculated for American Indian or Alaska Native and Asian or Pacific Islander mothers because rates based on fewer than 20 deaths are unreliable. See Appendix II for age-adjustment procedure. Data for additional years are available (see Appendix III).

SOURCES: Centers for Disease Control and Prevention, National Center for Health Statistics. *Vital statistics of the United States, vol II, mortality, part A*, for data years 1950–93. Public Health Service. Washington. U.S. Government Printing Office; for 1994–97, unpublished data; *Vital statistics of the United States, vol I, natality*, for data years 1950–93. Public Health Service. Washington. U.S. Government Printing Office; for 1994–97, unpublished data; data computed by the Division of Health and Utilization Analysis from numerator data compiled by the Division of Vital Statistics.

Table 45 (page 1 of 4). Death rates for motor vehicle-related injuries, according to sex, detailed race, Hispanic origin, and age: United States, selected years 1950–97

[Data are based on the National Vital Statistics System]

Sex, race, Hispanic origin, and age	1950[1]	1960[1]	1970	1980	1985	1990	1994	1995	1996	1997	1995–97[2]
All persons				Deaths per 100,000 resident population							
All ages, age adjusted	23.3	22.5	27.4	22.9	18.8	18.5	16.1	16.3	16.2	15.9	16.1
All ages, crude	23.1	21.3	26.9	23.5	19.3	18.8	16.3	16.5	16.5	16.2	16.4
Under 1 year	8.4	8.1	9.8	7.0	4.9	4.9	4.8	4.7	5.7	4.3	4.9
1–14 years	9.8	8.6	10.5	8.2	7.0	6.0	5.6	5.3	5.2	5.1	5.2
1–4 years	11.5	10.0	11.5	9.2	7.2	6.3	6.0	5.2	5.3	5.0	5.2
5–14 years	8.8	7.9	10.2	7.9	6.9	5.9	5.4	5.4	5.2	5.1	5.2
15–24 years	34.4	38.0	47.2	44.8	35.7	34.1	29.7	29.5	29.2	27.9	28.9
25–34 years	24.6	24.3	30.9	29.1	23.0	23.6	18.8	19.8	19.1	18.9	19.3
35–44 years	20.3	19.3	24.9	20.9	17.2	16.9	14.8	15.4	15.6	15.2	15.4
45–64 years	25.2	23.0	26.5	18.0	15.4	15.7	13.9	14.2	14.4	14.7	14.4
45–54 years	22.2	21.4	25.5	18.6	15.2	15.6	14.0	13.9	14.1	14.3	14.1
55–64 years	29.0	25.1	27.9	17.4	15.6	15.9	13.9	14.6	15.0	15.3	15.0
65 years and over	43.1	34.7	36.2	22.5	21.7	23.1	22.9	22.7	23.0	23.6	23.1
65–74 years	39.1	31.4	32.8	19.2	17.9	18.6	18.1	17.6	18.3	18.2	18.0
75–84 years	52.7	41.8	43.5	28.1	27.4	29.1	29.2	28.6	28.3	29.0	28.6
85 years and over	45.1	37.9	34.2	27.6	26.5	31.2	29.1	31.4	30.1	32.7	31.4
Male											
All ages, age adjusted	36.4	34.5	41.1	34.3	27.3	26.3	22.5	22.7	22.3	21.7	22.2
All ages, crude	35.4	31.8	39.7	35.3	28.0	26.7	22.5	22.7	22.4	22.0	22.4
Under 1 year	9.1	8.6	9.3	7.3	5.0	5.0	4.8	4.9	5.7	4.3	4.9
1–14 years	12.3	10.7	13.0	10.0	8.5	7.0	6.5	6.2	5.9	5.7	5.9
1–4 years	13.0	11.5	12.9	10.2	8.3	6.9	6.6	5.6	5.7	5.3	5.6
5–14 years	11.9	10.4	13.1	9.9	8.6	7.0	6.5	6.4	6.0	5.8	6.1
15–24 years	56.7	61.2	73.2	68.4	52.7	49.5	41.8	41.4	40.7	38.1	40.0
25–34 years	40.8	40.1	49.4	46.3	35.9	35.7	27.7	29.1	27.5	27.5	28.0
35–44 years	32.5	29.9	37.7	31.7	25.2	24.7	21.4	21.9	21.8	21.2	21.6
45–64 years	37.7	33.3	38.9	26.5	22.0	21.9	19.2	19.7	19.8	20.0	19.8
45–54 years	33.6	31.6	37.2	27.6	21.9	22.0	19.4	19.6	19.6	19.9	19.7
55–64 years	43.1	35.6	40.9	25.4	22.1	21.7	18.9	19.8	20.1	20.2	20.0
65 years and over	66.6	52.1	54.4	33.9	30.4	32.1	31.2	30.8	31.4	31.9	31.3
65–74 years	59.1	45.8	47.3	27.3	23.0	24.2	23.1	22.3	23.9	23.6	23.3
75–84 years	85.0	66.0	68.2	44.3	41.3	41.2	40.5	39.7	38.7	39.7	39.4
85 years and over	78.1	62.7	63.1	56.1	55.3	64.5	59.6	61.9	59.0	60.4	60.4
Female											
All ages, age adjusted	10.7	11.0	14.4	11.8	10.5	10.7	9.9	10.0	10.2	10.2	10.2
All ages, crude	10.9	11.0	14.7	12.3	11.0	11.3	10.4	10.6	10.7	10.8	10.7
Under 1 year	7.6	7.5	10.4	6.7	4.7	4.9	4.8	4.4	5.8	4.4	4.8
1–14 years	7.2	6.3	7.9	6.3	5.4	4.9	4.5	4.5	4.4	4.4	4.4
1–4 years	10.0	8.4	10.0	8.1	6.0	5.6	5.4	4.8	4.8	4.7	4.8
5–14 years	5.7	5.4	7.2	5.7	5.1	4.7	4.2	4.3	4.2	4.3	4.3
15–24 years	12.6	15.1	21.6	20.8	18.2	17.9	17.0	17.1	17.1	17.1	17.1
25–34 years	9.3	9.2	13.0	12.2	10.1	11.5	9.9	10.4	10.7	10.4	10.5
35–44 years	8.5	9.1	12.9	10.4	9.4	9.2	8.5	9.0	9.4	9.2	9.2
45–64 years	12.6	13.1	15.3	10.3	9.5	10.1	9.1	9.1	9.4	9.6	9.4
45–54 years	10.9	11.6	14.5	10.2	9.0	9.6	8.8	8.5	8.8	8.9	8.7
55–64 years	14.9	15.2	16.2	10.5	9.9	10.8	9.4	9.9	10.3	10.8	10.3
65 years and over	21.9	20.3	23.1	15.0	15.8	17.2	17.3	17.2	17.2	17.8	17.4
65–74 years	20.6	19.0	21.6	13.0	14.0	14.1	14.1	13.8	13.9	13.8	13.8
75–84 years	25.2	23.0	27.2	18.5	19.2	21.9	22.1	21.5	21.5	22.0	21.7
85 years and over	22.1	22.0	18.0	15.2	15.0	18.3	17.4	19.6	18.6	21.5	19.9
White male											
All ages, age adjusted	35.9	34.0	40.1	34.8	27.6	26.3	22.5	22.6	22.2	21.6	22.1
All ages, crude	35.1	31.5	39.1	35.9	28.3	26.7	22.5	22.6	22.4	21.9	22.3
Under 1 year	9.1	8.8	9.1	7.0	4.6	4.8	4.3	4.3	5.2	3.7	4.4
1–14 years	12.4	10.6	12.5	9.8	8.3	6.6	6.2	5.9	5.7	5.4	5.7
15–24 years	58.3	62.7	75.2	73.8	56.5	52.5	43.6	43.2	42.2	39.8	41.7
25–34 years	39.1	38.6	47.0	46.6	35.8	35.4	28.0	28.8	27.0	26.8	27.5
35–44 years	30.9	28.4	35.2	30.7	24.3	23.7	21.1	21.1	21.4	20.7	21.1
45–64 years	36.2	31.7	36.5	25.2	20.8	20.6	18.3	18.9	19.2	19.2	19.1
65 years and over	67.1	52.1	54.2	32.7	29.9	31.4	30.5	30.2	31.1	31.8	31.0

See footnotes at end of table.

Table 45 (page 2 of 4). **Death rates for motor vehicle-related injuries, according to sex, detailed race, Hispanic origin, and age: United States, selected years 1950–97**

[Data are based on the National Vital Statistics System]

Sex, race, Hispanic origin, and age	1950[1]	1960[1]	1970	1980	1985	1990	1994	1995	1996	1997	1995–97[2]
Black male				Deaths per 100,000 resident population							
All ages, age adjusted	39.8	38.2	50.1	32.9	28.0	28.9	24.7	25.3	24.9	24.9	25.0
All ages, crude	37.2	33.1	44.3	31.1	27.1	28.1	23.9	24.6	24.3	24.2	24.3
Under 1 year	---	*	10.6	7.8	*	*	8.0	8.3	7.6	7.8	7.9
1–14 years	---	11.2	16.3	11.4	9.7	8.9	8.7	7.8	7.6	7.6	7.7
15–24 years	41.6	46.4	58.1	34.9	32.0	36.1	35.0	34.3	35.2	32.7	34.1
25–34 years	57.4	51.0	70.4	44.9	37.7	39.5	29.1	32.9	32.5	33.2	32.9
35–44 years	45.9	43.6	59.5	41.2	34.7	33.5	25.3	28.9	26.6	27.0	27.5
45–64 years	54.6	47.8	61.7	39.5	32.9	33.3	27.3	26.9	26.8	28.9	27.6
65 years and over	52.6	48.2	53.4	42.4	35.2	36.3	37.7	36.3	35.6	32.3	34.7
American Indian or Alaska Native male[3]											
All ages, age adjusted	---	---	---	77.4	52.3	49.0	43.8	45.4	45.4	43.3	44.7
All ages, crude	---	---	---	74.6	51.7	47.6	41.8	43.8	44.2	42.2	43.4
1–14 years	---	---	---	15.1	16.2	11.6	9.5	8.5	13.5	8.2	10.1
15–24 years	---	---	---	126.1	77.3	75.2	68.0	76.6	69.6	67.6	71.2
25–34 years	---	---	---	107.0	84.0	78.2	58.4	73.1	70.5	64.3	69.3
35–44 years	---	---	---	82.8	55.8	57.0	52.9	50.4	48.8	54.7	51.3
45–64 years	---	---	---	77.4	52.2	45.9	49.5	42.5	39.8	37.8	40.0
65 years and over	---	---	---	97.0	*	43.0	*	*	43.5	50.1	41.0
Asian or Pacific Islander male[4]											
All ages, age adjusted	---	---	---	17.1	16.2	15.8	13.1	13.6	11.9	11.7	12.4
All ages, crude	---	---	---	17.1	16.0	15.8	12.5	13.1	11.5	11.4	12.0
1–14 years	---	---	---	8.2	5.2	6.3	3.8	4.3	2.9	2.7	3.3
15–24 years	---	---	---	27.2	28.1	25.7	22.3	20.6	22.4	15.7	19.6
25–34 years	---	---	---	18.8	18.4	17.0	11.0	13.2	13.3	15.7	14.1
35–44 years	---	---	---	13.1	12.0	12.2	8.5	10.4	9.9	8.5	9.6
45–64 years	---	---	---	13.7	13.4	15.1	13.0	15.0	9.7	12.1	12.2
65 years and over	---	---	---	37.3	37.3	33.6	39.3	34.4	23.9	31.0	29.6
Hispanic male[5]											
All ages, age adjusted	---	---	---	---	25.3	29.1	24.7	24.5	23.2	21.4	23.0
All ages, crude	---	---	---	---	25.6	29.2	23.9	23.5	22.3	20.8	22.2
1–14 years	---	---	---	---	7.7	7.2	6.9	5.8	5.6	5.1	5.5
15–24 years	---	---	---	---	44.9	48.2	42.4	42.4	37.5	35.3	38.2
25–34 years	---	---	---	---	31.2	41.0	31.0	31.6	28.0	27.4	29.0
35–44 years	---	---	---	---	26.3	28.0	24.8	23.8	23.9	22.9	23.5
45–64 years	---	---	---	---	25.9	28.9	23.0	23.0	23.8	21.3	22.7
65 years and over	---	---	---	---	22.9	35.3	33.2	35.1	35.2	28.6	32.8
White, non-Hispanic male[5]											
All ages, age adjusted	---	---	---	---	25.3	25.7	21.7	21.9	21.7	21.3	21.6
All ages, crude	---	---	---	---	25.9	26.0	21.8	22.0	21.9	21.7	21.9
1–14 years	---	---	---	---	7.8	6.4	6.0	5.8	5.5	5.4	5.6
15–24 years	---	---	---	---	53.3	52.3	42.6	42.3	42.0	40.1	41.5
25–34 years	---	---	---	---	33.2	34.0	26.7	27.5	26.1	26.2	26.6
35–44 years	---	---	---	---	21.6	23.1	20.1	20.3	20.5	20.0	20.3
45–64 years	---	---	---	---	18.0	19.8	17.5	18.2	18.4	18.8	18.5
65 years and over	---	---	---	---	27.6	31.1	30.0	29.6	30.5	31.7	30.6
White female											
All ages, age adjusted	10.6	11.1	14.4	12.3	10.8	11.0	10.0	10.3	10.4	10.3	10.3
All ages, crude	10.9	11.2	14.8	12.8	11.4	11.6	10.6	10.8	11.0	10.9	10.9
Under 1 year	7.8	7.5	10.2	7.1	3.9	4.7	3.9	4.5	5.7	4.3	4.8
1–14 years	7.2	6.2	7.5	6.2	5.4	4.8	4.3	4.3	4.3	4.1	4.3
15–24 years	12.6	15.6	22.7	23.0	20.0	19.5	18.3	18.4	18.1	18.4	18.3
25–34 years	9.0	9.0	12.7	12.2	10.1	11.6	9.8	10.4	10.8	10.3	10.5
35–44 years	8.1	8.9	12.3	10.6	9.4	9.2	8.4	9.0	9.3	9.0	9.1
45–64 years	12.7	13.1	15.1	10.4	9.5	9.9	8.8	8.9	9.3	9.4	9.2
65 years and over	22.2	20.8	23.7	15.3	16.2	17.4	17.6	17.7	17.4	17.9	17.7

See footnotes at end of table.

[Data are based on the National Vital Statistics System]

Sex, race, Hispanic origin, and age	1950[1]	1960[1]	1970	1980	1985	1990	1994	1995	1996	1997	1995–97[2]
Black female				Deaths per 100,000 resident population							
All ages, age adjusted	10.3	10.0	13.8	8.4	8.2	9.3	9.5	8.9	9.4	9.8	9.4
All ages, crude	10.2	9.7	13.4	8.3	8.3	9.4	9.5	9.0	9.5	9.9	9.5
Under 1 year	- - -	8.1	11.9	*	8.1	7.0	9.5	*	7.8	*	5.9
1–14 years	- - -	6.9	10.2	6.3	5.1	5.3	5.8	5.1	4.8	5.6	5.2
15–24 years	11.5	9.9	13.4	8.0	9.1	9.9	11.7	10.7	13.3	11.3	11.8
25–34 years	10.7	9.8	13.3	10.6	9.3	11.1	10.4	10.5	10.9	11.2	10.9
35–44 years	11.1	11.0	16.1	8.3	9.1	9.4	8.9	9.8	9.6	10.2	9.9
45–64 years	11.8	12.7	16.7	9.2	9.0	10.7	10.1	9.4	8.9	11.0	9.8
65 years and over	14.3	13.2	15.7	9.5	11.2	13.5	13.6	11.5	13.1	14.2	13.0
American Indian or Alaska Native female[3]											
All ages, age adjusted	- - -	- - -	- - -	32.5	20.9	17.8	19.3	21.0	22.6	21.3	21.6
All ages, crude	- - -	- - -	- - -	32.0	20.6	17.3	18.8	20.4	21.8	20.9	21.0
1–14 years	- - -	- - -	- - -	15.0	9.2	8.1	9.1	9.1	9.7	10.0	9.6
15–24 years	- - -	- - -	- - -	42.3	29.5	31.4	30.7	32.7	27.1	24.5	28.0
25–34 years	- - -	- - -	- - -	52.5	30.2	18.8	28.3	36.7	31.9	27.6	32.0
35–44 years	- - -	- - -	- - -	38.1	27.0	18.2	16.8	19.4	23.0	21.5	21.3
45–64 years	- - -	- - -	- - -	32.6	19.5	17.6	17.0	17.1	27.1	22.5	22.3
65 years and over	- - -	- - -	- - -	*	*	*	*	*	*	35.7	22.6
Asian or Pacific Islander female[4]											
All ages, age adjusted	- - -	- - -	- - -	8.4	8.0	9.2	7.7	8.2	7.2	8.0	7.8
All ages, crude	- - -	- - -	- - -	8.2	7.9	9.0	7.6	8.0	7.4	8.0	7.8
1–14 years	- - -	- - -	- - -	7.4	5.0	3.6	2.7	3.0	2.3	3.2	2.8
15–24 years	- - -	- - -	- - -	7.4	7.4	11.4	9.3	12.4	8.3	11.5	10.7
25–34 years	- - -	- - -	- - -	7.3	8.4	7.3	6.1	5.1	5.6	6.1	5.6
35–44 years	- - -	- - -	- - -	8.6	7.0	7.5	6.8	6.2	7.5	6.9	6.9
45–64 years	- - -	- - -	- - -	8.5	8.6	11.8	10.4	10.8	8.9	8.6	9.4
65 years and over	- - -	- - -	- - -	18.6	20.5	24.3	19.2	19.7	21.3	20.7	20.6
Hispanic female[5]											
All ages, age adjusted	- - -	- - -	- - -	- - -	8.3	9.2	8.3	8.5	8.7	8.5	8.6
All ages, crude	- - -	- - -	- - -	- - -	7.9	8.9	8.1	8.3	8.5	8.3	8.3
1–14 years	- - -	- - -	- - -	- - -	4.8	4.8	4.0	4.4	4.7	3.9	4.3
15–24 years	- - -	- - -	- - -	- - -	10.1	11.6	11.8	12.8	11.8	13.1	12.6
25–34 years	- - -	- - -	- - -	- - -	7.5	9.4	9.0	7.7	9.0	8.3	8.3
35–44 years	- - -	- - -	- - -	- - -	8.8	8.0	7.3	8.1	7.7	8.1	7.9
45–64 years	- - -	- - -	- - -	- - -	9.4	11.4	9.1	9.2	9.7	9.0	9.3
65 years and over	- - -	- - -	- - -	- - -	14.8	14.9	13.5	13.9	13.9	14.1	14.0

See footnotes at end of table.

Table 45 (page 4 of 4). Death rates for motor vehicle-related injuries, according to sex, detailed race, Hispanic origin, and age: United States, selected years 1950–97

[Data are based on the National Vital Statistics System]

Sex, race, Hispanic origin, and age	1950[1]	1960[1]	1970	1980	1985	1990	1994	1995	1996	1997	1995–97[2]
White, non-Hispanic female[5]					Deaths per 100,000 resident population						
All ages, age adjusted	---	---	---	---	10.4	11.1	10.1	10.3	10.4	10.4	10.4
All ages, crude	---	---	---	---	10.9	11.7	10.7	10.9	11.0	11.1	11.0
1–14 years	---	---	---	---	4.9	4.7	4.3	4.2	4.2	4.1	4.2
15–24 years	---	---	---	---	20.2	20.4	19.0	19.0	18.8	19.2	19.0
25–34 years	---	---	---	---	9.8	11.7	9.7	10.6	10.8	10.4	10.6
35–44 years	---	---	---	---	8.6	9.3	8.3	8.9	9.3	9.0	9.0
45–64 years	---	---	---	---	8.6	9.7	8.7	8.7	9.0	9.4	9.0
65 years and over	---	---	---	---	15.3	17.5	17.6	17.7	17.4	18.0	17.7

--- Data not available.

* Based on fewer than 20 deaths.

[1]Includes deaths of persons who were not residents of the 50 States and the District of Columbia.

[2]Average annual death rate.

[3]Interpretation of trends should take into account that population estimates for American Indians increased by 45 percent between 1980 and 1990, partly due to better enumeration techniques in the 1990 decennial census and to the increased tendency for people to identify themselves as American Indian in 1990.

[4]Interpretation of trends should take into account that the Asian population in the United States more than doubled between 1980 and 1990, primarily due to immigration.

[5]Excludes data from States lacking an Hispanic-origin item on their death certificates. See Appendix I, National Vital Statistics System.

NOTES: For data years shown, the code numbers for cause of death are based on the then current *International Classification of Diseases*, which are described in Appendix II, tables IV and V. Age groups were selected to minimize the presentation of unstable age-specific death rates based on small numbers of deaths and for consistency among comparison groups. The race groups, white, black, Asian or Pacific Islander, and American Indian or Alaska Native, include persons of Hispanic and non-Hispanic origin. Conversely, persons of Hispanic origin may be of any race. Consistency of race identification between the death certificate (source of data for numerator of death rates) and data from the Census Bureau (denominator) is high for individual white and black persons; however, persons identified as American Indian, Asian, or Hispanic origin in data from the Census Bureau are sometimes misreported as white or non-Hispanic on the death certificate, causing death rates to be underestimated by 22–30 percent for American Indians, about 12 percent for Asians, and about 7 percent for persons of Hispanic origin. (Sorlie PD, Rogot E, and Johnson NJ: Validity of demographic characteristics on the death certificate, *Epidemiology* 3(2):181–184, 1992.) See Appendix II for age-adjustment procedure. Data for additional years are available (see Appendix III).

SOURCES: Centers for Disease Control and Prevention, National Center for Health Statistics. Grove RD and Hetzel AM. *Vital statistics rates in the United States, 1940–60.* Washington: Public Health Service, 1968; *Vital statistics of the United States, vol II, mortality, part A,* for data years 1950–93. Public Health Service. Washington. U.S. Government Printing Office; for 1994–97, unpublished data; data computed by the Division of Health and Utilization Analysis from numerator data compiled by the Division of Vital Statistics and denominator data from national population estimates for race groups from table 1 and unpublished Hispanic population estimates prepared by the Housing and Household Economic Statistics Division, U.S. Bureau of the Census.

Table 46 (page 1 of 3). Death rates for homicide and legal intervention, according to sex, detailed race, Hispanic origin, and age: United States, selected years 1950–97

[Data are based on the National Vital Statistics System]

Sex, race, Hispanic origin, and age	1950[1]	1960[1]	1970	1980	1985	1990	1994	1995	1996	1997	1995–97[2]
All persons					Deaths per 100,000 resident population						
All ages, age adjusted	5.4	5.2	9.1	10.8	8.3	10.2	10.3	9.4	8.5	8.0	8.6
All ages, crude	5.3	4.7	8.3	10.7	8.4	10.0	9.6	8.7	7.9	7.4	8.0
Under 1 year	4.4	4.8	4.3	5.9	5.4	8.4	8.1	8.1	8.8	8.3	8.4
1–14 years	0.6	0.6	1.1	1.5	1.6	1.8	2.0	1.9	1.7	1.5	1.7
1–4 years	0.6	0.7	1.9	2.5	2.5	2.6	3.0	2.9	2.7	2.4	2.7
5–14 years	0.5	0.5	0.9	1.2	1.2	1.5	1.5	1.5	1.3	1.2	1.3
15–24 years	6.3	5.9	11.7	15.6	11.9	19.9	22.6	20.3	18.1	16.8	18.4
25–44 years	9.3	8.9	15.2	17.6	13.3	14.9	13.8	12.3	11.1	10.5	11.3
25–34 years	9.9	9.7	16.6	19.6	14.8	17.7	16.7	15.1	13.4	12.8	13.8
35–44 years	8.8	8.1	13.7	15.1	11.3	11.8	10.9	9.7	9.0	8.4	9.0
45–64 years	5.2	5.3	8.8	9.1	7.0	6.4	5.6	5.5	5.2	4.9	5.2
45–54 years	6.1	6.2	10.1	11.1	8.1	7.6	6.5	6.2	5.9	5.6	5.9
55–64 years	4.0	4.2	7.1	7.0	5.7	5.0	4.3	4.5	4.1	3.9	4.2
65 years and over	3.0	2.7	4.6	5.6	4.3	4.0	3.5	3.2	3.0	3.0	3.1
65–74 years	3.2	2.8	5.0	5.7	4.3	3.8	3.4	3.3	3.0	2.9	3.1
75–84 years	2.6	2.4	4.0	5.2	4.3	4.3	3.6	3.1	2.9	2.9	3.0
85 years and over	2.3	2.4	4.2	5.3	4.2	4.6	3.5	3.3	3.0	3.8	3.4
Male											
All ages, age adjusted	8.4	7.9	14.9	17.4	12.8	16.3	16.4	14.7	13.3	12.5	13.5
All ages, crude	8.1	7.1	13.4	17.3	13.0	16.2	15.5	13.8	12.5	11.8	12.7
Under 1 year	4.5	4.7	4.5	6.3	5.6	8.8	9.0	8.9	8.7	9.4	9.0
1–14 years	0.6	0.6	1.2	1.6	1.8	2.0	2.3	2.3	1.9	1.8	2.0
1–4 years	0.5	0.7	1.9	2.7	2.5	2.7	3.3	3.1	2.7	2.7	2.8
5–14 years	0.6	0.5	1.0	1.2	1.4	1.7	1.9	1.9	1.6	1.5	1.7
15–24 years	9.6	9.1	19.0	24.5	18.6	32.9	38.3	33.9	30.4	28.2	30.8
25–44 years	14.7	13.6	25.0	29.4	21.0	24.0	21.7	19.1	17.3	16.3	17.6
25–34 years	15.5	14.9	27.6	32.5	23.3	28.3	26.5	23.7	21.4	20.5	21.9
35–44 years	13.8	12.3	22.2	24.9	17.9	19.0	17.0	14.6	13.5	12.5	13.5
45–64 years	8.4	8.3	14.9	15.4	11.1	10.3	8.9	8.6	8.0	7.6	8.0
45–54 years	9.9	9.6	17.0	18.6	12.9	12.1	10.3	9.6	8.9	8.5	9.0
55–64 years	6.5	6.6	12.2	11.9	9.2	8.1	6.9	7.2	6.6	6.1	6.6
65 years and over	4.9	4.3	7.8	8.9	6.2	5.8	5.0	4.3	4.1	4.3	4.2
65–74 years	5.3	4.6	8.6	9.3	6.5	5.8	5.0	4.6	4.3	4.3	4.4
75–84 years	4.0	3.7	6.0	8.1	5.8	5.7	4.9	3.7	3.8	3.8	3.8
85 years and over	2.5	3.6	7.4	7.5	5.0	6.8	5.6	4.2	3.7	5.9	4.7
Female											
All ages, age adjusted	2.5	2.6	3.7	4.5	3.9	4.2	4.0	4.0	3.6	3.3	3.6
All ages, crude	2.4	2.4	3.4	4.5	4.0	4.2	3.9	3.8	3.5	3.2	3.5
Under 1 year	4.2	4.9	4.1	5.6	5.2	8.0	7.1	7.2	8.9	7.3	7.8
1–14 years	0.6	0.5	1.0	1.4	1.4	1.6	1.6	1.5	1.6	1.2	1.4
1–4 years	0.7	0.7	1.9	2.2	2.4	2.4	2.7	2.6	2.7	2.2	2.5
5–14 years	0.5	0.4	0.7	1.1	1.0	1.2	1.2	1.0	1.1	0.9	1.0
15–24 years	3.1	2.8	4.6	6.6	5.1	6.3	6.2	6.0	5.1	4.7	5.3
25–44 years	4.2	4.3	5.9	6.4	5.7	6.0	5.8	5.7	5.0	4.6	5.1
25–34 years	4.5	4.6	6.0	7.0	6.4	7.2	6.8	6.5	5.5	5.1	5.7
35–44 years	3.8	4.1	5.7	5.7	4.9	4.8	4.9	4.9	4.5	4.3	4.5
45–64 years	1.9	2.5	3.1	3.4	3.2	2.8	2.5	2.6	2.5	2.4	2.5
45–54 years	2.3	2.9	3.7	4.1	3.7	3.2	2.8	3.0	3.0	2.7	2.9
55–64 years	1.4	2.0	2.5	2.8	2.7	2.3	2.0	2.1	1.9	2.0	2.0
65 years and over	1.4	1.3	2.3	3.3	3.0	2.8	2.4	2.4	2.1	2.2	2.2
65–74 years	1.3	1.3	2.2	3.0	2.6	2.2	2.1	2.2	1.9	1.9	2.0
75–84 years	1.4	1.3	2.7	3.5	3.4	3.4	2.7	2.7	2.4	2.2	2.4
85 years and over	2.1	1.6	2.5	4.3	3.8	3.8	2.6	2.9	2.7	3.0	2.9
White male											
All ages, age adjusted	3.9	3.9	7.3	10.9	8.1	8.9	8.8	8.2	7.3	7.0	7.5
All ages, crude	3.9	3.6	6.8	10.9	8.2	9.0	8.5	7.8	7.0	6.7	7.2
Under 1 year	4.3	3.8	2.9	4.3	3.8	6.4	6.0	7.1	6.5	7.8	7.2
1–14 years	0.4	0.5	0.7	1.2	1.3	1.3	1.5	1.5	1.4	1.3	1.4
15–24 years	3.7	4.4	7.9	15.5	11.0	15.4	17.4	16.5	14.0	13.2	14.5
25–44 years	5.9	5.9	12.0	17.4	12.9	13.3	12.3	11.0	9.9	9.5	10.1
25–34 years	5.4	6.2	13.0	18.9	14.0	15.1	14.3	12.9	11.5	11.4	11.9
35–44 years	6.4	5.5	11.0	15.5	11.5	11.4	10.4	9.2	8.4	7.8	8.5
45–64 years	5.0	4.7	8.4	9.9	7.5	7.0	6.3	5.8	5.5	5.3	5.5
65 years and over	3.9	3.2	5.5	6.7	4.5	4.1	3.6	3.0	3.2	3.4	3.2

See footnotes at end of table.

[Data are based on the National Vital Statistics System]

Sex, race, Hispanic origin, and age	1950[1]	1960[1]	1970	1980	1985	1990	1994	1995	1996	1997	1995–97[2]
Black male				Deaths per 100,000 resident population							
All ages, age adjusted	51.1	44.9	82.1	71.9	50.2	68.7	66.2	57.6	52.6	48.3	52.8
All ages, crude	47.3	36.6	67.6	66.6	49.0	69.2	65.1	56.3	51.5	47.1	51.6
Under 1 year	---	10.3	14.3	18.6	16.7	21.4	23.9	19.4	23.1	18.1	20.2
1–14 years	---	1.5	4.4	4.1	4.2	5.8	6.4	6.1	4.8	4.7	5.2
15–24 years	58.9	46.4	102.5	84.3	65.9	138.3	157.6	132.0	123.1	113.3	122.7
25–44 years	97.8	84.9	143.3	130.1	87.5	106.2	90.9	77.9	71.0	65.0	71.3
25–34 years	110.5	92.0	158.5	145.1	95.6	125.4	112.1	98.3	89.5	82.9	90.2
35–44 years	83.7	77.5	126.2	110.3	74.9	82.3	67.6	56.2	52.0	47.1	51.7
45–64 years	47.6	45.4	83.0	70.8	46.3	41.7	33.4	34.6	30.5	27.4	30.8
65 years and over	16.7	17.9	33.7	31.1	26.2	25.9	22.1	19.9	15.6	14.4	16.6
American Indian or Alaska Native male[3]											
All ages, age adjusted	---	---	---	23.9	20.0	17.5	18.4	18.0	15.7	16.7	16.8
All ages, crude	---	---	---	23.4	19.0	17.3	18.3	17.8	15.3	16.4	16.5
15–24 years	---	---	---	36.0	27.1	27.7	32.5	32.2	26.6	27.7	28.8
25–44 years	---	---	---	39.7	30.2	26.0	27.9	28.4	23.6	23.9	25.3
45–64 years	---	---	---	22.1	21.2	15.5	*	13.2	12.7	13.3	13.1
Asian or Pacific Islander male[4]											
All ages, age adjusted	---	---	---	8.5	5.8	7.7	8.5	8.3	7.3	6.6	7.4
All ages, crude	---	---	---	8.3	6.0	7.9	8.5	8.0	7.2	6.5	7.2
15–24 years	---	---	---	9.3	8.6	14.9	19.6	19.4	15.6	13.4	16.1
25–44 years	---	---	---	11.3	8.9	9.7	9.9	8.1	8.4	7.6	8.0
45–64 years	---	---	---	10.4	5.4	7.0	6.3	8.4	7.6	6.5	7.4
Hispanic male[5]											
All ages, age adjusted	---	---	---	---	26.7	29.8	27.3	25.1	20.4	18.2	21.1
All ages, crude	---	---	---	---	27.6	31.5	27.8	25.2	20.9	18.6	21.5
Under 1 year	---	---	---	---	*	8.7	7.9	5.9	6.4	8.2	6.9
1–14 years	---	---	---	---	1.5	3.1	2.9	3.3	2.5	1.8	2.5
15–24 years	---	---	---	---	42.9	56.2	64.0	63.5	48.9	42.7	51.2
25–44 years	---	---	---	---	47.3	47.2	37.1	31.7	26.4	24.1	27.3
25–34 years	---	---	---	---	51.4	51.9	43.2	37.1	31.2	28.8	32.3
35–44 years	---	---	---	---	40.1	39.9	28.7	24.2	20.2	18.3	20.8
45–64 years	---	---	---	---	19.9	20.9	17.4	14.8	13.9	11.6	13.4
65 years and over	---	---	---	---	9.3	9.4	7.1	5.5	4.0	6.4	5.3
White, non-Hispanic male[5]											
All ages, age adjusted	---	---	---	---	6.2	5.8	5.7	5.1	4.7	4.8	4.9
All ages, crude	---	---	---	---	6.4	6.0	5.7	5.1	4.7	4.8	4.9
Under 1 year	---	---	---	---	4.6	5.4	5.4	6.7	6.4	7.4	6.8
1–14 years	---	---	---	---	1.2	0.9	1.1	1.1	1.1	1.1	1.1
15–24 years	---	---	---	---	7.7	7.7	8.3	7.3	6.4	6.5	6.7
25–44 years	---	---	---	---	9.5	9.0	8.5	7.6	6.9	6.9	7.1
25–34 years	---	---	---	---	9.6	9.6	9.0	8.2	7.3	7.6	7.7
35–44 years	---	---	---	---	9.3	8.3	7.9	7.1	6.6	6.3	6.6
45–64 years	---	---	---	---	6.4	5.8	5.2	4.8	4.6	4.7	4.7
65 years and over	---	---	---	---	4.4	3.7	3.4	2.7	3.1	3.1	3.0
White female											
All ages, age adjusted	1.4	1.5	2.2	3.2	2.9	2.8	2.7	2.8	2.5	2.3	2.5
All ages, crude	1.4	1.4	2.1	3.2	2.9	2.8	2.6	2.7	2.5	2.3	2.5
Under 1 year	3.9	3.5	2.9	4.3	4.3	5.1	5.1	5.0	6.8	4.6	5.5
1–14 years	0.4	0.4	0.7	1.1	1.1	1.0	1.1	1.1	1.1	0.9	1.0
15–24 years	1.3	1.5	2.7	4.7	3.6	4.0	3.9	4.0	3.3	3.2	3.5
25–44 years	2.0	2.1	3.3	4.2	4.1	3.8	3.7	3.8	3.3	3.1	3.4
45–64 years	1.5	1.7	2.1	2.6	2.6	2.3	1.9	2.2	2.1	1.9	2.1
65 years and over	1.2	1.2	1.9	2.9	2.6	2.2	1.9	2.0	1.8	1.9	1.9

See footnotes at end of table.

Table 46 (page 3 of 3). Death rates for homicide and legal intervention, according to sex, detailed race, Hispanic origin, and age: United States, selected years 1950–97

[Data are based on the National Vital Statistics System]

Sex, race, Hispanic origin, and age	1950[1]	1960[1]	1970	1980	1985	1990	1994	1995	1996	1997	1995–97[2]
Black female					Deaths per 100,000 resident population						
All ages, age adjusted	11.7	11.8	15.0	13.7	10.9	13.0	12.3	11.0	10.2	9.3	10.2
All ages, crude	11.5	10.4	13.3	13.5	11.1	13.5	12.4	11.1	10.2	9.3	10.2
Under 1 year	---	13.8	10.7	12.8	10.7	22.8	17.4	19.2	21.1	21.6	20.6
1–14 years	---	1.2	3.1	3.3	3.3	4.7	4.1	3.6	3.9	3.0	3.5
15–24 years	16.5	11.9	17.7	18.4	14.2	18.9	18.7	16.8	14.7	13.3	14.9
25–44 years	22.5	22.8	25.4	22.3	17.8	20.9	19.5	17.4	15.8	14.3	15.8
45–64 years	6.8	10.3	13.4	10.8	7.9	6.5	6.6	5.9	6.0	6.1	6.0
65 years and over	3.6	3.0	7.4	8.0	7.8	9.5	7.4	6.9	5.2	4.6	5.6
American Indian or Alaska Native female[3]											
All ages, age adjusted	---	---	---	8.3	4.8	4.9	5.4	5.6	4.5	5.2	5.1
All ages, crude	---	---	---	7.7	4.5	4.9	5.6	5.6	4.4	5.3	5.1
15–24 years	---	---	---	*	*	*	*	*	*	*	5.3
25–44 years	---	---	---	13.7	*	6.9	8.9	9.1	*	7.3	7.0
45–64 years	---	---	---	*	*	*	*	*	*	*	5.0
Asian or Pacific Islander female[4]											
All ages, age adjusted	---	---	---	3.0	2.7	2.7	2.4	2.6	2.1	2.2	2.3
All ages, crude	---	---	---	3.1	2.8	2.8	2.4	2.7	2.1	2.2	2.3
15–24 years	---	---	---	*	*	*	3.7	3.7	3.7	2.8	3.4
25–44 years	---	---	---	4.6	2.9	3.8	2.6	3.8	2.1	2.3	2.7
45–64 years	---	---	---	*	*	*	2.4	2.3	*	2.5	2.1
Hispanic female[5]											
All ages, age adjusted	---	---	---	---	4.2	4.6	4.2	4.4	3.4	3.1	3.6
All ages, crude	---	---	---	---	4.3	4.7	4.2	4.3	3.5	3.1	3.6
Under 1 year	---	---	---	---	*	*	7.1	*	7.7	*	6.2
1–14 years	---	---	---	---	1.5	1.9	1.9	1.8	1.5	1.2	1.5
15–24 years	---	---	---	---	5.7	8.1	6.5	6.9	5.1	4.8	5.6
25–44 years	---	---	---	---	6.8	6.1	5.8	5.8	4.8	4.5	5.1
45–64 years	---	---	---	---	3.2	3.3	3.0	3.4	2.7	2.5	2.9
65 years and over	---	---	---	---	*	*	*	2.3	*	*	1.6
White, non-Hispanic female[5]											
All ages, age adjusted	---	---	---	---	2.8	2.5	2.4	2.4	2.2	2.1	2.3
All ages, crude	---	---	---	---	2.9	2.6	2.4	2.4	2.3	2.1	2.3
Under 1 year	---	---	---	---	4.1	4.4	4.5	4.4	6.0	3.9	4.8
1–14 years	---	---	---	---	1.0	0.8	1.0	0.9	1.0	0.8	0.9
15–24 years	---	---	---	---	3.5	3.3	3.4	3.4	2.7	2.8	3.0
25–44 years	---	---	---	---	3.9	3.5	3.4	3.3	3.1	2.9	3.1
45–64 years	---	---	---	---	2.6	2.2	1.8	1.9	2.0	1.8	1.9
65 years and over	---	---	---	---	3.0	2.2	1.9	2.0	1.9	2.0	1.9

- - - Data not available.

* Based on fewer than 20 deaths.

[1]Includes deaths of persons who were not residents of the 50 States and the District of Columbia.

[2]Average annual death rate.

[3]Interpretation of trends should take into account that population estimates for American Indians increased by 45 percent between 1980 and 1990, partly due to better enumeration techniques in the 1990 decennial census and to the increased tendency for people to identify themselves as American Indian in 1990.

[4]Interpretation of trends should take into account that the Asian population in the United States more than doubled between 1980 and 1990, primarily due to immigration.

[5]Excludes data from States lacking an Hispanic-origin item on their death certificates. See Appendix I, National Vital Statistics System.

NOTES: For data years shown, the code numbers for cause of death are based on the then current *International Classification of Diseases*, which are described in Appendix II, tables IV and V. Age groups were selected to minimize the presentation of unstable age-specific death rates based on small numbers of deaths and for consistency among comparison groups. The race groups, white, black, Asian or Pacific Islander, and American Indian or Alaska Native, include persons of Hispanic and non-Hispanic origin. Conversely, persons of Hispanic origin may be of any race. Consistency of race identification between the death certificate (source of data for numerator of death rates) and data from the Census Bureau (denominator) is high for individual white and black persons; however, persons identified as American Indian, Asian, or Hispanic origin in data from the Census Bureau are sometimes misreported as white or non-Hispanic on the death certificate, causing death rates to be underestimated by 22–30 percent for American Indians, about 12 percent for Asians, and about 7 percent for persons of Hispanic origin. (Sorlie PD, Rogot E, and Johnson NJ: Validity of demographic characteristics on the death certificate, *Epidemiology* 3(2):181–184, 1992.) See Appendix II for age-adjustment procedure. Data for additional years are available (see Appendix III).

SOURCES: Centers for Disease Control and Prevention, National Center for Health Statistics. Grove RD and Hetzel AM. *Vital statistics rates in the United States, 1940–60*. Washington: Public Health Service, 1968; *Vital statistics of the United States, vol II, mortality, part A*, for data years 1950–93. Public Health Service. Washington. U.S. Government Printing Office; for 1994–97, unpublished data; data computed by the Division of Health and Utilization Analysis from numeratory data compiled by the Division of Vital Statistics and denominator data from national population estimates for race groups from table 1 and unpublished Hispanic population estimates prepared by the Housing and Household Economic Statistics Division, U.S. Bureau of the Census.

Table 47 (page 1 of 3). Death rates for suicide, according to sex, detailed race, Hispanic origin, and age: United States, selected years 1950–97

[Data are based on the National Vital Statistics System]

Sex, race, Hispanic origin, and age	1950[1]	1960[1]	1970	1980	1985	1990	1994	1995	1996	1997	1995–97[2]
All persons					Deaths per 100,000 resident population						
All ages, age adjusted	11.0	10.6	11.8	11.4	11.5	11.5	11.2	11.2	10.8	10.6	10.8
All ages, crude	11.4	10.6	11.6	11.9	12.4	12.4	12.0	11.9	11.6	11.4	11.7
Under 1 year	...	...	...	...	...	...	...	...	...	...	...
1–4 years	...	...	...	...	...	...	...	...	...	...	...
5–14 years	0.2	0.3	0.3	0.4	0.8	0.8	0.9	0.9	0.8	0.8	0.8
15–24 years	4.5	5.2	8.8	12.3	12.8	13.2	13.8	13.3	12.0	11.4	12.3
25–44 years	11.6	12.2	15.4	15.6	15.0	15.2	15.3	15.3	15.0	14.8	15.1
25–34 years	9.1	10.0	14.1	16.0	15.3	15.2	15.4	15.4	14.5	14.3	14.7
35–44 years	14.3	14.2	16.9	15.4	14.6	15.3	15.3	15.2	15.5	15.3	15.4
45–64 years	23.5	22.0	20.6	15.9	16.3	15.3	14.0	14.1	14.4	14.2	14.2
45–54 years	20.9	20.7	20.0	15.9	15.7	14.8	14.4	14.6	14.9	14.7	14.7
55–64 years	27.0	23.7	21.4	15.9	16.8	16.0	13.4	13.3	13.7	13.5	13.5
65 years and over	30.0	24.5	20.8	17.6	20.4	20.5	18.1	18.1	17.3	16.8	17.4
65–74 years	29.3	23.0	20.8	16.9	18.7	17.9	15.3	15.8	15.0	14.4	15.1
75–84 years	31.1	27.9	21.2	19.1	23.9	24.9	21.3	20.7	20.0	19.3	20.0
85 years and over	28.8	26.0	19.0	19.2	19.4	22.2	23.0	21.6	20.2	20.8	20.9
Male											
All ages, age adjusted	17.3	16.6	17.3	18.0	18.8	19.0	18.7	18.6	18.0	17.4	18.0
All ages, crude	17.8	16.5	16.8	18.6	20.0	20.4	19.8	19.8	19.3	18.7	19.2
Under 1 year	...	...	...	...	...	...	...	...	...	...	...
1–4 years	...	...	...	...	...	...	...	...	...	...	...
5–14 years	0.3	0.4	0.5	0.6	1.2	1.1	1.2	1.3	1.1	1.2	1.2
15–24 years	6.5	8.2	13.5	20.2	21.0	22.0	23.4	22.5	20.0	18.9	20.5
25–44 years	17.2	17.9	20.9	24.0	23.7	24.4	24.8	24.9	24.3	23.8	24.3
25–34 years	13.4	14.7	19.8	25.0	24.7	24.8	25.6	25.6	24.0	23.6	24.4
35–44 years	21.3	21.0	22.1	22.5	22.3	23.9	24.1	24.1	24.6	23.9	24.2
45–64 years	37.1	34.4	30.0	23.7	25.3	24.3	22.1	22.5	23.0	22.5	22.7
45–54 years	32.0	31.6	27.9	22.9	23.6	23.2	22.1	22.8	23.3	22.5	22.8
55–64 years	43.6	38.1	32.7	24.5	27.1	25.7	22.0	22.0	22.7	22.4	22.4
65 years and over	52.8	44.0	38.4	35.0	40.9	41.6	36.6	36.3	35.2	33.9	35.1
65–74 years	50.5	39.6	36.0	30.4	33.9	32.2	27.7	28.7	27.7	26.4	27.6
75–84 years	58.3	52.5	42.8	42.3	53.1	56.1	47.0	44.8	43.4	40.9	43.0
85 years and over	58.3	57.4	42.4	50.6	56.2	65.9	66.6	63.1	59.9	60.3	61.1
Female											
All ages, age adjusted	4.9	5.0	6.8	5.4	4.9	4.5	4.2	4.1	4.0	4.1	4.1
All ages, crude	5.1	4.9	6.6	5.5	5.2	4.8	4.5	4.4	4.4	4.4	4.4
Under 1 year	...	...	...	...	...	...	...	...	...	...	...
1–4 years	...	...	...	...	...	...	...	...	...	...	...
5–14 years	0.1	0.1	0.2	0.2	0.4	0.4	0.5	0.4	0.4	0.4	0.4
15–24 years	2.6	2.2	4.2	4.3	4.3	3.9	3.7	3.7	3.6	3.5	3.6
25–44 years	6.2	6.6	10.2	7.7	6.5	6.2	5.9	5.8	5.8	6.0	5.9
25–34 years	4.9	5.5	8.6	7.1	5.9	5.6	5.1	5.2	5.0	5.0	5.1
35–44 years	7.5	7.7	11.9	8.5	7.1	6.8	6.7	6.5	6.6	6.8	6.6
45–64 years	9.9	10.2	12.0	8.9	8.0	7.1	6.4	6.1	6.4	6.5	6.4
45–54 years	9.9	10.2	12.6	9.4	8.3	6.9	7.0	6.7	7.0	7.3	7.0
55–64 years	9.9	10.2	11.4	8.4	7.8	7.3	5.6	5.3	5.5	5.4	5.4
65 years and over	9.4	8.4	8.1	6.1	6.6	6.4	5.5	5.5	4.8	4.9	5.0
65–74 years	10.1	8.4	9.0	6.5	6.9	6.7	5.4	5.4	4.8	4.7	5.0
75–84 years	8.1	8.9	7.0	5.5	6.7	6.3	5.3	5.5	5.0	5.2	5.2
85 years and over	8.2	6.0	5.9	5.5	4.7	5.4	6.2	5.5	4.4	4.9	4.9
White male											
All ages, age adjusted	18.1	17.5	18.2	18.9	19.9	20.1	19.7	19.7	19.1	18.4	19.1
All ages, crude	19.0	17.6	18.0	19.9	21.6	22.0	21.3	21.4	20.9	20.2	20.8
15–24 years	6.6	8.6	13.9	21.4	22.3	23.2	24.1	23.5	20.9	19.5	21.3
25–44 years	17.9	18.5	21.5	24.6	24.8	25.4	26.1	26.3	25.7	25.3	25.8
45–64 years	39.3	36.5	31.9	25.0	27.0	26.0	23.8	24.2	24.9	24.2	24.4
65 years and over	55.8	46.7	41.1	37.2	43.7	44.2	38.9	38.7	37.8	36.1	37.5
65–74 years	53.2	42.0	38.7	32.5	35.8	34.2	29.3	30.3	29.6	28.0	29.3
75–84 years	61.9	55.7	45.5	45.5	57.0	60.2	50.0	47.5	46.1	43.4	45.6
85 years and over	61.9	61.3	45.8	52.8	60.9	70.3	71.4	68.2	65.4	65.0	66.1

See footnotes at end of table.

Table 47 (page 2 of 3). Death rates for suicide, according to sex, detailed race, Hispanic origin, and age: United States, selected years 1950–97

[Data are based on the National Vital Statistics System]

Sex, race, Hispanic origin, and age	1950[1]	1960[1]	1970	1980	1985	1990	1994	1995	1996	1997	1995–97[2]
Black male					Deaths per 100,000 resident population						
All ages, age adjusted	7.0	7.8	9.9	11.1	11.5	12.4	12.7	12.4	11.8	11.2	11.8
All ages, crude	6.3	6.4	8.0	10.3	11.0	12.0	12.4	11.9	11.4	10.9	11.4
15–24 years	4.9	4.1	10.5	12.3	13.3	15.1	20.6	18.0	16.7	16.0	16.9
25–44 years	9.8	12.6	16.1	19.2	17.8	19.6	18.9	18.6	17.8	17.0	17.8
45–64 years	12.7	13.0	12.4	11.8	12.9	13.1	10.3	11.8	11.8	10.5	11.3
65 years and over	9.0	9.9	8.7	11.4	15.8	14.9	15.4	14.3	12.6	13.6	13.5
65–74 years	10.0	11.3	8.7	11.1	16.7	14.7	15.0	13.5	12.7	12.9	13.0
75–84 years	- - -	6.6	8.9	10.5	15.6	14.4	14.9	16.6	12.5	14.1	14.4
85 years and over	- - -	6.9	*	*	*	*	*	*	*	*	14.1
American Indian or Alaska Native male[3]											
All ages, age adjusted	- - -	- - -	- - -	20.8	19.9	21.0	23.8	20.1	20.0	21.3	20.5
All ages, crude	- - -	- - -	- - -	20.9	20.3	20.9	23.3	19.6	19.9	20.9	20.2
15–24 years	- - -	- - -	- - -	45.3	42.0	49.1	45.8	34.2	32.1	38.4	34.9
25–44 years	- - -	- - -	- - -	31.2	30.2	27.8	38.4	31.8	34.8	32.6	33.1
45–64 years	- - -	- - -	- - -	*	*	*	14.8	15.0	11.5	15.5	14.0
65 years and over	- - -	- - -	- - -	*	*	*	*	*	*	*	13.5
Asian or Pacific Islander male[4]											
All ages, age adjusted	- - -	- - -	- - -	9.0	8.5	8.8	9.7	9.7	8.6	9.4	9.2
All ages, crude	- - -	- - -	- - -	8.8	8.4	8.7	9.6	9.4	8.6	9.2	9.0
15–24 years	- - -	- - -	- - -	10.8	14.2	13.5	15.1	16.0	11.9	12.2	13.3
25–44 years	- - -	- - -	- - -	11.0	9.3	10.6	12.7	11.5	11.5	10.6	11.2
45–64 years	- - -	- - -	- - -	13.0	10.4	9.7	9.1	9.1	8.6	12.3	10.1
65 years and over	- - -	- - -	- - -	18.6	16.7	16.8	18.3	20.3	16.0	21.0	19.1
Hispanic male[5]											
All ages, age adjusted	- - -	- - -	- - -	- - -	10.4	12.4	12.5	12.3	11.1	10.4	11.2
All ages, crude	- - -	- - -	- - -	- - -	9.8	11.4	11.8	11.5	10.6	9.8	10.6
15–24 years	- - -	- - -	- - -	- - -	13.8	14.7	18.7	18.3	15.5	14.4	16.0
25–44 years	- - -	- - -	- - -	- - -	14.8	16.2	16.8	15.5	14.6	13.9	14.6
45–64 years	- - -	- - -	- - -	- - -	12.3	16.1	13.6	14.2	13.3	11.6	13.0
65 years and over	- - -	- - -	- - -	- - -	14.7	23.4	17.8	19.9	17.7	17.7	18.4
White, non-Hispanic male[5]											
All ages, age adjusted	- - -	- - -	- - -	- - -	20.3	20.8	20.1	20.2	19.7	19.3	19.7
All ages, crude	- - -	- - -	- - -	- - -	22.3	23.1	22.2	22.3	22.0	21.5	22.0
15–24 years	- - -	- - -	- - -	- - -	22.6	24.4	24.4	23.8	21.4	20.2	21.8
25–44 years	- - -	- - -	- - -	- - -	25.1	26.4	26.9	27.3	27.1	26.8	27.0
45–64 years	- - -	- - -	- - -	- - -	27.3	26.8	24.4	24.8	25.6	25.1	25.1
65 years and over	- - -	- - -	- - -	- - -	46.4	45.4	39.7	39.2	38.6	36.8	38.2
White female											
All ages, age adjusted	5.3	5.3	7.2	5.7	5.3	4.8	4.5	4.4	4.4	4.4	4.4
All ages, crude	5.5	5.3	7.1	5.9	5.6	5.3	4.9	4.8	4.8	4.9	4.8
15–24 years	2.7	2.3	4.2	4.6	4.7	4.2	3.8	3.9	3.8	3.7	3.8
25–44 years	6.6	7.0	11.0	8.1	7.0	6.6	6.5	6.3	6.4	6.6	6.4
45–64 years	10.6	10.9	13.0	9.6	8.7	7.7	7.0	6.7	7.0	7.2	7.0
65 years and over	9.9	8.8	8.5	6.4	6.9	6.8	5.8	5.7	5.0	5.1	5.3

See footnotes at end of table.

Table 47 (page 3 of 3). Death rates for suicide, according to sex, detailed race, Hispanic origin, and age: United States, selected years 1950–97

[Data are based on the National Vital Statistics System]

Sex, race, Hispanic origin, and age	1950[1]	1960[1]	1970	1980	1985	1990	1994	1995	1996	1997	1995–97[2]
Black female				Deaths per 100,000 resident population							
All ages, age adjusted	1.7	1.9	2.9	2.4	2.1	2.4	2.1	2.0	2.0	1.9	2.0
All ages, crude	1.5	1.6	2.6	2.2	2.1	2.3	2.0	2.0	2.0	1.9	2.0
15–24 years	1.8	*	3.8	2.3	2.0	2.3	2.7	2.2	2.3	2.4	2.3
25–44 years	2.3	3.0	4.8	4.3	3.2	3.8	3.1	3.4	2.9	2.7	3.0
45–64 years	2.7	3.1	2.9	2.5	2.8	2.9	2.3	2.0	2.3	2.4	2.3
65 years and over	2.0	1.9	2.6	*	2.7	1.9	2.0	2.2	2.1	1.6	2.0
American Indian or Alaska Native female[3]											
All ages, age adjusted	---	---	---	5.0	4.4	3.8	4.3	4.4	5.9	4.4	4.9
All ages, crude	---	---	---	4.7	4.4	3.7	4.0	4.2	5.6	4.2	4.7
15–24 years	---	---	---	*	*	*	*	*	10.2	*	7.2
25–44 years	---	---	---	10.7	*	*	*	7.1	9.0	6.4	7.5
45–64 years	---	---	---	*	*	*	*	*	*	*	5.1
65 years and over	---	---	---	*	*	*	*	*	*	*	*
Asian or Pacific Islander female[4]											
All ages, age adjusted	---	---	---	4.7	4.4	3.4	3.8	3.7	3.6	3.4	3.6
All ages, crude	---	---	---	4.7	4.3	3.4	3.9	3.8	3.7	3.6	3.7
15–24 years	---	---	---	*	5.8	3.9	5.7	5.2	3.0	4.7	4.3
25–44 years	---	---	---	5.4	4.2	3.8	4.2	3.8	4.5	3.7	4.0
45–64 years	---	---	---	7.9	5.4	5.0	5.4	4.9	5.2	4.4	4.8
65 years and over	---	---	---	*	13.6	8.5	6.8	9.0	8.4	8.9	8.8
Hispanic female[5]											
All ages, age adjusted	---	---	---	---	1.8	2.3	1.9	2.0	2.2	1.7	2.0
All ages, crude	---	---	---	---	1.6	2.2	1.8	1.9	2.1	1.6	1.8
15–24 years	---	---	---	---	2.1	3.1	2.8	2.6	3.3	2.4	2.8
25–44 years	---	---	---	---	2.1	3.1	2.6	2.7	2.8	2.2	2.5
45–64 years	---	---	---	---	3.2	2.5	2.1	2.7	2.6	2.3	2.5
65 years and over	---	---	---	---	*	*	2.4	*	2.5	*	2.2
White, non-Hispanic female[5]											
All ages, age adjusted	---	---	---	---	5.7	5.0	4.7	4.6	4.5	4.7	4.6
All ages, crude	---	---	---	---	6.2	5.6	5.2	5.1	5.0	5.3	5.1
15–24 years	---	---	---	---	4.7	4.3	3.9	4.0	3.8	3.9	3.9
25–44 years	---	---	---	---	7.7	7.0	6.9	6.7	6.7	7.2	6.9
45–64 years	---	---	---	---	9.2	8.0	7.3	7.0	7.3	7.6	7.3
65 years and over	---	---	---	---	7.5	7.0	5.9	5.8	5.1	5.2	5.4

. . . Category not applicable.
- - - Data not available.
* Based on fewer than 20 deaths.
[1]Includes deaths of persons who were not residents of the 50 States and the District of Columbia.
[2]Average annual death rate.
[3]Interpretation of trends should take into account that population estimates for American Indians increased by 45 percent between 1980 and 1990, partly due to better enumeration techniques in the 1990 decennial census and to the increased tendency for people to identify themselves as American Indian in 1990.
[4]Interpretation of trends should take into account that the Asian population in the United States more than doubled between 1980 and 1990, primarily due to immigration.
[5]Excludes data from States lacking an Hispanic-origin item on their death certificates. See Appendix I, National Vital Statistics System.

NOTES: For data years shown, the code numbers for cause of death are based on the then current *International Classification of Diseases*, which are described in Appendix II, tables IV and V. Age groups chosen to show data for American Indians, Asians, Hispanics, and non-Hispanic whites were selected to minimize the presentation of unstable age-specific death rates based on small numbers of deaths and for consistency among comparison groups. The race groups, white, black, Asian or Pacific Islander, and American Indian or Alaska Native, include persons of Hispanic and non-Hispanic origin. Conversely, persons of Hispanic origin may be of any race. Consistency of race identification between the death certificate (source of data for numerator of death rates) and data from the Census Bureau (denominator) is high for individual white and black persons; however, persons identified as American Indian, Asian, or Hispanic origin in data from the Census Bureau are sometimes misreported as white or non-Hispanic on the death certificate, causing death rates to be underestimated by 22–30 percent for American Indians, about 12 percent for Asians, and about 7 percent for persons of Hispanic origin. (Sorlie PD, Rogot E, and Johnson NJ: Validity of demographic characteristics on the death certificate, *Epidemiology* 3(2):181–184, 1992.) See Appendix II for age-adjustment procedure. Data for additional years are available (see Appendix III).

SOURCES: Centers for Disease Control and Prevention, National Center for Health Statistics. Grove RD and Hetzel AM. *Vital statistics rates in the United States, 1940–60.* Washington: Public Health Service, 1968; *Vital statistics of the United States, vol II, mortality, part A,* for data years 1950–93. Public Health Service. Washington. U.S. Government Printing Office; for 1994–97, unpublished data; data computed by the Division of Health and Utilization Analysis from numerator data compiled by the Division of Vital Statistics and denominator data from national population estimates for race groups from table 1 and unpublished Hispanic population estimates prepared by the Housing and Household Economic Statistics Division, U.S. Bureau of the Census.

Table 48 (page 1 of 3). Death rates for firearm-related injuries, according to sex, detailed race, Hispanic origin, and age: United States, selected years 1970–97

[Data are based on the National Vital Statistics System]

Sex, race, Hispanic origin, and age	1970	1980	1985	1988	1990	1993	1994	1995	1996	1997	1995–97[1]
All persons					Deaths per 100,000 resident population						
All ages, age adjusted	14.0	14.8	12.8	13.4	14.6	15.6	15.1	13.9	12.9	12.2	13.0
All ages, crude	13.0	14.9	13.3	13.9	14.9	15.4	14.8	13.7	12.8	12.1	12.9
Under 1 year	*	*	*	*	*	*	*	*	*	*	0.2
1–14 years	1.6	1.4	1.4	1.5	1.5	1.8	1.6	1.6	1.3	1.1	1.3
1–4 years	1.0	0.7	0.7	0.6	0.6	0.6	0.6	0.6	0.5	0.5	0.5
5–14 years	1.7	1.6	1.8	1.9	1.9	2.3	2.0	2.0	1.6	1.4	1.6
15–24 years	15.5	20.6	17.2	20.6	25.8	31.1	30.8	27.2	24.2	22.3	24.6
25–44 years	20.9	22.5	17.9	18.3	19.3	19.3	18.8	17.2	16.1	15.4	16.2
25–34 years	22.2	24.3	19.3	20.4	21.8	22.4	21.9	20.1	18.3	17.8	18.8
35–44 years	19.6	20.0	16.0	15.8	16.3	16.0	15.6	14.4	14.0	13.2	13.9
45–64 years	17.6	15.2	14.3	13.4	13.6	13.2	12.2	11.8	11.9	11.3	11.7
45–54 years	18.1	16.4	14.7	13.5	13.9	13.7	12.8	12.1	12.3	11.5	12.0
55–64 years	17.0	13.9	13.9	13.3	13.3	12.5	11.4	11.4	11.2	11.0	11.2
65 years and over	13.8	13.5	15.6	16.2	16.0	15.1	14.3	14.2	13.9	13.2	13.8
65–74 years	14.5	13.8	15.1	14.9	14.4	13.5	12.6	12.9	12.6	11.9	12.5
75–84 years	13.4	13.4	17.7	19.3	19.4	17.7	16.9	16.4	15.9	14.9	15.7
85 years and over	10.2	11.6	12.2	13.6	14.7	15.4	15.1	14.6	14.5	14.3	14.5
Male											
All ages, age adjusted	23.8	25.3	21.9	23.0	25.4	26.9	26.2	24.1	22.4	21.1	22.5
All ages, crude	22.2	25.7	22.8	24.1	26.2	26.8	26.0	23.9	22.5	21.2	22.5
Under 1 year	*	*	*	*	*	*	*	*	*	*	*
1–14 years	2.3	2.0	2.1	2.2	2.2	2.6	2.3	2.3	1.8	1.7	1.9
1–4 years	1.2	0.9	0.8	0.8	0.7	0.8	0.7	0.8	0.5	0.5	0.6
5–14 years	2.7	2.5	2.7	2.8	2.9	3.4	3.0	2.9	2.4	2.1	2.5
15–24 years	26.4	34.8	29.1	35.5	44.7	54.0	54.0	47.6	42.2	38.9	42.9
25–44 years	34.1	38.1	29.7	30.5	32.6	32.2	31.7	28.9	27.0	25.8	27.2
25–34 years	36.5	41.4	32.1	34.2	37.0	37.8	37.4	34.3	31.4	30.5	32.1
35–44 years	31.6	33.2	26.6	26.0	27.4	26.4	26.0	23.7	22.9	21.5	22.7
45–64 years	31.0	25.9	24.5	22.9	23.4	22.7	21.0	20.2	20.4	19.4	20.0
45–54 years	30.7	27.3	24.4	22.4	23.2	23.1	21.3	20.4	20.5	19.3	20.1
55–64 years	31.3	24.5	24.6	23.5	23.7	22.2	20.5	20.0	20.2	19.7	19.9
65 years and over	29.7	29.7	34.2	35.5	35.3	32.8	31.2	30.9	30.2	28.5	29.8
65–74 years	29.5	27.8	30.0	29.4	28.2	26.2	24.6	25.3	24.8	23.1	24.4
75–84 years	31.0	33.0	42.7	47.0	46.9	41.9	39.9	37.7	36.4	34.1	36.0
85 years and over	26.2	34.9	38.2	43.1	49.3	50.5	49.7	47.4	46.7	45.8	46.6
Female											
All ages, age adjusted	4.8	4.8	4.2	4.2	4.3	4.6	4.2	4.0	3.6	3.4	3.7
All ages, crude	4.4	4.7	4.2	4.2	4.3	4.5	4.1	3.9	3.6	3.4	3.6
Under 1 year	*	*	*	*	*	*	*	*	*	*	*
1–14 years	0.8	0.7	0.7	0.8	0.8	0.9	0.9	0.8	0.7	0.6	0.7
1–4 years	0.9	0.5	0.5	0.5	0.5	0.5	0.5	0.5	0.4	0.5	0.5
5–14 years	0.8	0.7	0.8	0.9	1.0	1.1	1.0	0.9	0.8	0.7	0.8
15–24 years	4.8	6.1	5.0	5.1	6.0	7.1	6.5	6.0	5.1	4.8	5.3
25–44 years	8.3	7.4	6.2	6.3	6.1	6.4	6.0	5.6	5.2	5.0	5.3
25–34 years	8.4	7.5	6.6	6.7	6.7	7.1	6.5	5.9	5.2	5.1	5.4
35–44 years	8.2	7.2	5.8	5.8	5.4	5.8	5.5	5.3	5.1	4.9	5.1
45–64 years	5.4	5.4	5.0	4.7	4.5	4.4	4.1	4.0	3.9	3.7	3.8
45–54 years	6.4	6.2	5.6	5.1	4.9	4.8	4.6	4.3	4.4	4.1	4.3
55–64 years	4.2	4.6	4.5	4.3	4.0	3.8	3.3	3.5	3.1	3.0	3.2
65 years and over	2.4	2.5	3.2	3.2	3.1	3.0	2.7	2.8	2.6	2.5	2.6
65–74 years	2.8	3.1	3.6	3.7	3.6	3.4	3.0	3.0	2.8	2.9	2.9
75–84 years	1.7	1.7	3.0	2.9	2.9	2.8	2.5	2.8	2.6	2.3	2.6
85 years and over	*	1.3	1.8	2.1	1.3	1.9	1.8	1.8	1.7	1.7	1.7
White male											
All ages, age adjusted	18.2	21.1	19.4	19.3	20.5	20.7	20.4	19.3	18.0	17.1	18.1
All ages, crude	17.6	21.8	20.7	20.7	21.8	21.5	21.1	20.1	19.0	18.1	19.0
1–14 years	1.8	1.9	2.1	1.9	1.9	2.0	1.8	1.9	1.5	1.4	1.6
15–24 years	16.9	28.4	24.1	25.3	29.5	33.0	34.2	31.4	26.9	24.8	27.7
25–44 years	24.2	29.5	25.0	24.4	25.7	25.1	24.9	23.6	22.0	21.2	22.3
25–34 years	24.3	31.1	26.3	26.0	27.8	27.9	27.6	26.1	23.6	23.1	24.3
35–44 years	24.1	27.1	23.3	22.5	23.3	22.2	22.3	21.2	20.6	19.5	20.4
45–64 years	27.4	23.3	23.6	22.5	22.8	22.0	20.6	19.7	20.2	19.4	19.8
65 years and over	29.9	30.1	35.4	37.0	36.8	34.4	32.5	32.3	31.8	30.0	31.4

See footnotes at end of table.

[Data are based on the National Vital Statistics System]

Sex, race, Hispanic origin, and age	1970	1980	1985	1988	1990	1993	1994	1995	1996	1997	1995–97[1]
Black male					Deaths per 100,000 resident population						
All ages, age adjusted	73.4	61.8	42.2	51.0	61.5	68.8	65.1	55.6	52.0	47.4	51.6
All ages, crude	60.6	57.7	41.3	51.7	61.9	67.6	63.8	54.0	50.6	46.1	50.2
1–14 years	5.3	3.0	2.7	4.0	4.4	6.1	5.2	4.6	3.6	3.1	3.7
15–24 years	97.3	77.9	61.3	99.0	138.0	179.0	169.6	140.2	131.6	119.9	130.5
25–44 years	126.2	114.1	71.8	82.1	90.3	88.2	84.5	71.2	67.0	61.8	66.6
25–34 years	145.6	128.4	79.8	97.1	108.6	110.7	109.0	94.4	88.6	84.0	89.0
35–44 years	104.2	92.3	59.2	60.7	66.1	62.3	57.7	46.6	44.7	39.5	43.5
45–64 years	71.1	55.6	36.9	30.7	34.5	33.4	29.1	29.1	27.0	23.3	26.4
65 years and over	30.6	29.7	26.3	24.8	23.9	22.0	23.2	21.4	19.1	17.8	19.4
American Indian or Alaska Native male[2]											
All ages, age adjusted	---	26.5	24.9	24.0	20.8	21.8	24.6	23.4	19.4	20.7	21.1
All ages, crude	---	27.5	24.4	24.1	20.5	21.2	24.1	22.9	19.1	20.1	20.7
15–24 years	---	55.3	39.8	48.1	49.1	37.3	54.6	45.5	40.0	39.4	41.5
25–44 years	---	43.9	40.3	34.4	25.4	32.7	33.8	34.1	26.7	29.3	30.0
45–64 years	---	*	21.2	*	*	18.5	13.6	15.6	13.8	13.9	14.4
65 years and over	---	*		*	*	*	*	*	*	*	13.0
Asian or Pacific Islander male[3]											
All ages, age adjusted	---	8.1	7.1	8.4	9.2	11.9	10.9	10.8	8.7	9.0	9.5
All ages, crude	---	8.2	7.3	8.6	9.4	11.7	10.8	10.4	8.6	8.7	9.2
15–24 years	---	10.8	12.6	14.2	21.0	27.6	26.9	27.1	19.6	19.7	22.0
25–44 years	---	12.8	9.8	11.0	10.9	13.5	13.0	11.3	10.0	9.6	10.3
45–64 years	---	10.4	6.7	9.3	8.1	9.7	7.4	8.6	7.7	8.7	8.3
65 years and over	---	*	*	*	*	*	*	*	*	7.7	6.2
Hispanic male[4]											
All ages, age adjusted	---	---	25.3	23.8	28.9	30.5	29.9	28.0	22.5	19.9	23.3
All ages, crude	---	---	26.0	24.5	29.9	30.8	30.0	27.6	22.6	19.9	23.2
1–14 years	---	---	1.4	1.4	2.6	2.7	2.3	2.9	1.9	1.4	2.0
15–24 years	---	---	42.0	40.4	55.5	70.3	72.0	70.7	54.4	47.9	57.1
25–44 years	---	---	43.2	37.4	42.7	40.0	38.8	33.5	27.5	24.5	28.4
25–34 years	---	---	47.3	39.9	47.3	46.0	45.5	39.9	32.8	29.3	33.9
35–44 years	---	---	35.9	33.0	35.4	31.2	29.5	24.9	20.8	18.7	21.3
45–64 years	---	---	19.2	20.6	21.4	21.1	19.2	17.2	16.2	13.7	15.6
65 years and over	---	---	12.4	15.3	19.1	16.7	14.7	15.6	11.7	12.3	13.1
White, non-Hispanic male[4]											
All ages, age adjusted	---	---	18.4	17.9	18.7	18.3	18.1	17.2	16.4	15.9	16.5
All ages, crude	---	---	19.9	19.7	20.4	19.8	19.5	18.6	18.0	17.5	18.1
1–14 years	---	---	2.0	1.8	1.6	1.8	1.6	1.6	1.4	1.4	1.5
15–24 years	---	---	22.0	22.1	24.1	25.3	26.3	23.3	20.4	19.4	21.0
25–44 years	---	---	23.0	22.0	23.3	22.4	22.4	21.6	20.6	20.3	20.8
25–34 years	---	---	23.7	23.0	24.7	24.1	23.9	22.9	21.2	21.4	21.9
35–44 years	---	---	22.0	20.8	21.6	20.6	20.9	20.4	20.1	19.4	19.9
45–64 years	---	---	23.0	21.9	22.7	21.7	20.5	19.7	20.2	19.8	19.9
65 years and over	---	---	37.3	38.6	37.4	34.7	33.2	32.7	32.6	30.8	32.0
White female											
All ages, age adjusted	4.0	4.2	3.9	3.7	3.7	3.9	3.6	3.5	3.1	3.1	3.3
All ages, crude	3.7	4.1	4.0	3.8	3.8	3.9	3.6	3.5	3.2	3.2	3.3
15–24 years	3.4	5.1	4.4	4.1	4.8	5.2	4.9	4.6	3.8	3.8	4.1
25–44 years	6.9	6.2	5.6	5.3	5.3	5.5	5.2	5.0	4.6	4.7	4.7
45–64 years	5.0	5.1	5.0	4.7	4.5	4.5	4.1	4.0	3.9	3.8	3.9
65 years and over	2.2	2.5	3.2	3.3	3.1	3.0	2.7	2.9	2.6	2.6	2.7

See footnotes at end of table.

Table 48 (page 3 of 3). Death rates for firearm-related injuries, according to sex, detailed race, Hispanic origin, and age: United States, selected years 1970–97

[Data are based on the National Vital Statistics System]

Sex, race, Hispanic origin, and age	1970	1980	1985	1988	1990	1993	1994	1995	1996	1997	1995–97[1]
Black female					Deaths per 100,000 resident population						
All ages, age adjusted	11.4	9.1	6.6	7.6	7.8	8.8	8.0	6.8	6.5	5.6	6.3
All ages, crude	10.0	8.8	6.5	7.7	7.8	8.6	7.8	6.6	6.4	5.4	6.1
15–24 years	15.2	12.3	8.3	11.2	13.3	18.3	15.5	13.5	12.0	10.6	12.0
25–44 years	19.4	16.1	11.4	13.1	12.4	12.9	11.9	10.0	9.8	8.0	9.2
45–64 years	10.2	8.2	5.8	5.2	4.8	4.0	4.6	4.1	4.1	3.4	3.8
65 years and over	4.3	3.1	3.7	2.8	3.1	3.0	2.9	2.6	3.0	2.2	2.6
American Indian or Alaska Native female[2]											
All ages, age adjusted	- - -	6.1	4.3	3.6	3.6	4.5	4.5	4.5	3.8	3.2	3.8
All ages, crude	- - -	5.8	4.1	3.8	3.4	4.5	4.4	4.4	3.7	3.0	3.7
15–24 years	- - -	*	*	*	*	*	*	*	*	*	5.5
25–44 years	- - -	10.2	*	6.9	*	7.8	7.5	7.7	5.9	*	5.6
45–64 years	- - -	*	*	*	*	*	*	*	*	*	3.7
65 years and over	- - -	*	*	*	*	*	*	*	*	*	*
Asian or Pacific Islander female[3]											
All ages, age adjusted	- - -	2.0	1.7	1.8	2.0	2.6	2.1	2.2	1.7	1.8	1.9
All ages, crude	- - -	2.1	1.7	2.0	2.1	2.6	2.1	2.2	1.7	1.7	1.9
15–24 years	- - -	*	*	*	*	3.8	4.0	4.2	3.7	3.2	3.7
25–44 years	- - -	3.2	2.2	3.4	2.7	3.5	2.6	2.9	2.1	1.9	2.3
45–64 years	- - -	*	*	*	*	2.9	*	*	*	*	1.8
65 years and over	- - -	*	*	*	*	*	*	*	*	*	*
Hispanic female[4]											
All ages, age adjusted	- - -	- - -	3.2	3.1	3.6	4.0	3.5	3.5	2.8	2.4	2.9
All ages, crude	- - -	- - -	3.2	3.1	3.6	3.9	3.4	3.4	2.7	2.3	2.8
15–24 years	- - -	- - -	5.1	5.5	6.9	7.8	6.9	6.6	5.0	4.5	5.3
25–44 years	- - -	- - -	5.5	4.7	5.1	5.2	5.0	4.9	4.1	3.3	4.1
45–64 years	- - -	- - -	2.2	2.1	2.4	2.6	2.4	2.4	2.3	2.2	2.3
65 years and over	- - -	- - -	*	*	*	*	*	*	*	*	0.9
White, non-Hispanic female[4]											
All ages, age adjusted	- - -	- - -	3.9	3.7	3.6	3.7	3.5	3.4	3.1	3.2	3.2
All ages, crude	- - -	- - -	4.1	3.8	3.7	3.8	3.6	3.5	3.2	3.3	3.3
15–24 years	- - -	- - -	4.5	3.9	4.3	4.6	4.5	4.1	3.5	3.6	3.7
25–44 years	- - -	- - -	5.6	5.3	5.1	5.4	5.1	4.8	4.5	4.8	4.7
45–64 years	- - -	- - -	5.1	4.9	4.6	4.5	4.1	4.1	4.0	3.9	4.0
65 years and over	- - -	- - -	3.4	3.6	3.2	3.0	2.7	2.9	2.7	2.7	2.7

* Based on fewer than 20 deaths.

- - - Data not available.

[1]Average annual death rate.

[2]Interpretation of trends should take into account that population estimates for American Indians increased by 45 percent between 1980 and 1990, partly due to better enumeration techniques in the 1990 decennial census and to the increased tendency for people to identify themselves as American Indian in 1990.

[3]Interpretation of trends should take into account that the Asian population in the United States more than doubled between 1980 and 1990, primarily due to immigration.

[4]Excludes data from States lacking an Hispanic-origin item on their death certificates. See Appendix I, National Vital Statistics System.

NOTES: For data years shown, the code numbers for cause of death are based on the then current *International Classification of Diseases*, which are described in Appendix II, tables IV and V. Age groups chosen to show data for American Indians, Asians, Hispanics, and non-Hispanic whites were selected to minimize the presentation of unstable age-specific death rates based on small numbers of deaths and for consistency among comparison groups. The race groups, white, black, Asian or Pacific Islander, and American Indian or Alaska Native, include persons of Hispanic and non-Hispanic origin. Conversely, persons of Hispanic origin may be of any race. Consistency of race identification between the death certificate (source of data for numerator of death rates) and data from the Census Bureau (denominator) is high for individual white and black persons; however, persons identified as American Indian, Asian, or Hispanic origin in data from the Census Bureau are sometimes misreported as white or non-Hispanic on the death certificate, causing death rates to be underestimated by 22–30 percent for American Indians, about 12 percent for Asians, and about 7 percent for persons of Hispanic origin. (Sorlie PD, Rogot E, and Johnson NJ: Validity of demographic characteristics on the death certificate, *Epidemiology* 3(2):181–184, 1992.) See Appendix II for age-adjustment procedure. Data for additional years are available (see Appendix III).

SOURCES: Centers for Disease Control and Prevention, National Center for Health Statistics. *Vital statistics of the United States, vol II, mortality, part A*, for data years 1950–93. Public Health Service. Washington. U.S. Government Printing Office; for 1994–97, unpublished data; data computed by the Division of Health and Utilization Analysis from numerator data compiled by the Division of Vital Statistics and denominator data from national population estimates for race groups from table 1 and unpublished Hispanic population estimates prepared by the Housing and Household Economic Statistics Division, U.S. Bureau of the Census.

Table 49. Deaths from selected occupational diseases for males, according to age: United States, selected years 1970–97

[Data are based on the National Vital Statistics System]

Age and cause of death	1970	1975	1980	1985	1989	1990	1991	1992	1993	1994	1995	1996	1997
25 years and over						Number of deaths[1]							
Malignant neoplasm of peritoneum and pleura (mesothelioma)	602	591	552	571	565	629	607	618	551	511	546	574	557
Coalworkers' pneumoconiosis	1,155	973	977	947	725	727	692	631	564	491	531	533	483
Asbestosis.	25	43	96	130	261	282	247	270	308	325	342	345	387
Silicosis	351	243	202	138	130	146	150	110	123	113	110	95	93
25–64 years													
Malignant neoplasm of peritoneum and pleura (mesothelioma)	308	280	241	210	179	199	190	193	164	161	163	146	154
Coalworkers' pneumoconiosis	294	188	136	89	50	49	48	32	34	21	40	20	25
Asbestosis.	17	22	30	29	31	50	35	34	32	35	32	33	33
Silicosis	90	64	49	30	21	35	29	25	25	25	15	19	19
65 years and over													
Malignant neoplasm of peritoneum and pleura (mesothelioma)	294	311	311	361	386	430	417	425	387	350	383	428	403
Coalworkers' pneumoconiosis	861	785	841	858	675	678	644	599	530	470	491	513	458
Asbestosis.	8	21	66	101	230	232	212	236	276	290	310	312	354
Silicosis	261	179	153	108	109	111	121	85	98	88	95	76	74

[1]This table classifies deaths according to underlying cause. Additional deaths for which occupational diseases are classified as nonunderlying causes can be identified from multiple cause of death data from the National Vital Statistics System. The numbers of such deaths are shown below for males 25 years of age and over.

Nonunderlying cause of death	1980	1985	1989	1990	1991	1992	1993	1994	1995	1996	1997
Malignant neoplasm of peritoneum and pleura (mesothelioma)	135	102	83	105	96	87	84	103	83	74	81
Coalworkers' pneumoconiosis	1,587	1,652	1,402	1,248	1,227	1,130	1,052	974	876	874	800
Asbestosis.	228	382	588	619	660	653	661	701	796	778	741
Silicosis	232	187	156	152	155	130	145	109	122	111	96

NOTES: Selection of occupational diseases based on definitions in D. Rutstein et al.: Sentinel health events (occupational): A basis for physician recognition and public health surveillance, *Am. J. Public Health* 73(9):1054–1062, Sept. 1983. For data years shown, the code numbers for cause of death are based on the then current *International Classification of Diseases*, which are described in Appendix II, tables IV and V. Data for additional years are available (see Appendix III).

SOURCE: Data computed by the Centers for Disease Control and Prevention, National Center for Health Statistics, Office of Analysis, Epidemiology, and Health Promotion from numerator data compiled by the Division of Vital Statistics.

Table 50. Occupational injury deaths, according to industry: United States, selected years 1980–94

[Data are based on information from death certificates]

Industry	1980	1985	1987	1988	1989	1990	1991	1992	1993	1994
	Deaths per 100,000 workers[1]									
Total civilian work force.	7.6	5.8	5.2	5.0	4.9	4.6	4.5	4.3	4.4	4.4
Agriculture, forestry, and fishing.	24.4	23.7	21.5	20.7	20.6	18.0	18.1	17.7	18.7	16.4
Mining.	43.8	30.0	23.2	23.4	26.7	30.0	23.9	22.3	25.4	25.1
Construction	21.3	16.6	15.9	14.9	14.3	14.0	12.6	12.7	12.2	12.3
Manufacturing	4.7	4.0	4.0	3.8	3.7	4.0	3.9	3.7	3.7	3.6
Transportation, communication, and public utilities.	21.2	15.7	12.9	13.2	12.9	10.4		10.1	10.9	10.3
Wholesale trade.	4.4	2.8	2.6		2.3	3.6	3.7	3.2	3.7	3.8
Retail trade	3.7	2.7	2.4	.3	2.2	2.8	3.0	2.9	3.1	3.0
Finance, insurance, and real estate.	1.4	1.0	1.2	0.9	1.0	0.9	1.1	1.0	1.1	1.1
Services	2.4	1.8	1.6	1.7	1.6	1.5	1.7	1.5	1.5	1.6
Public administration	7.7	6.4	6.8	6.1	5.3	3.8	3.2	4.4	4.6	4.7
Not classified.	- - -	- - -	- - -	- - -	- - -	- - -	- - -	- - -	- - -	- - -
	Number of deaths									
Total civilian work force.	7,405	6,250	5,884	5,751	5,714	5,384	5,219	5,034	5,291	5,406
Agriculture, forestry, and fishing.	848	791	730	687	695	603	615	598	608	587
Mining.	412	282	190	176	192	219	175	148	170	168
Construction	1,294	1,160	1,188	1,130	1,096	1,077	891	889	884	920
Manufacturing	1,014	834	831	810	791	838	793	737	715	726
Transportation, communication, and public utilities.	1,355	1,184	1,013	1,068	1,046	847	847	829	927	898
Wholesale trade.	167	122	120	135	107	168	170	152	169	177
Retail trade	595	489	449	443	430	543	581	573	635	632
Finance, insurance, and real estate.	84	69	94	72	81	75	89	76	84	87
Services	663	603	563	642	606	592	656	590	641	669
Public administration	401	319	359	333	292	213	183	247	263	274
Not classified.	572	397	347	255	378	209	219	195	195	268

- - - Data not available.

[1]Denominators are from the U.S. Bureau of Labor Statistics' annual average employment data.

NOTES: Includes deaths to United States workers, 16 years of age and over, that resulted from an "external" cause and the item "injury at work" was checked on the death certificate. Industry is coded based on *Standard Industrial Classification Manual*, 1987 Edition (see Appendix II, table VI). Data for additional years are available (see Appendix III). Data for 1991–93 have been revised and differ from the previous edition of *Health, United States*.

SOURCE: Centers for Disease Control and Prevention, National Institute for Occupational Safety and Health, Division of Safety Research. National Traumatic Occupational Fatalities (NTOF) surveillance system. Morgantown, West Virginia.

Table 51. Vaccinations of children 19–35 months of age for selected diseases, according to race, Hispanic origin, poverty status, and residence in metropolitan statistical area (MSA): United States, 1994–97

[Data are based on telephone interviews of a sample of the civilian noninstitutionalized population supplemented by a survey of immunization providers for interview participants]

Vaccination and year	All	Race and Hispanic origin					Poverty status[1]		Location of residence		
		White, non-Hispanic	Black, non-Hispanic	Hispanic[2]	American Indian or Alaska Native[3]	Asian or Pacific Islander[3]	Below poverty	At or above poverty	Inside MSA		Outside MSA
									Central city	Remaining areas	
				Percent of children 19–35 months of age							
Combined series (4:3:1:3):[4]											
1994	69	72	67	62	82	60	61	72	68	70	70
1995	74	77	70	69	70	75	67	77	73	76	75
1996	77	79	74	71	80	78	69	80	74	78	77
1997	76	79	73	72	72	70	71	79	74	78	77
DTP (4 doses or more):[5]											
1994	76	80	72	70	84	84	69	79	75	77	78
1995	79	81	74	75	73	82	71	81	77	80	79
1996	81	83	79	77	83	84	73	84	80	83	81
1997	81	84	78	77	80	80	76	84	80	83	81
Polio (3 doses or more):											
1994	83	85	79	81	90	92	78	85	83	84	83
1995	88	89	84	87	87	89	84	89	87	88	89
1996	91	92	90	89	89	90	88	92	89	92	92
1997	91	92	90	90	91	88	90	92	90	91	92
Measles-containing:[6]											
1994	89	90	86	88	90	95	87	90	90	90	87
1995	90	91	86	88	88	95	85	91	89	91	90
1996	91	92	89	88	87	94	87	92	90	92	91
1997	91	92	90	88	92	89	86	92	90	91	90
Hib (3 doses or more):[7]											
1994	86	87	85	84	90	70	81	88	86	87	86
1995	92	93	89	90	92	91	88	93	91	92	92
1996	92	93	90	89	90	92	88	93	90	93	92
1997	93	94	92	90	87	89	90	94	92	94	94
Hepatitis B (3 doses or more):											
1994	37	40	29	33	43	39	25	41	36	40	28
1995	68	68	65	69	55	80	64	69	68	71	60
1996	82	82	82	80	78	84	78	83	81	83	80
1997	84	85	83	81	83	88	80	85	82	85	85

Vaccination and year	Race and Hispanic origin and poverty status[1]					
	White, non-Hispanic		Black, non-Hispanic		Hispanic[2]	
	Below poverty	At or above poverty	Below poverty	At or above poverty	Below poverty	At or above poverty
	Percent of children 19–35 months of age					
Combined series (4:3:1:3):[4]						
1995	68	79	66	75	65	72
1996	68	81	70	78	68	74
1997	70	76	72	80	71	77

[1]Poverty status is based on family income and family size using Bureau of the Census poverty thresholds. Children missing information about poverty status were omitted from analysis by poverty level. In 1997, 18.4 percent of all children, 24.2 percent of Hispanic, 16.0 percent of non-Hispanic white, and 21.3 percent of non-Hispanic black children were missing information about poverty status and were omitted. See Appendix II.
[2]Persons of Hispanic origin may be of any race.
[3]Excludes persons of Hispanic origin.
[4]The 4:3:1:3 combined series consists of 4 doses of diphtheria-tetanus-pertussis (DTP) vaccine, 3 doses of polio vaccine, 1 dose of a measles-containing vaccine, and 3 doses of *Haemophilus influenzae* type b (Hib) vaccine.
[5]Diphtheria-tetanus-pertussis vaccine.
[6]Respondents were asked about measles-containing or MMR (measles-mumps-rubella) vaccines.
[7]*Haemophilus influenzae* type b (Hib) vaccine.

NOTE: Final estimates of data from the National Immunization Survey include an adjustment for children with missing immunization provider data.

SOURCE: Centers for Disease Control and Prevention, National Center for Health Statistics and National Immunization Program. Data from the National Immunization Survey.

Table 52 (page 1 of 2). Vaccination coverage among children 19–35 months of age acccrding to geographic division, State, and selected urban areas: United States, 1994–97

[Data are based on telephone interviews of a sample of the civilian noninstitutionalized population supplemented by a survey of immunization providers for interview participants]

Geographic division and State	1994	1995	1996	1997
	Percent of children 19–35 months of age with 4:3:1:3 series[1]			
United States	69	74	77	76
New England:				
Maine	75	87	85	84
New Hampshire	78	86	83	84
Vermont	82	84	85	84
Massachusetts	77	80	86	86
Rhode Island	78	82	85	81
Connecticut	81	83	87	85
Middle Atlantic:				
New York	72	77	79	76
New Jersey	67	72	77	76
Pennsylvania	71	76	79	80
East North Central:				
Ohio	70	73	77	73
Indiana	69	75	70	72
Illinois	60	79	75	74
Michigan	55	67	74	75
Wisconsin	70	74	76	79
West North Central:				
Minnesota	74	76	83	78
Iowa	75	82	80	76
Missouri	59	75	74	77
North Dakota	73	81	81	82
South Dakota	67	79	80	76
Nebraska	62	75	80	75
Kansas	76	70	73	82
South Atlantic:				
Delaware	77	72	80	79
Maryland	75	78	78	80
District of Columbia	67	67	78	73
Virginia	76	71	77	72
West Virginia	62	71	71	80
North Carolina	75	80	77	80
South Carolina	78	80	84	79
Georgia	75	77	80	79
Florida	72	75	77	77
East South Central:				
Kentucky	74	79	76	79
Tennessee	68	73	77	77
Alabama	70	75	75	85
Mississippi	79	81	79	80
West South Central:				
Arkansas	64	73	72	77
Louisiana	66	76	79	76
Oklahoma	70	73	73	71
Texas	65	73	72	74
Mountain:				
Montana	69	71	77	74
Idaho	58	64	66	70
Wyoming	71	71	77	72
Colorado	66	77	76	72
New Mexico	66	76	79	75
Arizona	70	70	70	73
Utah	62	66	63	69
Nevada	63	65	70	71
Pacific:				
Washington	68	77	78	79
Oregon	64	72	70	72
California	67	69	76	74
Alaska	65	72	69	75
Hawaii	78	78	77	79

See footnotes at end of table.

[Data are based on telephone interviews of a sample of the civilian noninstitutionalized population supplemented by a survey of immunization providers for interview participants]

Geographic division and urban areas	1994	1995	1996	1997
	Percent of children 19–35 months of age with 4:3:1:3 series[1]			
New England:				
Boston, Massachusetts	87	87	84	86
Middle Atlantic:				
New York City, New York.	73	78	75	75
Newark, New Jersey.	46	67	62	66
Philadelphia, Pennsylvania	67	67	75	78
East North Central:				
Cuyahoga County (Cleveland), Ohio.	82	71	80	73
Franklin County (Columbus), Ohio	71	74	78	74
Marion County (Indianapolis), Indiana.	72	75	72	81
Chicago, Illinois	55	69	74	68
Detroit, Michigan	45	57	63	65
Milwaukee County (Milwaukee), Wisconsin	72	68	70	70
South Atlantic:				
Baltimore, Maryland	74	75	81	83
District of Columbia	67	67	78	73
Fulton/DeKalb Counties (Atlanta), Georgia	72	79	74	75
Dade County (Miami), Florida	73	77	76	75
Duval County (Jacksonville), Florida.	69	71	76	70
East South Central:				
Davidson County (Nashville), Tennessee	65	73	77	77
Shelby County (Memphis), Tennessee	67	68	70	70
Jefferson County (Birmingham), Alabama	72	85	77	82
West South Central:				
Orleans Parish (New Orleans), Louisiana	59	75	71	69
Bexar County (San Antonio), Texas	60	74	74	79
Dallas County (Dallas), Texas	62	70	71	74
El Paso County (El Paso), Texas	78	77	62	65
Houston, Texas	57	70	68	64
Mountain:				
Maricopa County (Phoenix), Arizona.	71	69	71	72
Pacific:				
King County (Seattle), Washington.	70	82	81	77
Los Angeles County (Los Angeles), California . .	65	70	79	71
San Diego County (San Diego), California	68	73	77	78
Santa Clara County (Santa Clara), California . .	78	74	79	73

[1]The 4:3:1:3 combined series consists of 4 doses of diphtheria-tetanus-pertussis (DTP) vaccine, 3 doses of polio vaccine, 1 dose of a measles-containing vaccine, and 3 doses of Haemophilus influenzae type b (Hib) vaccine.

NOTES: Urban areas were chosen because they were high risk for under-vaccination. Final estimates of data from the National Immunization Survey include an adjustment for children with missing immunization provider data.

SOURCES: Centers for Disease Control and Prevention, National Center for Health Statistics and National Immunization Program. National, State, and Urban Area Vaccination Coverage Levels Among Children Aged 19–35 Months—United States, 1997. *Morbidity and mortality weekly report* 1998; 47(26). Atlanta, Georgia: Centers for Disease Control and Prevention.

Table 53. Selected notifiable disease rates, according to disease: United States, selected years 1950–97

[Data are based on reporting by State health departments]

Disease	1950	1960	1970	1980	1990	1994	1995	1996	1997
					Cases per 100,000 population				
Diphtheria	3.83	0.51	0.21	0.00	0.00	0.00	–	0.01	0.01
Haemophilus influenzae, invasive	---	---	---	---	---	0.45	0.45	0.45	0.44
Hepatitis A	---	---	27.87	12.84	12.64	10.29	12.13	11.70	11.22
Hepatitis B	---	---	4.08	8.39	8.48	4.81	4.19	4.01	3.90
Lyme disease	---	---	---	---	---	5.01	4.49	6.21	4.79
Meningococcal disease	---	---	---	---	0.99	1.11	1.25	1.30	1.24
Mumps	---	---	55.55	3.86	2.17	0.60	0.35	0.29	0.27
Pertussis (whooping cough)	79.82	8.23	2.08	0.76	1.84	1.77	1.97	2.94	2.46
Poliomyelitis, total	22.02	1.77	0.02	0.00	0.00	0.00	0.00	0.01	0.01
Paralytic[1]	---	1.40	0.02	0.00	0.00	0.00	0.00	0.01	0.01
Rocky Mountain spotted fever	---	---	---	---	0.26	0.18	0.23	0.32	0.16
Rubella (German measles)	---	---	27.75	1.72	0.45	0.09	0.05	0.10	0.07
Rubeola (measles)	211.01	245.42	23.23	5.96	11.17	0.37	0.12	0.20	0.06
Salmonellosis, excluding typhoid fever	---	3.85	10.84	14.88	19.54	16.64	17.66	17.15	15.66
Shigellosis	15.45	6.94	6.79	8.41	10.89	11.44	12.32	9.80	8.64
Tuberculosis[2]	80.45	30.83	18.28	12.25	10.33	9.36	8.70	8.04	7.42
Sexually transmitted diseases:[3]									
Syphilis[4]	146.02	68.78	45.26	30.51	54.30	31.40	26.40	20.10	17.50
Primary and secondary	16.73	9.06	10.89	12.06	20.30	7.90	6.30	4.30	3.20
Early latent	39.71	10.11	8.08	9.00	22.30	12.30	10.10	7.60	6.30
Late and late latent	70.22	45.91	24.94	9.30	10.40	10.30	9.20	7.70	7.70
Congenital[5]	8.97	2.48	0.97	0.12	1.60	0.90	0.70	0.50	0.40
Chlamydia[6]	---	---	---	---	160.80	194.50	190.40	192.60	207.00
Gonorrhea[7]	192.50	145.40	297.22	445.10	277.40	165.60	149.40	123.10	122.50
Chancroid	3.34	0.94	0.70	0.30	1.70	0.30	0.20	0.10	0.10
					Number of cases				
Diphtheria	5,796	918	435	3	4	2	–	2	4
Haemophilus influenzae, invasive	---	---	---	---	---	1,174	1,180	1,170	1,162
Hepatitis A	---	---	56,797	29,087	31,441	26,796	31,582	31,032	30,021
Hepatitis B	---	---	8,310	19,015	21,102	12,517	10,805	10,637	10,416
Lyme disease	---	---	---	---	---	13,043	11,700	16,455	12,801
Meningococcal disease	---	---	---	---	2,451	2,886	3,243	3,437	3,308
Mumps	---	---	104,953	8,576	5,292	1,537	906	751	683
Pertussis (whooping cough)	120,718	14,809	4,249	1,730	4,570	4,617	5,137	7,796	6,564
Poliomyelitis, total	33,300	3,190	33	9	6	8	6	5	3
Paralytic[1]	---	2,525	31	8	6	8	6	5	3
Rocky Mountain spotted fever	---	---	---	---	651	465	590	831	409
Rubella (German measles)	---	---	56,552	3,904	1,125	227	128	238	181
Rubeola (measles)	319,124	441,703	47,351	13,506	27,786	963	281	508	138
Salmonellosis, excluding typhoid fever	---	6,929	22,096	33,715	48,603	43,323	45,970	45,471	41,901
Shigellosis	23,367	12,487	13,845	19,041	27,077	29,769	32,080	25,978	23,117
Tuberculosis[2]	121,742	55,494	37,137	27,749	25,701	24,361	22,860	21,337	19,851
Sexually transmitted diseases:[3]									
Syphilis[4]	217,558	122,538	91,382	68,832	135,043	81,696	69,320	53,215	46,537
Primary and secondary	23,939	16,145	21,982	27,204	50,578	20,627	16,542	11,390	8,550
Early latent	59,256	18,017	16,311	20,297	55,397	32,012	26,655	20,186	16,617
Late and late latent	113,569	81,798	50,348	20,979	25,750	26,840	24,272	20,356	20,321
Congenital[5]	13,377	4,416	1,953	277	3,865	2,217	1,860	1,283	1,049
Chlamydia[6]	---	---	---	---	323,663	451,705	478,533	490,047	526,653
Gonorrhea[7]	286,746	258,933	600,072	1,004.029	690,042	419,470	392,622	326,522	324,901
Chancroid	4,977	1,680	1,416	788	4,212	773	607	386	243

0.00 Rate greater than zero but less than 0.005.
– Quantity zero.
- - - Data not available.
[1]Data beginning in 1986 may be updated due to retrospective case evaluations or late reports.
[2]Data after 1974 are not comparable to prior years because of changes in reporting criteria effective in 1975.
[3]Newly reported civilian cases prior to 1991; includes military cases beginning in 1991 and adjustments to the number of cases through June 16, 1998. For 1950 data for Alaska and Hawaii not included.
[4]Includes stage of syphilis not stated.
[5]Data reported for 1989 and later years reflect change in case definition introduced in 1988. Through 1994, all cases of congenitally acquired syphilis; as of 1995, congenital syphilis less than 1 year of age.
[6]Chlamydia was non-notifiable in 1994 and earlier years (see Appendix I).
[7]Data for 1994 do not include cases from Georgia.

NOTES: The total resident population was used to calculate all rates except sexually transmitted diseases, for which the civilian resident population was used prior to 1991. Population data from those States where diseases were not notifiable or not available were excluded from rate calculation. See Appendix I for information on underreporting of notifiable diseases. Some numbers for 1990–96 have been revised and differ from the previous edition of *Health, United States*. Data for additional years are available (see Appendix III).

SOURCES: Centers for Disease Control and Prevention. Summary of notifiable diseases, United States, 1997. Morbidity and mortality weekly report; 46(53). Atlanta, Georgia: Public Health Service. 1998; National Center for HIV, STD, and TB Prevention, Division of STD Prevention. Sexually transmitted disease surveillance, 1997. Atlanta, Georgia: Public Health Service. Centers for Disease Control and Prevention, 1998.

Table 54. Acquired immunodeficiency syndrome (AIDS) cases, according to age at diagnosis, sex, detailed race, and Hispanic origin: United States, selected years 1985–98

[Data are based on reporting by State health departments]

Age at diagnosis, sex, race, and Hispanic origin	All years[1]	All years[1]	1985	1990	1993	1994	1995	1996	1997	January–June 1998	12 months ending June 30, 1998
	Percent distribution[2]	Number, by year of report									Cases per 100,000 population[3]
All races	...	643,350	8,161	41,540	102,082	77,092	70,839	66,398	58,254	24,014	19.6
Male											
All males, 13 years and over	100.0	536,198	7,510	36,283	85,266	62,811	57,061	52,553	45,291	18,423	38.5
White, non-Hispanic	50.6	271,446	4,755	20,881	43,256	29,497	26,206	23,173	17,557	7,181	20.0
Black, non-Hispanic	33.1	177,356	1,708	10,267	28,354	22,446	20,945	20,069	18,785	7,595	145.3
Hispanic[4]	15.1	80,987	991	4,762	12,624	10,083	9,172	8,581	8,248	3,326	67.2
American Indian or Alaska Native[5] ...	0.3	1,527	7	81	310	207	197	169	165	51	18.1
Asian or Pacific Islander[5]	0.8	4,184	49	263	662	525	486	481	380	168	10.0
13–19 years.................	0.4	1,924	28	107	361	226	228	204	183	81	1.1
20–29 years.................	16.5	88,475	1,504	6,943	14,629	9,691	8,426	7,071	5,791	2,223	27.2
30–39 years.................	45.8	245,361	3,588	16,718	38,909	28,942	25,842	23,842	20,185	7,992	82.2
40–49 years.................	26.6	142,559	1,634	8,854	22,863	17,197	16,273	15,479	13,627	5,702	57.6
50–59 years.................	8.0	42,793	597	2,650	6,407	5,060	4,721	4,432	4,124	1,783	29.4
60 years and over..............	2.8	15,086	159	1,011	2,097	1,695	1,571	1,525	1,381	642	7.0
Female											
All females, 13 years and over	100.0	99,259	523	4,534	15,943	13,310	13,032	13,192	12,515	5,401	10.2
White, non-Hispanic	23.6	23,448	142	1,225	4,043	3,081	3,060	2,867	2,474	1,012	2.6
Black, non-Hispanic	59.0	58,523	279	2,546	9,105	7,851	7,624	8,104	7,845	3,447	54.1
Hispanic[4]	16.4	16,299	99	732	2,629	2,284	2,230	2,074	2,040	859	17.6
American Indian or Alaska Native[5] ...	0.3	294	2	8	61	40	38	43	35	15	4.5
Asian or Pacific Islander[5]	0.5	537	1	19	97	50	71	80	64	31	1.6
13–19 years.................	1.2	1,230	4	66	200	174	156	177	176	84	1.3
20–29 years.................	22.1	21,958	178	1,117	3,721	2,944	2,678	2,684	2,427	990	12.0
30–39 years.................	45.6	45,260	232	2,079	7,526	6,001	5,966	5,907	5,496	2,297	22.5
40–49 years.................	21.9	21,718	45	781	3,217	3,081	3,080	3,265	3,248	1,466	15.2
50–59 years.................	6.0	5,936	26	272	848	768	816	833	818	414	5.9
60 years and over..............	3.2	3,157	38	219	431	342	336	326	350	150	1.3
Children											
All children, under 13 years	100.0	7,893	128	723	873	971	746	653	448	190	0.7
White, non-Hispanic	18.5	1,463	26	158	153	143	117	95	63	36	0.2
Black, non-Hispanic	60.9	4,810	84	388	535	633	483	428	292	116	3.1
Hispanic[4]	19.4	1,533	18	168	175	180	135	125	86	37	0.9
American Indian or Alaska Native[5] ...	0.3	27	–	5	3	2	2	3	2	–	0.2
Asian or Pacific Islander[5]	0.6	45	–	4	4	11	5	1	3	1	0.2
Under 1 year	39.7	3,134	63	316	352	350	271	219	131	55	2.7
1–12 years	60.3	4,759	65	407	521	621	475	434	317	135	0.6

... Category not applicable.
– Quantity zero.
[1]Includes cases prior to 1985 and through June 30, 1998.
[2]Percents may not sum to 100 percent due to rounding.
[3]Computed using official postcensus resident population estimates for 1997 from the U.S. Bureau of the Census.
[4]Persons of Hispanic origin may be of any race.
[5]Excludes persons of Hispanic origin.

NOTES: The AIDS case reporting definitions were expanded in 1985, 1987, and 1993. See Appendix II. Excludes data for U.S. dependencies and possessions and independent nations in free association with the United States. Data are updated periodically because of reporting delays. Data for all years have been updated through June 30, 1998, and may differ from previous editions of *Health, United States*. Similar data as of December 31, 1998, are available in the Centers for Disease Control and Prevention, HIV/AIDS Surveillance Report, Year-end edition Vol 10 No 2. 1998.

SOURCE: Centers for Disease Control and Prevention, National Center for HIV, STD, and TB Prevention, Division of HIV/AIDS Prevention, 1998 special data run.

Table 55 (page 1 of 2). Acquired immunodeficiency syndrome (AIDS) cases, according to race, Hispanic origin, sex, and transmission category for persons 13 years of age and over at diagnosis: United States, selected years 1985–98

[Data are based on reporting by State health departments]

Race, Hispanic origin, sex, and transmission category	All years[1]	All years[1]	1985	1990	1993	1994	1995	1996	1997	January–June 1998
Race and Hispanic origin	Percent distribution[2]	Number, by year of report								
All races	100.0	635,457	8,033	40,817	101,209	76,121	70,093	65,745	57,806	23,824
Men who have sex with men	49.5	314,241	5,355	23,785	49,514	35,269	30,978	27,538	21,163	8,388
Injecting drug use	24.7	156,964	1,389	9,289	28,127	21,088	18,676	16,610	14,110	5,193
Men who have sex with men and injecting drug use	6.4	40,460	656	2,833	7,393	4,593	3,892	3,239	2,357	908
Hemophilia/coagulation disorder. . .	0.7	4,718	71	348	1,084	509	457	332	206	74
Heterosexual contact[3]	9.1	57,811	151	2,254	9,053	8,235	8,242	8,949	7,869	2,953
Sex with injecting drug user	3.7	23,323	107	1,490	3,965	2,982	2,763	2,725	2,180	852
Transfusion[4]	1.3	8,093	166	780	1,082	673	606	525	393	145
Undetermined[5]	8.4	53,170	245	1,528	4,956	5,754	7,242	8,552	11,708	6,163
White, non-Hispanic	100.0	294,894	4,897	22,106	47,299	32,578	29,266	26,040	20,031	8,193
Men who have sex with men	69.3	204,293	3,982	16,565	31,970	21,714	18,917	16,424	11,832	4,669
Injecting drug use	11.7	34,595	246	2,058	6,438	4,537	4,136	3,696	2,945	1,147
Men who have sex with men and injecting drug use	7.4	21,795	409	1,586	3,902	2,335	1,992	1,654	1,114	446
Hemophilia/coagulation disorder. . .	1.2	3,652	59	280	878	372	324	215	139	50
Heterosexual contact[3]	4.6	13,632	34	648	2,295	1,940	1,917	1,893	1,583	567
Sex with injecting drug user	1.9	5,528	19	350	981	749	691	645	486	174
Transfusion[4]	1.6	4,842	125	507	590	317	286	213	146	55
Undetermined[5]	4.1	12,085	42	462	1,226	1,363	1,694	1,945	2,272	1,259
Black, non-Hispanic	100.0	235,879	1,987	12,813	37,459	30,297	28,569	28,173	26,630	11,042
Men who have sex with men	28.5	67,290	784	4,474	10,697	8,248	7,423	6,934	5,878	2,289
Injecting drug use	37.5	88,435	741	5,175	15,748	12,033	10,568	9,492	8,198	3,008
Men who have sex with men and injecting drug use	5.7	13,330	162	906	2,482	1,619	1,382	1,168	933	316
Hemophilia/coagulation disorder. . .	0.2	587	5	34	125	71	78	69	39	15
Heterosexual contact[3]	14.2	33,595	91	1,221	5,142	4,753	4,678	5.458	4,773	1,880
Sex with injecting drug user	5.6	13,302	65	854	2,210	1,689	1,515	1,571	1,269	526
Transfusion[4]	0.9	2,160	30	167	325	242	226	215	178	60
Undetermined[5]	12.9	30,482	174	836	2,940	3,331	4,214	4,837	6,631	3,474
Hispanic[6]	100.0	97,286	1,090	5,494	15,253	12,367	11,402	10,655	10,288	4,185
Men who have sex with men	39.4	38,353	547	2,461	6,106	4,770	4,155	3,733	3,087	1,294
Injecting drug use	34.0	33,070	395	2,021	5,789	4,415	3,847	3,319	2,838	995
Men who have sex with men and injecting drug use	5.1	4,915	83	319	922	577	471	373	277	131
Hemophilia/coagulation disorder. . .	0.4	378	7	28	60	53	47	38	21	6
Heterosexual contact[3]	10.3	10,002	26	374	1,509	1,480	1,565	1,496	1,412	478
Sex with injecting drug user	4.4	4,304	23	281	730	520	536	480	405	145
Transfusion[4]	0.9	867	6	83	138	90	75	82	57	25
Undetermined[5]	10.0	9,701	26	208	729	982	1,242	1,614	2,596	1,256

See footnotes at end of table.

Table 55 (page 2 of 2). Acquired immunodeficiency syndrome (AIDS) cases, according to race, Hispanic origin, sex, and transmission category for persons 13 years of age and over at diagnosis: United States, selected years 1985–98

[Data are based on reporting by State health departments]

Race, Hispanic origin, sex, and transmission category	All years[1]	All years[1]	1985	1990	1993	1994	1995	1996	1997	January–June 1998
Sex	Percent distribution[2]	Number, by year of report								
Male	100.0	536,198	7,510	36,283	85,266	62,811	57,061	52,553	45,291	18,423
Men who have sex with men	58.6	314,241	5,355	23,785	49,514	35,269	30,978	27,538	21,163	8,388
Injecting drug use	21.2	113,705	1,103	6,958	20,066	15,148	13,353	11,838	9,950	3,652
Men who have sex with men and injecting drug use	7.5	40,460	656	2,833	7,393	4,593	3,892	3,239	2,357	908
Hemophilia/coagulation disorder	0.8	4,504	68	332	1,052	481	430	309	182	70
Heterosexual contact[3]	3.7	19,832	32	715	2,997	2,776	2,826	3,202	2,939	1,147
Sex with injecting drug user	1.3	7,235	25	455	1,183	934	882	831	747	327
Transfusion[4]	0.9	4,650	103	446	598	367	337	265	214	74
Undetermined[5]	7.2	38,806	193	1,214	3,646	4,177	5,245	6,162	8,486	4,184
Female	100.0	99,259	523	4,534	15,943	13,310	13,032	13,192	12,515	5,401
Injecting drug use	43.6	43,259	286	2,331	8,061	5,940	5,323	4,772	4,160	1,541
Hemophilia/coagulation disorder	0.2	214	3	16	32	28	27	23	24	4
Heterosexual contact[3]	38.3	37,979	119	1,539	6,056	5,459	5,416	5,747	4,930	1,806
Sex with injecting drug user	16.2	16,088	82	1,035	2,782	2,048	1,881	1,894	1,433	525
Transfusion[4]	3.5	3,443	63	334	484	306	269	260	179	71
Undetermined[5]	14.5	14,364	52	314	1,310	1,577	1,997	2,390	3,222	1,979

[1]Includes cases prior to 1985 and through June 30, 1998.
[2]Percents may not sum to 100 percent due to rounding.
[3]Includes persons who have had heterosexual contact with a person with human immunodeficiency virus (HIV) infection or at risk of HIV infection.
[4]Receipt of blood transfusion, blood components, or tissue.
[5]Includes persons for whom risk information is incomplete (because of death, refusal to be interviewed, or loss to followup), persons still under investigation, men reported to have had heterosexual contact only with prostitutes, and interviewed persons for whom no specific risk is identified.
[6]Persons of Hispanic origin may be of any race.

NOTES: The AIDS case reporting definitions were expanded in 1985, 1987, and 1993. See Appendix II. Excludes data for U.S. dependencies and possessions and independent nations in free association with the United States. Data are updated periodically because of reporting delays. Data for all years have been updated through June 30, 1998, and may differ from previous editions of *Health, United States*. Similar data as of December 31, 1998, are available in the Centers for Disease Control and Prevention, HIV/AIDS Surveillance Report, Year-end edition Vol 10 No 2. 1998.

SOURCE: Centers for Disease Control and Prevention, National Center for HIV, STD, and TB Prevention, Division of HIV/AIDS Prevention, 1998 special data run.

Table 56. Acquired immunodeficiency syndrome (AIDS) cases, according to geographic division and State: United States, selected years 1985–98

[Data are based on reporting by State health departments]

Geographic division and State of residence	All years[1]	1985	1990	1993	1994	1995	1996	1997	January–June 1998	12 months ending June 30, 1998
				Number, by year of report						Cases per 100,000 population[2]
United States[3]	643,350	8,161	41,540	102,082	77,092	70,839	66,398	58,254	24,014	19.6
New England	27,108	282	1,513	5,132	2,816	3,578	2,758	2,368	830	14.5
Maine	824	11	65	149	116	129	50	51	18	3.3
New Hampshire	789	3	65	122	94	110	93	55	22	5.1
Vermont	338	2	22	71	38	44	25	29	10	3.6
Massachusetts	13,295	170	845	2,697	1,376	1,436	1,303	860	386	12.8
Rhode Island	1,801	11	89	338	274	221	176	151	67	14.3
Connecticut	10,061	85	427	1,755	918	1,638	1,111	1,222	327	27.3
Middle Atlantic	182,401	3,153	11,946	25,526	22,072	19,122	18,262	18,298	6,951	41.2
New York	124,793	2,481	8,279	16,990	14,700	12,363	12,351	13,154	4,759	62.5
New Jersey	37,34.	474	2,447	5,368	4,864	4,395	3,578	3,233	1,232	31.1
Pennsylvania	20,266	198	1,220	3,168	2,508	2,364	2,333	1,911	960	15.8
East North Central	48,940	354	3,041	7,963	6,216	5,363	5,166	4,345	1,768	9.9
Ohio	9,899	53	694	1,530	1,172	1,096	1,158	851	331	7.0
Indiana	5,263	26	294	945	615	524	589	521	326	8.3
Illinois	21,086	190	1,262	2,947	3,039	2,208	2,191	1,835	706	15.0
Michigan	9,559	61	579	1,817	1,020	1,193	958	883	305	8.2
Wisconsin	3,133	24	212	724	370	342	270	255	100	4.3
West North Central	15,609	127	1,055	3,126	1,598	1,695	1,621	1,151	444	5.8
Minnesota	3,269	41	203	655	410	364	304	211	65	3.8
Iowa	1,121	12	68	197	129	115	109	100	49	3.4
Missouri	8,019	50	579	1,716	701	781	855	569	209	10.1
North Dakota	94	–	1	11	21	5	13	12	4	1.6
South Dakota	138	1	9	29	20	18	14	11	9	2.3
Nebraska	918	7	58	178	88	115	99	91	39	4.6
Kansas	2,050	16	137	340	229	297	227	157	69	5.7
South Atlantic	145,274	1,286	8,789	22,712	18,609	17,836	16,536	13,790	5,900	25.5
Delaware	2,082	12	93	370	268	316	284	230	75	22.0
Maryland	17,790	149	987	2,500	2,659	2,543	2,231	1,851	718	32.0
District of Columbia	10,887	177	733	1,588	1,397	1,028	1,255	998	481	178.3
Virginia	10,694	107	745	1,619	1,152	1,601	1,195	1,175	425	14.8
West Virginia	930	6	61	106	93	124	121	130	57	7.2
North Carolina	8,553	67	570	1,372	1,186	997	899	851	390	10.9
South Carolina	7,402	37	373	1,472	1,146	967	852	773	386	20.7
Georgia	19,324	194	1,229	2,843	2,270	2,305	2,409	1,715	616	18.2
Florida	67,612	537	3,998	10,842	8,438	7,955	7,290	6,067	2,752	37.5
East South Central	17,852	73	1,058	2,690	2,077	2,261	2,274	2,051	936	12.1
Kentucky	2,707	18	191	320	316	296	398	362	127	8.0
Tennessee	6,633	19	340	1,197	752	890	820	775	333	12.9
Alabama	5,108	28	239	732	582	636	607	568	274	14.0
Mississippi	3,404	8	288	441	427	439	449	346	202	13.1
West South Central	62,927	612	4,424	9,951	7,585	6,083	6,780	6,299	2,899	20.4
Arkansas	2,492	10	209	398	286	275	266	241	104	8.9
Louisiana	10,708	104	700	1,414	1,223	1,079	1,456	1,092	512	24.4
Oklahoma	3,185	20	206	721	269	295	273	282	170	9.0
Texas	46,542	478	3,309	7,418	5,807	4,434	4,785	4,684	2,113	23.0
Mountain	20,051	158	1,127	3,862	2,275	2,253	2,004	1,844	831	10.9
Montana	283	–	17	32	29	25	34	41	15	3.9
Idaho	432	4	28	71	61	48	38	52	15	3.2
Wyoming	159	–	6	38	19	19	7	16	2	1.0
Colorado	6,277	62	366	1,322	810	671	518	380	147	8.1
New Mexico	1,742	14	108	295	214	164	206	169	130	12.7
Arizona	5,786	49	315	1,217	609	669	583	445	329	12.0
Utah	1,599	17	98	264	153	163	194	152	65	7.3
Nevada	3,773	12	189	623	380	494	424	589	128	28.9
Pacific	122,749	2,115	8,567	21,047	13,781	12,578	10,961	8,072	3,370	16.9
Washington	8,448	107	747	1,567	924	881	794	633	236	9.4
Oregon	4,254	33	336	773	605	457	460	303	93	7.2
California	107,468	1,942	7,304	18,283	11,978	10,913	9,472	6,990	2,962	19.6
Alaska	423	4	24	67	58	69	36	51	12	6.7
Hawaii	2,156	29	156	357	216	258	199	95	67	10.8

– Quantity zero.

[1]Includes cases prior to 1985 and through June 30, 1998.
[2]Computed using official postcensus resident population estimates for 1997 from the U.S. Bureau of the Census.
[3]Includes unknown State of residence.
NOTES: The AIDS case reporting definitions were expanded in 1985, 1987, and 1993. See Appendix II. Excludes data for U.S. dependencies and possessions and independent nations in free association with the United States. Data are updated periodically because of reporting delays. Data for all years have been updated through June 30, 1998, and may differ from previous editions of *Health, United States*. Similar data as of December 31, 1998, are available in the Centers for Disease Control and Prevention, HIV/AIDS Surveillance Report, Year-end edition Vol 10, No 2. 1998.
SOURCE: Centers for Disease Control and Prevention, National Center for HIV, STD, and TB Prevention, Division of HIV/AIDS Prevention, 1998 special data run.

Table 57. Age-adjusted cancer incidence rates for selected cancer sites, according to sex and race: Selected geographic areas, selected years 1973–95

[Data are based on the Surveillance, Epidemiology, and End Results Program's population-based registries in Atlanta, Detroit, Seattle-Puget Sound, San Francisco-Oakland, Connecticut, Iowa, New Mexico, Utah, and Hawaii]

Race, sex, and site	1973	1975	1980	1985	1990	1991	1992	1993	1994	1995
White male	\multicolumn{10}{c}{Number of new cases per 100,000 population[1]}
All sites	364.3	379.7	407.5	431.2	481.9	518.9	535.3	502.1	475.0	452.3
Oral cavity and pharynx	17.6	18.3	17.0	16.8	16.4	16.1	15.7	16.0	14.7	14.2
Esophagus	4.8	4.8	4.9	5.3	6.1	5.7	6.2	5.9	6.0	5.6
Stomach	14.0	12.5	12.3	10.5	9.4	9.7	9.4	9.1	9.4	8.8
Colon and rectum	54.2	55.1	58.7	63.4	59.0	58.0	56.5	54.2	53.0	49.7
Colon	34.8	36.1	39.3	43.4	40.3	40.6	39.1	38.1	37.1	34.6
Rectum	19.5	19.0	19.4	20.1	18.7	17.4	17.4	16.1	15.9	15.1
Pancreas	12.8	12.5	11.1	10.7	10.1	10.0	10.4	9.6	9.8	9.3
Lung and bronchus	72.4	75.9	82.2	82.0	80.9	80.4	79.5	77.2	74.5	71.5
Prostate gland	62.6	68.9	78.8	87.1	133.0	169.1	188.3	163.4	140.0	129.8
Urinary bladder	27.3	28.8	31.5	31.2	32.4	32.4	32.0	32.0	31.7	30.6
Non-Hodgkin's lymphoma	10.3	11.4	12.6	15.9	19.6	20.5	19.6	20.0	20.6	20.7
Leukemia	14.3	14.2	14.6	14.8	14.4	14.2	14.5	13.6	13.3	13.4
Black male										
All sites	441.4	438.0	510.4	532.7	575.8	622.5	659.7	665.3	637.1	584.1
Oral cavity and pharynx	16.6	17.2	23.1	22.6	24.8	21.3	22.7	23.0	25.1	20.6
Esophagus	13.3	17.6	16.4	19.4	19.9	15.3	15.8	15.3	13.3	12.4
Stomach	25.9	19.9	21.4	18.8	18.2	20.2	16.2	18.7	19.4	14.3
Colon and rectum	42.8	47.6	63.5	60.8	59.7	62.6	62.4	62.1	59.8	54.0
Colon	31.7	34.7	45.8	47.0	46.2	46.6	47.1	47.2	44.5	41.1
Rectum	11.1	12.9	17.7	13.8	13.5	16.0	15.3	14.9	15.3	12.9
Pancreas	15.9	15.6	17.6	19.7	15.4	14.7	16.0	15.5	17.4	15.6
Lung and bronchus	104.8	101.0	131.0	131.3	118.6	126.0	128.7	115.7	113.3	114.7
Prostate gland	106.3	111.5	126.7	133.6	173.3	223.3	256.9	270.6	245.7	211.6
Urinary bladder	10.6	13.4	14.5	16.3	15.5	15.1	16.7	18.2	15.8	14.6
Non-Hodgkin's lymphoma	8.8	7.0	9.3	10.0	14.2	15.9	15.4	15.7	17.9	18.2
Leukemia	12.0	12.5	13.1	13.0	12.1	10.0	11.7	12.1	9.8	9.4
White female										
All sites	295.1	310.5	311.3	343.8	356.3	359.5	356.8	349.9	354.6	351.9
Colon and rectum	41.7	42.9	44.7	45.9	40.2	38.9	38.5	37.8	37.0	36.6
Colon	30.3	30.9	32.9	34.0	30.1	29.0	28.7	28.0	27.8	27.5
Rectum	11.5	12.0	11.8	12.0	10.1	9.9	9.8	9.8	9.3	9.0
Pancreas	7.5	7.1	7.3	8.1	7.7	7.6	8.0	7.3	7.6	7.3
Lung and bronchus	17.8	21.8	28.2	35.9	42.5	44.2	44.4	43.8	44.5	44.2
Melanoma of skin	5.9	6.9	9.4	10.5	11.4	12.2	11.9	11.7	12.1	12.9
Breast	84.4	90.0	87.8	107.2	114.4	116.4	114.4	112.2	114.8	115.0
Cervix uteri	12.8	11.1	9.1	7.6	8.3	7.7	7.9	7.7	7.2	6.5
Corpus uteri	29.5	33.7	25.3	23.1	23.1	22.5	22.8	22.2	22.8	22.7
Ovary	14.6	14.4	14.0	15.1	16.1	16.3	15.8	15.7	14.9	15.2
Non-Hodgkin's lymphoma	7.6	8.5	9.2	11.4	12.9	12.5	12.9	12.8	13.5	12.6
Black female										
All sites	283.7	296.5	304.8	323.7	342.7	344.5	345.3	338.5	345.5	330.0
Colon and rectum	41.8	43.5	49.6	45.9	49.5	46.3	46.1	44.8	46.9	43.9
Colon	30.0	32.7	41.2	36.0	38.6	37.8	36.2	36.6	37.1	35.3
Rectum	11.8	10.8	8.5	9.9	10.9	8.5	9.9	8.2	9.7	8.6
Pancreas	11.6	11.6	13.0	11.3	10.3	12.6	13.0	12.1	12.0	12.3
Lung and bronchus	20.9	20.6	33.8	40.2	46.9	49.8	49.1	46.0	49.3	42.9
Breast	69.0	78.5	74.3	92.5	97.7	98.1	102.6	101.0	101.9	101.3
Cervix uteri	29.9	28.0	19.0	15.9	13.9	13.4	11.3	11.3	11.6	11.4
Corpus uteri	15.0	17.1	14.1	15.4	14.6	14.7	14.6	14.8	15.8	15.7
Ovary	10.5	10.1	10.1	10.1	10.2	10.1	10.7	11.1	12.5	9.7
Non-Hodgkin's lymphoma	5.5	4.2	6.0	7.1	9.3	8.6	8.4	8.1	7.2	9.1

[1]Age adjusted by the direct method to the 1970 U.S. population. See Appendix II for age-adjustment procedure.

NOTE: Numbers have been revised and differ from previous editions of *Health, United States*.

SOURCE: National Institutes of Health, National Cancer Institute, Cancer Statistics Branch, Bethesda, Maryland 20892.

Table 58. Five-year relative cancer survival rates for selected cancer sites, according to race and sex: Selected geographic areas, 1974–79, 1980–82, 1983–85, 1986–88, and 1989–94

[Data are based on the Surveillance, Epidemiology, and End Results Program's population-based registries in Atlanta, Detroit, Seattle-Puget Sound, San Francisco-Oakland, Connecticut, Iowa, New Mexico, Utah, and Hawaii]

Sex and site	White					Black				
	1974–79	1980–82	1983–85	1986–88	1989–94	1974–79	1980–82	1983–85	1986–88	1989–94
Male					Percent of patients					
All sites	43.3	46.6	49.1	52.8	60.0	31.9	34.2	34.7	37.7	45.1
Oral cavity and pharynx	54.0	54.3	54.9	53.0	52.0	31.2	26.2	30.2	29.8	27.4
Esophagus	5.0	6.7	7.9	11.7	12.5	2.3	4.6	5.2	7.1	8.2
Stomach	13.8	15.4	14.7	16.5	16.1	15.1	18.5	17.9	14.3	20.5
Colon	50.8	56.0	59.9	64.1	64.6	44.9	46.4	48.3	52.0	51.4
Rectum	48.9	51.5	56.0	60.3	61.0	36.6	36.1	42.8	47.1	53.3
Pancreas	2.7	2.6	2.5	3.0	3.7	2.4	3.7	4.8	6.6	3.3
Lung and bronchus	11.6	12.2	12.2	12.4	13.0	9.9	11.0	10.4	11.9	9.7
Prostate gland	70.0	74.5	77.7	85.2	95.1	60.5	64.7	64.0	69.2	81.2
Urinary bladder	75.7	79.9	80.7	84.4	86.3	58.6	62.4	64.3	67.5	66.5
Non-Hodgkin's lymphoma	47.0	50.9	53.9	50.9	48.5	44.1	47.9	43.6	47.1	37.3
Leukemia	35.4	39.3	41.6	45.3	45.3	31.1	30.2	32.3	35.3	27.5
Female										
All sites	57.2	57.0	59.1	61.9	63.1	46.7	45.9	45.5	47.8	48.8
Colon	52.4	55.4	58.5	61.7	63.1	48.6	51.3	50.0	53.4	53.1
Rectum	50.6	54.6	57.1	60.2	61.6	43.6	40.8	45.3	55.2	53.2
Pancreas	2.2	3.1	3.3	3.2	4.2	4.1	5.7	5.8	5.6	4.0
Lung and bronchus	16.7	16.2	17.1	15.9	16.5	15.4	15.4	14.2	11.6	13.9
Melanoma of skin	85.7	88.2	89.4	91.4	91.2	68.9	- - -	71.6	- - -	77.3
Breast	75.2	77.1	79.7	84.6	86.7	63.1	65.9	63.7	69.6	70.6
Cervix uteri	69.4	67.8	70.5	71.9	71.5	63.0	61.1	60.0	55.0	59.0
Corpus uteri	87.5	82.8	84.9	85.1	86.5	59.2	54.1	54.2	56.7	54.4
Ovary	37.1	38.6	40.4	42.2	50.1	40.4	38.6	42.0	38.7	46.3
Non-Hodgkin's lymphoma	49.1	52.8	55.7	56.5	57.3	56.9	53.3	46.8	54.3	46.9

- - - Data not available.

NOTES: Rates are based on followup of patients through 1994. The rate is the ratio of the observed survival rate for the patient group to the expected survival rate for persons in the general population similar to the patient group with respect to age, sex, race, and calendar year of observation. It estimates the chance of surviving the effects of cancer. Numbers have been revised and differ from previous editions of *Health, United States.*

SOURCE: National Institutes of Health, National Cancer Institute, Cancer Statistics Branch, Bethesda, Maryland 20892.

Table 59. Limitation of activity caused by chronic conditions, according to selected characteristics: United States, 1990 and 1996

[Data are based on household interviews of a sample of the civilian noninstitutionalized population]

Characteristic	Total with limitation of activity		Limited but not in major activity		Limited in amount or kind of major activity		Unable to carry on major activity	
	1990	1996	1990	1996	1990	1996	1990	1996
	Percent of population							
Total[1,2]	12.9	13.6	4.1	4.1	5.0	5.2	3.9	4.4
Age								
Under 15 years	4.7	5.7	1.2	1.5	3.1	3.8	0.4	0.5
Under 5 years	2.2	2.6	0.6	0.6	1.0	1.5	0.6	0.5
5–14 years	6.1	7.3	1.6	1.9	4.1	4.9	0.4	0.5
15–44 years	8.5	9.6	2.6	2.7	3.5	3.7	2.4	3.2
45–64 years	21.8	22.0	5.7	5.5	7.5	7.2	8.6	9.4
65 years and over	37.5	36.3	15.4	14.8	11.9	11.0	10.2	10.5
65–74 years	33.7	31.4	13.2	12.0	9.9	9.2	10.6	10.1
75 years and over	43.3	43.1	18.8	18.7	14.9	13.5	9.6	10.9
Sex and age								
Male[1]	12.9	13.7	3.8	4.0	4.7	5.0	4.4	4.7
Under 15 years	5.5	7.0	1.4	1.8	3.6	4.7	0.5	0.6
15–44 years	8.4	9.5	2.3	2.5	3.5	3.6	2.7	3.5
45–64 years	21.4	21.2	4.7	4.5	6.6	6.4	10.1	10.4
65–74 years	34.0	31.1	13.0	12.6	8.4	7.7	12.7	10.8
75 years and over	38.8	41.6	20.3	22.6	10.2	9.5	8.3	9.5
Female[1]	13.0	13.5	4.3	4.2	5.3	5.2	3.4	4.1
Under 15 years	3.9	4.4	1.0	1.2	2.5	2.8	0.4	0.4
15–44 years	8.7	9.6	2.9	2.9	3.6	3.8	2.2	2.9
45–64 years	22.2	22.8	6.6	6.4	8.4	7.9	7.2	8.4
65–74 years	33.5	31.7	13.4	11.6	11.1	10.4	8.9	9.6
75 years and over	46.0	44.0	17.9	16.3	17.7	16.0	10.4	11.7
Race and age								
White[1]	12.8	13.1	4.2	4.1	5.0	5.0	3.6	4.0
Under 15 years	4.7	5.3	1.3	1.4	3.0	3.6	0.4	0.3
15–44 years	8.5	9.3	2.7	2.7	3.6	3.7	2.2	2.9
45–64 years	21.2	21.2	5.8	5.5	7.6	7.0	7.9	8.6
65–74 years	33.2	30.5	13.4	12.1	9.8	9.0	10.0	9.5
75 years and over	42.9	42.7	19.2	19.2	14.7	13.0	9.0	10.4
Black[1]	15.5	17.6	3.8	4.0	5.3	6.5	6.5	7.0
Under 15 years	5.3	8.6	1.2	2.2	3.4	5.3	0.7	1.1
15–44 years	9.4	12.1	2.2	2.7	3.4	4.2	3.9	5.2
45–64 years	28.1	29.3	5.7	5.6	7.7	8.9	14.8	14.7
65–74 years	41.6	39.5	12.4	12.1	11.5	11.7	17.6	15.7
75 years and over	50.9	47.8	16.2	11.5	17.6	19.6	17.0	16.7
Family income[1,3]								
Less than $16,000	22.9	26.4	5.2	5.8	8.1	8.8	9.6	11.8
$16,000–$24,999	14.8	15.7	4.3	4.2	5.7	6.3	4.8	5.2
$25,000–$34,999	11.6	13.2	3.8	4.3	4.7	5.0	3.0	3.8
$35,000–$49,999	10.4	10.6	3.7	3.8	4.4	4.1	2.3	2.6
$50,000 or more	8.4	8.5	3.4	3.5	3.3	3.4	1.7	1.6
Geographic region[1]								
Northeast	11.9	12.8	3.9	4.1	4.5	5.0	3.6	3.8
Midwest	12.9	13.1	3.9	3.8	5.5	5.3	3.4	4.0
South	14.0	14.2	4.1	3.8	5.3	5.5	4.6	4.9
West	12.5	14.0	4.4	4.8	4.5	4.6	3.7	4.5
Location of residence[1]								
Within MSA[4]	12.4	13.1	4.0	4.1	4.7	4.9	3.7	4.0
Outside MSA[4]	14.9	15.5	4.3	4.2	6.1	5.7	4.5	5.5

[1] Age adjusted. See Appendix II for age-adjustment procedure.
[2] Includes all other races not shown separately and unknown family income.
[3] Family income categories for 1996. In 1990 the two lowest income categories are less than $14,000 and $14,000–$24,999; the three higher income categories are as shown.
[4] Metropolitan statistical area.

SOURCE: Centers for Disease Control and Prevention, National Center for Health Statistics, Division of Health Interview Statistics. Data from the National Health Interview Survey.

Table 60. Respondent-assessed health status, according to selected characteristics: United States, 1991–96

[Data are based on household interviews of a sample of the civilian noninstitutionalized population]

	Percent with fair or poor health								
	Both sexes			Male			Female		
Characteristic	1991	1995	1996	1991	1995	1996	1991	1995	1996
Total[1,2]	9.2	9.3	9.2	8.9	8.9	8.7	9.6	9.8	9.7
Age									
Under 18 years	2.6	2.6	2.6	2.7	2.7	2.5	2.6	2.4	2.7
Under 6 years	2.7	2.7	2.6	2.9	3.1	2.6	2.4	2.2	2.5
6–17 years	2.6	2.5	2.6	2.5	2.4	2.4	2.6	2.6	2.8
18–44 years	6.1	6.6	6.7	5.2	5.5	5.6	6.9	7.7	7.7
45–54 years	13.4	13.4	13.1	12.5	12.5	12.3	14.2	14.3	13.9
55–64 years	20.7	21.4	21.2	20.7	20.6	21.4	20.8	22.2	21.1
65 years and over	29.0	28.3	27.0	29.2	28.8	26.6	28.9	28.0	27.4
65–74 years......................	26.0	25.6	23.8	26.7	26.3	23.2	25.5	25.0	24.4
75–84 years......................	32.6	31.4	30.2	33.2	31.7	31.3	32.3	31.2	29.4
85 years and over	37.3	35.3	36.2	36.5	38.5	34.9	37.6	33.8	36.8
Race[1,3]									
White	8.5	8.6	8.4	8.3	8.3	8.0	8.7	8.8	8.7
Black	15.0	15.3	15.0	14.0	13.7	13.7	15.9	16.6	16.0
American Indian or Alaska Native	16.8	15.9	18.9	16.1	16.1	19.2	17.0	16.0	17.8
Asian or Pacific Islander.............	6.7	8.2	8.3	5.9	7.0	6.5	7.3	9.2	10.0
Race and Hispanic origin[1]									
White, non-Hispanic..................	8.0	8.0	7.9	7.9	7.8	7.6	8.1	8.1	8.1
Black, non-Hispanic..................	15.0	15.4	14.9	14.1	13.8	13.7	15.9	16.6	15.9
Hispanic[3]	13.7	13.6	12.9	12.3	12.3	11.8	14.9	14.8	14.1
Mexican[3]	14.9	14.9	13.7	13.0	13.9	11.9	16.8	16.0	15.4
Poverty status[1,4]									
Poor.............................	21.8	22.5	22.2	22.4	22.1	21.6	21.5	23.0	22.8
Near poor	13.5	14.2	14.1	13.5	14.9	14.4	13.5	13.8	14.0
Nonpoor	5.5	5.6	5.5	5.4	5.3	5.3	5.7	5.8	5.6
Race and Hispanic origin and poverty status[1,4]									
White, non-Hispanic:									
Poor	21.1	21.4	21.6	22.7	21.6	22.5	20.2	21.5	21.1
Near poor	12.9	13.6	13.8	13.5	15.0	14.7	12.5	12.5	13.2
Nonpoor	5.2	5.2	5.1	5.2	5.1	5.0	5.3	5.3	5.1
Black, non-Hispanic:									
Poor	24.9	26.7	26.9	25.2	26.2	26.0	24.8	27.1	27.8
Near poor	15.5	17.2	16.6	14.6	15.9	15.2	16.3	18.1	17.6
Nonpoor	8.5	8.1	8.5	7.6	7.3	7.6	9.5	8.9	9.3
Hispanic:[3]									
Poor	21.1	21.2	19.9	20.2	20.1	17.7	21.7	22.3	21.8
Near poor	15.8	15.5	14.7	14.3	14.1	14.3	17.4	16.9	15.5
Nonpoor	7.9	7.0	7.7	7.1	6.4	7.6	8.7	7.6	7.5
Geographic region[1]									
Northeast	7.4	8.0	8.2	7.2	7.7	7.7	7.6	8.3	8.7
Midwest	8.0	8.5	8.1	7.7	8.3	7.7	8.3	8.7	8.6
South.............................	11.6	10.9	10.7	11.3	10.3	10.1	11.9	11.4	11.3
West	8.6	8.9	8.7	8.1	8.2	8.4	9.1	9.6	9.2
Location of residence[1]									
Within MSA[5]	8.8	8.9	8.4	8.3	8.4	7.8	9.3	9.4	9.0
Outside MSA[5]	10.6	11.1	11.8	10.9	10.8	11.5	10.4	11.4	12.1

[1]Age adjusted. See Appendix II for age-adjustment procedure.
[2]Includes all other races not shown separately and unknown family income.
[3]The race groups, white, black, American Indian or Alaska Native, and Asian or Pacific Islander, include persons of Hispanic and non-Hispanic origin; persons of Hispanic origin may be of any race.
[4]Poverty status is based on family income and family size using Bureau of the Census poverty thresholds. Poor persons are defined as below the poverty threshold. Near poor persons have incomes of 100 percent to less than 200 percent of poverty threshold. Nonpoor persons have incomes of 200 percent or greater than the poverty threshold. See Appendix II, Poverty level.
[5]Metropolitan statistical area.

SOURCE: Centers for Disease Control and Prevention, National Center for Health Statistics, Division of Health Interview Statistics. Data from the National Health Interview Survey.

Table 61. Current cigarette smoking by persons 18 years of age and over, according to sex, race, and age: United States, selected years 1965–95

[Data are based on household interviews of a sample of the civilian noninstitutionalized population]

Sex, race, and age	1965	1974	1979	1983	1985	1990	1991	1992	1993	1994	1995
18 years and over, age adjusted					Percent of persons						
All persons	42.3	37.2	33.5	32.2	30.0	25.4	25.4	26.4	25.0	25.5	24.7
Male	51.6	42.9	37.2	34.7	32.1	28.0	27.5	28.2	27.5	27.8	26.7
Female	34.0	32.5	30.3	29.9	28.2	23.1	23.6	24.8	22.7	23.3	22.8
White male	50.8	41.7	36.5	34.1	31.3	27.6	27.0	28.0	27.0	27.5	26.4
Black male	59.2	54.0	44.1	41.3	39.9	32.2	34.7	32.0	33.2	33.5	28.5
White female	34.3	32.3	30.6	30.1	28.3	23.9	24.2	25.7	23.7	24.3	23.6
Black female	32.1	35.9	30.8	31.8	30.7	20.4	23.1	23.9	19.8	21.1	22.8
18 years and over, crude											
All persons	42.4	37.1	33.5	32.1	30.1	25.5	25.6	26.5	25.0	25.5	24.7
Male	51.9	43.1	37.5	35.1	32.6	28.4	28.1	28.6	27.7	28.2	27.0
Female	33.9	32.1	29.9	29.5	27.9	22.8	23.5	24.6	22.5	23.1	22.6
White male	51.1	41.9	36.8	34.5	31.7	28.0	27.4	28.2	27.0	27.7	26.6
Black male	60.4	54.3	44.1	40.6	39.9	32.5	35.0	32.2	32.7	33.7	28.5
White female	34.0	31.7	30.1	29.4	27.7	23.4	23.7	25.1	23.1	23.7	23.1
Black female	33.7	36.4	31.1	32.2	31.0	21.2	24.4	24.2	20.8	21.7	23.5
All males											
18–24 years	54.1	42.1	35.0	32.9	28.0	26.6	23.5	28.0	28.8	29.8	27.8
25–34 years	60.7	50.5	43.9	38.8	38.2	31.6	32.8	32.8	30.2	31.4	29.5
35–44 years	58.2	51.0	41.8	41.0	37.6	34.5	33.1	32.9	32.0	33.2	31.5
45–64 years	51.9	42.6	39.3	35.9	33.4	29.3	29.3	28.6	29.2	28.3	27.1
65 years and over	28.5	24.8	20.9	22.0	19.6	14.6	15.1	16.1	13.5	13.2	14.9
White male											
18–24 years	53.0	40.8	34.3	32.5	28.4	27.4	25.1	30.0	30.4	31.8	28.4
25–34 years	60.1	49.5	43.6	38.6	37.3	31.6	32.1	33.5	29.9	32.5	29.9
35–44 years	57.3	50.1	41.3	40.8	36.6	33.5	32.1	30.9	31.2	32.0	31.2
45–64 years	51.3	41.2	38.3	35.0	32.1	28.7	28.0	28.1	27.8	26.9	26.3
65 years and over	27.7	24.3	20.5	20.6	18.9	13.7	14.2	14.9	12.5	11.9	14.1
Black male											
18–24 years	62.8	54.9	40.2	34.2	27.2	21.3	15.0	16.2	19.9	18.7	14.6
25–34 years	68.4	58.5	47.5	39.9	45.6	33.8	39.4	29.5	30.7	29.8	25.1
35–44 years	67.3	61.5	48.6	45.5	45.0	42.0	44.4	47.5	36.9	44.5	36.3
45–64 years	57.9	57.8	50.0	44.8	46.1	36.7	42.0	35.4	42.4	41.2	33.9
65 years and over	36.4	29.7	26.2	38.9	27.7	21.5	24.3	28.3	27.9	25.6	28.5
All females											
18–24 years	38.1	34.1	33.8	35.5	30.4	22.5	22.4	24.9	22.9	25.2	21.8
25–34 years	43.7	38.8	33.7	32.6	32.0	28.2	28.4	30.1	27.3	28.8	26.4
35–44 years	43.7	39.8	37.0	33.8	31.5	24.8	27.6	27.3	27.4	26.8	27.1
45–64 years	32.0	33.4	30.7	31.0	29.9	24.8	24.6	26.1	23.0	22.8	24.0
65 years and over	9.6	12.0	13.2	13.1	13.5	11.5	12.0	12.4	10.5	11.1	11.5
White female											
18–24 years	38.4	34.0	34.5	36.5	31.8	25.4	25.1	28.5	26.8	28.5	24.9
25–34 years	43.4	38.6	34.1	32.2	32.0	28.5	28.4	31.5	28.4	30.2	27.3
35–44 years	43.9	39.3	37.2	34.8	31.0	25.0	27.0	27.6	27.3	27.1	27.0
45–64 years	32.7	33.0	30.6	30.6	29.7	25.4	25.3	25.8	23.4	23.2	24.3
65 years and over	9.8	12.3	13.8	13.2	13.3	11.5	12.1	12.6	10.5	11.1	11.7
Black female											
18–24 years	37.1	35.6	31.8	32.0	23.7	10.0	11.8	10.3	8.2	11.8	8.8
25–34 years	47.8	42.2	35.2	38.0	36.2	29.1	32.4	26.9	24.7	24.8	26.7
35–44 years	42.8	46.4	37.7	32.7	40.2	25.5	35.3	32.4	31.5	28.2	31.9
45–64 years	25.7	38.9	34.2	36.3	33.4	22.6	23.4	30.9	21.3	23.5	27.5
65 years and over	7.1	8.9	8.5	13.1	14.5	11.1	9.6	11.1	10.2	13.6	13.3

NOTES: The definition of current smoker was revised in 1992 and 1993. See discussion of current smoker in Appendix II. See Appendix II for age-adjustment procedure. Data for additional years are available (see Appendix III).

SOURCE: Centers for Disease Control and Prevention, National Center for Health Statistics, Division of Health Interview Statistics: Data from the National Health Interview Survey; data computed by the Division of Health and Utilization Analysis from data compiled by the Division of Health Interview Statistics.

Table 62. Age-adjusted prevalence of current cigarette smoking by persons 25 years of age and over, according to sex, race, and education: United States, selected years 1974–95

[Data are based on household interviews of a sample of the civilian noninstitutionalized population]

Sex, race, and education	1974	1979	1983	1985	1990	1991	1992	1993	1994	1995
25 years and over, age adjusted					Percent of persons					
All persons[1]	37.1	33.3	31.7	30.2	25.6	26.0	26.5	24.8	25.1	24.6
Less than 12 years	43.8	41.1	40.8	41.0	36.7	37.4	36.7	35.8	37.5	35.7
12 years	36.4	33.7	33.6	32.1	29.3	29.7	30.7	28.3	29.2	29.0
13–15 years	35.8	33.2	30.3	29.7	23.5	24.7	24.6	24.5	24.9	22.9
16 or more years	27.5	22.8	20.7	18.6	14.1	13.9	15.3	13.6	11.9	13.6
All males[1]	43.0	37.6	35.1	32.9	28.3	28.4	28.2	27.2	27.4	26.4
Less than 12 years	52.4	48.1	47.2	46.0	41.8	42.4	41.2	41.0	43.9	39.7
12 years	42.6	39.1	37.4	35.6	33.2	32.9	33.3	30.5	31.7	32.6
13–15 years	41.6	36.5	33.0	33.0	25.9	27.2	26.1	27.4	27.3	24.0
16 or more years	28.6	23.1	21.8	19.7	14.6	14.8	15.8	14.6	13.2	13.9
White males[1]	41.9	36.9	34.5	31.9	27.7	27.3	27.6	26.3	26.6	26.0
Less than 12 years	51.6	48.0	47.9	45.2	41.7	41.8	41.4	39.7	42.6	38.8
12 years	42.2	38.6	37.1	34.8	33.0	32.4	32.9	29.7	31.7	32.7
13–15 years	41.4	36.4	32.6	32.3	25.4	26.0	25.9	26.9	26.9	23.6
16 or more years	28.1	22.8	21.1	19.2	14.5	14.7	15.0	14.1	12.7	13.4
Black males[1]	53.8	44.9	42.8	42.5	34.5	38.8	35.3	36.0	36.5	31.4
Less than 12 years	58.3	50.1	46.0	51.1	41.4	47.8	44.5	47.2	51.6	41.4
12 years	*51.2	48.4	47.2	41.9	37.4	39.6	38.7	36.4	37.1	36.4
13–15 years	*45.7	39.3	44.7	42.3	28.3	32.7	27.0	30.1	29.7	26.4
16 or more years	*41.8	*37.9	*31.3	*32.0	20.6	18.3	*26.9	*16.0	*25.9	*16.9
All females[1]	32.2	29.6	28.8	27.8	23.2	23.9	24.8	22.7	22.9	23.0
Less than 12 years	36.8	35.0	35.3	36.7	32.1	33.0	32.4	31.0	31.6	32.1
12 years	32.5	29.9	30.9	29.6	26.3	27.1	28.7	26.7	27.3	26.3
13–15 years	30.2	30.0	27.5	26.7	21.1	22.5	23.3	21.8	22.5	22.0
16 or more years	26.1	22.5	19.2	17.4	13.6	12.8	14.6	12.4	10.3	13.3
White females[1]	31.9	29.8	28.8	27.6	23.6	24.0	25.1	23.1	23.5	23.3
Less than 12 years	37.0	36.1	35.5	37.1	33.6	33.7	33.1	31.7	33.0	33.1
12 years	32.1	29.9	30.9	29.4	26.8	27.5	29.5	27.6	28.4	26.7
13–15 years	30.5	30.6	28.0	27.1	21.4	22.3	23.6	21.9	22.3	22.5
16 or more years	25.8	21.9	18.9	16.8	13.7	13.3	14.2	12.5	10.8	13.5
Black females[1]	35.9	30.6	31.8	32.1	22.6	25.5	26.8	22.2	23.0	25.7
Less than 12 years	36.4	31.9	36.9	39.2	26.8	33.3	33.2	29.8	30.1	31.6
12 years	41.9	33.0	35.2	32.3	24.0	26.0	25.9	23.9	22.5	27.9
13–15 years	33.2	*28.8	26.5	23.7	23.1	24.8	27.0	22.7	28.1	21.0
16 or more years	*35.2	*43.4	*38.7	27.5	16.9	14.4	*25.8	*13.3	*11.3	*18.0

* These age-adjusted percents should be considered unreliable because of small sample size. For age groups where percent smoking was 0 or 100, the age-adjustment procedure was modified to substitute the percent from the next lower education group.
[1]Includes unknown education.

NOTES: The definition of current smoker was revised in 1992 and 1993. See discussion of current smoker in Appendix II. See Appendix II for age-adjustment procedure. Data for additional years are available (see Appendix III).

SOURCE: Data computed by the Centers for Disease Control and Prevention, National Center for Health Statistics, Division of Health and Utilization Analysis from data compiled by the Division of Health Interview Statistics.

Table 63. Current cigarette smoking by adults according to sex, race, Hispanic origin, age, and education: United States, average annual 1990–92 and 1993–95

[Data are based on household interviews of a sample of the civilian noninstitutionalized population]

Race, Hispanic origin, and age	Male		Female	
	1990–92	1993–95	1990–92	1993–95
18 years of age and over, age adjusted	Percent of persons			
All races[1,2]	27.9	27.3	23.8	22.9
White	27.5	26.9	24.6	23.9
Black	33.0	31.8	22.5	21.3
American Indian or Alaska Native[3]	34.5	39.9	36.4	32.9
Asian or Pacific Islander	24.4	24.8	6.2	7.4
White, non-Hispanic	27.9	27.5	25.6	25.1
Black, non-Hispanic	33.0	31.7	22.7	21.5
Hispanic[2]	25.4	23.0	15.7	13.7
Mexican	25.8	24.0	14.7	12.0
18 years of age and over, crude				
All races[1,2]	28.4	27.6	23.6	22.7
White	27.8	27.1	24.1	23.3
Black	33.2	31.6	23.3	22.0
American Indian or Alaska Native	35.5	40.7	37.3	35.4
Asian or Pacific Islander	24.9	25.8	6.3	7.5
White, non-Hispanic	28.0	27.4	24.8	24.2
Black, non-Hispanic	33.3	31.6	23.3	22.2
Hispanic[2]	26.5	24.6	16.6	14.4
Mexican	27.1	25.4	15.0	12.6
18–24 years:				
White, non-Hispanic	28.9	31.4	28.7	29.1
Black, non-Hispanic	17.7	17.4	10.8	9.4
Hispanic[2]	19.3	23.8	12.8	13.2
25–34 years:				
White, non-Hispanic	32.7	31.5	30.9	30.7
Black, non-Hispanic	34.6	28.0	29.2	25.8
Hispanic[2]	29.9	27.4	19.2	15.1
35–44 years:				
White, non-Hispanic	32.3	32.0	27.3	27.9
Black, non-Hispanic	44.1	39.9	31.3	30.8
Hispanic[2]	32.1	25.3	19.9	19.5
45–64 years:				
White, non-Hispanic	28.4	27.3	26.1	24.5
Black, non-Hispanic	38.0	39.1	26.1	24.5
Hispanic[2]	26.6	23.8	17.1	12.9
65 years and over:				
White, non-Hispanic	14.2	12.9	12.3	11.3
Black, non-Hispanic	25.2	27.5	10.7	12.6
Hispanic[2]	16.1	12.1	6.6	7.1
Education, race, and Hispanic origin				
25 years of age and over, age adjusted				
Less than 12 years:				
White, non-Hispanic	46.0	46.7	40.5	41.0
Black, non-Hispanic	45.2	47.3	31.6	31.5
Hispanic[2]	30.3	24.7	15.9	13.9
12 years:				
White, non-Hispanic	33.1	32.0	28.6	28.6
Black, non-Hispanic	38.4	36.9	25.4	24.8
Hispanic[2]	29.8	25.2	18.6	16.2
13 years or more:				
White, non-Hispanic	19.4	18.7	18.3	17.6
Black, non-Hispanic	25.3	24.4	22.8	20.3
Hispanic[2]	20.0	18.0	14.4	9.8

[1]Includes all other races not shown separately.
[2]The race groups white, black, American Indian or Alaska Native, and Asian or Pacific Islander include persons of Hispanic and non-Hispanic origin; persons of Hispanic origin may be of any race.
[3]In 1993–95 the percent of American Indian males 65 years of age and over who smoked was 0. The age-adjustment procedure was modified to replace the 0 with the percent of American Indian males in this age group who smoked in 1990–92.

NOTES: See Appendix II for age-adjustment procedure. The definition of current smoker was revised in 1992 and 1993. See discussion of current smoker in Appendix II .

SOURCE: Centers for Disease Control and Prevention, National Center for Health Statistics. Data computed by the Division of Health and Utilization Analysis from the National Health Interview Survey.

Table 64 (page 1 of 2). Use of selected substances in the past month by persons 12 years of age and over, according to age, sex, race, and Hispanic origin: United States, selected years 1979–97

[Data are based on household interviews of a sample of the population 12 years of age and over]

Substance, age, sex, race, and Hispanic origin	1979	1985	1990	1991	1992	1993	1994	1995	1996	1997
Cigarettes					Percent of population					
12–17 years.	---	29	22	21	18	19	19	20	18	20
12–13 years	---	---	---	---	---	---	9	11	7	10
14–15 years	---	---	---	---	---	---	20	21	18	20
16–17 years	---	---	---	---	---	---	29	30	28	30
12–17 years:										
Male	---	31	24	23	18	18	20	21	18	19
Female	---	28	21	19	18	19	18	20	19	21
White, non-Hispanic	---	33	26	24	22	21	22	23	21	22
Black, non-Hispanic	---	17	*	8	6	8	12	12	12	15
Hispanic[1]	---	21	21	17	14	16	14	16	15	16
18–25 years:										
Male	---	---	---	---	---	---	37	38	43	47
Female	---	---	---	---	---	---	32	32	33	35
White, non-Hispanic	---	---	---	---	---	---	39	39	43	45
Black, non-Hispanic	---	---	---	---	---	---	25	24	29	30
Hispanic[1]	---	---	---	---	---	---	28	28	30	31
Alcohol										
12 years and over	63	60	53	52	49	51	54	52	51	51
12–17 years	50	41	33	27	21	24	22	21	19	21
12–13 years	---	---	---	---	---	---	9	8	5	7
14–15 years	---	---	---	---	---	---	22	21	19	21
16–17 years	---	---	---	---	---	---	36	34	31	33
18–25 years	75	70	63	63	59	59	63	61	60	58
26–34 years	72	71	64	63	62	64	65	63	62	60
35 years and over	60	58	50	50	47	50	54	53	52	53
12–17 years:										
Male	52	44	34	30	22	24	22	22	19	21
Female	47	38	31	24	19	23	21	20	18	20
White, non-Hispanic	53	46	37	27	22	26	24	23	20	22
Black, non-Hispanic	---	30	21	28	18	18	18	15	15	16
Hispanic[1]	---	27	24	28	20	22	18	19	20	19
18–25 years:										
Male	---	---	---	---	---	---	71	68	67	66
Female	---	---	---	---	---	---	55	55	54	51
White, non-Hispanic	---	---	---	---	---	---	68	67	65	64
Black, non-Hispanic	---	---	---	---	---	---	52	48	50	47
Hispanic[1]	---	---	---	---	---	---	54	49	50	49
Heavy alcohol[2]										
12 years and over	---	20	14	16	15	15	17	16	15	15
12–17 years	---	22	15	13	10	11	8	8	7	8
12–13 years	---	---	---	---	---	---	2	2	1	1
14–15 years	---	---	---	---	---	---	8	8	6	8
16–17 years	---	---	---	---	---	---	16	15	15	16
18–25 years	---	34	30	31	30	29	34	30	32	28
26–34 years	---	28	21	22	23	22	24	24	23	23
35 years and over	---	13	8	10	9	10	12	12	11	12
12–17 years:										
Male	---	29	19	17	13	15	10	9	9	10
Female	---	14	12	9	7	7	7	6	6	7
White, non-Hispanic	---	26	18	16	11	13	10	9	8	9
Black, non-Hispanic	---	6	*	6	6	3	4	3	4	4
Hispanic[1]	---	15	11	11	9	12	5	7	8	7
18–25 years:										
Male	---	---	---	---	---	---	47	41	44	39
Female	---	---	---	---	---	---	21	19	21	17
White, non-Hispanic	---	---	---	---	---	---	40	34	37	33
Black, non-Hispanic	---	---	---	---	---	---	17	16	19	13
Hispanic[1]	---	---	---	---	---	---	26	23	25	22

See footnotes at end of table.

Table 64 (page 2 of 2). Use of selected substances in the past month by persons 12 years of age and over, according to age, sex, race, and Hispanic origin: United States, selected years 1979–97

[Data are based on household interviews of a sample of the population 12 years of age and over]

Substance, age, sex, race, and Hispanic origin	1979	1985	1990	1991	1992	1993	1994	1995	1996	1997
Marijuana					Percent of population					
12 years and over	13	10	5	5	5	5	5	5	5	5
12–17 years	14	10	4	4	3	4	6	8	7	9
12–13 years	---	---	---	---	---	---	2	2	1	3
14–15 years	---	---	---	---	---	---	5	10	7	9
16–17 years	---	---	---	---	---	---	12	13	13	16
18–25 years	36	22	13	13	11	11	12	12	13	13
26–34 years	20	19	10	8	9	8	7	7	6	6
35 years and over	3	3	2	3	2	2	2	2	2	3
12–17 years:										
Male	16	11	5	4	4	4	7	9	8	10
Female	12	9	4	3	3	4	5	7	7	8
White, non-Hispanic	16	12	5	4	4	4	6	8	7	10
Black, non-Hispanic	10	6	2	3	2	3	6	8	7	9
Hispanic[1]	8	6	3	3	3	4	6	8	7	8
18–25 years:										
Male	---	---	---	---	---	---	16	15	17	17
Female	---	---	---	---	---	---	9	9	9	8
White, non-Hispanic	---	---	---	---	---	---	13	13	14	13
Black, non-Hispanic	---	---	---	---	---	---	12	12	14	14
Hispanic[1]	---	---	---	---	---	---	8	7	8	8
Cocaine										
12 years and over	2.6	3.0	0.9	1.0	0.7	0.7	0.7	0.7	0.8	0.7
12–17 years	1.5	1.5	0.6	0.4	0.3	0.4	0.3	0.8	0.6	1.0
18–25 years	9.9	8.1	2.3	2.2	2.0	1.6	1.2	1.3	2.0	1.2
26–34 years	3.0	6.3	1.9	1.9	1.5	1.0	1.3	1.2	1.5	0.9
35 years and over	0.2	0.5	0.5	0.5	0.2	0.4	0.4	0.4	0.4	0.5
12–17 years:										
Male	2.2	1.9	0.8	0.5	0.3	0.5	0.3	0.8	0.4	0.9
Female	0.8	1.1	0.5	0.3	0.3	0.4	0.3	0.7	0.8	1.1
White, non-Hispanic	1.4	1.5	0.4	0.3	0.2	0.4	0.3	0.9	0.5	1.1
Black, non-Hispanic	*	1.3	0.8	0.5	0.3	0.3	0.1	0.1	0.1	0.1
Hispanic[1]	2.1	2.6	2.0	1.4	1.3	1.1	0.8	0.8	1.1	1.0
18–25 years:										
Male	---	---	---	---	---	---	0.9	1.7	2.7	1.9
Female	---	---	---	---	---	---	0.6	0.9	1.4	0.5
White, non-Hispanic	---	---	---	---	---	---	1.2	1.5	2.3	1.2
Black, non-Hispanic	---	---	---	---	---	---	0.7	0.7	1.1	0.9
Hispanic[1]	---	---	---	---	---	---	2.2	1.1	2.1	1.5

- - - Data not available.
* Estimates with relative standard error greater than 17.5 percent of the log transformation of the proportion are not shown.
[1]Persons of Hispanic origin may be of any race.
[2]Five or more drinks on the same occasion at least once in the past month.

NOTES: In 1994 the survey underwent major changes. Estimates for 1993 and earlier years are adjusted to be comparable with data from the redesigned survey. See Appendix I, Substance Abuse and Mental Health Services Administration. Estimates of the use of substances from the National Household Survey on Drug Abuse and the Monitoring the Future Study differ because of different methodologies, sampling frames, and tabulation categories. Data for additional years are available (see Appendix III).

SOURCES: National Household Survey on Drug Abuse Series H–6: Preliminary Results from the 1997 National Household Survey on Drug Abuse; and H–7: National Household Survey on Drug Abuse: Population Estimates 1997.

Table 65 (page 1 of 2). Use of selected substances in the past month and heavy alcohol use in the past 2 weeks by high school seniors and eighth-graders, according to sex and race: United States, selected years 1980–98

[Data are based on a survey of high school seniors and eighth-graders in the coterminous United States]

Substance, sex, race, and grade in school	1980	1985	1989	1990	1991	1992	1993	1994	1995	1996	1997	1998
Cigarettes					Percent using substance in the past month							
All seniors	30.5	30.1	28.6	29.4	28.3	27.8	29.9	31.2	33.5	34.0	36.5	35.1
Male	26.8	28.2	27.7	29.1	29.0	29.2	30.7	32.9	34.5	34.9	37.3	36.3
Female	33.4	31.4	29.0	29.2	27.5	26.1	28.7	29.2	32.0	32.4	35.2	33.3
White	31.0	31.7	32.1	32.5	31.8	31.8	34.6	35.9	37.3	38.9	42.5	41.0
Black	25.2	18.7	12.4	12.0	9.4	8.2	10.9	11.0	15.0	13.5	14.9	14.9
All eighth-graders	---	---	---	---	14.3	15.5	16.7	18.6	19.1	21.0	19.4	19.1
Male	---	---	---	---	15.5	14.9	17.2	19.3	18.8	20.6	19.1	18.0
Female	---	---	---	---	13.1	15.9	16.3	17.9	19.0	21.1	19.5	19.8
White	---	---	---	---	15.0	17.4	18.1	19.8	21.7	23.8	22.0	21.1
Black	---	---	---	---	5.3	5.3	7.7	9.6	8.2	11.3	10.4	10.8
Marijuana												
All seniors	33.7	25.7	16.7	14.0	13.8	11.9	15.5	19.0	21.2	21.9	23.7	22.8
Male	37.8	28.7	19.5	16.1	16.1	13.4	18.2	23.0	24.6	25.1	26.4	26.5
Female	29.1	22.4	13.8	11.5	11.2	10.2	12.5	15.1	17.2	18.3	20.3	18.8
White	34.2	26.4	18.6	15.6	15.0	13.1	16.7	20.1	21.5	22.5	24.6	24.2
Black	26.5	21.7	9.4	5.2	6.5	5.6	10.8	15.9	17.8	18.8	18.2	18.3
All eighth-graders	---	---	---	---	3.2	3.7	5.1	7.8	9.1	11.3	10.2	9.7
Male	---	---	---	---	3.8	3.8	6.1	9.5	9.8	12.1	11.4	10.3
Female	---	---	---	---	2.6	3.5	4.1	6.0	8.2	10.2	8.9	8.8
White	---	---	---	---	3.0	3.5	4.6	6.7	9.0	11.0	10.2	8.9
Black	---	---	---	---	2.1	1.9	3.7	6.2	7.0	9.3	8.7	9.4
Cocaine												
All seniors	5.2	6.7	2.8	1.9	1.4	1.3	1.3	1.5	1.8	2.0	2.3	2.4
Male	6.0	7.7	3.6	2.3	1.7	1.5	1.7	1.9	2.2	2.6	2.8	3.0
Female	4.3	5.6	2.0	1.3	0.9	0.9	0.9	1.1	1.3	1.4	1.6	1.7
White	5.4	7.0	2.9	1.8	1.3	1.2	1.2	1.5	1.7	2.1	2.4	2.7
Black	2.0	2.7	1.2	0.5	0.8	0.5	0.4	0.6	0.4	0.4	0.7	0.4
All eighth-graders	---	---	---	---	0.5	0.7	0.7	1.0	1.2	1.3	1.1	1.4
Male	---	---	---	---	0.7	0.6	0.9	1.2	1.1	1.2	1.2	1.5
Female	---	---	---	---	0.4	0.8	0.6	0.9	1.2	1.4	1.0	1.2
White	---	---	---	---	0.4	0.6	0.5	0.9	1.0	1.4	1.0	1.0
Black	---	---	---	---	0.4	0.4	0.3	0.3	0.4	0.4	0.3	0.6
Inhalants												
All seniors	1.4	2.2	2.3	2.7	2.4	2.3	2.5	2.7	3.2	2.5	2.5	2.3
Male	1.8	2.8	3.1	3.5	3.3	3.0	3.2	3.6	3.9	3.1	3.3	2.9
Female	1.0	1.7	1.5	2.0	1.6	1.6	1.7	1.9	2.5	2.0	1.8	1.7
White	1.4	2.4	2.4	3.0	2.4	2.4	2.7	2.9	3.7	2.9	3.1	2.6
Black	1.0	0.8	1.1	1.5	1.5	1.5	1.3	1.8	1.1	0.9	0.9	1.0
All eighth-graders	---	---	---	---	4.4	4.7	5.4	5.6	6.1	5.8	5.6	4.8
Male	---	---	---	---	4.1	4.4	4.9	5.4	5.6	4.8	5.1	4.8
Female	---	---	---	---	4.7	4.9	6.0	5.8	6.6	6.6	5.8	4.7
White	---	---	---	---	4.5	5.0	5.8	6.1	7.0	6.6	6.4	5.3
Black	---	---	---	---	2.3	2.4	2.9	2.6	2.3	1.7	2.2	2.2

See footnotes at end of table.

Table 65 (page 2 of 2). Use of selected substances in the past month and heavy alcohol use in the past 2 weeks by high school seniors and eighth-graders, according to sex and race: United States, selected years 1980–98

[Data are based on a survey of high school seniors and eighth-graders in the coterminous United States]

Substance, sex, race, and grade in school	1980	1985	1989	1990	1991	1992	1993	1994	1995	1996	1997	1998
Alcohol[1]					Percent using substance in the past month							
All seniors	72.0	65.9	60.0	57.1	54.0	51.3	48.6	50.1	51.3	50.8	52.7	52.0
Male	77.4	69.8	65.1	61.3	58.4	55.8	54.2	55.5	55.7	54.8	56.2	57.3
Female	66.8	62.1	54.9	52.3	49.0	46.8	43.4	45.2	47.0	46.9	48.9	46.9
White	75.8	70.2	65.3	62.2	57.7	56.0	53.4	54.8	54.8	54.7	57.9	57.6
Black	47.7	43.6	38.1	32.9	34.4	29.5	35.1	33.1	37.4	35.7	33.1	33.6
All eighth-graders	---	---	---	---	25.1	26.1	24.3	25.5	24.6	26.2	24.5	23.0
Male	---	---	---	---	26.3	26.3	25.3	26.5	25.0	26.6	25.2	24.0
Female	---	---	---	---	23.8	25.9	28.7	24.7	24.0	25.8	23.9	21.9
White	---	---	---	---	26.0	27.3	25.1	25.4	25.4	27.7	25.7	24.0
Black	---	---	---	---	17.8	19.2	17.7	20.2	17.3	19.0	16.9	15.4
Heavy alcohol[2]					Percent in last 2 weeks							
All seniors	41.2	36.7	33.0	32.2	29.8	27.9	27.5	28.2	29.8	30.2	31.3	31.5
Male	52.1	45.3	41.2	39.1	37.8	35.6	34.6	37.0	36.9	37.0	37.9	39.2
Female	30.5	28.2	24.9	24.4	21.2	20.3	20.7	20.2	23.0	23.5	24.4	24.0
White	44.6	40.1	36.9	36.2	32.9	31.3	31.3	31.7	32.9	34.0	36.1	36.6
Black	17.0	16.7	16.6	11.6	11.8	10.8	14.6	14.2	15.5	15.1	12.0	12.7
All eighth-graders	---	---	---	---	12.9	13.4	13.5	14.5	14.5	15.6	14.5	13.7
Male	---	---	---	---	14.3	13.9	14.8	16.0	15.1	16.5	15.3	14.4
Female	---	---	---	---	11.4	12.8	12.3	13.0	13.9	14.5	13.5	12.7
White	---	---	---	---	12.6	12.9	12.4	13.4	14.5	15.7	14.6	13.5
Black	---	---	---	---	9.9	9.3	11.9	11.8	10.0	10.9	8.8	9.1

- - - Data not available.

[1]In 1993 the alcohol question was changed to indicate that a "drink" meant "more than a few sips." 1993 data based on a half sample.
[2]Five or more drinks in a row at least once in the prior 2-week period.

NOTES: Monitoring the Future Study excludes high school dropouts (see Appendix I) and absentees (about 16–17 percent of high school seniors, about 9–10 percent of eighth-graders). High school dropouts and absentees have higher drug usage than those included in the survey. Estimates of the use of substances from the National Household Survey on Drug Abuse and the Monitoring the Future Study differ because of different methodologies, sampling frames, and tabulation categories. See Appendix I. Data for additional years are available (see Appendix III).

SOURCE: National Institute on Drug Abuse. Monitoring the Future Study. Annual surveys.

Table 66. Cocaine-related emergency room episodes, according to age, sex, race, and Hispanic origin: United States, selected years 1985–96

[Data are weighted national estimates based on a sample of emergency rooms]

Age, sex, race, and Hispanic origin	1985	1990	1991	1992	1993	1994	1995	1996
All races, both sexes[1]				Number of episodes				
All ages[2]	28,801	80,355	101,189	119,843	123,423	142,878	135,801	152,433
6–17 years	1,004	1,877	2,210	1,546	1,578	2,068	2,058	2,595
18–25 years	9,356	19,614	21,766	23,883	22,159	25,392	21,116	22,065
26–34 years	12,895	35,639	46,137	52,760	52,658	60,500	54,953	58,732
35 years and over	5,495	23,054	30,582	41,288	46,614	54,238	57,348	68,723
White, non-Hispanic male								
All ages[2]	7,540	15,512	19,385	21,360	21,193	27,216	25,634	28,647
6–17 years	354	527	486	264	371	409	493	604
18–25 years	2,785	3,810	5,284	5,297	5,155	5,877	5,458	4,968
26–34 years	3,236	6,724	8,777	9,175	8,828	11,908	10,426	11,406
35 years and over	1,149	4,432	4,747	6,585	6,818	8,985	9,228	11,647
Black, non-Hispanic male								
All ages[2]	8,159	27,745	36,597	46,064	46,218	51,622	48,875	51,687
6–17 years	94	241	244	246	213	273	304	348
18–25 years	1,714	5,104	5,743	6,308	5,661	6,698	4,735	3,886
26–34 years	3,888	12,160	16,232	19,952	18,542	20,978	18,756	18,559
35 years and over	2,444	10,202	14,110	19,416	21,709	23,533	25,019	28,742
Hispanic male[3]								
All ages[2]	2,041	4,821	6,571	8,683	9,195	9,566	7,889	12,577
6–17 years	38	144	201	336	206	518	181	431
18–25 years	720	1,774	1,831	2,535	2,184	2,165	1,892	3,725
26–34 years	849	1,758	2,723	3,457	3,893	3,652	2,904	4,342
35 years and over	432	1,125	1,801	2,332	2,885	3,222	2,907	4,056
White, non-Hispanic female								
All ages[2]	4,111	8,331	9,541	10,132	11,263	13,230	13,634	15,594
6–17 years	338	486	529	204	323	357	495	542
18–25 years	1,690	2,663	2,765	2,817	2,832	3,400	2,966	3,344
26–34 years	1,757	3,636	4,427	4,571	5,472	5,905	6,041	6,540
35 years and over	323	1,539	1,808	2,531	2,562	3,566	4,126	5,156
Black, non-Hispanic female								
All ages[2]	3,959	14,833	19,149	22,687	22,186	25,066	24,138	25,713
6–17 years	91	177	210	100	134	102	153	89
18–25 years	1,249	3,820	3,892	4,247	3,674	3,908	3,307	2,803
26–34 years	1,927	7,418	9,481	11,078	10,381	11,551	10,831	11,082
35 years and over	686	3,369	5,512	7,198	7,953	9,472	9,823	11,712
Hispanic female[3]								
All ages[2]	781	1,719	2,356	3,074	3,466	3,595	3,519	5,044
6–17 years	38	64	183	193	166	79	131	250
18–25 years	349	634	616	815	697	955	901	1,297
26–34 years	298	663	1,044	1,324	1,529	1,559	1,280	2,116
35 years and over	95	357	513	732	1,072	998	1,203	1,378

[1]Includes other races and unknown race, Hispanic origin, and/or sex.
[2]Includes unknown age.
[3]Persons of Hispanic origin may be of any race.

NOTES: Data for additional years are available (see Appendix II!). Data for 1994 and 1995 were revised and differ from the previous edition of *Health, United States*.

SOURCE: Substance Abuse and Mental Health Services Administration, Office of Applied Studies, Drug Abuse Warning Network.

Table 67. Alcohol consumption by persons 18 years of age and over, according to sex, race, Hispanic origin, and age: United States, 1985 and 1990

[Data are based on household interviews of a sample of the civilian noninstitutionalized population]

Alcohol consumption, race, Hispanic origin, and age	Both sexes		Male		Female	
	1985	1990	1985	1990	1985	1990
Drinking status			Percent distribution			
All	100.0	100.0	100.0	100.0	100.0	100.0
Abstainer	26.9	29.7	14.4	16.6	38.0	41.5
Former drinker	7.5	9.6	9.2	11.6	6.1	7.8
Current drinker	65.6	60.7	76.4	71.8	55.9	50.7
Race, Hispanic origin, and age			Percent current drinkers among all persons			
All persons:						
18–44 years	72.8	67.5	82.4	77.1	63.8	58.3
18–24 years	71.8	63.7	79.5	71.7	64.5	56.1
25–44 years	73.2	68.8	83.5	78.9	63.5	59.0
45 years and over	55.5	51.3	67.4	63.8	45.6	40.8
45–64 years	62.2	57.6	72.2	68.4	53.0	47.6
65 years and over	44.3	41.4	58.2	55.6	34.7	31.3
White, non-Hispanic:						
18–44 years	76.9	72.7	85.0	80.4	68.9	65.1
18–24 years	77.9	71.5	84.9	77.5	71.0	65.7
25–44 years	76.5	73.1	85.0	81.2	68.2	65.0
45 years and over	57.6	53.8	69.0	65.5	48.2	44.0
45–64 years	65.2	61.0	74.1	70.6	56.9	52.2
65 years and over	45.8	43.3	59.6	57.1	36.2	33.3
Black, non-Hispanic:						
18–44 years	59.0	51.5	72.2	68.1	48.2	37.9
45 years and over	41.5	36.0	57.1	51.3	29.9	24.5
Hispanic:[1]						
18–44 years	58.7	55.7	73.2	71.3	45.6	42.0
45 years and over	48.5	43.4	64.3	63.3	35.4	27.8
Level of alcohol consumption in past 2 weeks for current drinkers			Percent distribution of current drinkers			
All drinking levels	100.0	100.0	100.0	100.0	100.0	100.0
None	21.6	24.1	18.0	20.3	26.1	29.1
Light	37.1	39.4	30.9	33.9	44.7	46.4
Moderate	29.5	27.4	34.0	32.3	24.0	21.1
Heavier	11.8	9.1	17.2	13.6	5.3	3.4
Race, Hispanic origin, and age			Percent heavier drinkers among current drinkers			
All persons:						
18–44 years	11.0	8.5	16.6	13.0	4.2	2.8
18–24 years	12.2	8.8	18.3	13.8	5.0	2.7
25–44 years	10.6	8.4	16.0	12.7	3.8	2.9
45 years and over	13.3	10.3	18.2	14.7	7.4	4.6
45–64 years	13.2	9.9	18.1	14.4	7.2	4.1
65 years and over	13.6	11.0	18.4	15.3	7.9	5.5
White, non-Hispanic:						
18–44 years	11.2	8.5	17.1	13.2	4.0	2.8
18–24 years	13.3	9.9	20.4	16.0	5.2	3.0
25–44 years	10.4	8.1	16.0	12.4	3.6	2.7
45 years and over	13.4	10.4	18.2	15.0	7.6	4.7
45–64 years	13.2	10.0	18.0	14.6	7.3	4.2
65 years and over	13.9	11.3	18.7	15.8	8.3	5.7
Black, non-Hispanic:						
18–44 years	9.6	10.3	13.4	14.7	5.1	3.9
45 years and over	10.3	7.7	16.2	10.1	*	*
Hispanic:[1]						
18–44 years	10.6	7.9	15.2	11.3	*	*
45 years and over	15.7	12.1	*	17.2	*	*

* Estimates based on fewer than 30 subjects are not shown.
[1] Persons of Hispanic origin may be of any race.

NOTES: Abstainers consumed fewer than 12 drinks in any single year. Former drinkers consumed 12 or more drinks in any single year, but no drinks in the past year. Current drinkers consumed 12 or more drinks in a single year and at least 1 drink in the past year. For current drinkers, drinking levels are classified according to the average daily consumption of absolute alcohol (ethanol), in ounces, in the previous 2-week period, assuming 0.5 ounce of ethanol per drink, as follows: none; light, .01–.21; moderate, .22–.99; and heavier, 1.00 or more. This corresponds to up to 3, 4–13, and 14 or more drinks per week for light, moderate, and heavier drinkers.

SOURCE: Data computed by the Alcohol Epidemiologic Data System of the National Institute on Alcohol Abuse and Alcoholism from data in the National Health Interview Survey compiled by the Division of Health Interview Statistics, National Center for Health Statistics, Centers for Disease Control and Prevention.

Table 68. Hypertension among persons 20 years of age and over, according to sex, age, race, and Hispanic origin: United States, 1960–62, 1971–74, 1976–80, and 1988–94

[Data are based on physical examinations of a sample of the civilian noninstitutionalized population]

Sex, age, race, and Hispanic origin[1]	1960–62	1971–74	1976–80[2]	1988–94
20–74 years, age adjusted[3]		Percent of population		
Both sexes[4]	36.9	38.3	39.0	23.1
Male	40.0	42.4	44.0	25.3
Female[4]	33.7	34.3	34.0	20.8
White male	39.3	41.7	43.5	24.3
White female[4]	31.7	32.4	32.3	19.3
Black male	48.1	51.8	48.7	34.9
Black female[4]	50.8	50.3	47.5	33.8
White, non-Hispanic male	- - -	- - -	43.9	24.4
White, non-Hispanic female[4]	- - -	- - -	32.1	19.3
Black, non-Hispanic male	- - -	- - -	48.7	35.0
Black, non-Hispanic female[4]	- - -	- - -	47.6	34.2
Mexican male	- - -	- - -	25.0	25.2
Mexican female[4]	- - -	- - -	21.8	22.0
20–74 years, crude				
Both sexes[4]	39.0	39.7	39.7	23.1
Male	41.7	43.3	44.0	24.7
Female[4]	36.6	36.5	35.6	21.5
White male	41.0	42.8	43.8	24.3
White female[4]	34.9	34.9	34.2	20.4
Black male	50.5	52.1	47.4	31.5
Black female[4]	52.0	50.2	46.1	30.6
White, non-Hispanic male	- - -	- - -	44.3	25.0
White, non-Hispanic female[4]	- - -	- - -	34.4	20.9
Black, non-Hispanic male	- - -	- - -	47.5	31.6
Black, non-Hispanic female[4]	- - -	- - -	46.1	31.2
Mexican male	- - -	- - -	18.8	18.0
Mexican female[4]	- - -	- - -	16.7	15.8
Male				
20–34 years	22.8	24.8	28.9	8.6
35–44 years	37.7	39.1	40.5	20.9
45–54 years	47.6	55.0	53.6	34.1
55–64 years	60.3	62.5	61.8	42.9
65–74 years	68.8	67.2	67.1	57.3
75 years and over	- - -	- - -	- - -	64.2
Female[4]				
20–34 years	9.3	11.2	11.1	3.4
35–44 years	24.0	28.2	28.8	12.7
45–54 years	43.4	43.6	47.1	25.1
55–64 years	66.4	62.5	61.1	44.2
65–74 years	81.5	78.3	71.8	60.8
75 years and over	- - -	- - -	- - -	77.3

- - - Data not available.

[1] The race groups, white and black, include persons of Hispanic and non-Hispanic origin. Conversely, persons of Hispanic origin may be of any race.
[2] Data for Mexicans are for 1982–84. See Appendix I.
[3] See Appendix II for age-adjustment procedure.
[4] Excludes pregnant women.

NOTES: A person with hypertension is defined by either having elevated blood pressure (systolic pressure of at least 140 mmHg or diastolic pressure of at least 90 mmHg) or taking antihypertensive medication. Percents are based on a single measurement of blood pressure to provide comparable data across the 4 time periods. In 1976–80, 31.3 percent of persons 20–74 years of age had hypertension, based on the average of 3 blood pressure measurements, in contrast to 39.7 percent when a single measurement is used.

SOURCE: Centers for Disease Control and Prevention, National Center for Health Statistics, Division of Health Examination Statistics. Unpublished data.

Table 69. Serum cholesterol levels among persons 20 years of age and over, according to sex, age, race, and Hispanic origin: United States, 1960–62, 1971–74, 1976–80, and 1988–94

[Data are based on physical examinations of a sample of the civilian noninstitutionalized population]

Sex, age, race, and Hispanic origin[1]	Percent of population with high serum cholesterol				Mean serum cholesterol level, mg/dL			
	1960–62	1971–74	1976–80[2]	1988–94	1960–62	1971–74	1976–80[2]	1988–94
20–74 years, age adjusted[3]								
Both sexes	31.8	27.2	26.3	18.9	220	214	213	203
Male	28.7	25.8	24.6	17.5	217	213	211	202
Female	34.5	28.2	27.6	20.0	222	215	214	204
White male	29.4	25.9	24.6	17.8	218	213	211	202
White female	35.1	28.1	28.0	20.2	223	215	214	205
Black male	24.5	25.1	24.1	15.7	210	212	208	199
Black female	30.7	29.2	24.9	19.4	216	217	213	203
White, non-Hispanic male	- - -	- - -	24.7	17.3	- - -	- - -	211	202
White, non-Hispanic female	- - -	- - -	28.3	20.2	- - -	- - -	214	205
Black, non-Hispanic male	- - -	- - -	24.0	15.7	- - -	- - -	208	200
Black, non-Hispanic female	- - -	- - -	24.9	19.8	- - -	- - -	214	203
Mexican male	- - -	- - -	18.8	17.8	- - -	- - -	207	204
Mexican female	- - -	- - -	20.0	17.5	- - -	- - -	207	203
20–74 years, crude								
Both sexes	33.6	28.2	26.8	18.7	222	216	213	203
Male	30.7	26.8	24.9	17.6	220	214	211	202
Female	36.3	29.6	28.5	19.9	225	217	215	204
White male	31.4	26.9	25.0	18.1	221	215	211	203
White female	37.5	29.8	29.2	20.5	227	217	216	205
Black male	26.7	25.1	23.9	14.4	214	212	208	198
Black female	29.9	28.8	23.7	16.8	216	216	212	199
White, non-Hispanic male	- - -	- - -	25.1	17.9	- - -	- - -	211	203
White, non-Hispanic female	- - -	- - -	29.8	20.9	- - -	- - -	216	206
Black, non-Hispanic male	- - -	- - -	23.7	14.5	- - -	- - -	208	198
Black, non-Hispanic female	- - -	- - -	23.7	17.2	- - -	- - -	212	200
Mexican male	- - -	- - -	16.6	15.5	- - -	- - -	203	200
Mexican female	- - -	- - -	16.5	14.0	- - -	- - -	202	197
Male								
20–34 years	15.1	12.4	11.9	8.2	198	194	192	186
35–44 years	33.9	31.8	27.9	19.4	227	221	217	206
45–54 years	39.2	37.5	36.9	26.6	231	229	227	216
55–64 years	41.6	36.2	36.8	28.0	233	229	229	216
65–74 years	38.0	34.7	31.7	21.9	230	226	221	212
75 years and over	- - -	- - -	- - -	20.4	- - -	- - -	- - -	205
Female								
20–34 years	12.4	10.9	9.8	7.3	194	191	189	184
35–44 years	23.1	19.3	20.7	12.3	214	207	207	195
45–54 years	46.9	38.7	40.5	26.7	237	232	232	217
55–64 years	70.1	53.1	52.9	40.9	262	245	249	235
65–74 years	68.5	57.7	51.6	41.3	266	250	246	233
75 years and over	- - -	- - -	- - -	38.2	- - -	- - -	- - -	229

- - - Data not available.

[1] The race groups, white and black, include persons of Hispanic and non-Hispanic origin. Conversely, persons of Hispanic origin may be of any race.
[2] Data for Mexicans are for 1982–84. See Appendix I.
[3] See Appendix II for age-adjustment procedure.

NOTES: High serum cholesterol is defined as greater than or equal to 240 mg/dL (6.20 mmol/L). Risk levels have been defined by the Second report of the National Cholesterol Education Program Expert Panel on Detection, Evaluation and Treatment of High Blood Cholesterol in Adults. National Heart, Lung, and Blood Institute, National Institutes of Health. September 1993. (Summarized in *JAMA* 269 (23): 3015–23. June 16, 1993.)

SOURCE: Centers for Disease Control and Prevention, National Center for Health Statistics, Division of Health Examination Statistics. Unpublished data.

Table 70. Healthy weight, overweight, and obesity among persons 20 years of age and over, according to sex, age, race, and Hispanic origin: United States, 1960–62, 1971–74, 1976–80, and 1988–94

[Data are based on measured height and weight of a sample of the civilian noninstitutionalized population]

Sex, age, race, and Hispanic origin[1]	Healthy weight[2]				Overweight[3]				Obesity[4]			
	1960–62	1971–74	1976–80[5]	1988–94	1960–62	1971–74	1976–80[5]	1988–94	1960–62	1971–74	1976–80[5]	1988–94
20–74 years, age adjusted[6]					Percent of population							
Both sexes[7,8]	50.1	48.2	49.1	41.7	43.5	46.0	46.0	54.6	12.8	14.1	14.5	22.6
Male	48.1	44.0	46.0	39.1	48.4	52.7	51.3	59.4	10.4	11.8	12.2	19.9
Female[7]	52.1	52.2	52.1	44.3	38.6	39.7	40.8	49.9	14.9	16.1	16.5	25.1
White male	47.3	43.5	45.2	38.0	49.1	53.4	52.3	60.5	10.1	11.5	12.0	20.3
White female[7]	54.5	54.3	54.3	46.2	36.1	37.6	38.3	48.0	13.6	14.7	14.9	23.5
Black male	53.6	47.4	48.4	40.2	42.7	49.1	48.4	57.0	13.6	15.9	15.1	20.9
Black female[7]	34.3	34.4	34.0	28.9	56.9	57.6	60.6	66.6	24.8	28.6	30.2	37.6
White, non-Hispanic male	- - -	- - -	45.5	38.7	- - -	- - -	52.0	59.9	- - -	- - -	11.9	20.1
White, non-Hispanic female[7] . .	- - -	- - -	54.9	48.0	- - -	- - -	37.6	45.7	- - -	- - -	14.8	22.5
Black, non-Hispanic male	- - -	- - -	48.5	40.0	- - -	- - -	48.3	57.2	- - -	- - -	15.0	21.1
Black, non-Hispanic female[7] . . .	- - -	- - -	34.4	29.2	- - -	- - -	60.2	66.8	- - -	- - -	29.9	37.7
Mexican male	- - -	- - -	38.3	31.6	- - -	- - -	59.6	67.0	- - -	- - -	15.5	23.1
Mexican female[7]	- - -	- - -	37.0	29.8	- - -	- - -	60.1	67.8	- - -	- - -	25.4	34.6
20–74 years, crude												
Both sexes[7,8]	49.0	47.5	48.7	41.4	45.2	47.0	46.4	55.0	13.5	14.4	14.7	22.7
Male	47.1	43.3	45.8	38.8	49.4	53.5	51.5	59.6	10.7	12.0	12.3	19.9
Female[7]	50.7	51.3	51.5	43.9	41.2	41.0	41.6	50.5	16.1	16.7	16.8	25.5
White male	46.3	42.6	45.0	37.5	50.2	54.3	52.5	61.1	10.4	11.7	12.1	20.4
White female[7]	53.0	53.3	53.6	45.4	38.9	39.1	39.4	49.0	14.7	15.4	15.3	24.0
Black male	53.0	47.3	48.3	40.6	43.9	49.3	48.5	56.7	14.1	16.0	15.0	20.9
Black female[7]	33.2	34.2	34.5	29.7	58.8	58.2	60.0	65.9	26.6	28.7	29.8	37.0
White, non-Hispanic male	- - -	- - -	45.3	37.9	- - -	- - -	52.2	60.8	- - -	- - -	12.0	20.3
White, non-Hispanic female[7] . .	- - -	- - -	54.0	46.9	- - -	- - -	38.9	47.1	- - -	- - -	15.2	23.1
Black, non-Hispanic male	- - -	- - -	48.4	40.4	- - -	- - -	48.4	57.0	- - -	- - -	14.9	21.1
Black, non-Hispanic female[7] . . .	- - -	- - -	35.0	29.9	- - -	- - -	59.4	66.2	- - -	- - -	29.5	37.2
Mexican male	- - -	- - -	41.0	34.4	- - -	- - -	57.0	64.0	- - -	- - -	14.6	20.7
Mexican female[7]	- - -	- - -	39.4	31.2	- - -	- - -	57.4	66.2	- - -	- - -	23.8	33.6
Male												
20–34 years	54.2	53.9	55.7	50.3	42.7	42.8	41.2	47.5	9.2	9.7	8.9	14.1
35–44 years	44.1	34.5	40.5	33.3	53.5	63.2	57.2	65.5	12.1	13.5	13.5	21.5
45–54 years	43.9	36.7	37.9	33.5	53.9	59.7	60.2	66.1	12.5	13.7	16.7	23.2
55–64 years	43.5	38.1	37.9	28.1	52.2	58.5	60.2	70.5	9.2	14.1	14.1	27.2
65–74 years	44.0	41.4	41.1	29.8	47.8	54.6	54.2	68.5	10.4	10.9	13.2	24.1
75 years and over	- - -	- - -	- - -	40.6	- - -	- - -	- - -	56.5	- - -	- - -	- - -	13.2
Female[7]												
20–34 years	62.6	61.7	61.0	54.3	21.2	25.8	27.9	37.0	7.2	9.7	11.0	18.5
35–44 years	56.2	53.5	53.4	45.5	37.2	40.5	40.7	49.6	14.7	17.7	17.8	25.5
45–54 years	46.1	47.7	47.2	35.6	49.3	49.0	48.7	60.3	20.3	18.9	19.6	32.4
55–64 years	37.2	39.2	42.7	31.2	59.9	54.5	53.7	66.3	24.4	24.1	22.9	33.7
65–74 years	35.5	39.6	36.5	36.0	60.9	55.9	59.5	60.3	23.2	22.0	21.5	26.9
75 years and over	- - -	- - -	- - -	41.0	- - -	- - -	- - -	52.3	- - -	- - -	- - -	19.2

- - - Data not available.

[1] The race groups, white and black, include persons of Hispanic and non-Hispanic origin.

[2] Body mass index (BMI) of 19 to less than 25 kilograms/meter[2] (see Appendix II, Body mass index).

[3] BMI greater than or equal to 25.

[4] BMI greater than or equal to 30.

[5] Data for Mexicans are for 1982–84. See Appendix I.

[6] See Appendix II for age-adjustment procedure.

[7] Excludes pregnant women.

[8] Includes persons of all races and Hispanic origins, not just those shown separately.

NOTES: Percents do not sum to 100 because the percent of persons with BMI less than 19 is not shown and the percent of persons with obesity is a subset of the percent with overweight. Height was measured without shoes; two pounds are deducted from data for 1960–62 to allow for weight of clothing.

SOURCE: Centers for Disease Control and Prevention, National Center for Health Statistics, Division of Health Examination Statistics. Unpublished data.

Table 71. Overweight children and adolescents 6–17 years of age, according to sex, age, race, and Hispanic origin: United States, selected years 1963–65 through 1988–94

[Data are based on physical examinations of a sample of the civilian noninstitutionalized population]

Age, sex, race, and Hispanic origin[1]	1963–65 1966–70[2]	1971–74	1976–80[3]	1988–94[4]
6–11 years of age, age adjusted		Percent of population		
Both sexes	5.0	5.5	7.6	13.6
Boys	4.9	6.5	8.1	14.7
White	5.4	6.6	8.1	14.6
Black	1.7	5.6	8.6	15.1
White, non-Hispanic	- - -	- - -	7.4	13.1
Black, non-Hispanic	- - -	- - -	8.6	14.7
Mexican	- - -	- - -	14.5	18.8
Girls	5.2	4.4	7.1	12.6
White	5.1	4.4	6.5	11.7
Black	5.3	4.5	11.5	17.4
White, non-Hispanic	- - -	- - -	6.2	11.9
Black, non-Hispanic	- - -	- - -	11.6	17.7
Mexican	- - -	- - -	10.7	15.8
12–17 years of age, age adjusted				
Both sexes	5.0	6.2	5.6	11.4
Boys	5.0	5.3	5.3	12.4
White	5.2	5.5	5.3	13.1
Black	3.6	4.4	6.0	12.1
White, non-Hispanic	- - -	- - -	4.5	11.8
Black, non-Hispanic	- - -	- - -	6.1	12.5
Mexican	- - -	- - -	7.7	14.8
Girls[5]	5.0	7.2	6.0	10.5
White	4.8	6.6	5.4	10.0
Black	6.4	10.5	10.2	16.1
White, non-Hispanic	- - -	- - -	5.4	9.3
Black, non-Hispanic	- - -	- - -	10.5	16.0
Mexican	- - -	- - -	9.3	14.1
Boys				
6–8 years	5.1	6.3	8.1	15.4
9–11 years	4.8	6.7	8.1	14.0
12–14 years	5.2	5.4	5.4	11.5
15–17 years	4.8	5.2	5.1	13.1
Girls[5]				
6–8 years	5.1	4.1	7.1	14.6
9–11 years	5.2	4.7	7.1	10.8
12–14 years	5.0	8.6	7.8	13.9
15–17 years	4.9	6.0	4.5	7.5

- - - Data not available.

[1]The race groups, white and black, include persons of Hispanic and non-Hispanic origin. Conversely, persons of Hispanic origin may be of any race.
[2]Data for children 6–11 years of age are for 1963–65; data for adolescents 12–17 years of age are for 1966–70.
[3]Data for Mexicans are for 1982–84. See Appendix I.
[4]Excludes one non-Hispanic white adolescent boy age 12–14 years with an outlier sample weight.
[5]Excludes pregnant women starting with 1971–74. Pregnancy status not available for 1963–65/1966–70.

NOTES: Overweight is defined as body mass index (BMI) at or above the sex- and age-specific 95th percentile BMI cutoff points calculated at 6-month age intervals for children 6–11 years of age from the 1963–65 National Health Examination Survey (NHES) and for adolescents 12–17 years of age from the 1966–70 NHES. Age is at time of examination at mobile examination center. Some data for 1988–94 have been revised and differ from the previous edition of Health, United States. See Appendix II for age-adjustment procedure.

SOURCE: Centers for Disease Control and Prevention, National Center for Health Statistics, Division of Health Examination Statistics. Unpublished data.

Table 72. Untreated dental caries among children 2–17 years of age according to age, sex, race and Hispanic origin, and poverty status: United States, 1971–74, 1982–84, and 1988–94

[Data are based on dental examinations of a sample of the civilian noninstitutionalized population]

Sex, race and Hispanic origin[1], and poverty status	2–5 years			6–17 years		
	1971–74	1982–84	1988–94	1971–74	1982–84	1988–94
	Percent of children with at least one untreated dental caries					
Total[2]	24.4	- - -	18.7	55.0	- - -	23.1
Sex						
Male	26.1	- - -	19.2	54.8	- - -	22.6
Female	22.7	- - -	18.1	55.2	- - -	23.7
Race and Hispanic origin[3]						
White, non-Hispanic	23.7	- - -	14.4	52.3	- - -	18.9
Black, non-Hispanic	28.2	- - -	25.1	70.9	- - -	33.0
Mexican	- - -	23.1	34.9	- - -	42.8	37.2
Poverty status[4,5]						
Poor	30.7	- - -	28.8	70.4	- - -	36.3
Near poor	29.8	- - -	24.3	60.2	- - -	29.2
Nonpoor	17.5	- - -	9.7	46.3	- - -	14.5
Race, Hispanic origin, and poverty status[3,4,5]						
White, non-Hispanic:						
Below poverty	31.9	- - -	25.4	68.1	- - -	32.5
At or above poverty	22.1	- - -	12.4	50.3	- - -	16.7
Black, non-Hispanic:						
Below poverty	29.0	- - -	27.5	73.4	- - -	35.6
At or above poverty	26.5	- - -	23.0	67.4	- - -	31.2
Mexican:						
Below poverty	- - -	22.6	38.5	- - -	46.4	45.8
At or above poverty	- - -	22.0	30.5	- - -	39.3	27.6

- - - Data not available.

[1]Persons of Hispanic origin may be of any race.

[2]Includes all other races not shown separately and unknown family income.

[3]In 1971–74, data are for white children and black children.

[4]Poverty status is based on family income and family size. Poor children are defined as in families whose incomes are below the poverty threshold. Near poor children are in families whose incomes are 100 percent to less than 200 percent of poverty threshold. Nonpoor children are in families whose incomes are 200 percent or greater than the poverty threshold. See Appendix II, Poverty level.

[5]Data for children with unknown poverty status are not included in the analysis. In 1971–74, 2–3 percent of white children and black children; in 1982–84, 7–10 percent of Mexican children; and in 1988–94, 4 percent of non-Hispanic white children, 8 percent of non-Hispanic black children, and 12 percent of Mexican children have unknown poverty status.

NOTE: Age is at time of dental examination at mobile examination center.

SOURCES: Centers for Disease Control and Prevention, National Center for Health Statistics: data computed by the Division of Epidemiology from data compiled by the Division of Health Examination Statistics. Unpublished data.

Table 73. Persons residing in counties that met national ambient air quality standards throughout the year, by race and Hispanic origin: United States, 1988–96

[Data are based on air quality measurements in counties with monitoring devices]

Type of pollutant, race, and Hispanic origin	1988	1989	1990	1991	1992	1993	1994	1995	1996
All pollutants				Percent of population					
All persons	49.7	65.3	71.0	65.2	78.4	76.5	75.1	67.9	81.3
White	---	---	71.8	66.0	79.1	76.9	76.4	69.7	81.9
Black	---	---	71.5	63.4	76.5	75.2	70.4	59.4	80.8
American Indian or Alaska Native	---	---	76.8	75.2	83.0	82.4	80.0	77.9	83.2
Asian or Pacific Islander	---	---	49.6	46.7	64.4	62.8	55.6	48.2	64.4
Hispanic	---	---	49.3	45.2	56.8	57.7	54.8	44.5	56.3
Ozone									
All persons	53.6	72.6	76.3	71.9	81.9	79.5	79.9	71.6	83.3
White	---	---	76.9	72.7	82.7	79.9	80.0	73.0	83.9
Black	---	---	77.0	69.7	79.8	79.3	75.4	66.1	82.9
American Indian or Alaska Native	---	---	83.0	84.8	88.4	85.5	84.3	81.2	99.9
Asian or Pacific Islander	---	---	58.0	55.2	67.0	64.5	58.5	51.4	65.6
Hispanic	---	---	57.1	53.4	61.2	60.2	58.3	48.5	59.7
Carbon monoxide									
All persons	87.8	86.2	90.8	92.0	94.3	95.4	93.9	95.2	94.9
White	---	---	91.0	92.3	94.4	95.6	94.3	96.4	95.1
Black	---	---	93.4	93.5	95.5	96.0	92.6	96.1	96.0
American Indian or Alaska Native	---	---	88.7	89.9	92.9	95.1	93.2	94.2	93.8
Asian or Pacific Islander	---	---	73.7	78.0	84.7	85.8	84.6	85.9	85.5
Hispanic	---	---	72.5	75.6	79.8	82.2	81.4	82.6	80.9
Particulates (PM–10)[1]									
All persons	89.4	88.8	92.6	91.9	89.6	97.5	94.8	90.2	97.1
White	---	---	92.7	92.1	90.2	97.6	95.6	91.0	97.1
Black	---	---	94.2	93.6	87.9	96.8	94.0	87.1	96.8
American Indian or Alaska Native	---	---	92.4	90.6	89.9	97.4	96.2	90.4	96.8
Asian or Pacific Islander	---	---	82.7	80.8	79.3	98.5	93.2	80.7	96.9
Hispanic	---	---	76.1	76.3	71.3	97.4	91.0	75.2	92.7
Sulfur dioxide									
All persons	99.3	99.9	99.4	97.9	100.0	99.4	100.0	100.0	99.9
White	---	---	99.4	98.3	100.0	99.4	100.0	100.0	99.9
Black	---	---	99.5	95.6	100.0	99.5	100.0	100.0	100.0
American Indian or Alaska Native	---	---	99.8	99.4	100.0	100.0	100.0	100.0	100.0
Asian or Pacific Islander	---	---	99.8	97.4	100.0	99.8	100.0	100.0	100.0
Hispanic	---	---	99.9	96.9	100.0	100.0	100.0	100.0	100.0
Nitrogen dioxide									
All persons	96.6	96.5	96.4	96.4	100.0	100.0	100.0	100.0	100.0
White	---	---	96.8	96.8	100.0	100.0	100.0	100.0	100.0
Black	---	---	96.6	96.6	100.0	100.0	100.0	100.0	100.0
American Indian or Alaska Native	---	---	97.2	97.2	100.0	100.0	100.0	100.0	100.0
Asian or Pacific Islander	---	---	86.7	86.7	100.0	100.0	100.0	100.0	100.0
Hispanic	---	---	85.0	85.0	100.0	100.0	100.0	100.0	100.0
Lead									
All persons	99.3	99.4	94.1	94.1	98.1	97.8	98.3	98.1	98.3
White	---	---	94.9	94.8	98.5	98.2	98.7	98.3	98.6
Black	---	---	91.5	91.1	95.3	94.8	95.9	96.2	96.1
American Indian or Alaska Native	---	---	96.4	96.4	99.4	99.3	99.4	99.3	99.4
Asian or Pacific Islander	---	---	85.5	85.5	99.0	98.9	99.1	98.9	99.1
Hispanic	---	---	83.6	84.0	99.4	99.5	99.5	98.9	99.0

--- Data not available.

[1] Particulate matter smaller than 10 microns.

NOTES: The race groups, white, black, American Indian or Alaska Native, and Asian or Pacific Islander, include persons of Hispanic and non-Hispanic origin. Conversely, persons of Hispanic origin may be of any race. Standard is met if the concentration of the pollutant does not exceed the criterion value more than once per calendar year. See Appendix II, National ambient air quality standards. 1988–89 data based on 1987 county population estimates; 1990–96 data based on 1990 county population estimates.

SOURCES: U.S. Environmental Protection Agency, Aerometric Information Retrieval System; data computed by the National Center for Health Statistics, Division of Health Promotion Statistics from data compiled by the U.S. Environmental Protection Agency, Office of Air Quality and Standards.

Table 74. Occupational injuries with lost workdays in the private sector, according to industry: United States, selected years 1980–97

[Data are based on employer records from a sample of business establishments]

Industry	1980	1985	1989	1990	1991	1992	1993	1994	1995	1996	1997
	Number of injuries with lost workdays in thousands										
Total private sector[1]	2,491.0	2,484.7	2,955.5	2,987.3	2,794.0	2,776.1	2,772.5	2,848.3	2,767.6	2,646.3	2,682.6
Agriculture, fishing, and forestry[1]	39.3	45.2	52.2	57.2	54.3	52.3	51.2	48.5	51.7	49.0	53.8
Mining	66.2	43.9	33.9	35.6	31.4	25.6	24.2	24.0	22.8	19.5	22.6
Construction	242.6	272.8	301.2	296.3	239.9	226.8	226.5	241.7	217.9	216.8	227.4
Manufacturing	1,009.5	825.1	1,007.4	975.0	886.0	833.7	819.5	859.4	838.1	782.9	785.4
Transportation, communication, and public utilities	263.0	243.5	273.9	293.3	283.5	266.1	284.1	301.5	289.2	293.0	281.3
Wholesale trade	191.1	188.4	230.3	211.5	204.1	205.3	205.3	214.0	214.7	203.9	200.7
Retail trade	330.2	399.9	480.6	483.9	457.0	476.7	480.4	477.7	459.6	433.9	456.9
Finance, insurance, and real estate	38.1	45.5	52.6	63.7	62.2	64.4	61.7	58.8	52.2	49.5	47.6
Services	311.1	420.6	523.4	570.8	575.6	625.1	619.6	622.8	621.4	597.8	606.9
	Injuries with lost workdays per 100 full-time equivalents[2]										
Total private sector[1]	3.9	3.6	3.9	3.9	3.7	3.6	3.5	3.5	3.4	3.1	3.1
Agriculture, fishing, and forestry[1]	5.6	5.6	5.6	5.7	5.2	5.2	4.8	4.6	4.2	3.8	4.0
Mining	6.4	4.7	4.8	4.9	4.4	4.0	3.8	3.8	3.8	3.2	3.7
Construction	6.5	6.8	6.7	6.6	6.0	5.7	5.4	5.4	4.8	4.4	4.4
Manufacturing	5.2	4.4	5.3	5.3	5.0	4.7	4.6	4.7	4.6	4.3	4.2
Transportation, communication, and public utilities	5.4	4.9	5.2	5.4	5.3	4.9	5.2	5.3	5.0	5.0	4.7
Wholesale trade	3.8	3.5	3.9	3.6	3.6	3.6	3.6	3.6	3.5	3.3	3.1
Retail trade	2.9	3.1	3.4	3.4	3.3	3.3	3.2	3.2	2.9	2.7	2.8
Finance, insurance, and real estate	0.8	0.9	0.9	1.1	1.0	1.1	1.0	0.9	0.9	0.8	0.8
Services	2.3	2.5	2.6	2.7	2.8	2.9	2.7	2.7	2.7	2.5	2.4

[1]Excludes farms with fewer than 11 employees.
[2]Incidence rate calculated as (N/EH) x 200,000, where N = total number of injuries with lost workdays in a calendar year, EH = total hours worked by all full-time and part-time employees in a calendar year, and 200,000 = base for 100 full-time equivalent employees working 40 hours per week, 50 weeks per year.

NOTES: Industry is coded based on various editions of the *Standard Industrial Classification Manual* as follows: data for 1980–87 are based on the 1972 edition, 1977 supplement; and data for 1988–97 are based on the 1987 edition (see Appendix II, Industry). Data for additional years are available (see Appendix III).

SOURCE: U.S. Department of Labor, Bureau of Labor Statistics. Workplace injuries and illnesses, 1980–97 editions. 1982–98.

Table 75. Physician contacts, according to selected patient characteristics: United States, 1987–96

[Data are based on household interviews of a sample of the civilian noninstitutionalized population]

Characteristic	1987	1988	1989	1990	1991	1992	1993	1994	1995	1996
					Physician contacts per person					
Total[1,2]	5.4	5.3	5.3	5.5	5.6	5.9	6.0	6.0	5.8	5.8
Age										
Under 15 years	4.5	4.6	4.6	4.5	4.7	4.6	4.9	4.6	4.5	4.4
Under 5 years	6.7	7.0	6.7	6.9	7.1	6.9	7.2	6.8	6.5	6.5
5–14 years	3.3	3.3	3.5	3.2	3.4	3.4	3.6	3.4	3.4	3.3
15–44 years	4.6	4.7	4.6	4.8	4.7	5.0	5.0	5.0	4.8	4.6
45–64 years	6.4	6.1	6.1	6.4	6.6	7.2	7.1	7.3	7.1	7.2
65 years and over	8.9	8.7	8.9	9.2	10.4	10.6	10.9	11.3	11.1	11.7
65–74 years	8.4	8.4	8.2	8.5	9.2	9.7	9.9	10.3	9.8	10.2
75 years and over	9.7	9.2	9.9	10.1	12.3	12.1	12.3	12.7	12.9	13.7
Sex and age										
Male[1]	4.6	4.6	4.8	4.7	4.9	5.1	5.2	5.2	4.9	5.0
Under 5 years	6.7	7.3	7.5	7.2	7.6	7.1	7.5	7.0	6.8	7.1
5–14 years	3.4	3.4	3.7	3.3	3.5	3.5	3.8	3.5	3.6	3.6
15–44 years	3.3	3.3	3.4	3.4	3.4	3.7	3.6	3.7	3.3	3.2
45–64 years	5.5	5.2	5.2	5.6	5.8	6.1	6.1	6.3	6.0	6.0
65–74 years	8.1	7.9	8.5	8.0	8.6	9.2	9.3	10.1	9.5	9.4
75 years and over	9.2	9.6	9.9	10.0	11.6	12.2	11.7	11.6	11.9	13.5
Female[1]	6.0	6.0	5.9	6.1	6.3	6.6	6.7	6.7	6.5	6.5
Under 5 years	6.7	6.8	5.9	6.5	6.6	6.7	6.9	6.5	6.3	5.9
5–14 years	3.1	3.3	3.3	3.2	3.2	3.3	3.4	3.3	3.1	3.0
15–44 years	5.8	6.0	5.9	6.0	5.9	6.2	6.4	6.2	6.2	6.0
45–64 years	7.2	6.9	7.0	7.1	7.4	8.2	8.1	8.3	8.1	8.4
65–74 years	8.6	8.8	7.9	9.0	9.7	10.1	10.4	10.5	10.1	10.9
75 years and over	10.0	9.0	9.9	10.2	12.7	12.1	12.8	13.4	13.5	13.7
Race and age										
White[1]	5.5	5.5	5.5	5.6	5.8	6.0	6.0	6.1	5.9	5.8
Under 5 years	7.1	7.6	7.1	7.1	7.4	7.3	7.5	7.1	6.7	6.6
5–14 years	3.5	3.6	3.8	3.5	3.7	3.7	3.9	3.7	3.6	3.5
15–44 years	4.7	4.8	4.8	4.9	4.9	5.0	5.1	5.1	4.9	4.7
45–64 years	6.4	6.1	6.2	6.4	6.6	7.2	7.0	7.4	7.0	7.2
65–74 years	8.4	8.3	8.0	8.5	9.4	9.6	9.7	10.5	9.9	10.2
75 years and over	9.7	9.3	9.7	10.1	12.1	12.0	12.2	12.4	13.1	13.2
Black[1]	5.1	4.8	4.9	5.1	5.2	5.9	6.0	5.7	5.5	5.7
Under 5 years	5.1	4.6	5.3	5.6	6.0	5.6	6.2	5.2	5.8	5.6
5–14 years	2.3	2.2	2.3	2.2	2.1	2.3	2.4	2.5	2.5	2.7
15–44 years	4.2	4.2	3.9	4.2	4.0	5.3	4.7	4.8	4.3	4.5
45–64 years	7.3	6.6	6.3	7.1	7.5	7.8	8.7	7.7	8.0	7.3
65–74 years	8.6	9.1	10.0	9.2	7.3	10.9	11.5	9.3	9.9	10.2
75 years and over	10.8	8.7	12.7	10.4	15.7	13.7	13.1	16.3	11.5	19.8
Family income[1,3]										
Less than $16,000	6.8	6.2	6.3	6.3	6.8	7.3	7.3	7.6	7.4	7.5
$16,000–$24,999	5.6	5.3	5.2	5.6	5.6	6.0	5.7	5.9	6.1	5.5
$25,000–$34,999	5.2	5.0	5.5	5.2	5.5	5.7	6.0	5.8	5.3	5.6
$35,000–$49,999	5.2	5.5	5.2	5.7	5.8	5.9	6.0	6.2	5.7	5.9
$50,000 or more	5.4	5.5	6.0	5.6	5.8	5.8	5.8	6.0	5.6	5.3
Geographic region[1]										
Northeast	5.2	5.0	5.3	5.2	5.4	5.9	5.9	5.9	5.6	5.7
Midwest	5.6	5.4	5.4	5.3	5.8	5.9	6.2	6.0	5.8	5.7
South	5.1	5.2	5.3	5.6	5.5	5.8	5.7	5.6	5.8	6.1
West	5.5	5.9	5.5	5.6	5.9	6.1	6.0	6.4	5.8	5.3
Location of residence[1]										
Within MSA[4]	5.5	5.5	5.4	5.6	5.8	6.0	6.1	6.0	5.9	5.8
Outside MSA[4]	4.8	4.9	5.2	4.9	5.1	5.6	5.6	5.7	5.3	5.7

[1]Age adjusted. See Appendix II for age-adjustment procedure.
[2]Includes all other races not shown separately and unknown family income.
[3]Family income categories for 1996. In 1995 the two lowest income categories are less than $15,000 and $15,000–$24,999; the three higher income categories are as shown. In 1989–94 the two lowest income categories are less than $14,000 and $14,000–$24,999; the three higher income categories are as shown. Income categories for 1988 are less than $13,000; $13,000–$18,999; $19,000–$24,999; $25,000–$44,999; and $45,000 or more. Income categories for 1987 are less than $10,000; $10,000–$14,999; $15,000–$19,999; $20,000–$34,999; and $35,000 or more.
[4]Metropolitan statistical area.

NOTE: Data for additional years are available (see Appendix III).

SOURCE: Centers for Disease Control and Prevention, National Center for Health Statistics, Division of Health Interview Statistics. Data from the National Health Interview Survey.

Table 76. Physician contacts, according to place of contact and selected patient characteristics: United States, 1990 and 1996

[Data are based on household interviews of a sample of the civilian noninstitutionalized population]

Characteristic	Total	Doctor's office 1990	Doctor's office 1996	Hospital outpatient department[1] 1990	Hospital outpatient department[1] 1996	Telephone 1990	Telephone 1996	Home 1990	Home 1996	Other[2] 1990	Other[2] 1996
					Percent distribution						
Total[3,4]	100.0	59.9	55.7	13.7	12.3	12.7	13.1	2.1	3.3	11.6	15.6
Age											
Under 15 years	100.0	60.7	57.4	13.6	11.1	14.9	14.6	0.9	2.4	9.9	14.5
Under 5 years	100.0	59.1	57.0	14.0	11.3	15.9	14.7	*1.1	*2.3	9.8	14.7
5–14 years.............	100.0	62.6	57.8	13.1	11.0	13.7	14.4	*0.6	*2.6	10.0	14.2
15–44 years	100.0	59.4	56.6	14.3	12.9	12.0	13.2	0.6	*0.6	13.7	16.7
45–64 years	100.0	60.4	54.6	14.1	13.7	12.2	12.3	2.0	2.7	11.4	16.7
65 years and over	100.0	58.7	49.4	11.1	10.1	9.9	9.5	11.8	19.2	8.4	11.9
65–74 years.............	100.0	60.2	54.7	13.7	9.8	9.7	10.9	7.0	9.9	9.4	14.7
75 years and over.............	100.0	56.8	43.9	7.8	10.5	10.2	8.0	18.1	28.8	7.0	8.9
Sex[3]											
Male.............	100.0	57.6	54.7	16.1	13.9	11.3	12.1	2.1	3.8	12.9	15.4
Female	100.0	61.6	56.5	12.2	11.2	13.4	13.6	2.0	2.9	10.9	15.9
Race[3]											
White	100.0	61.7	57.2	12.3	11.3	13.1	13.9	1.9	2.9	11.0	14.8
Black	100.0	48.2	48.7	24.3	18.9	9.1	8.3	2.8	5.0	15.6	19.1
Family income[3,5]											
Less than $16,000	100.0	48.9	45.8	19.9	16.5	11.5	11.0	3.2	5.7	16.4	20.9
$16,000–$24,999	100.0	56.9	50.3	16.0	15.3	11.8	12.1	1.7	2.1	13.5	20.2
$25,000–$34,999.............	100.0	60.9	56.0	13.8	12.9	13.2	14.3	1.6	2.4	10.4	14.4
$35,000–$49,999	100.0	62.0	60.3	11.5	10.7	14.6	13.7	1.1	3.1	10.9	12.1
$50,000 or more	100.0	66.1	61.5	8.9	8.9	14.1	15.2	1.5	2.1	9.5	12.3
Geographic region[3]											
Northeast	100.0	62.6	61.1	13.0	11.9	11.7	13.8	1.9	2.4	10.8	10.9
Midwest	100.0	55.8	50.2	14.7	12.4	15.4	16.2	1.9	4.1	12.3	17.1
South	100.0	61.1	56.6	13.6	12.9	11.3	11.6	2.6	3.7	11.3	15.1
West.............	100.0	60.4	55.8	13.6	11.8	12.8	10.8	1.4	2.1	12.0	19.5
Location of residence[3]											
Within MSA[6]	100.0	59.6	56.2	13.7	11.9	13.1	13.3	1.9	3.3	11.7	15.4
Outside MSA[6]	100.0	61.4	54.1	14.1	13.8	10.7	12.4	2.6	3.2	11.2	16.5

* Relative standard error greater than 30 percent.
[1]Includes hospital outpatient clinic, emergency room, and other hospital contacts.
[2]Includes clinics or other places outside a hospital.
[3]Age adjusted. See Appendix II for age-adjustment procedure.
[4]Includes all other races not shown separately and unknown family income.
[5]Family income categories for 1996. In 1990 the two lowest income categories are less than $14,000 and $14,000–$24,999; the three higher income categories are as shown.
[6]Metropolitan statistical area.

SOURCE: Centers for Disease Control and Prevention, National Center for Health Statistics, Division of Health Interview Statistics. Data from the National Health Interview Survey.

Table 77. Physician contacts, according to respondent-assessed health status, age, sex, and poverty status: United States, average annual 1987–89 and 1994–96

[Data are based on household interviews of a sample of the civilian noninstitutionalized population]

| Age, sex, and poverty status[1] | Respondent-assessed health status | | | | | |
| | All | | Good to excellent | | Fair or poor | |
	1987–89	1994–96	1987–89	1994–96	1987–89	1994–96
Total[2]	Physician contacts per person per ···					
Male:						
Poor	5.2	6.1	3.4	4.1	11.1	14.7
Near poor	4.9	5.3	3.7	3.6	13.4	14.3
Nonpoor	4.8	5.1	4.2	4.5	16.8	16.2
Female:						
Poor	7.0	8.1	4.7	5.4	13.6	15.9
Near poor	5.9	6.7	4.6	4.9	14.9	17.4
Nonpoor	6.2	6.6	5.6	5.7	19.4	21.9
Under 15 years						
Poor	4.0	4.5	3.6	3.9	10.8	14.9
Near poor	4.2	4.1	3.8	3.8	15.2	15.4
Nonpoor	5.3	4.9	5.0	4.7	22.6	19.7
15–44 years						
Male:						
Poor	3.6	4.3	2.8	2.9	9.8	13.5
Near poor	3.5	3.4	2.9	2.6	11.7	13.2
Nonpoor	3.4	3.4	3.1	3.1	14.0	13.6
Female:						
Poor	6.4	6.9	5.1	5.2	14.0	15.6
Near poor	5.6	5.9	4.7	4.9	16.0	15.5
Nonpoor	6.1	6.4	5.6	5.8	20.4	23.5
45–64 years						
Male:						
Poor	7.5	8.8	3.1	5.2	11.4	12.8
Near poor	6.5	7.5	3.5	3.5	12.8	15.6
Nonpoor	5.1	5.8	4.1	4.7	13.8	15.4
Female:						
Poor	10.9	12.7	4.6	6.4	17.3	18.6
Near poor	7.6	9.2	4.7	5.3	14.5	18.5
Nonpoor	6.8	7.8	5.7	6.3	16.1	21.2
65 years and over						
Male:						
Poor	9.7	11.6	5.5	7.3	13.2	16.2
Near poor	8.9	11.6	6.5	7.4	12.9	18.5
Nonpoor	8.5	10.5	6.5	8.0	15.5	20.5
Female:						
Poor	10.6	15.0	6.5	9.4	16.0	22.8
Near poor	9.2	12.5	6.6	8.2	14.3	22.0
Nonpoor	8.8	11.0	7.1	8.4	14.9	21.7

[1]Poverty status is based on family income and family size using Bureau of the Census poverty thresholds. Poor persons are defined as below the poverty threshold. Near poor persons have incomes of 100 percent to less than 200 percent of poverty threshold. Nonpoor persons have incomes of 200 percent or greater than the poverty threshold. See Appendix II.
[2]Age adjusted. See Appendix II for age-adjustment procedure.

NOTES: Persons with unknown family income or unknown health status were eliminated from the analysis. Persons who reported their health to be good, very good, or excellent were categorized as good to excellent health. See Appendix II. Data for additional years are available (see Appendix III).

SOURCE: Centers for Disease Control and Prevention, National Center for Health Statistics. Data computed by the Division of Health and Utilization Analysis from data compiled by the Division of Health Interview Statistics.

Table 78. Interval since last physician contact, according to selected patient characteristics: United States, 1964, 1990, and 1996

[Data are based on household interviews of a sample of the civilian noninstitutionalized population]

Characteristic	Total	Less than 1 year			1 year–less than 2 years			2 years or more[1]		
		1964	1990	1996	1964	1990	1996	1964	1990	1996
					Percent distribution[2]					
Total[3,4]	100.0	66.9	78.2	80.1	14.0	10.1	9.5	19.1	11.7	10.4
Age										
Under 15 years	100.0	68.4	82.9	85.6	14.8	10.7	9.4	16.7	6.4	5.0
Under 5 years	100.0	80.7	93.6	94.9	11.1	5.0	4.2	8.2	1.4	0.9
5–14 years	100.0	61.7	77.2	81.0	16.9	13.7	12.0	21.4	9.1	7.0
15–44 years	100.0	66.3	73.3	74.2	15.0	11.6	11.6	18.7	15.0	14.2
45–64 years	100.0	64.5	77.3	79.3	13.0	8.6	8.3	22.5	14.1	12.4
65 years and over	100.0	69.7	87.1	90.1	9.3	4.7	4.0	21.0	8.2	5.9
65–74 years	100.0	68.8	85.7	88.3	9.4	5.1	4.5	21.8	9.1	7.1
75 years and over	100.0	71.3	89.3	92.4	9.3	4.1	3.3	19.5	6.6	4.3
Sex and age										
Male[3]	100.0	63.5	73.3	74.9	15.0	11.3	10.8	21.5	15.4	14.3
Under 15 years	100.0	- - -	82.8	85.7	- - -	10.7	9.4	- - -	6.5	4.9
15–44 years	100.0	- - -	64.2	64.9	- - -	13.8	13.8	- - -	22.0	21.3
45–64 years	100.0	- - -	72.4	72.7	- - -	9.8	10.1	- - -	17.8	17.2
65–74 years	100.0	- - -	84.2	87.7	- - -	5.8	4.8	- - -	10.0	7.6
75 years and over	100.0	- - -	86.9	91.8	- - -	4.7	3.5	- - -	8.4	4.7
Female[3]	100.0	69.9	82.9	85.1	13.1	9.0	8.3	17.0	8.1	6.7
Under 15 years	100.0	- - -	83.0	85.5	- - -	10.7	9.4	- - -	6.4	5.1
15–44 years	100.0	- - -	82.1	83.3	- - -	9.5	9.4	- - -	8.3	7.4
45–64 years	100.0	- - -	81.9	85.5	- - -	7.6	6.6	- - -	10.6	7.9
65–74 years	100.0	- - -	86.9	88.9	- - -	4.6	4.4	- - -	8.4	6.8
75 years and over	100.0	- - -	90.7	92.8	- - -	3.7	3.2	- - -	5.6	4.0
Race and age										
White[3]	100.0	68.1	78.7	80.3	13.8	9.9	9.3	18.1	11.5	10.4
Under 15 years	100.0	- - -	83.6	86.0	- - -	10.3	9.0	- - -	6.1	5.0
15–44 years	100.0	- - -	73.9	74.5	- - -	11.4	11.3	- - -	14.8	14.1
45–64 years	100.0	- - -	77.3	79.1	- - -	8.7	8.2	- - -	14.1	12.6
65–74 years	100.0	- - -	86.0	88.1	- - -	5.0	4.6	- - -	9.0	7.3
75 years and over	100.0	- - -	89.3	92.7	- - -	4.2	3.1	- - -	6.5	4.1
Black[3,5]	100.0	58.3	77.5	81.3	15.1	11.0	9.8	26.6	11.6	8.8
Under 15 years	100.0	- - -	79.9	84.9	- - -	12.6	10.8	- - -	7.5	4.3
15–44 years	100.0	- - -	72.3	75.9	- - -	12.7	11.6	- - -	15.0	12.5
45–64 years	100.0	- - -	80.2	82.9	- - -	8.0	7.7	- - -	11.8	9.3
65–74 years	100.0	- - -	84.4	90.2	- - -	5.9	*3.9	- - -	9.7	5.9
75 years and over	100.0	- - -	89.4	89.6	- - -	*3.4	*4.2	- - -	7.3	*6.2
Family income[3,6]										
Less than $16,000	100.0	58.6	77.3	77.6	13.2	9.8	10.1	28.2	12.9	12.2
$16,000–$24,999	100.0	62.5	76.7	75.4	14.2	10.2	10.9	23.3	13.2	13.7
$25,000–$34,999	100.0	66.8	78.7	78.9	14.5	10.0	9.9	18.7	11.4	11.2
$35,000–$49,999	100.0	70.2	80.1	81.0	14.0	9.4	9.3	15.7	10.4	9.7
$50,000 or more	100.0	73.6	81.7	84.3	12.9	8.9	8.2	13.5	9.4	7.5
Geographic region[3]										
Northeast	100.0	68.0	81.6	83.7	14.1	9.1	8.0	17.9	9.3	8.4
Midwest	100.0	66.6	79.5	80.1	14.2	9.6	9.9	19.2	10.9	10.0
South	100.0	65.2	76.0	79.2	13.9	11.3	10.1	20.9	12.7	10.7
West	100.0	69.0	77.5	78.2	13.7	9.4	9.5	17.3	13.1	12.3
Location of residence[3]										
Within MSA[7]	100.0	68.2	79.0	80.4	14.0	9.7	9.4	17.8	11.3	10.2
Outside MSA[7]	100.0	64.0	75.7	78.8	14.1	11.4	10.1	21.9	12.9	11.1

- - - Data not available.
* Relative standard error greater than 30 percent.
[1] Includes persons who never visited a physician.
[2] Denominator excludes persons with unknown interval.
[3] Age adjusted. See Appendix II for age-adjustment procedure.
[4] Includes all other races not shown separately and unknown family income.
[5] 1964 data include all other races.
[6] Family income categories for 1996. In 1990 the two lowest income categories are less than $14,000 and $14,000–$24,999; the three higher income categories are as shown. Income categories in 1964 are less than $2,000; $2,000–$3,999; $4,000–$6,999; $7,000–$9,999; and $10,000 or more.
[7] Metropolitan statistical area.

SOURCE: Centers for Disease Control and Prevention, National Center for Health Statistics, Division of Health Interview Statistics. Data from the National Health Interview Survey.

Table 79. No physician contact within the past 12 months among children under 6 years of age according to selected characteristics: United States, average annual 1993–94 and 1995–96

[Data are based on household interviews of a sample of the civilian noninstitutionalized population]

Characteristic	1993–94	1995–96
	Percent of children without a physician contact within the past 12 months	
All children[1]	8.3	9.2
Race[2]		
White	7.8	8.9
Black	10.1	9.9
American Indian or Alaska Native	12.7	16.4
Asian or Pacific Islander	8.9	11.5
Race and Hispanic origin		
White, non-Hispanic	7.3	8.1
Black, non-Hispanic	10.3	10.0
Hispanic[2]	9.9	11.7
Poverty status[3]		
Poor	10.6	11.6
Near poor	9.9	10.7
Nonpoor	5.0	6.2
Race and Hispanic origin and poverty status[3]		
White, non-Hispanic:		
Poor	8.8	11.8
Near poor	10.0	9.3
Nonpoor	4.8	5.9
Black, non-Hispanic:		
Poor	12.2	9.5
Near poor	8.7	11.8
Nonpoor	5.0	8.7
Hispanic:[2]		
Poor	10.7	12.8
Near poor	10.3	12.3
Nonpoor	5.7	6.5
Health insurance status[4]		
Insured	6.8	7.3
Private	6.6	6.9
Medicaid	7.2	7.9
Uninsured	15.6	18.5
Poverty status and health insurance status[3,4]		
Poor:		
Insured	7.9	9.3
Uninsured	21.7	22.1
Near poor:		
Insured	8.6	8.9
Uninsured	13.7	18.4
Nonpoor:		
Insured	4.8	5.5
Uninsured	8.7	15.2
Geographic region		
Northeast	4.4	5.5
Midwest	8.0	9.4
South	11.0	10.5
West	7.8	10.3
Location of residence		
Within MSA[5]	7.6	8.9
Outside MSA[5]	10.8	10.9

[1]Includes all other races not shown separately and unknown poverty status and unknown health insurance status.
[2]The race groups white, black, American Indian or Alaska Native, and Asian or Pacific Islander include persons of Hispanic and non-Hispanic origin; persons of Hispanic origin may be of any race.
[3]Poverty status is based on family income and family size using Bureau of the Census poverty thresholds. Poor persons are defined as below the poverty threshold. Near poor persons have incomes of 100 percent to less than 200 percent of poverty threshold. Nonpoor persons have incomes of 200 percent or greater than the poverty threshold. See Appendix II, Poverty level.
[4]Health insurance categories are mutually exclusive. Persons who reported more than one type of health insurance coverage were classified to a single type of coverage according to the following hierarchy: Medicaid, private, other. Other health insurance includes Medicare or military coverage. See Appendix II, Health insurance coverage.
[5]MSA is metropolitan statistical area.
NOTES: Some numbers in this table differ from previous editions of Health, United States. See Appendix II for definition of physician contact. In 1993–94 and 1995–96 between 8–9 percent of children have unknown health insurance status and 13 percent of children have unknown poverty status.
SOURCE: Centers for Disease Control and Prevention, National Center for Health Statistics, data computed by the Division of Health and Utilization Analysis from the National Health Interview Survey health insurance supplements.

Table 80. No usual source of health care among children under 18 years of age according to selected characteristics: United States, average annual 1993–94 and 1995–96

[Data are based on household interviews of a sample of the civilian noninstitutionalized population]

Characteristic	Under 6 years of age		6–17 years of age	
	1993–94	1995–96	1993–94	1995–96
	Percent of children without a usual source of health care[1]			
All children[2]	5.0	4.3	8.7	7.2
Race[3]				
White	4.5	4.2	8.0	6.8
Black	7.4	5.1	11.6	8.4
American Indian or Alaska Native	*	*	8.1	6.6
Asian or Pacific Islander	3.3	*	13.4	10.8
Race and Hispanic origin				
White, non-Hispanic	3.5	3.0	6.4	5.1
Black, non-Hispanic	7.5	5.2	11.3	8.5
Hispanic[3]	8.8	8.6	17.1	15.6
Poverty status[4]				
Poor	8.8	7.0	15.5	12.1
Near poor	6.4	5.9	10.9	10.1
Nonpoor	1.6	1.8	4.0	3.7
Race and Hispanic origin and poverty status[4]				
White, non-Hispanic:				
Poor	6.8	7.0	11.5	10.4
Near poor	6.2	4.3	9.6	7.5
Nonpoor	1.4	1.6	3.6	3.2
Black, non-Hispanic:				
Poor	10.0	6.6	14.7	8.1
Near poor	6.3	6.5	10.5	12.1
Nonpoor	*	2.2	5.4	5.0
Hispanic:[3]				
Poor	11.1	7.9	22.6	18.7
Near poor	8.0	11.9	16.8	18.2
Nonpoor	*	4.0	6.1	6.9
Health insurance status[5]				
Insured	3.1	2.4	5.6	4.3
Private	1.9	1.6	4.3	3.5
Medicaid	5.7	4.2	10.3	7.4
Uninsured	17.6	17.4	25.6	24.1
Poverty status and health insurance status[4,5]				
Poor:				
Insured	5.4	4.5	10.0	6.7
Uninsured	24.8	21.4	30.3	28.1
Near poor:				
Insured	4.0	3.1	7.1	5.7
Uninsured	16.0	18.1	23.0	23.8
Nonpoor:				
Insured	1.3	1.3	3.3	3.0
Uninsured	6.5	10.3	15.2	16.3
Geographic region				
Northeast	2.5	2.1	4.4	3.6
Midwest	3.9	3.2	5.5	4.6
South	7.1	5.0	12.3	8.9
West	5.2	6.2	10.3	10.6
Location of residence				
Within MSA[6]	4.8	4.3	8.8	7.3
Outside MSA[6]	5.7	3.9	8.2	6.8

* Relative standard error greater than 30 percent.

[1]Persons who report multiple sources of care are defined as having a usual source of care. Persons who report the emergency department as the place of their usual source of care are defined as having no usual source of care. See Appendix II for definition of usual source of care.

[2]Includes all other races not shown separately and unknown poverty status and unknown health insurance status.

[3]The race groups white, black, American Indian or Alaska Native, and Asian or Pacific Islander include persons of Hispanic and non-Hispanic origin; persons of Hispanic origin may be of any race.

[4]Poverty status is based on family income and family size using Bureau of the Census poverty thresholds. Poor persons are defined as below the poverty threshold. Near poor persons have incomes of 100 percent to less than 200 percent of poverty threshold. Nonpoor persons have incomes of 200 percent or greater than the poverty threshold. See Appendix II, Poverty level.

[5]Health insurance categories are mutually exclusive. Persons who reported more than one type of health insurance coverage were classified to a single type of coverage according to the following hierarchy: Medicaid, private, other. Other health insurance includes Medicare or military coverage. See Appendix II, Health insurance coverage. [6]MSA is metropolitan statistical area.

NOTES: Numbers in this table have been revised and differ from the previous editions of Health, United States. In 1993–94 and 1995–96 between 7–9 percent of children have unknown health insurance status and 14 percent of children have unknown poverty status.

SOURCE: Centers for Disease Control and Prevention, National Center for Health Statistics, data computed by the Division of Health and Utilization Analysis from the National Health Interview Survey access to care and health insurance supplements.

Table 81 (page 1 of 2). No usual source of health care among adults 18–64 years of age according to selected characteristics: United States, average annual 1990, 1993–94, and 1995–96

[Data are based on household interviews of a sample of the civilian noninstitutionalized population]

Characteristic	Both sexes			Male			Female		
	1990	1993–94	1995–96	1990	1993–94	1995–96	1990	1993–94	1995–96
Age[2]	Percent of adults without a usual source of health care[1]								
18–64 years, age adjusted	23.6	18.2	17.1	32.2	23.3	21.2	15.5	13.4	13.1
18–24 years	33.1	25.9	23.1	44.7	32.3	27.4	22.1	19.7	18.8
25–44 years	25.1	19.6	18.6	35.2	25.8	24.0	15.4	13.6	13.5
45–64 years	16.1	12.2	11.8	20.3	14.6	13.8	12.2	10.0	10.0
18–64 years, age adjusted									
Race[3]									
White	22.8	17.8	16.4	30.4	22.5	20.2	15.5	13.2	12.6
Black	23.9	18.6	19.3	35.9	24.5	24.2	13.9	13.7	15.3
American Indian or Alaska Native	23.3	18.9	21.7	37.7	25.8	24.4	10.2	13.1	19.1
Asian or Pacific Islander	35.1	23.1	21.8	41.1	27.5	25.0	27.6	19.1	18.8
Race and Hispanic origin									
White, non-Hispanic	21.6	16.5	14.9	28.9	21.0	18.4	14.4	12.1	11.5
Black, non-Hispanic	23.7	18.3	19.1	35.7	24.1	23.8	13.9	13.5	15.2
Hispanic[3]	34.5	28.1	27.2	45.5	34.9	32.8	25.0	21.8	21.5
Mexican	37.1	29.7	28.7	46.2	36.0	34.7	28.7	23.4	22.2
Poverty status[4]									
Poor	29.7	26.6	26.6	41.4	35.5	33.1	22.2	20.3	21.8
Near poor	28.1	23.4	22.4	38.7	29.1	27.1	18.8	18.1	18.2
Nonpoor	21.2	14.2	13.4	28.4	18.5	17.0	13.6	9.7	9.7
Race and Hispanic origin and poverty status[4]									
White, non-Hispanic:									
Poor	27.9	25.5	23.0	39.0	33.0	28.7	20.1	19.7	18.6
Near poor	25.6	21.4	20.2	35.3	26.7	24.3	17.5	16.5	16.5
Nonpoor	20.2	13.9	12.8	26.9	18.1	16.3	13.1	9.5	9.2
Black, non-Hispanic:									
Poor	24.8	22.5	24.4	39.4	33.1	31.6	16.8	16.7	20.6
Near poor	25.8	21.7	23.3	38.1	28.8	29.7	14.4	15.9	18.0
Nonpoor	21.1	13.3	14.6	31.0	17.4	18.6	11.5	8.8	10.3
Hispanic:[3]									
Poor	42.1	36.4	34.3	52.7	47.9	42.1	35.6	27.7	27.7
Near poor	39.7	33.6	32.2	52.2	40.6	37.5	27.9	26.5	26.5
Nonpoor	28.7	17.6	17.5	39.6	22.6	22.3	18.2	12.5	12.2
Health insurance status[5]									
Insured	19.7	12.7	11.7	27.0	16.5	14.6	13.0	9.3	9.0
Uninsured	42.0	40.8	40.9	52.9	47.2	46.0	30.3	33.7	35.1
Poverty status and health insurance status[4,5]									
Poor:									
Insured	21.5	15.0	16.3	31.8	20.0	20.2	15.5	12.2	14.1
Uninsured	41.9	44.8	42.2	53.3	53.9	48.0	32.6	36.4	36.4
Near poor:									
Insured	21.8	15.0	14.0	31.0	19.6	17.2	14.6	11.2	11.5
Uninsured	43.8	40.8	40.5	56.1	46.4	46.3	30.8	34.7	34.4
Nonpoor:									
Insured	19.1	11.7	10.8	25.9	15.4	13.8	12.3	8.0	7.7
Uninsured	41.7	35.7	38.8	50.8	41.6	42.6	29.2	27.7	33.0

See footnotes at end of table.

Table 81 (page 2 of 2). No usual source of health care among adults 18–64 years of age according to selected characteristics: United States, average annual 1990, 1993–94, and 1995–96

[Data are based on household interviews of a sample of the civilian noninstitutionalized population]

Characteristic	Both sexes			Male			Female		
	1990	1993–94	1995–96	1990	1993–94	1995–96	1990	1993–94	1995–96
Geographic region	Percent of adults without a usual source of health care[1]								
Northeast	20.5	14.1	13.3	27.4	17.9	16.3	13.8	10.6	10.4
Midwest	19.6	15.3	15.9	27.5	19.9	19.4	12.0	10.9	12.5
South	25.8	21.0	18.0	34.6	26.3	22.6	17.6	15.9	13.7
West	26.3	20.3	20.1	35.0	25.4	24.3	18.0	15.3	16.0
Location of residence									
Within MSA[6]	24.0	18.5	17.5	32.1	23.4	21.4	16.3	13.8	13.6
Outside MSA[6]	20.9	16.8	15.1	29.2	21.3	18.6	12.9	12.4	11.6

[1]Persons who report multiple sources of care are defined as having a usual source of care. Persons who report the emergency department as the place of their usual source of care are defined as having no usual source of care. See Appendix II for definition of usual source of care.
[2]Includes all other races not shown separately and unknown poverty status and unknown health insurance status.
[3]The race groups white, black, American Indian or Alaska Native, and Asian or Pacific Islander include persons of Hispanic and non-Hispanic origin; persons of Hispanic origin may be of any race.
[4]Poverty status is based on family income and family size using Bureau of the Census poverty thresholds. Poor persons are defined as below the poverty threshold. Near poor persons have incomes of 100 percent to less than 200 percent of poverty threshold. Nonpoor persons have incomes of 200 percent or greater than the poverty threshold. See Appendix II, Poverty level.
[5]See Appendix II, Health insurance coverage.
[6]MSA is metropolitan statistical area.

NOTES: In 1990, 1993–94, and 1995–96 between 16–17 percent of adults have unknown health insurance status and 11–13 percent of adults have unknown poverty status. Data for 1991 not included in this trend table due to a slightly different question in that year on usual source of care.

SOURCE: Centers for Disease Control and Prevention, National Center for Health Statistics, data computed by the Division of Health Utilization Analysis from the National Health Interview Survey access to care and health insurance supplements.

Table 82 (page 1 of 2). Use of mammography for women 40 years of age and over according to selected characteristics: United States, selected years 1987–94

[Data are based on household interviews of a sample of the civilian noninstitutionalized population]

Characteristic	1987	1990	1991	1993	1994
Age	Percent of women having a mammogram within the past 2 years[1]				
40 years and over................	28.7	51.4	54.6	59.7	60.9
40–49 years..................	31.9	55.1	55.6	59.9	61.3
50 years and over	27.4	49.7	54.1	59.7	60.6
50–64 years..................	31.7	56.0	60.3	65.1	66.5
65 years and over.............	22.8	43.4	48.1	54.2	55.0
Age, race, and Hispanic origin					
40 years and over:					
White, non-Hispanic.............	30.3	52.7	56.0	60.6	61.3
Black, non-Hispanic.............	23.8	46.0	47.7	59.2	64.4
Hispanic[2]	18.3	45.2	49.2	50.9	51.9
40–49 years:					
White, non-Hispanic.............	34.3	57.0	58.1	61.6	62.0
Black, non-Hispanic	27.9	48.4	48.0	55.6	67.2
Hispanic[2]	15.3	45.1	44.0	52.6	47.5
50 years and over:					
White, non-Hispanic	28.8	50.7	55.1	60.2	61.0
Black, non-Hispanic	21.5	44.6	47.6	61.4	62.4
Hispanic[2]	20.0	45.2	53.7	49.7	54.7
50–64 years:					
White, non-Hispanic..........	33.6	58.1	61.5	66.2	67.5
Black, non-Hispanic..........	26.4	48.4	52.4	65.5	63.6
Hispanic[2]	23.0	47.5	61.7	59.2	60.1
65 years and over:					
White, non-Hispanic..........	24.0	43.8	49.1	54.7	54.9
Black, non-Hispanic..........	14.1	39.7	41.6	56.3	61.0
Hispanic[2]	*13.7	41.1	40.9	35.7	48.0
Age and poverty status[3]					
40 years and over:					
Below poverty	15.0	28.7	36.5	40.8	44.4
At or above poverty	31.0	54.8	58.4	62.7	64.8
40–49 years:					
Below poverty.................	19.0	33.2	33.7	35.8	44.0
At or above poverty............	33.4	57.3	58.8	62.6	64.7
50 years and over:					
Below poverty.................	13.8	27.0	37.6	42.9	44.5
At or above poverty............	29.9	53.5	58.2	62.8	64.9
50–64 years:					
Below poverty	14.5	25.6	39.6	45.3	47.0
At or above poverty	34.1	59.5	64.3	67.8	70.3
65 years and over:					
Below poverty	13.4	28.0	36.0	41.2	43.2
At or above poverty	25.0	46.6	51.5	57.3	58.7

See footnotes at end of table.

Table 82 (page 2 of 2). Use of mammography for women 40 years of age and over according to selected characteristics: United States, selected years 1987–94

[Data are based on household interviews of a sample of the civilian noninstitutionalized population]

Characteristic	1987	1990	1991	1993	1994
Age and education	Percent of women having a mammogram within the past 2 years[1]				
40 years of age and over:					
Less than 12 years	17.8	36.4	40.0	46.4	48.2
12 years	31.3	52.7	55.8	59.0	61.0
13 years or more	37.7	62.8	65.2	69.5	69.7
40–49 years of age:					
Less than 12 years	15.1	38.5	40.8	43.6	50.4
12 years	32.6	53.1	52.0	56.6	55.8
13 years or more	39.2	62.3	63.7	66.1	68.7
50 years of age and over:					
Less than 12 years	18.4	36.0	39.9	46.9	47.7
12 years	30.6	52.6	57.7	60.1	63.6
13 years or more	36.8	63.2	66.3	72.5	70.5
50–64 years of age:					
Less than 12 years	21.2	41.0	43.6	51.4	51.6
12 years	33.8	56.5	60.8	62.4	67.8
13 years or more.............	40.5	68.0	72.7	78.5	74.7
65 years of age and over:					
Less than 12 years	16.5	33.0	37.7	44.2	45.6
12 years	25.9	47.5	54.0	57.4	59.1
13 years or more.............	32.3	56.7	57.9	64.8	64.3

* Relative standard error greater than 30 percent.

[1]Questions concerning use of mammography differed slightly on the National Health Interview Survey across the years for which data are shown. In 1987 and 1990 women were asked to report when they had their last mammogram. In 1991 women were asked whether they had a mammogram in the past 2 years. In 1993 and 1994 women were asked whether they had a mammogram within the past year, between 1 and 2 years ago, or over 2 years ago.

[2]Persons of Hispanic origin may be of any race.

[3]Poverty status is based on family income and family size using Bureau of the Census poverty thresholds (see Appendix II).

SOURCE: Centers for Disease Control and Prevention, National Center for Health Statistics, Division of Health Interview Statistics. Data from the National Health Interview Survey.

Table 83 (page 1 of 2). Ambulatory care visits to physician offices and hospital outpatient and emergency departments by selected patient characteristics: United States, 1995–97

[Data are based on reporting by a sample of office-based physician visits and hospital outpatient department and emergency department visits]

Age, sex, and race	All places[1]			Physician offices		
	1995	1996	1997	1995	1996	1997
	Number of visits in thousands					
Total	860,858	892,025	959,300	697,082	734,493	787,372
Age						
Under 15 years	169,297	176,919	176,294	131,548	140,851	137,361
15–44 years	310,530	312,794	339,428	237,868	243,535	266,188
45–64 years	188,319	198,885	226,064	159,531	170,229	192,753
45–54 years	104,891	112,393	124,377	88,266	95,689	105,511
55–64 years	83,429	86,492	101,687	71,264	74,540	87,243
65 years and over	192,712	203,427	217,514	168,135	179,878	191,069
65–74 years	102,605	105,624	112,593	90,544	93,879	99,714
75 years and over	90,106	97,803	104,922	77,591	85,999	91,355
	Number of visits per 100 persons					
Total, age adjusted	322	330	350	260	271	286
Total, crude	329	337	360	266	278	295
Age						
Under 15 years	285	298	295	221	237	230
15–44 years	260	261	283	200	203	222
45–64 years	364	374	412	309	320	351
45–54 years	339	349	372	286	297	316
55–64 years	401	411	473	343	354	406
65 years and over	612	639	678	534	565	596
65–74 years	560	579	623	494	515	552
75 years and over	683	719	750	588	632	653
Sex and age						
Male, age adjusted	280	289	304	223	235	245
Male, crude	277	285	301	220	232	243
Under 15 years	288	303	311	220	240	243
15–44 years	191	183	194	140	135	144
45–54 years	275	284	302	229	240	251
55–64 years	351	374	433	300	325	370
65–74 years	508	558	583	445	497	516
75 years and over	711	767	744	616	683	653
Female, age adjusted	362	371	395	296	306	326
Female, crude	378	387	416	310	321	345
Under 15 years	281	292	279	222	233	216
15–44 years	329	338	370	258	270	299
45–54 years	400	411	438	339	352	377
55–64 years	446	445	510	382	382	439
65–74 years	603	597	656	534	530	581
75 years and over	666	689	753	571	600	652
Race and age						
White, age adjusted	329	329	355	272	277	297
White, crude	338	339	368	281	286	310
Under 15 years	305	309	312	247	255	253
15–44 years	265	256	286	209	205	230
45–54 years	334	339	372	286	294	324
55–64 years	397	404	469	345	356	410
65–74 years	557	574	613	496	515	547
75 years and over	689	716	745	598	634	653
Black, age adjusted	294	368	357	190	255	242
Black, crude	281	354	342	178	242	228
Under 15 years	198	276	257	103	172	151
15–44 years	249	307	284	150	197	177
45–54 years	387	461	422	281	346	294
55–64 years	414	481	542	294	350	396
65–74 years	553	613	711	429	492	582
75 years and over	534	804	764	395	651	607

See notes at end of table.

Table 83 (page 2 of 2). Ambulatory care visits to physician offices and hospital outpatient and emergency departments by selected patient characteristics: United States, 1995–97

[Data are based on reporting by a sample of office-based physician visits and hospital outpatient department and emergency department visits]

Age, sex, and race	Hospital outpatient departments			Hospital emergency departments		
	1995	1996	1997	1995	1996	1997
	Number of visits in thousands					
Total	67,232	67,186	76,993	96,545	90,347	94,936
Age						
Under 15 years	15,039	15,196	18,240	22,709	20,872	20,693
15–44 years	26,895	26,857	29,430	45,767	42,402	43,809
45–64 years	14,811	14,911	17,682	13,978	13,745	15,629
45–54 years	8,029	8,496	9,597	8,595	8,207	9,270
55–64 years	6,782	6,415	8,085	5,383	5,538	6,359
65 years and over	10,487	10,222	11,640	14,090	13,328	14,805
65–74 years	6,004	5,799	6,677	6,057	5,945	6,201
75 years and over	4,482	4,422	4,963	8,033	7,382	8,604
	Number of visits per 100 persons					
Total, age adjusted	26	25	29	36	34	35
Total, crude	26	25	29	37	34	36
Age						
Under 15 years	25	26	31	38	35	35
15–44 years	23	22	25	38	35	36
45–64 years	29	28	32	27	26	28
45–54 years	26	26	29	28	25	28
55–64 years	33	31	38	26	26	30
65 years and over	33	32	36	45	42	46
65–74 years	33	32	37	33	33	34
75 years and over	34	32	35	61	54	61
Sex and age						
Male, age adjusted	21	21	24	36	33	34
Male, crude	21	20	24	36	33	34
Under 15 years	27	26	31	41	36	36
15–44 years	14	14	16	37	33	34
45–54 years	20	20	23	26	24	27
55–64 years	26	24	33	25	26	30
65–74 years	29	29	33	34	32	34
75 years and over	34	30	31	61	54	60
Female, age adjusted	30	30	33	36	35	36
Female, crude	31	31	34	37	35	37
Under 15 years	24	25	30	36	34	33
15–44 years	31	31	33	40	38	39
45–54 years	32	32	34	29	27	28
55–64 years	38	37	42	26	27	30
65–74 years	36	34	40	32	33	34
75 years and over	34	34	38	61	55	62
Race and age						
White, age adjusted	23	21	26	34	31	32
White, crude	23	21	26	34	31	33
Under 15 years	23	21	27	35	33	32
15–44 years	21	19	22	36	32	33
45–54 years	23	22	23	25	23	25
55–64 years	28	25	33	24	24	26
65–74 years	29	28	33	32	31	32
75 years and over	31	29	31	60	53	61
Black, age adjusted	47	56	56	57	57	60
Black, crude	45	54	54	58	58	60
Under 15 years	40	52	52	56	52	54
15–44 years	38	48	43	62	63	64
45–54 years	55	62	72	51	54	55
55–64 years	73	79	83	47	51	63
65–74 years	77	74	75	47	47	54
75 years and over	66	73	81	73	80	76

[1] All places includes visits to physician offices and hospital outpatient and emergency departments.

NOTES: Rates are based on the civilian noninstitutionalized population as of July 1. Population figures are adjusted for net underenumeration using the 1990 National Population Adjustment Matrix from the U.S. Bureau of the Census. Rates will be overestimated to the extent that visits by institutionalized persons are counted in the numerator (for example, hospital emergency department visits by nursing home residents) and institutionalized persons are omitted from the denominator. Data for additional years are available (see Appendix III).

SOURCES: Centers for Disease Control and Prevention, National Center for Health Statistics, Division of Health Care Statistics. Data from the National Ambulatory Medical Care Survey and the National Hospital Ambulatory Medical Care Survey.

Table 84. Ambulatory care visits to physician offices, percent distribution according to selected patient characteristics and physician specialty: United States, 1975, 1985, and 1997

[Data are based on reporting by a sample of office-based physicians]

Age, sex, and race	All specialties	General and family practice			Internal medicine			Pediatrics			Obstetrics and gynecology		
		1975	1985	1997	1975	1985	1997	1975	1985	1997	1975	1985	1997
						Percent distribution							
Total	100.0	41.3	30.5	25.5	10.9	11.6	15.4	8.2	11.4	11.7	8.5	8.9	9.0
Age													
Under 15 years.	100.0	34.1	25.0	20.6	2.1	2.2	1.9	43.7	55.2	62.2	*	*	*
15–44 years	100.0	40.9	33.0	28.7	8.1	8.3	14.0	1.4	2.6	2.2	17.5	19.1	20.8
45–64 years	100.0	44.4	32.0	27.1	16.2	15.7	18.7	*	*	*	3.9	4.7	5.9
45–54 years	100.0	44.5	32.9	28.6	15.0	14.3	17.1	*	*	*	5.3	6.5	7.3
55–64 years	100.0	44.2	31.3	25.3	17.5	16.9	20.6	*	*	*	2.3	3.2	4.3
65 years and over.	100.0	45.5	29.1	22.7	19.3	22.1	23.7	*	*	*	1.2	1.4	2.0
65–74 years	100.0	46.0	28.8	23.4	18.6	22.1	23.1	*	*	*	1.4	2.0	2.5
75 years and over	100.0	44.6	29.4	22.0	20.5	22.1	24.5	*	*	*	*	*	*
Sex and age													
Male:													
Under 15 years	100.0	34.8	24.7	20.0	2.0	1.9	1.5	43.2	53.9	63.0	. . .	. . .	. . .
15–44 years	100.0	45.9	36.4	36.7	10.0	9.9	15.6	1.9	2.5	3.2	. . .	. . .	. . .
45–64 years	100.0	43.4	31.0	26.7	17.3	16.0	22.5	*	*	*	. . .	. . .	. . .
65 years and over	100.0	45.7	28.1	22.0	17.5	20.8	22.1	*	*	*	. . .	. . .	. . .
Female:													
Under 15 years	100.0	33.3	25.3	21.3	2.2	2.5	2.3	44.3	56.5	61.2	*	*	*
15–44 years	100.0	38.3	31.3	24.9	7.1	7.5	13.2	1.1	2.6	1.7	26.4	28.4	30.7
45–64 years	100.0	45.0	32.7	27.4	15.5	15.5	16.0	*	*	*	6.4	7.7	10.0
65 years and over	100.0	45.4	29.7	23.2	20.4	23.0	24.8	*	*	*	1.9	2.3	3.4
Race													
White.	100.0	40.8	30.0	26.3	11.1	11.8	14.5	8.2	11.4	11.6	8.2	8.7	8.6
Black	100.0	46.9	35.4	23.0	9.9	10.4	21.9	8.0	11.3	12.9	11.9	9.9	12.0

Age, sex, and race	General surgery			Ophthalmology			Orthopedic surgery			All others		
	1975	1985	1997	1975	1985	1997	1975	1985	1997	1975	1985	1997
					Percent distribution							
Total	7.3	4.7	2.7	4.4	6.3	5.8	3.4	5.0	4.4	16.0	21.7	25.5
Age												
Under 15 years. . . . . :.	2.6	1.4	0.7	3.4	2.6	2.3	3.4	2.9	2.4	9.6	10.4	9.7
15–44 years	7.5	4.4	2.7	3.4	3.9	2.8	3.9	6.1	4.9	17.4	22.5	23.9
45–64 years	9.7	6.6	3.6	4.9	7.1	6.2	3.7	6.1	5.2	17.3	27.4	33.2
45–54 years	10.0	6.6	3.5	4.3	6.0	5.3	4.1	6.6	5.3	16.7	26.7	32.9
55–64 years	9.3	6.6	3.7	5.4	7.9	7.3	3.3	5.7	5.0	17.9	28.0	33.7
65 years and over.	7.9	6.2	3.3	6.9	13.5	12.2	1.9	3.4	4.3	17.3	24.2	31.5
65–74 years	7.9	6.4	3.5	6.4	11.2	10.3	2.1	3.6	4.4	17.4	25.9	32.8
75 years and over	7.8	6.0	3.1	7.8	16.6	14.4	1.4	3.1	4.3	17.0	21.9	30.0
Sex and age												
Male:												
Under 15 years	2.9	1.7	*	2.7	2.5	2.0	3.7	3.3	2.6	10.1	11.9	10.1
15–44 years	8.8	5.0	3.6	4.1	5.2	3.2	7.1	11.0	8.3	21.9	29.8	29.3
45–64 years	9.1	6.2	3.2	5.1	7.2	5.9	4.3	7.0	5.8	20.7	32.2	35.7
65 years and over	7.7	6.7	3.5	6.4	11.8	11.5	1.6	2.6	3.4	20.9	29.8	37.2
Female:												
Under 15 years	2.3	*	*	4.3	2.6	2.7	3.0	2.4	2.2	9.1	8.9	9.2
15–44 years	6.9	4.1	2.3	3.0	3.3	2.5	2.2	3.8	3.2	15.1	19.0	21.4
45–64 years	10.1	6.9	3.8	4.8	7.0	6.5	3.2	5.5	4.7	15.0	24.2	31.5
65 years and over	8.0	5.9	3.1	7.2	14.5	12.7	2.1	3.8	4.9	15.0	20.7	27.6
Race												
White.	7.5	4.6	2.9	4.3	6.4	5.9	3.5	5.0	4.5	16.5	22.3	25.7
Black	6.1	6.2	1.4	3.2	4.7	4.7	2.8	4.8	3.5	11.0	17.2	20.5

* Relative standard error greater than 50 percent.
. . . Category not applicable.

NOTES: In 1975 and 1985 the survey excluded Alaska and Hawaii. Beginning in 1989 the survey included all 50 States. Specialty information based on the physician's self-designated primary area of practice. General and family practice includes general practice, family practice, and beginning in 1992 general and family practice includes subspecialties also. Internal medicine includes general internal medicine and excludes all subspecialties. Pediatrics and obstetrics and gynecology include physicians practicing in the general field and subspecialties.

SOURCE: Centers for Disease Control and Prevention, National Center for Health Statistics, Division of Health Care Statistics. Data from the National Ambulatory Medical Care Survey.

Table 85. Persons with a dental visit within the past year among persons 25 years of age and over, according to selected patient characteristics: United States, selected years 1983–93

[Data are based on household interviews of a sample of the civilian noninstitutionalized population]

Characteristic	1983[1]	1989[1]	1990	1991	1993
	Percent of persons with a visit within the past year				
Total[2,3]	53.9	58.9	62.3	58.2	60.8
Age					
25–34 years	59.0	60.9	65.1	59.1	60.3
35–44 years	60.3	65.9	69.1	64.8	66.9
45–64 years	54.1	59.9	62.8	59.2	62.0
65 years and over	39.3	45.8	49.6	47.2	51.7
65–74 years....................	43.8	50.0	53.5	51.1	56.3
75 years and over...............	31.8	39.0	43.4	41.3	44.9
Sex[3]					
Male.........................	51.7	56.2	58.8	55.5	58.2
Female.......................	55.9	61.4	65.6	60.8	63.4
Poverty status[3,4]					
Below poverty	30.4	33.3	38.2	33.0	35.9
At or above poverty	55.8	62.1	65.4	61.9	64.3
Race and Hispanic origin[3]					
White, non-Hispanic.............	56.6	61.8	64.9	61.5	64.0
Black, non-Hispanic.............	39.1	43.3	49.1	44.3	47.3
Hispanic[5]	42.1	48.9	53.8	43.1	46.2
Education[3]					
Less than 12 years	35.1	36.9	41.2	35.2	38.0
12 years	54.8	58.2	61.3	56.7	58.7
13 years or more	70.9	73.9	75.7	72.2	73.8
Education, race, and Hispanic origin[3]					
Less than 12 years:					
White, non-Hispanic	36.1	39.1	41.8	38.1	41.2
Black, non-Hispanic	31.7	32.0	37.9	33.0	33.1
Hispanic[5]....................	33.8	36.5	42.7	28.9	33.0
12 years:					
White, non-Hispanic	56.6	59.8	62.8	58.8	60.4
Black, non-Hispanic	40.5	44.8	51.1	43.1	48.2
Hispanic[5]....................	48.7	56.5	59.9	49.5	54.6
13 years or more:					
White, non-Hispanic	72.6	75.8	77.3	74.2	75.8
Black, non-Hispanic	54.4	57.2	64.4	61.7	61.3
Hispanic[5]....................	58.4	66.2	67.9	61.2	61.8

[1]Data for 1983 and 1989 are not strictly comparable with data for later years. Data for 1983 and 1989 are based on responses to the question "About how long has it been since you last went to a dentist?" Starting in 1990 data are based on the question "During the past 12 months, how many visits did you make to a dentist?"
[2]Includes all other races not shown separately and unknown poverty status and education level.
[3]Age adjusted. See Appendix II for age-adjustment procedure.
[4]Poverty status is based on family income and family size using Bureau of the Census poverty thresholds. See Appendix II.
[5]Persons of Hispanic origin may be of any race.

NOTES: Denominators exclude persons with unknown dental data. Estimates for 1983 and 1989 are based on data for all members of the sample household. Beginning in 1990 estimates are based on one adult member per sample household. Estimates for 1993 are based on responses during the last half of the year only.

SOURCE: Centers for Disease Control and Prevention, National Center for Health Statistics, Division of Health Interview Statistics. Data from the National Health Interview Survey.

Table 86. Substance abuse clients in specialty treatment units according to substance abused, geographic division, and State: United States, 1996–97

[Data are based on a 1-day census of treatment providers]

Geographic division and State	All clients		Clients with both alcoholism and drug abuse		Alcoholism only clients		Drug abuse only clients	
	1996	1997	1996	1997	1996	1997	1996	1997
	Clients per 100,000 population							
United States	423.0	415.3	183.7	170.7	117.5	109.0	121.8	135.7
New England	517.9	589.9	253.2	245.2	124.5	153.1	140.2	191.6
Maine	574.6	776.3	280.9	374.3	203.2	260.2	90.5	141.8
New Hampshire	367.5	255.3	203.7	104.7	132.8	103.3	31.0	47.4
Vermont	370.3	326.5	169.9	143.7	151.0	139.9	49.4	42.9
Massachusetts	568.8	647.6	310.3	272.6	126.5	175.5	132.0	199.5
Rhode Island	635.6	616.1	207.2	229.5	173.1	156.1	255.3	230.6
Connecticut	445.4	570.3	181.7	217.6	68.1	89.4	195.6	263.3
Middle Atlantic	547.5	578.2	221.0	195.4	101.1	124.1	225.4	258.6
New York	773.6	849.1	298.9	234.7	127.5	185.7	347.2	428.7
New Jersey	364.1	308.4	145.5	137.0	61.9	52.7	156.8	118.7
Pennsylvania	331.6	356.7	154.8	176.0	87.4	80.3	89.3	100.3
East North Central	456.0	452.0	201.1	195.1	147.1	147.0	107.8	109.9
Ohio	453.5	432.2	240.3	223.2	134.1	123.9	79.0	85.0
Indiana	341.8	375.3	128.6	154.5	126.6	132.7	86.5	88.1
Illinois	433.9	398.6	202.6	183.5	109.5	104.5	121.8	110.7
Michigan	598.7	627.4	228.7	228.4	213.2	220.9	156.8	178.1
Wisconsin	377.6	381.4	144.0	146.1	161.4	174.0	72.2	61.3
West North Central	262.1	261.4	130.2	126.7	85.2	86.7	46.7	48.0
Minnesota	182.5	195.1	94.8	93.0	58.4	69.3	29.3	32.8
Iowa	219.7	223.1	112.2	107.1	78.7	79.9	28.8	36.1
Missouri	246.7	246.3	136.6	128.6	52.2	56.9	57.8	60.8
North Dakota	313.9	384.1	135.0	157.6	143.8	181.9	35.1	44.6
South Dakota	419.1	305.5	159.4	120.1	238.7	148.2	21.0	37.2
Nebraska	309.6	304.6	139.5	155.3	123.3	117.1	46.8	32.2
Kansas	398.3	384.8	185.7	181.4	127.3	127.5	85.3	76.0
South Atlantic	341.5	365.8	155.4	164.0	97.0	93.1	89.1	108.8
Delaware	552.9	580.4	293.6	367.1	110.4	111.8	148.9	101.5
Maryland	572.2	559.3	274.4	237.1	109.8	113.7	187.9	208.4
District of Columbia	974.1	1,806.2	403.5	599.5	220.7	318.5	349.9	888.2
Virginia	286.4	371.5	138.3	191.4	78.5	95.2	69.6	84.9
West Virginia	287.6	299.2	65.8	73.7	182.1	177.9	39.6	47.6
North Carolina	324.8	280.4	155.0	134.9	108.9	90.3	60.9	55.3
South Carolina	427.8	349.0	145.7	126.7	188.9	141.6	93.2	80.7
Georgia	158.7	262.4	63.4	118.8	46.9	64.1	48.4	79.5
Florida	336.9	339.6	165.9	157.9	80.3	68.4	90.7	113.3
East South Central	304.6	301.7	107.6	110.4	121.6	84.4	75.5	106.9
Kentucky	697.6	368.8	217.7	124.5	348.6	141.8	131.3	102.4
Tennessee	211.2	290.3	66.5	134.8	66.4	65.8	78.3	89.7
Alabama	159.3	295.1	81.4	66.0	29.6	68.4	48.4	160.7
Mississippi	149.1	237.4	70.3	111.9	46.9	63.6	31.9	61.9
West South Central	264.4	270.2	128.6	106.3	50.3	72.3	85.6	91.5
Arkansas	212.0	194.8	109.3	77.9	43.5	41.9	59.1	74.9
Louisiana	343.0	340.8	180.1	175.5	58.2	64.8	104.7	100.6
Oklahoma	312.8	275.0	121.6	91.2	76.4	96.1	114.8	87.7
Texas	244.9	263.4	120.6	97.0	44.7	74.0	79.6	92.4
Mountain	438.1	432.1	182.4	166.3	159.3	139.1	96.4	126.8
Montana	263.9	305.5	131.3	150.9	95.2	90.5	37.3	64.1
Idaho	382.9	244.3	180.8	170.3	134.0	38.4	68.1	35.7
Wyoming	509.3	506.7	265.2	204.7	192.8	232.9	51.3	69.1
Colorado	608.1	418.2	275.3	136.3	224.6	149.4	108.2	132.5
New Mexico	522.2	456.4	217.9	174.7	217.1	201.7	87.2	80.1
Arizona	334.3	340.7	82.3	119.0	137.8	94.1	114.3	127.7
Utah	467.4	846.9	234.2	358.8	137.2	257.5	96.0	230.6
Nevada	310.4	380.4	141.7	122.3	72.0	102.6	96.7	155.5
Pacific	558.8	436.1	233.3	195.8	166.6	92.6	158.8	147.7
Washington	775.1	671.6	425.8	371.6	250.5	205.7	98.8	94.4
Oregon	619.8	830.9	337.4	394.1	150.1	247.6	132.3	189.3
California	522.7	347.4	191.0	142.4	153.3	50.1	178.3	155.0
Alaska	703.8	1,070.1	309.8	427.4	340.9	460.9	53.1	181.8
Hawaii	251.5	218.9	116.4	89.8	82.1	50.3	53.0	78.8

NOTES: Rates are based on the resident population 12 years of age and over as of July 1. Client data are as of October 1. Beginning in 1997, two changes were implemented causing a discontinuity with earlier years. First, the scope of the universe was expanded to include all substance abuse treatment facilities whereas previously only State-sanctioned facilities were included. Second, facilities that served only DUI/DWI clients were excluded whereas previously they had been included. The effects of these changes vary from State to State. Treatment rates at the State level can vary from year to year for a variety of reasons, including failure of large facilities to respond to the survey in some years, and normal variation in the number of people in treatment on a given day.

SOURCE: Substance Abuse and Mental Health Services Administration, Office of Applied Studies. Uniform Facility Data Set (UFDS) Survey, 1996–97.

Table 87. Additions to mental health organizations according to type of service and organization: United States, selected years 1983–94

[Data are based on inventories of mental health organizations]

Service and organization	Additions in thousands				Additions per 100,000 civilian population			
	1983	1990	1992	1994	1983	1990	1992	1994
Inpatient and residential treatment								
All organizations	1,633	2,036	2,092	2,197	701.4	833.5	830.0	840.3
State and county mental hospitals	339	276	275	236	146.0	113.2	109.3	91.2
Private psychiatric hospitals	165	407	470	480	70.9	166.5	186.4	185.5
Non-Federal general hospital psychiatric services	786	960	951	1,067	336.8	393.2	377.4	411.9
Department of Veterans Affairs psychiatric services[1]	149	198	181	172	64.3	81.2	71.6	61.5
Residential treatment centers for emotionally disturbed children	17	42	36	39	7.1	17.0	14.4	15.0
All other[2]	177	153	179	203	76.3	62.4	70.9	75.2
Outpatient treatment								
All organizations	2,665	3,005	2,883	3,242	1,147.5	1,230.9	1,180.6	1,252.8
State and county mental hospitals	84	43	46	38	36.3	17.5	18.6	14.8
Private psychiatric hospitals	78	121	141	145	33.4	49.7	57.7	56.1
Non-Federal general hospital psychiatric services	469	605	429	443	202.1	247.8	175.8	171.0
Department of Veterans Affairs psychiatric services[1]	103	164	145	120	44.5	67.2	59.2	46.5
Residential treatment centers for emotionally disturbed children	33	86	113	156	14.1	35.3	46.2	60.3
Freestanding psychiatric outpatient clinics	538	462	464	567	231.7	189.3	190.3	218.9
All other[2]	1,360	1,524	1,545	1,773	585.4	624.1	632.8	685.2
Partial care treatment								
All organizations	177	293	281	273	76.3	120.2	115.8	105.3
State and county mental hospitals	4	5	4	3	1.6	2.2	1.7	1.3
Private psychiatric hospitals	6	42	65	68	2.4	17.2	26.8	26.4
Non-Federal general hospital psychiatric services	46	54	50	55	19.8	21.9	20.7	21.1
Department of Veterans Affairs psychiatric services[1]	10	19	14	12	4.4	8.0	5.9	4.6
Residential treatment centers for emotionally disturbed children	3	13	8	12	1.5	5.5	3.5	4.3
Freestanding psychiatric outpatient clinics[3]	5	...	...	...	2.3	...	...	...
All other[2,3,4]	103	160	140	123	44.3	65.4	57.2	47.6

... Category not applicable.
[1]Includes Department of Veterans Affairs neuropsychiatric hospitals, general hospital psychiatric services, and psychiatric outpatient clinics.
[2]Includes other multiservice mental health organizations with inpatient and residential treatment services that are not elsewhere classified.
[3]Beginning in 1986 outpatient psychiatric clinics providing partial care are counted as multiservice mental health organizations in the "all other" category.
[4]Includes freestanding psychiatric partial care organizations.

NOTES: See Appendix II for definition of Addition. Outpatient and partial care treatment exclude office-based mental health care (psychiatrists, psychologists, licensed clinical social workers, and psychiatric nurses). Data for additional years are available (see Appendix III).

SOURCES: Survey and Analysis Branch, Division of State and Community Systems Development, Center for Mental Health Services. Manderscheid RW, Sonnenschein MA. *Mental health, United States, 1996.* DHHS. 1996. Unpublished data.

Table 88. Home health care and hospice patients, according to selected characteristics: United States, 1992–96

[Data are based on a survey of current home health care and hospice patients]

Type of patient and characteristic	1992	1994	1996
Home health care patients	**Number of current patients**		
Total..	1,232,200	1,879,510	2,427,483
Age at admission[1]:	**Percent distribution**		
Under 65 years............................	24.1	27.2	27.5
65 years and over.........................	75.9	72.8	72.5
65–74 years..............................	24.5	22.0	21.8
75–84 years..............................	34.0	31.1	33.9
85 years and over	17.5	19.7	16.7
Sex:			
Male..	33.2	32.5	32.9
Female.....................................	66.8	67.5	67.1
Primary admission diagnosis[2]:			
Malignant neoplasms.....................	5.7	5.7	4.8
Diabetes....................................	7.7	8.1	8.5
Diseases of the nervous system and sense organs...........	6.3	8.0	5.8
Diseases of the circulatory system	25.9	27.2	25.6
Diseases of heart........................	12.6	14.3	10.9
Cerebrovascular diseases..............	5.8	6.1	7.8
Diseases of the respiratory system ...	6.6	6.1	7.7
Decubitus ulcers	1.9	1.1	1.0
Diseases of the musculoskeletal system and connective tissue ...	9.4	8.3	8.8
Osteoarthritis............................	2.5	2.8	3.2
Fractures, all sites........................	3.8	3.7	3.3
Fracture of neck of femur (hip).........	1.4	1.7	1.3
Other..	32.7	31.8	34.6
Hospice patients	**Number of current patients**		
Total...	52,100	60,783	59,363
Age at admission[1]:	**Percent distribution**		
Under 65 years............................	20.4	31.2	22.1
65 years and over.........................	79.6	68.8	77.9
65–74 years..............................	27.4	23.1	24.6
75–84 years..............................	39.1	29.0	31.9
85 years and over	13.0	16.7	21.4
Sex:			
Male..	46.1	44.7	44.9
Female.....................................	53.9	55.3	55.1
Primary admission diagnosis[2]:			
Malignant neoplasms.....................	65.7	57.2	58.3
Malignant neoplasms of large intestine and rectum	9.0	8.0	4.0
Malignant neoplasms of trachea, bronchus, and lung.........	21.1	12.5	15.8
Malignant neoplasm of breast	3.9	4.8	6.2
Malignant neoplasm of prostate	6.0	5.9	6.6
Diseases of heart	10.2	9.3	8.3
Diseases of the respiratory system	4.3	6.6	7.3
Other..	19.8	27.0	26.1

[1]Denominator excludes persons with unknown age.
[2]Denominator excludes persons with unknown diagnosis.

NOTES: Current home health care and hospice patients are those who were under the care of their agency on any given day during the survey period. Diagnostic categories are based on the *International Classification of Diseases, 9th Revision, Clinical Modification.* For a listing of the code numbers, see Appendix II, table VII.

SOURCE: Centers for Disease Control and Prevention, National Center for Health Statistics, Division of Health Care Statistics. Data from the National Home and Hospice Care Survey.

Table 89. Discharges, days of care, and average length of stay in short-stay hospitals, according to selected characteristics: United States, 1964, 1990, and 1996

[Data are based on household interviews of a sample of the civilian noninstitutionalized population]

Characteristic	Discharges			Days of care			Average length of stay		
	1964	1990	1996	1964	1990	1996	1964	1990	1996
	Number per 1,000 population						Number of days		
Total[1,2]	109.1	91.0	82.4	970.9	607.1	469.9	8.9	6.7	5.7
Age									
Under 15 years	67.6	46.7	37.3	405.7	271.3	212.3	6.0	5.8	5.7
Under 5 years	94.3	79.9	73.6	731.1	496.4	480.7	7.8	6.2	6.5
5–14 years	53.1	29.0	19.0	229.1	150.8	76.6	4.3	5.2	4.0
15–44 years	100.6	62.6	54.6	760.7	340.5	258.3	7.6	5.4	4.7
45–64 years	146.2	135.7	113.7	1,559.3	911.5	621.4	10.7	6.7	5.5
65 years and over	190.0	248.8	268.7	2,292.7	2,092.4	1,818.0	12.1	8.4	6.8
65–74 years	181.2	215.4	228.8	2,150.4	1,719.3	1,491.6	11.9	8.0	6.5
75 years and over	206.7	300.6	323.7	2,560.4	2,669.9	2,267.6	12.4	8.9	7.0
Sex[1]									
Male	103.8	91.0	82.5	1,010.2	622.7	487.6	9.7	6.8	5.9
Female	113.7	91.7	83.1	933.4	592.9	458.0	8.2	6.5	5.5
Race[1]									
White	112.4	89.5	79.9	961.4	580.9	423.0	8.6	6.5	5.3
Black[3]	84.0	112.0	104.6	1,062.9	875.9	800.3	12.7	7.8	7.7
Family income[1,4]									
Less than $16,000	102.4	142.2	146.0	1,051.2	1,141.2	960.8	10.3	8.0	6.6
$16,000–$24,999	116.4	98.4	97.7	1,213.9	594.5	572.2	10.4	6.0	5.9
$25,000–$34,999	110.7	85.1	76.7	939.8	560.6	429.1	8.5	6.6	5.6
$35,000–$49,999	109.2	73.2	62.3	882.6	380.3	272.0	8.1	5.2	4.4
$50,000 or more	110.7	72.5	54.2	918.9	446.2	257.7	8.3	6.2	4.8
Geographic region[1]									
Northeast	98.5	84.9	67.0	993.8	623.4	405.2	10.1	7.3	6.0
Midwest	109.2	91.5	91.3	944.9	570.8	524.8	8.7	6.2	5.7
South	117.8	106.4	95.3	968.0	713.6	549.5	8.2	6.7	5.8
West	110.5	70.5	66.2	985.9	444.6	339.5	8.9	6.3	5.1
Location of residence[1]									
Within MSA[5]	107.5	85.9	75.7	1,015.4	599.6	444.2	9.4	7.0	5.9
Outside MSA[5]	113.3	109.5	105.7	871.9	636.0	556.3	7.7	5.8	5.3

[1] Age adjusted. See Appendix II for age-adjustment procedure.
[2] Includes all other races not shown separately and unknown family income.
[3] 1964 data include all other races.
[4] Family income categories for 1996. In 1990 the two lowest income categories are less than $14,000 and $14,000–$24,999; the three higher income categories are as shown. Income categories in 1964 are less than $2,000; $2,000–$3,999; $4,000–$6,999; $7,000–$9,999; and $10,000 or more.
[5] Metropolitan statistical area.

NOTES: Estimates of hospital utilization from the National Health Interview Survey (NHIS) and the National Hospital Discharge Survey (NHDS) may differ because NHIS data are based on household interviews of the civilian noninstitutionalized population and exclude deliveries, whereas NHDS data are based on hospital discharge records of all persons. NHDS includes records for persons discharged alive or deceased and institutionalized persons, and excludes newborn infants. Differences in hospital utilization estimated by the two surveys are particularly evident for the elderly and for women. See Appendix I.

SOURCE: Centers for Disease Control and Prevention, National Center for Health Statistics, Division of Health Interview Statistics. Data from the National Health Interview Survey.

Table 90. Discharges, days of care, and average length of stay in non-Federal short-stay hospitals, according to selected characteristics: United States, selected years 1980–96

[Data are based on a sample of hospital records]

Characteristic	1980[1]	1985[1]	1990	1992	1993[2]	1994	1995	1996
	Discharges per 1,000 population							
Total[3]	158.5	137.7	113.0	110.5	107.6	106.5	104.7	102.3
Sex[3]								
Male	140.3	124.4	100.9	98.6	95.2	94.2	92.3	89.7
Female	177.0	151.8	126.0	123.2	120.5	119.1	117.4	115.3
Age								
Under 15 years	71.6	57.7	44.6	45.2	37.7	39.2	41.7	38.2
15–44 years	150.1	125.0	101.6	96.0	95.4	93.2	89.8	87.0
45–64 years	194.8	170.8	135.0	131.0	126.8	124.1	118.2	117.2
65 years and over	383.7	369.8	330.9	336.5	341.6	341.6	344.6	346.1
65–74 years	315.8	297.2	259.1	264.5	262.2	261.6	257.6	257.3
75 years and over	489.3	475.6	429.9	432.7	446.3	445.3	455.2	455.2
Geographic region[3]								
Northeast	147.6	129.1	121.0	123.9	118.3	121.3	120.0	112.6
Midwest	175.4	143.4	115.1	105.3	102.2	102.6	99.5	99.6
South	165.1	143.5	119.2	116.3	116.9	111.8	110.9	105.7
West	136.9	130.3	92.1	93.7	87.6	87.6	86.0	90.3
	Days of care per 1,000 population							
Total[3]	1,129.0	872.1	705.0	659.3	626.9	594.0	544.3	520.6
Sex[3]								
Male	1,076.0	848.2	690.4	656.3	616.3	580.8	533.1	511.8
Female	1,187.1	902.0	725.3	667.5	640.5	609.5	556.7	531.6
Age								
Under 15 years	315.7	263.0	215.4	219.6	195.5	189.2	185.6	174.4
15–44 years	786.8	603.3	465.3	416.1	399.3	390.4	346.0	333.9
45–64 years	1,596.9	1,201.6	911.5	827.1	785.0	727.5	655.6	624.3
65 years and over	4,098.4	3,228.0	2,867.7	2,771.7	2,676.2	2,516.3	2,352.4	2,263.7
65–74 years	3,147.0	2,437.3	2,067.7	2,040.8	1,927.1	1,798.8	1,669.0	1,603.8
75 years and over	5,578.7	4,381.4	3,970.7	3,747.8	3,664.6	3,445.7	3,220.1	3,074.7
Geographic region[3]								
Northeast	1,204.7	953.5	878.0	838.6	787.2	774.9	722.1	666.9
Midwest	1,296.2	952.0	713.4	626.2	600.5	553.9	502.9	484.4
South	1,105.5	848.9	704.1	676.2	655.1	618.0	564.9	532.2
West	836.2	713.2	509.9	483.1	445.2	420.3	385.2	402.5
	Average length of stay in days							
Total[3]	7.1	6.3	6.2	6.0	5.8	5.6	5.2	5.1
Sex[3]								
Male	7.7	6.8	6.8	6.7	6.5	6.2	5.8	5.7
Female	6.7	5.9	5.8	5.4	5.3	5.1	4.7	4.6
Age								
Under 15 years	4.4	4.6	4.8	4.9	5.2	4.8	4.5	4.6
15–44 years	5.2	4.8	4.6	4.3	4.2	4.2	3.9	3.8
45–64 years	8.2	7.0	6.8	6.3	6.2	5.9	5.5	5.3
65 years and over	10.7	8.7	8.7	8.2	7.8	7.4	6.8	6.5
65–74 years	10.0	8.2	8.0	7.7	7.3	6.9	6.5	6.2
75 years and over	11.4	9.2	9.2	8.7	8.2	7.7	7.1	6.8
Geographic region[3]								
Northeast	8.2	7.4	7.3	6.8	6.7	6.4	6.0	5.9
Midwest	7.4	6.6	6.2	5.9	5.9	5.4	5.1	4.9
South	6.7	5.9	5.9	5.8	5.6	5.5	5.1	5.0
West	6.1	5.5	5.5	5.2	5.1	4.8	4.5	4.5

[1]Comparisons of data from 1980–85 with data from later years should be made with caution as estimates of change may reflect improvements in the design (see Appendix I) rather than true changes in hospital use.

[2]In 1993 children's hospitals had a high rate of nonresponse that may have resulted in underestimates of hospital utilization by children.

[3]Age adjusted. See Appendix II for age-adjustment procedure.

NOTES: Rates are based on the civilian population as of July 1. Estimates of hospital utilization from the National Health Interview Survey (NHIS) and the National Hospital Discharge Survey (NHDS) may differ because NHIS data are based on household interviews of the civilian noninstitutionalized population and exclude deliveries, whereas NHDS data are based on hospital discharge records of all persons. NHDS includes records for persons discharged alive or deceased and institutionalized persons, and excludes newborn infants. Differences in hospital utilization estimated by the two surveys are particularly evident for the elderly and for women. See Appendix I. Data for additional years are available (see Appendix III).

SOURCE: Centers for Disease Control and Prevention, National Center for Health Statistics, Division of Health Care Statistics. Data from the National Hospital Discharge Survey.

Table 91. Discharges, days of care, and average length of stay in non-Federal short-stay hospitals for discharges with the diagnosis of human immunodeficiency virus (HIV) and for all discharges: United States, selected years 1986–97

[Data are based on a sample of hospital records]

Type of discharge, sex, and age	1986[1]	1987[1]	1988	1990	1992	1993	1995[2]	1996[2]	1997[2]
	Discharges in thousands								
Discharges with diagnosis of HIV	44	67	95	146	194	225	249	227	178
Male, 20–49 years	35	51	73	102	141	158	162	141	107
Female, 20–49 years	*	*	13	27	31	44	55	52	46
All discharges	34,256	33,387	31,146	30,788	30,951	30,825	30,722	30,545	30,914
Male, 20–49 years	4,300	4,075	3,670	3,649	3,529	3,619	3,360	3,248	3,116
Female, 20–49 years	9,027	8,980	8,169	8,228	7,942	7,901	7,593	7,457	7,322
	Discharges per 1,000 population								
Discharges with diagnosis of HIV	0.18	0.28	0.39	0.59	0.76	0.88	0.92	0.84	0.66
Male, 20–49 years	0.67	0.96	1.36	1.84	2.47	2.76	2.69	2.35	1.77
Female, 20–49 years	*	*	0.23	0.47	0.54	0.74	0.91	0.86	0.76
All discharges	143.7	138.8	128.3	124.3	122.1	120.2	115.7	114.0	114.3
Male, 20–49 years	82.2	76.8	68.2	65.8	62.0	63.1	56.5	54.0	51.8
Female, 20–49 years	166.7	163.6	147.1	144.5	136.1	134.6	125.9	122.8	120.8
	Days of care in thousands								
Discharges with diagnosis of HIV	714	936	1,277	2,188	2,136	2,561	2,326	2,123	1,448
Male, 20–49 years	573	724	914	1,645	1,422	1,696	1,408	1,401	855
Female, 20–49 years	*	*	233	341	455	619	559	457	364
All discharges	218,496	214,942	203,678	197,422	190,386	184,601	164,627	159,883	157,458
Male, 20–49 years	26,488	26,295	22,697	22,539	21,614	21,348	17,984	17,818	15,529
Female, 20–49 years	40,620	39,356	34,800	34,473	30,886	29,555	26,596	25,368	24,955
	Days of care per 1,000 population								
Discharges with diagnosis of HIV	2.99	3.89	5.26	8.83	8.43	9.99	8.60	7.85	5.35
Male, 20–49 years	10.95	13.64	16.97	29.68	24.97	29.57	23.42	23.30	14.22
Female, 20–49 years	*	*	4.19	5.99	7.80	10.54	9.22	7.53	6.00
All discharges	916.5	893.6	838.8	796.9	751.0	719.9	620.2	596.5	582.3
Male, 20–49 years	506.4	495.2	421.5	406.6	379.5	372.2	302.7	296.2	258.3
Female, 20–49 years	750.2	717.1	626.5	605.4	529.3	503.4	441.0	417.8	411.7
	Average length of stay in days								
Discharges with diagnosis of HIV	16.4	14.1	13.4	14.9	11.0	11.4	9.3	9.4	8.1
Male, 20–49 years	16.4	14.1	12.5	16.2	10.1	10.7	8.7	9.9	8.0
Female, 20–49 years	*	*	18.0	12.6	14.6	14.2	10.2	8.7	7.9
All discharges	6.4	6.4	6.5	6.4	6.2	6.0	5.4	5.2	5.1
Male, 20–49 years	6.2	6.5	6.2	6.2	6.1	5.9	5.4	5.5	5.0
Female, 20–49 years	4.5	4.4	4.3	4.2	3.9	3.7	3.5	3.4	3.4

* Statistics based on fewer than 5,000 estimated discharges are not shown.
[1]Comparisons of data from 1986 and 1987 with data from later years should be made with caution as estimates of change may reflect improvements in the design (see Appendix I) rather than true changes in hospital use.
[2]Beginning with data year 1995, population figures are adjusted for net underenumeration using the 1990 National Population Adjustment Matrix from the U.S. Bureau of the Census. Rates for 1995 differ from those published in the previous edition of *Health, United States*.

NOTES: Excludes newborn infants. Rates are based on the civilian population as of July 1. Discharges with diagnosis of HIV have at least one HIV diagnosis listed on the face sheet of the medical record and are not limited to the first-listed diagnosis. See Appendix II, Human immunodeficiency virus (HIV) infection. Data for additional years are available (see Appendix III).

SOURCE: Centers for Disease Control and Prevention, National Center for Health Statistics, Division of Health Care Statistics. Data from the National Hospital Discharge Survey.

Table 92 (page 1 of 3). Rates of discharges and days of care in non-Federal short-stay hospitals, according to sex, age, and selected first-listed diagnoses: United States, 1985, 1990, 1995, and 1996

[Data are based on a sample of hospital records]

Sex, age, and first-listed diagnosis	Discharges				Days of care			
	1985[1]	1990	1995	1996	1985[1]	1990	1995	1996
Both sexes				Number per 1,000 population				
Total[2,3]	137.7	113.0	104.7	102.3	872.1	705.0	544.3	520.6
Male								
All ages[2,3]	124.4	100.9	92.3	89.7	848.2	690.4	533.1	511.8
Under 15 years[3]	64.4	49.2	46.6	42.0	289.9	234.1	212.8	193.2
Bronchitis	1.7	0.8	0.7	0.5	5.4	2.4	2.1	1.6
Pneumonia	5.7	6.3	7.8	6.0	23.6	26.3	28.1	21.8
Asthma	3.5	3.9	4.5	4.2	12.0	11.0	12.1	11.6
Injuries and poisoning	9.3	5.9	4.9	4.8	36.8	26.0	21.5	17.1
Fracture, all sites	3.2	2.0	1.6	1.7	16.7	7.9	7.6	6.1
15–44 years[3]	75.3	57.8	50.2	47.7	458.2	353.6	269.5	263.2
Psychoses	3.0	3.5	4.9	4.7	43.7	50.3	49.5	44.6
Diseases of heart	3.0	2.9	2.7	2.8	16.6	15.4	11.3	10.5
Intervertebral disc disorders	2.9	2.4	1.6	1.5	18.7	10.0	4.0	4.3
Injuries and poisoning	17.9	13.4	9.9	9.3	98.7	66.7	47.3	43.9
Fracture, all sites	5.2	4.1	3.3	3.1	34.6	22.9	17.9	15.0
45–64 years[3]	177.6	140.2	121.2	120.8	1,229.0	943.6	682.2	658.7
Malignant neoplasms	13.1	10.6	7.6	7.7	120.6	99.1	53.4	55.8
Trachea, bronchus, lung	3.6	2.7	1.5	1.4	31.9	19.1	10.2	9.7
Diabetes	3.4	2.9	3.4	3.2	26.5	21.2	22.3	24.4
Diseases of heart	36.9	31.7	29.7	30.5	239.2	185.0	143.7	139.3
Ischemic heart disease	27.1	22.6	21.3	21.8	171.1	128.2	99.0	97.7
Acute myocardial infarction	9.2	7.4	7.5	7.7	82.4	55.8	42.5	42.9
Congestive heart failure	2.5	3.0	2.9	3.2	18.9	19.7	16.3	18.5
Cerebrovascular diseases	5.0	4.1	3.8	4.1	51.0	40.7	25.7	25.1
Pneumonia	3.4	3.5	3.0	3.2	27.4	27.4	20.6	22.1
Injuries and poisoning	15.0	11.6	10.2	10.4	99.1	82.6	56.2	56.1
Fracture, all sites	4.0	3.3	2.9	2.9	29.9	24.2	18.4	15.9
65–74 years[3]	325.5	285.9	274.5	270.6	2,622.0	2,237.2	1,759.0	1,675.3
Malignant neoplasms	38.8	27.7	24.3	23.5	352.8	275.8	190.7	171.0
Large intestine and rectum	3.9	3.0	2.6	2.8	54.9	34.0	27.8	26.3
Trachea, bronchus, lung	10.8	6.3	5.2	4.7	89.5	55.4	39.8	33.6
Prostate	6.6	5.0	5.0	4.8	48.2	32.9	26.5	21.3
Diabetes	4.3	4.3	5.3	4.6	42.6	39.6	46.8	36.0
Diseases of heart	69.9	69.0	74.1	73.5	520.2	484.1	416.7	396.2
Ischemic heart disease	43.2	41.7	43.7	44.8	317.2	283.4	244.6	240.2
Acute myocardial infarction	17.6	13.9	15.4	16.4	160.4	121.7	101.7	105.1
Congestive heart failure	9.8	11.3	14.8	11.9	76.4	89.6	87.0	73.6
Cerebrovascular diseases	18.5	13.7	17.0	15.3	182.0	114.0	111.9	92.0
Pneumonia	10.9	11.3	12.6	13.0	104.9	107.1	86.8	89.2
Hyperplasia of prostate	13.5	14.3	7.5	5.0	84.8	64.6	22.4	14.6
Osteoarthritis	3.4	5.0	5.9	6.7	36.9	44.6	33.4	31.4
Injuries and poisoning	16.0	17.5	16.0	15.8	131.7	138.1	106.4	103.3
Fracture, all sites	4.5	4.5	4.4	3.5	42.8	45.6	32.1	25.6
Fracture of neck of femur (hip)	1.4	1.5	1.8	1.4	21.6	18.0	14.6	10.6
75 years and over[3]	529.1	476.3	472.8	476.6	4,682.0	4,211.9	3,248.8	3,160.4
Malignant neoplasms	55.7	40.8	30.1	28.0	545.9	406.4	250.2	199.5
Large intestine and rectum	6.9	5.4	4.9	4.2	84.7	80.3	52.9	41.0
Trachea, bronchus, lung	10.4	5.3	3.5	5.6	99.0	53.1	31.2	43.2
Prostate	15.3	9.7	4.3	3.5	116.5	65.3	17.5	13.9
Diabetes	6.4	4.6	6.9	6.7	66.6	50.9	41.9	55.6
Diseases of heart	108.6	105.7	113.4	114.3	841.2	851.7	674.6	616.5
Ischemic heart disease	51.3	48.9	51.6	53.2	413.2	396.2	320.6	299.4
Acute myocardial infarction	23.8	23.0	22.2	22.4	230.5	226.5	168.6	153.1
Congestive heart failure	27.8	30.9	31.2	31.4	220.5	241.2	192.6	172.0
Cerebrovascular diseases	37.9	30.0	31.9	33.4	380.7	296.9	214.4	228.3
Pneumonia	30.1	38.4	40.2	38.3	305.7	391.8	323.8	291.7
Hyperplasia of prostate	19.7	17.8	9.4	7.8	141.0	108.7	32.7	34.0
Osteoarthritis	4.4	5.7	6.5	7.7	49.4	60.4	54.1	43.9
Injuries and poisoning	31.8	31.1	32.5	33.2	358.8	339.7	222.6	239.2
Fracture, all sites	14.3	13.7	16.1	14.2	223.9	144.4	114.5	116.7
Fracture of neck of femur (hip)	8.4	8.5	9.0	9.2	161.3	97.4	68.6	77.3

See footnotes at end of table.

Table 92 (page 2 of 3). Rates of discharges and days of care in non-Federal short-stay hospitals, according to sex, age, and selected first-listed diagnoses: United States, 1985, 1990, 1995, and 1996

[Data are based on a sample of hospital records]

Sex, age, and first-listed diagnosis	Discharges				Days of care			
	1985[1]	1990	1995	1996	1985[1]	1990	1995	1996
Female	Number per 1,000 population							
All ages[2,3]	151.8	126.0	117.4	115.3	902.0	725.3	556.7	531.6
Under 15 years[3]	50.6	39.7	36.5	34.3	234.8	195.8	157.1	154.6
Bronchitis	1.2	0.7	0.4	0.4	3.6	3.0	1.2	1.2
Pneumonia	4.7	4.8	5.4	5.0	20.9	20.5	20.0	18.5
Asthma	2.1	2.3	2.8	2.5	7.5	7.2	7.8	6.4
Injuries and poisoning	6.1	3.9	3.4	2.9	23.0	15.1	12.1	12.4
Fracture, all sites	1.9	1.3	0.9	0.7	8.9	6.0	4.0	2.7
15–44 years[3]	173.5	144.7	129.0	126.1	744.8	575.4	421.8	404.4
Delivery	67.9	68.5	63.3	64.2	222.6	191.0	135.0	140.2
Psychoses	3.2	3.8	5.3	5.0	50.7	56.3	51.5	48.2
Diseases of heart	1.5	1.3	1.9	1.4	8.8	6.8	9.1	6.2
Intervertebral disc disorders	1.8	1.4	1.1	1.1	13.5	6.8	2.9	3.2
Injuries and poisoning	9.2	6.9	5.8	5.3	48.0	36.5	24.8	20.1
Fracture, all sites	1.9	1.6	1.4	1.3	13.8	10.8	5.9	5.5
45–64 years[3]	164.6	130.2	115.4	113.8	1,176.5	881.9	630.9	592.0
Malignant neoplasms	15.4	12.6	9.6	9.0	128.8	106.8	60.5	53.3
Trachea, bronchus, lung	2.4	1.7	1.5	1.3	22.3	14.7	8.0	7.9
Breast	3.9	2.8	2.1	1.9	25.2	12.0	7.5	5.3
Diabetes	3.8	2.9	3.2	2.8	31.6	25.7	19.3	17.8
Diseases of heart	18.0	16.5	14.9	16.4	121.4	100.5	70.5	75.8
Ischemic heart disease	10.6	9.9	8.3	9.7	71.1	57.1	37.8	40.9
Acute myocardial infarction	3.0	2.8	2.5	2.9	33.5	21.5	15.0	16.6
Congestive heart failure	1.8	2.1	2.5	2.5	12.7	15.8	14.4	14.4
Cerebrovascular diseases	3.7	3.0	3.2	2.9	44.9	31.9	21.3	21.9
Pneumonia	3.3	3.3	3.3	3.4	29.2	26.4	21.8	20.9
Injuries and poisoning	12.2	9.4	8.4	7.8	82.4	62.9	45.1	39.8
Fracture, all sites	4.1	3.1	2.7	2.8	30.0	24.8	14.0	13.7
65–74 years[3]	275.5	238.2	244.0	246.6	2,294.9	1,935.3	1,597.0	1,546.3
Malignant neoplasms	29.1	20.6	20.1	19.8	274.8	187.5	146.9	133.9
Large intestine and rectum	3.2	2.4	2.2	2.4	41.8	34.5	19.7	22.4
Trachea, bronchus, lung	3.6	2.6	2.8	3.0	34.9	26.6	25.0	22.2
Breast	5.1	3.9	3.2	3.3	44.6	17.4	9.9	9.6
Diabetes	6.8	5.8	4.7	6.0	65.5	46.3	35.8	38.2
Diseases of heart	49.4	44.6	47.8	53.4	375.1	313.1	273.6	298.5
Ischemic heart disease	27.5	24.1	24.0	27.0	205.1	151.9	133.8	148.9
Acute myocardial infarction	8.6	7.4	7.9	9.0	88.7	57.3	57.9	57.1
Congestive heart failure	8.2	9.1	10.2	11.2	67.9	80.8	66.8	72.6
Cerebrovascular diseases	15.0	11.2	10.4	12.0	155.1	94.8	71.1	76.9
Pneumonia	7.0	8.6	10.5	10.8	65.2	80.8	79.2	79.5
Osteoarthritis	4.3	6.8	8.5	9.5	45.2	68.1	48.4	47.7
Injuries and poisoning	19.7	17.6	17.9	20.2	178.8	164.2	112.5	135.3
Fracture, all sites	9.3	8.3	7.0	9.7	97.7	96.2	43.4	61.6
Fracture of neck of femur (hip)	3.5	3.5	2.8	4.7	48.0	58.8	21.2	34.4

See footnotes at end of table.

Table 92 (page 3 of 3). Rates of discharges and days of care in non-Federal short-stay hospitals, according to sex, age, and selected first-listed diagnoses: United States, 1985, 1990, 1995, and 1996

[Data are based on a sample of hospital records]

Sex, age, and first-listed diagnosis	Discharges				Days of care			
	1985[1]	1990	1995	1996	1985[1]	1990	1995	1996
Female—Con.	Number per 1,000 population							
75 years and over[3]	446.8	404.6	445.1	442.8	4,219.1	3,838.9	3,203.8	3,025.3
Malignant neoplasms	26.1	21.8	20.3	18.8	282.9	254.1	173.3	148.7
Large intestine and rectum	5.3	4.6	3.6	3.8	69.3	68.9	48.0	43.4
Trachea, bronchus, lung	1.8	2.1	1.8	2.2	24.9	20.3	16.0	16.6
Breast	4.1	3.8	3.0	2.2	37.0	21.7	8.9	6.6
Diabetes	6.6	4.6	6.2	6.3	69.7	54.6	43.5	40.8
Diseases of heart	91.6	83.5	95.1	95.7	773.1	664.4	594.6	576.8
Ischemic heart disease	40.9	33.3	36.8	36.8	341.4	250.0	218.4	220.0
Acute myocardial infarction	17.0	12.9	15.0	15.2	170.3	124.3	114.7	112.6
Congestive heart failure	24.5	27.6	31.9	30.8	208.3	233.7	221.5	198.3
Cerebrovascular diseases	33.7	29.2	30.0	30.0	368.1	298.3	205.2	207.6
Pneumonia	18.4	23.6	27.7	28.1	184.8	256.9	224.8	199.5
Osteoarthritis	4.8	5.2	8.7	9.9	64.4	53.4	57.9	56.2
Injuries and poisoning	47.8	45.8	47.7	47.0	541.4	483.2	368.7	315.0
Fracture, all sites	31.9	31.1	31.2	32.6	402.9	348.4	248.7	226.8
Fracture of neck of femur (hip)	18.9	18.6	19.3	21.3	270.8	233.4	169.5	156.6

[1]Comparisons of data from 1985 with data from later years should be made with caution as estimates of change may reflect improvements in the design (see Appendix I) rather than true changes in hospital use.
[2]Age adjusted. See Appendix II for age-adjustment procedure.
[3]Includes discharges with first-listed diagnoses not shown in table.

NOTES: Excludes newborn infants. Rates are based on the civilian population as of July 1. Diagnostic categories are based on the *International Classification of Diseases, Ninth Revision, Clinical Modification*. For a listing of the code numbers, see Appendix II, table VII.

SOURCE: Centers for Disease Control and Prevention, National Center for Health Statistics, Division of Health Care Statistics. Data computed by the Division of Health and Utilization Analysis from the National Hospital Discharge Survey.

Table 93 (page 1 of 3). Discharges and average length of stay in non-Federal short-stay hospitals, according to sex, age, and selected first-listed diagnoses: United States, 1985, 1990, 1995, and 1996

[Data are based on a sample of hospital records]

Sex, age, and first-listed diagnosis	Discharges				Average length of stay			
	1985[1]	1990	1995	1996	1985[1]	1990	1995	1996
Both sexes	Number in thousands				Number of days			
Total[2,3]	35,056	30,788	30,722	30,545	6.3	6.2	5.2	5.1
Male								
All ages[2,3]	14,160	12,280	12,198	12,110	6.8	6.8	5.8	5.7
Under 15 years[3]	1,698	1,362	1,377	1,240	4.5	4.8	4.6	4.6
Bronchitis	45	22	21	15	3.2	3.1	3.0	3.2
Pneumonia	150	174	231	178	4.2	4.2	3.6	3.6
Asthma	93	107	134	123	3.4	2.8	2.7	2.8
Injuries and poisoning	245	164	144	142	4.0	4.4	4.4	3.6
Fracture, all sites	85	54	47	51	5.2	4.0	4.8	3.6
15–44 years[3]	4,153	3,330	2,949	2,831	6.1	6.1	5.4	5.5
Psychoses	167	200	287	277	14.4	14.5	10.1	9.5
Diseases of heart	165	166	159	166	5.5	5.3	4.2	3.7
Intervertebral disc disorders	161	138	95	90	6.4	4.2	2.5	2.8
Injuries and poisoning	988	772	581	550	5.5	5.0	4.8	4.7
Fracture, all sites	290	238	195	185	6.6	5.5	5.4	4.8
45–64 years[3]	3,776	3,115	3,053	3,138	6.9	6.7	5.6	5.5
Malignant neoplasms	279	235	191	200	9.2	9.4	7.0	7.3
Trachea, bronchus, lung	76	60	37	36	8.9	7.1	6.9	6.9
Diabetes	71	65	86	83	7.9	7.3	6.5	7.6
Diseases of heart	784	704	749	793	6.5	5.8	4.8	4.6
Ischemic heart disease	577	502	537	567	6.3	5.7	4.6	4.5
Acute myocardial infarction	197	165	188	200	8.9	7.5	5.7	5.6
Congestive heart failure	53	66	73	84	7.6	6.7	5.6	5.7
Cerebrovascular diseases	107	91	96	105	10.2	10.0	6.8	6.2
Pneumonia	73	77	75	82	8.0	7.9	6.9	7.0
Injuries and poisoning	320	257	257	269	6.6	7.2	5.5	5.4
Fracture, all sites	85	74	74	76	7.5	7.2	6.3	5.4
65–74 years[3]	2,389	2,268	2,290	2,253	8.1	7.8	6.4	6.2
Malignant neoplasms	284	220	203	196	9.1	9.9	7.8	7.3
Large intestine and rectum	29	24	22	23	14.0	11.4	10.7	9.4
Trachea, bronchus, lung	79	50	44	39	8.3	8.7	7.6	7.2
Prostate	49	40	41	40	7.3	6.5	5.3	4.4
Diabetes	31	34	44	38	9.9	9.1	8.8	7.8
Diseases of heart	513	547	618	612	7.4	7.0	5.6	5.4
Ischemic heart disease	317	331	365	373	7.3	6.8	5.6	5.4
Acute myocardial infarction	129	110	129	137	9.1	8.8	6.6	6.4
Congestive heart failure	72	90	123	99	7.8	7.9	5.9	6.2
Cerebrovascular diseases	136	108	141	127	9.8	8.3	6.6	6.0
Pneumonia	80	90	105	108	9.6	9.5	6.9	6.9
Hyperplasia of prostate	99	113	62	42	6.3	4.5	3.0	2.9
Osteoarthritis	25	39	49	56	10.9	9.0	5.7	4.7
Injuries and poisoning	118	139	133	132	8.2	7.9	6.7	6.5
Fracture, all sites	33	36	36	29	9.5	10.2	7.4	7.2
Fracture of neck of femur (hip)	10	12	15	12	15.2	11.8	8.1	7.6
75 years and over[3]	2,144	2,203	2,528	2,648	8.8	8.8	6.9	6.6
Malignant neoplasms	226	189	161	155	9.8	10.0	8.3	7.1
Large intestine and rectum	28	25	26	23	12.3	15.0	10.8	9.8
Trachea, bronchus, lung	42	25	19	31	9.5	10.0	8.9	7.8
Prostate	62	45	23	20	7.6	6.8	4.1	4.0
Diabetes	26	21	37	37	10.5	11.0	6.1	8.3
Diseases of heart	440	489	606	635	7.7	8.1	5.9	5.4
Ischemic heart disease	208	226	276	296	8.1	8.1	6.2	5.6
Acute myocardial infarction	97	106	119	125	9.7	9.9	7.6	6.8
Congestive heart failure	113	143	167	174	7.9	7.8	6.2	5.5
Cerebrovascular diseases	154	139	171	186	10.0	9.9	6.7	6.8
Pneumonia	122	178	215	213	10.2	10.2	8.0	7.6
Hyperplasia of prostate	80	82	50	43	7.2	6.1	3.5	4.4
Osteoarthritis	18	27	35	43	11.3	10.5	8.3	5.7
Injuries and poisoning	129	144	174	184	11.3	10.9	6.8	7.2
Fracture, all sites	58	63	86	79	15.6	10.6	7.1	8.2
Fracture of neck of femur (hip)	34	39	48	51	19.2	11.5	7.7	8.4

See footnotes at end of table.

Table 93 (page 2 of 3). Discharges and average length of stay in non-Federal short-stay hospitals, according to sex, age, and selected first-listed diagnoses: United States, 1985, 1990, 1995, and 1996

[Data are based on a sample of hospital records]

Sex, age, and first-listed diagnosis	Discharges				Average length of stay			
	1985[1]	1990	1995	1996	1985[1]	1990	1995	1996
Female	Number in thousands				Number of days			
All ages[2,3]	20,896	18,508	18,525	18,435	5.9	5.8	4.7	4.6
Under 15 years[3]	1,274	1,049	1,028	967	4.6	4.9	4.3	4.5
Bronchitis	30	19	13	11	3.0	4.0	2.7	2.9
Pneumonia	119	125	152	142	4.4	4.3	3.7	3.7
Asthma	52	62	78	72	3.6	3.1	2.8	2.5
Injuries and poisoning	153	102	97	81	3.8	3.9	3.5	4.3
Fracture, all sites	47	33	27	21	4.8	4.8	4.2	3.6
15–44 years[3]	9,813	8,469	7,644	7,495	4.3	4.0	3.3	3.2
Delivery	3,838	4,008	3,752	3,817	3.3	2.8	2.1	2.2
Psychoses	180	222	316	299	15.9	14.9	9.7	9.6
Diseases of heart	85	73	110	86	5.8	5.4	4.9	4.3
Intervertebral disc disorders	104	85	63	66	7.4	4.7	2.7	2.9
Injuries and poisoning	521	402	344	315	5.2	5.3	4.3	3.8
Fracture, all sites	108	93	84	78	7.2	6.8	4.2	4.2
45–64 years[3]	3,834	3,129	3,115	3,156	7.1	6.8	5.5	5.2
Malignant neoplasms	359	303	258	249	8.4	8.5	6.3	5.9
Trachea, bronchus, lung	56	41	39	36	9.3	8.6	5.5	6.0
Breast	91	67	56	54	6.5	4.3	3.6	2.7
Diabetes	88	70	86	78	8.3	8.9	6.0	6.3
Diseases of heart	420	397	403	455	6.7	6.1	4.7	4.6
Ischemic heart disease	248	237	225	268	6.7	5.8	4.5	4.2
Acute myocardial infarction	71	68	68	82	11.0	7.6	6.0	5.7
Congestive heart failure	43	51	68	69	6.9	7.4	5.7	5.8
Cerebrovascular diseases	85	72	86	82	12.2	10.7	6.7	7.5
Pneumonia	76	80	88	93	8.9	7.9	6.7	6.2
Injuries and poisoning	283	225	225	215	6.8	6.7	5.4	5.1
Fracture, all sites	96	75	72	78	7.3	7.9	5.2	4.9
65–74 years[3]	2,623	2,421	2,542	2,551	8.3	8.1	6.5	6.3
Malignant neoplasms	277	210	209	205	9.4	9.1	7.3	6.8
Large intestine and rectum	31	24	23	25	13.0	14.5	8.8	9.3
Trachea, bronchus, lung	35	26	29	31	9.6	10.2	8.9	7.3
Breast	49	40	33	34	8.7	4.5	3.1	2.9
Diabetes	64	59	49	62	9.7	8.0	7.7	6.4
Diseases of heart	470	453	497	553	7.6	7.0	5.7	5.6
Ischemic heart disease	262	245	250	280	7.5	6.3	5.6	5.5
Acute myocardial infarction	82	75	82	93	10.3	7.8	7.4	6.4
Congestive heart failure	78	92	106	116	8.3	8.9	6.5	6.5
Cerebrovascular diseases	143	114	109	125	10.3	8.5	6.8	6.4
Pneumonia	66	87	109	111	9.4	9.4	7.6	7.4
Osteoarthritis	40	69	89	98	10.6	10.0	5.7	5.0
Injuries and poisoning	188	179	187	209	9.1	9.3	6.3	6.7
Fracture, all sites	88	85	72	100	10.6	11.5	6.2	6.4
Fracture of neck of femur (hip)	33	36	29	49	13.9	16.7	7.5	7.3

See footnotes at end of table.

Table 93 (page 3 of 3). Discharges and average length of stay in non-Federal short-stay hospitals, according to sex, age, and selected first-listed diagnoses: United States, 1985, 1990, 1995, and 1996

[Data are based on a sample of hospital records]

Sex, age, and first-listed diagnosis	Discharges				Average length of stay			
	1985[1]	1990	1995	1996	1985[1]	1990	1995	1996
Female—Con.	Number in thousands				Number of days			
75 years and over[3]	3,352	3,440	4,196	4,266	9.4	9.5	7.2	6.8
Malignant neoplasms	196	185	191	181	10.8	11.7	8.5	7.9
Large intestine and rectum	40	39	34	37	13.1	15.1	13.3	11.3
Trachea, bronchus, lung	13	18	17	21	13.9	9.9	8.7	7.6
Breast	31	33	29	21	9.1	5.7	2.9	3.0
Diabetes	49	39	58	60	10.6	11.9	7.1	6.5
Diseases of heart	688	711	896	922	8.4	8.0	6.3	6.0
Ischemic heart disease	307	283	347	354	8.3	7.5	5.9	6.0
Acute myocardial infarction	127	110	142	146	10.0	9.6	7.6	7.4
Congestive heart failure	184	235	301	296	8.5	8.5	6.9	6.4
Cerebrovascular diseases	253	249	283	289	10.9	10.2	6.8	6.9
Pneumonia	138	201	261	270	10.1	10.9	8.1	7.1
Osteoarthritis	36	45	82	95	13.5	10.2	6.6	5.7
Injuries and poisoning	358	389	449	453	11.3	10.6	7.7	6.7
Fracture, all sites	240	265	294	314	12.6	11.2	8.0	7.0
Fracture of neck of femur (hip)	142	158	182	205	14.3	12.5	8.8	7.4

[1]Comparisons of data from 1985 with data from later years should be made with caution as estimates of change may reflect improvements in the design (see Appendix I) rather than true changes in hospital use.
[2]Average length of stay is age-adjusted. See Appendix II for age-adjustment procedure.
[3]Includes discharges with first-listed diagnoses not shown in table.

NOTES: Excludes newborn infants. Diagnostic categories are based on the *International Classification of Diseases, Ninth Revision, Clinical Modification*. For a listing of the code numbers, see Appendix II, table VII.

SOURCE: Centers for Disease Control and Prevention, National Center for Health Statistics, Division of Health Care Statistics. Data computed by the Division of Health and Utilization Analysis from the National Hospital Discharge Survey.

Table 94 (page 1 of 2). Ambulatory and inpatient procedures among males according to place, age, and type of procedure: United States, 1994, 1995, and 1996

[Data are based on a sample of inpatient and ambulatory surgery records]

Age and procedure category	Procedures per 1,000 population								
	Total			Ambulatory[1]			Inpatient[2]		
	1994	1995	1996	1994	1995	1996	1994	1995	1996
Both sexes, age adjusted[3]	239.2	239.1	244.8	98.8	103.3	109.0	140.5	135.8	135.8
Male, age adjusted[3]	214.7	215.6	222.3	93.5	97.8	104.0	121.2	117.8	118.3
Under 15 years[4]	85.3	85.2	86.3	48.7	45.9	48.0	36.6	39.3	38.3
Myringotomy with insertion of tube	11.6	10.8	10.5	11.0	10.3	10.1	0.5	0.4	0.4
Tonsillectomy, with or without adenoidectomy	4.6	5.3	4.6	4.1	4.8	4.2	0.5	0.5	0.4
Reduction of fracture	2.2	1.8	2.3	0.9	0.8	1.1	1.3	1.0	1.3
15–44 years[4]	119.9	118.9	119.4	57.9	60.3	62.4	62.1	58.6	57.0
Cardiac catheterization	1.5	1.4	1.7	0.5	*0.3	0.5	1.1	1.1	1.1
Endoscopy of small or large intestine with or without biopsy	6.8	6.7	7.0	4.9	4.9	5.5	1.9	1.7	1.5
Cholecystectomy	0.7	0.8	0.8	*0.2	*0.3	0.4	0.5	0.5	0.4
Reduction of fracture	3.6	3.7	3.9	1.1	1.1	1.5	2.5	2.5	2.5
Arthroscopy of the knee	4.2	4.3	3.6	3.6	4.0	3.4	0.5	0.4	0.2
Excision or destruction of intervertebral disc	1.7	1.6	1.6	*	*	*0.2	1.5	1.4	1.3
Angiocardiography with contrast material	2.3	2.1	2.2	0.7	0.4	0.6	1.6	1.7	1.6
45–64 years[4]	321.7	327.4	341.8	132.7	146.7	155.9	189.0	180.7	185.9
Coronary angioplasty	5.9	5.8	6.7	*	*	*	5.6	5.6	6.4
Coronary artery bypass graft[5]	6.7	7.6	7.2	–	–	–	6.7	7.6	7.2
Cardiac catheterization	14.9	15.5	18.1	3.3	3.8	5.4	11.7	11.7	12.7
Endoscopy of small or large intestine with or without biopsy	27.4	27.7	28.3	20.2	21.1	21.8	7.2	6.5	6.4
Cholecystectomy	2.6	2.6	3.2	*0.5	*0.7	1.1	2.1	1.8	2.1
Prostatectomy	2.7	2.5	2.1	*	*	*	2.5	2.2	1.9
Reduction of fracture	2.9	3.1	2.8	*0.6	*0.8	0.8	2.3	2.3	2.0
Arthroscopy of the knee	3.9	4.6	4.6	3.7	4.5	4.4	*0.3	*	*
Excision or destruction of intervertebral disc	2.8	2.3	3.0	*	*	*	2.6	2.2	2.6
Angiocardiography with contrast material	20.6	20.8	24.2	4.6	5.1	6.4	16.0	15.8	17.7
65–74 years[4]	693.7	697.7	729.6	269.9	280.8	314.5	423.8	416.9	415.1
Coronary angioplasty	10.1	9.8	12.4	*	*	*	9.9	9.3	11.6
Extraction of lens	32.5	34.1	37.2	31.4	33.2	36.7	*	*	*
Insertion of prosthetic lens (pseudophakos)	26.7	26.7	30.0	25.6	25.8	29.4	*	*	*
Coronary artery bypass graft[5]	15.3	18.1	19.1	–	–	–	15.3	18.1	19.1
Cardiac catheterization	27.9	30.5	33.1	5.7	7.1	10.2	22.2	23.4	22.9
Pacemaker insertion or replacement	5.7	5.0	6.3	*	*	*	5.6	4.7	5.7
Carotid endarterectomy	3.2	4.2	3.9	*	–	*	3.2	4.2	3.9
Endoscopy of small or large intestine with or without biopsy	60.6	58.9	56.5	42.4	42.5	40.0	18.2	16.4	16.5
Cholecystectomy	5.0	5.3	4.9	*	*	*	4.4	4.4	3.9
Prostatectomy	14.9	13.2	11.7	*	*	*1.5	14.1	12.3	10.2
Reduction of fracture	3.3	2.8	3.1	*	*	*	2.7	2.4	2.4
Total hip replacement	1.6	2.5	2.3	–	–	–	1.6	2.5	2.3
Angiocardiography with contrast material	39.8	39.5	43.0	9.0	9.2	13.4	30.8	30.3	29.5

See footnotes at end of table.

Table 94 (page 2 of 2). Ambulatory and inpatient procedures among males according to place, age, and type of procedure: United States, 1994, 1995, and 1996

[Data are based on a sample of inpatient and ambulatory surgery records]

	Procedures per 1,000 population								
	Total			Ambulatory[1]			Inpatient[2]		
Age and procedure category	1994	1995	1996	1994	1995	1996	1994	1995	1996
75 years and over[4]	919.6	918.6	953.9	337.9	353.7	377.2	581.8	564.9	576.7
Coronary angioplasty	6.6	8.1	8.5	*	–	*	6.4	8.1	7.4
Extraction of lens	62.6	73.0	72.1	61.5	71.3	71.3	*	*	*
Insertion of prosthetic lens (pseudophakos)	48.8	55.0	55.5	47.7	53.4	54.9	*	*	*
Coronary artery bypass graft[5]	10.7	12.5	11.5	–	–	–	10.7	12.5	11.5
Cardiac catheterization	21.8	23.8	26.6	*3.8	4.7	7.0	18.0	19.1	19.6
Pacemaker insertion or replacement	16.0	16.3	18.1	*	*	*	15.3	15.3	16.3
Carotid endarterectomy	3.6	4.6	4.6	*	–	–	3.6	4.6	4.6
Endoscopy of small or large intestine with or without biopsy	78.7	79.4	83.8	43.0	43.2	48.7	35.7	36.2	35.1
Cholecystectomy	6.5	6.5	6.7	*	*	*	6.2	5.5	5.7
Prostatectomy	18.1	17.4	14.5	*2.1	*2.2	*2.2	16.1	15.2	12.3
Reduction of fracture	6.5	6.9	6.8	*	*	*	6.4	6.3	6.5
Total hip replacement	2.2	2.1	2.2	–	–	–	2.2	2.1	2.2
Angiocardiography with contrast material	27.9	29.4	36.0	*3.8	5.5	10.3	24.1	23.9	25.8

* Rates for all places or inpatient hospitals based on fewer than 5,000 estimated procedures are unreliable and are not shown; those based on 5,000–9,999 estimated procedures are preceded by an asterisk and may have low reliability. Rates for ambulatory surgery based on fewer than 10,000 estimated procedures are unreliable and are not shown; those based on 10,000–19,999 estimated procedures are preceded by an asterisk.

– Quantity zero.

[1]Data are from the National Survey of Ambulatory Surgery and exclude ambulatory surgery procedures for patients who became inpatients. See Appendix II, Ambulatory surgery.

[2]Data are from the National Hospital Discharge Survey and exclude newborn infants.

[3]See Appendix II for age-adjustment procedure.

[4]Includes procedures not listed in table.

[5]Data in the main body of the table are for all-listed coronary artery bypass grafts. Often, more than one coronary bypass procedure is performed during a single operation. The following table gives information based on the number of inpatient discharges with one or more coronary artery bypass grafts.

Sex and age	1994	1995	1996
	Inpatient discharges per 1,000 population		
Males:			
45–64 years	4.1	4.5	4.2
65–74 years	9.3	11.2	11.4
75 years and over	7.6	8.9	7.6

NOTES: Data in this table are for up to four procedures for inpatients and for up to six procedures for ambulatory surgery patients. See Appendix II, Procedure. Procedure categories are based on the International Classification of Diseases, Ninth Revision, Clinical Modification. For a listing of the code numbers, see Appendix II, table VIII. Rates are based on the civilian population as of July 1.

SOURCES: Centers for Disease Control and Prevention, National Center for Health Statistics, Division of Health Care Statistics. Data computed by the Division of Health and Utilization Analysis from the National Hospital Discharge Survey and the National Survey of Ambulatory Surgery.

Table 95 (page 1 of 2). Ambulatory and inpatient procedures among females according to place, age, and type of procedure: United States, 1994, 1995, and 1996

[Data are based on a sample of inpatient and ambulatory surgery records]

	Procedures per 1,000 population								
	Total			Ambulatory[1]			Inpatient[2]		
Age and procedure category	1994	1995	1996	1994	1995	1996	1994	1995	1996
Both sexes, age adjusted[3]	239.2	239.1	244.8	98.8	103.3	109.0	140.5	135.8	135.8
Female, age adjusted[3]	265.8	264.3	269.4	104.5	109.1	114.4	161.2	155.2	155.0
Under 15 years[4]	64.0	64.5	63.2	35.0	33.9	34.2	29.0	30.5	29.0
Myringotomy with insertion of tube	8.6	8.0	7.1	8.2	7.6	6.8	0.4	*0.3	*0.3
Tonsillectomy, with or without adenoidectomy	5.4	5.3	5.3	4.9	4.8	4.9	0.5	0.4	0.4
Reduction of fracture	1.2	1.3	1.3	*0.6	0.7	0.8	0.7	0.6	0.5
15–44 years[4]	290.7	282.8	287.4	92.0	93.7	98.6	198.7	189.2	188.9
Cardiac catheterization	0.6	0.6	0.6	*	*0.2	*0.2	0.4	0.4	0.4
Endoscopy of small or large intestine with or without biopsy	8.3	8.8	9.8	6.3	7.1	7.9	1.9	1.8	1.8
Cholecystectomy	3.5	4.0	4.0	1.4	1.7	2.1	2.1	2.3	1.9
Bilateral destruction or occlusion of fallopian tubes	11.3	11.5	11.0	5.2	6.0	5.3	6.1	5.5	5.7
Hysterectomy	5.2	5.7	5.4	*	*0.3	*0.2	5.0	5.5	5.2
Cesarean section[5]	14.5	13.2	14.0	–	–	–	14.5	13.2	14.0
Repair of current obstetrical laceration	15.3	16.2	17.8	*	*	*	15.3	16.2	17.8
Reduction of fracture	1.5	1.7	1.6	0.4	0.5	0.5	1.1	1.2	1.1
Arthroscopy of the knee	2.1	2.2	2.2	1.9	2.1	2.0	0.2	*0.1	*0.1
Excision or destruction of intervertebral disc	1.2	0.9	1.0	*	*	*	1.1	0.8	0.9
Lumpectomy	2.5	2.0	2.1	2.4	1.9	2.1	*0.1	*0.1	*
Mastectomy	0.3	0.3	0.2	*	*	*	0.2	0.2	0.2
45–64 years[4]	327.1	326.7	333.7	154.7	165.0	172.3	172.4	161.7	161.4
Coronary angioplasty	2.1	2.1	2.3	*	*	*	2.1	2.0	2.0
Coronary artery bypass graft[6]	2.0	1.7	2.0	–	–	–	2.0	1.7	2.0
Cardiac catheterization	8.2	7.4	8.4	2.2	2.0	2.4	6.0	5.3	6.0
Endoscopy of small or large intestine with or without biopsy	28.5	30.3	28.3	22.0	24.2	22.8	6.5	6.2	5.5
Cholecystectomy	5.5	5.8	6.7	1.8	2.3	3.3	3.7	3.5	3.4
Hysterectomy	7.4	7.3	8.1	*	*	*	7.1	7.1	7.8
Reduction of fracture	2.8	2.9	3.1	*0.7	*0.7	0.8	2.2	2.2	2.3
Arthroscopy of the knee	2.9	3.5	3.6	2.8	3.4	3.5	*	*	*
Excision or destruction of intervertebral disc	2.1	1.7	2.0	*	*	*	2.0	1.6	1.8
Lumpectomy	5.4	5.4	4.9	4.9	5.0	4.5	0.5	0.4	*0.4
Mastectomy	1.8	1.8	1.7	*	*	*0.4	1.6	1.5	1.3
Angiocardiography with contrast material	11.5	10.8	11.7	3.0	2.7	3.3	8.5	8.1	8.4
65–74 years[4]	576.0	591.6	618.8	251.5	269.3	288.4	324.4	322.3	330.4
Coronary angioplasty	5.0	4.7	5.9	*	*	*	4.8	4.6	5.6
Extraction of lens	42.4	48.6	47.7	41.3	47.7	47.2	*	*	*
Insertion of prosthetic lens (pseudophakos)	34.1	36.1	35.9	33.1	35.3	35.4	*	*	*
Coronary artery bypass graft[6]	5.0	6.1	6.6	–	*	–	5.0	6.1	6.6
Cardiac catheterization	15.8	15.8	19.9	3.3	3.6	5.4	12.5	12.2	14.6
Pacemaker insertion or replacement	4.5	3.9	3.8	*	*	*	4.2	3.8	3.6
Carotid endarterectomy	1.7	2.3	2.1	–	–	–	1.7	2.3	2.1
Endoscopy of small or large intestine with or without biopsy	54.5	58.5	59.4	38.6	40.6	44.9	15.9	17.9	14.5
Cholecystectomy	6.4	6.1	6.9	*1.3	*1.6	2.3	5.1	4.5	4.6
Hysterectomy	4.7	4.3	3.8	*	*	*	4.6	4.3	3.7
Reduction of fracture	5.3	5.1	5.9	*	*	*	4.6	4.3	5.0
Total hip replacement	2.6	2.6	2.9	–	–	*	2.6	2.6	2.8
Lumpectomy	4.8	5.1	5.5	4.4	4.6	4.9	*	*	*0.6
Mastectomy	3.0	2.7	2.7	*	*	*	2.7	2.3	2.3
Angiocardiography with contrast material	22.6	22.3	26.9	4.8	4.9	6.8	17.8	17.3	20.1

See footnotes at end of table.

Table 95 (page 2 of 2). Ambulatory and inpatient procedures among females according to place, age, and type of procedure: United States, 1994, 1995, and 1996

[Data are based on a sample of inpatient and ambulatory surgery records]

	Procedures per 1,000 population								
	Total			Ambulatory[1]			Inpatient[2]		
Age and procedure category	1994	1995	1996	1994	1995	1996	1994	1995	1996
75 years and over[4]	742.5	764.0	779.1	271.1	301.2	315.8	471.4	462.8	463.3
Coronary angioplasty	4.0	4.3	4.8	*	*	*	3.9	4.2	4.3
Extraction of lens	72.1	83.4	82.4	69.8	81.1	81.7	*	*	*
Insertion of prosthetic lens (pseudophakos)	56.1	62.8	61.4	53.9	60.6	60.7	*	*	*
Coronary artery bypass graft[6]	3.3	4.1	4.6	–	–	–	3.3	4.1	4.6
Cardiac catheterization	11.8	12.9	15.0	*1.5	*1.8	3.5	10.3	11.1	11.5
Pacemaker insertion or replacement	11.9	10.6	12.3	*	*	*1.1	11.4	10.0	11.2
Carotid endarterectomy	2.0	2.0	2.3	–	*	–	2.0	2.0	2.3
Endoscopy of small or large intestine with or without biopsy . . .	69.7	73.4	71.0	34.1	38.8	38.2	35.6	34.6	32.8
Cholecystectomy	4.9	6.4	6.1	*	*	*1.2	4.2	5.5	5.0
Hysterectomy	2.4	2.4	2.8	–	*	*	2.4	2.4	2.6
Reduction of fracture	14.6	15.5	17.3	*	*	*	13.8	14.5	16.7
Total hip replacement	3.2	3.3	3.6	*	*	*	3.2	3.3	3.5
Lumpectomy	3.2	3.2	3.2	2.7	2.5	2.8	*	*0.7	*
Mastectomy	2.6	2.9	2.1	*	*	*	2.4	2.5	1.8
Angiocardiography with contrast material	16.6	17.5	20.8	2.3	*2.1	5.4	14.4	15.4	15.4

* Rates for all places or inpatient hospitals based on fewer than 5,000 estimated procedures are unreliable and are not shown; those based on 5,000–9,999 estimated procedures are preceded by an asterisk and may have low reliability. Rates for ambulatory surgery based on fewer than 10,000 estimated procedures are unreliable and are not shown; those based on 10,000–19,999 estimated procedures are preceded by an asterisk.
– Quantity zero.
[1]Data are from the National Survey of Ambulatory Surgery and exclude ambulatory surgery procedures for patients who became inpatients. See Appendix II, Ambulatory surgery.
[2]Data are from the National Hospital Discharge Survey and exclude newborn infants.
[3]See Appendix II for age-adjustment procedure.
[4]Includes procedures not listed in table.
[5]Cesarean sections accounted for 22.0 percent of deliveries in 1994, 20.8 percent in 1995, and 21.8 percent in 1996.
[6]Data in the main body of the table are for all-listed coronary artery bypass grafts. Often, more than one coronary bypass procedure is performed during a single operation. The following table gives information based on the number of inpatient discharges with one or more coronary artery bypass grafts.

Sex and age	1994	1995	1996
	Inpatient discharges per 1,000 population		
Female:			
45–64 years	1.3	1.0	1.2
65–74 years	3.3	3.8	4.1
75 years and over	2.3	3.0	3.3

NOTES: Data in this table are for up to four procedures for inpatients and for up to six procedures for ambulatory surgery patients. See Appendix II, Procedure. Procedure categories are based on the *International Classification of Diseases, Ninth Revision, Clinical Modification*. For a listing of the code numbers, see Appendix II, table VIII. Rates are based on the civilian population as of July 1.

SOURCES: Centers for Disease Control and Prevention, National Center for Health Statistics, Division of Health Care Statistics. Data computed by the Division of Health and Utilization Analysis from the National Hospital Discharge Survey and the National Survey of Ambulatory Surgery.

Table 96. Hospital admissions, average length of stay, and outpatient visits, according to type of ownership and size of hospital, and percent outpatient surgery: United States, selected years 1975–97

[Data are based on reporting by a census of hospitals]

Type of ownership and size of hospital	1975	1980	1985	1990	1994	1995	1996	1997
Admissions				Number in thousands				
All hospitals	36,157	38,892	36,304	33,774	33,125	33,282	33,307	33,624
Federal	1,913	2,044	2,103	1,759	1,588	1,559	1,422	1,249
Non-Federal[1]	34,243	36,848	34,201	32,015	31,538	31,723	31,885	32,375
Community[2]	33,435	36,143	33,449	31,181	30,718	30,945	31,099	31,577
Nonprofit	23,722	25,566	24,179	22,878	22,704	22,557	22,542	22,905
For profit	2,646	3,165	3,242	3,066	3,035	3,428	3,684	3,953
State-local government	7,067	7,413	6,028	5,236	4,979	4,961	4,873	4,720
6–24 beds	174	159	102	95	98	124	117	139
25–49 beds	1,431	1,254	1,009	870	881	944	925	933
50–99 beds	3,675	3,700	2,953	2,474	2,212	2,299	2,280	2,311
100–199 beds	7,017	7,162	6,487	5,833	5,983	6,288	6,456	6,416
200–299 beds	6,174	6,596	6,371	6,333	6,501	6,495	6,426	6,352
300–399 beds	4,739	5,358	5,401	5,091	4,843	4,693	4,856	5,099
400–499 beds	3,689	4,401	3,723	3,644	3,505	3,413	3,481	3,360
500 beds or more	6,537	7,513	7,401	6,840	6,695	6,690	6,558	6,967
Average length of stay				Number of days				
All hospitals	11.4	9.9	9.1	9.1	8.2	7.8	7.5	7.3
Federal	20.3	16.8	14.8	14.9	14.4	13.1	13.4	14.3
Non-Federal[1]	10.9	9.6	8.8	8.8	7.9	7.5	7.2	7.0
Community[2]	7.7	7.6	7.1	7.2	6.7	6.5	6.2	6.1
Nonprofit	7.8	7.7	7.2	7.3	6.6	6.4	6.1	6.0
For profit	6.6	6.5	6.1	6.4	6.1	5.8	5.6	5.5
State-local government	7.6	7.3	7.2	7.7	7.6	7.4	7.2	7.1
6–24 beds	5.6	5.3	5.0	5.4	5.2	5.5	4.9	4.8
25–49 beds	6.0	5.8	5.3	6.1	5.7	5.7	5.3	5.2
50–99 beds	6.8	6.7	6.5	7.2	7.3	7.0	6.9	6.8
100–199 beds	7.1	7.0	6.7	7.1	6.7	6.4	6.2	6.0
200–299 beds	7.5	7.4	6.8	6.9	6.4	6.2	5.9	5.9
300–399 beds	7.8	7.6	7.0	7.0	6.4	6.1	5.9	5.7
400–499 beds	8.1	7.9	7.3	7.3	6.7	6.3	6.1	6.1
500 beds or more	9.1	8.7	8.1	8.1	7.4	7.1	6.7	6.6
Outpatient visits[3]				Number in thousands				
All hospitals	254,844	262,951	282,140	368,184	453,584	483,195	505,455	520,600
Federal	51,957	50,566	52,342	58,527	61,103	59,934	56,593	60,757
Non-Federal[1]	202,887	212,385	229,798	309,657	392,481	423,261	448,861	459,843
Community[2]	190,672	202,310	218,716	301,329	382,924	414,345	439,863	450,140
Nonprofit	131,435	142,156	158,953	221,073	282,653	303,851	320,746	330,215
For profit	7,713	9,696	12,378	20,110	26,443	31,940	37,347	40,919
State-local government	51,525	50,459	47,386	60,146	73,828	78,554	81,770	79,007
6–24 beds	915	1,155	829	1,471	2,354	3,644	3,622	3,920
25–49 beds	5,855	6,227	6,623	10,812	16,749	19,465	20,960	21,682
50–99 beds	16,303	17,976	18,716	27,582	34,907	38,597	41,003	40,882
100–199 beds	35,156	36,453	41,049	58,940	79,420	91,312	99,999	100,838
200–299 beds	32,772	36,073	40,515	60,561	79,364	84,080	86,958	83,826
300–399 beds	29,169	30,495	33,773	43,699	54,324	54,277	60,190	64,741
400–499 beds	22,127	25,501	23,950	33,394	40,152	44,284	47,241	46,579
500 beds or more	48,375	48,430	53,262	64,870	75,654	78,685	79,891	87,672
Outpatient surgery				Percent of total surgeries[4]				
Community hospitals[2]	- - -	16.3	34.6	50.5	57.2	58.1	59.5	60.7

- - - Data not available.

[1]The category of non-Federal hospitals is comprised of psychiatric, tuberculosis and other respiratory diseases hospitals, and long-term and short-term hospitals.

[2]Community hospitals are short-term hospitals excluding hospital units in institutions such as prison and college infirmaries, facilities for the mentally retarded, and alcoholism and chemical dependency hospitals.

[3]Outpatient visits include visits to the emergency department, outpatient department, referred visits (pharmacy, EKG, radiology), and outpatient surgery.

[4]The American Hospital Association defines surgery as a surgical episode in the operating or procedure room. During a single episode, multiple surgical procedures may be performed. In contrast the National Hospital Discharge Survey codes up to 4 procedures and the National Survey of Ambulatory Surgery codes up to 6 procedures that are performed in a single surgical episode. See Appendix II, Ambulatory surgery and Outpatient surgery.

NOTE: Data for additional years are available (see Appendix III).

SOURCES: American Hospital Association: Hospital Statistics, 1976, 1981, 1986, 1991–99 Editions. Chicago, 1976, 1981, 1986, 1991–99. (Copyrights 1976, 1981, 1986, 1991–99: Used with the permission of the American Hospital Association (AHA) and Health Forum, an AHA company.)

Table 97. Nursing home residents 65 years of age and over according to age, sex, and race: United States, 1973–74, 1985, 1995, and 1997

[Data are based on a sample of nursing home residents]

Age, sex, and race	Residents				Residents per 1,000 population			
	1973–74	1985	1995	1997	1973–74	1985	1995	1997
Age								
65 years and over	961,500	1,318,300	1,422,600	1,465,000	44.7	46.2	42.4	43.4
65–74 years	163,100	212,100	190,200	198,400	12.3	12.5	10.1	10.8
75–84 years	384,900	509,000	511,900	528,300	57.7	57.7	45.9	45.5
85 years and over	413,600	597,300	720,400	738,300	257.3	220.3	198.6	192.0
Male								
65 years and over	265,700	334,400	356,800	372,100	30.0	29.0	26.1	26.7
65–74 years	65,100	80,600	79,300	80,800	11.3	10.8	9.5	9.8
75–84 years	102,300	141,300	144,300	159,300	39.9	43.0	33.3	34.6
85 years and over	98,300	112,600	133,100	132,000	182.7	145.7	130.8	119.0
Female								
65 years and over	695,800	983,900	1,065,800	1,092,900	54.9	57.9	53.7	55.1
65–74 years	98,000	131,500	110,900	117,700	13.1	13.8	10.6	11.6
75–84 years	282,600	367,700	367,600	368,900	68.9	66.4	53.9	52.7
85 years and over	315,300	484,700	587,300	606,300	294.9	250.1	224.9	221.6
White								
65 years and over	920,600	1,227,400	1,271,200	1,294,900	46.9	47.7	42.3	43.0
65–74 years	150,100	187,800	154,400	160,800	12.5	12.3	9.3	10.0
75–84 years	369,700	473,600	453,800	464,400	60.3	59.1	44.9	44.2
85 years and over	400,800	566,000	663,000	669,700	270.8	228.7	200.7	192.4
Black								
65 years and over	37,700	82,000	122,900	137,400	22.0	35.0	45.2	49.4
65–74 years	12,200	22,500	29,700	31,400	11.1	15.4	18.4	19.2
75–84 years	13,400	30,600	47,300	51,900	26.7	45.3	57.2	60.6
85 years and over	12,100	29,000	45,800	54,100	105.7	141.5	167.1	186.0

NOTES: Excludes residents in personal care or domiciliary care homes. Age refers to age at time of interview. Rates are based on the resident population as of July 1. In 1997 population figures are adjusted for net underenumeration using the 1990 National Population Adjustment Matrix from the U.S. Bureau of the Census.

SOURCES: Centers for Disease Control and Prevention: Hing E, Sekscenski E, Strahan G. The National Nursing Home Survey: 1985 summary for the United States. National Center for Health Statistics. Vital Health Stat 13(97). 1989; and unpublished data from the 1995 and 1997 National Nursing Home Surveys.

Table 98. Nursing home residents 65 years of age and over, according to selected functional status and age, sex, and race: United States, 1985, 1995, and 1997

[Data are based on a sample of nursing home residents]

| | Functional status[1] | | | | | | | | | | | |
| | Dependent mobility | | | Incontinent | | | Dependent eating | | | Dependent mobility, eating, and incontinent | | |
Age, sex, and race	1985	1995	1997	1985	1995	1997	1985	1995	1997	1985	1995	1997
All persons						Percent						
65 years and over, age adjusted[2]	75.7	79.0	79.3	55.0	63.8	64.9	40.9	44.9	45.1	32.5	36.5	35.7
65 years and over, crude	74.8	79.0	79.4	54.5	63.8	64.9	40.5	44.9	45.1	32.1	36.5	35.6
65–74 years	61.2	73.0	73.1	42.9	61.9	59.2	33.5	43.8	42.1	25.7	35.8	30.7
75–84 years	70.5	76.5	77.1	55.1	62.5	64.3	39.4	45.2	44.8	30.6	35.3	34.5
85 years and over	83.3	82.4	82.6	58.1	65.3	66.9	43.9	45.0	46.1	35.6	37.5	37.8
Male												
65 years and over, age adjusted[2]	71.2	⁻6.6	76.3	54.2	63.8	65.0	36.0	42.1	42.8	28.0	34.3	33.6
65 years and over, crude	67.8	75.8	75.6	51.9	63.9	64.5	34.9	42.7	42.9	26.9	34.8	33.7
65–74 years	55.8	70.6	72.3	38.8	63.4	60.1	32.8	44.2	42.7	24.1	36.9	32.9
75–84 years	65.7	76.6	75.1	54.4	64.6	65.9	32.6	44.1	43.7	25.5	35.5	34.6
85 years and over	79.2	78.2	78.3	58.1	63.4	65.6	39.2	40.2	42.1	30.9	32.7	33.0
Female												
65 years and over, age adjusted[2]	77.3	79.7	80.2	55.4	63.6	64.8	42.4	45.6	45.6	33.9	36.9	35.9
65 years and over, crude	77.1	80.1	80.6	55.4	63.8	65.1	42.4	45.6	45.8	33.8	37.0	36.3
65–74 years	64.5	74.8	73.7	45.4	60.9	58.6	34.0	43.6	41.6	26.7	35.0	29.2
75–84 years	72.3	76.5	78.0	55.3	61.7	63.6	42.0	45.7	45.3	32.6	35.2	34.4
85 years and over	84.3	83.3	83.5	58.1	65.7	67.2	45.0	46.0	46.9	36.7	38.6	38.8
White												
65 years and over, age adjusted[2]	75.2	78.5	78.9	54.6	63.2	64.4	40.4	44.2	44.2	32.1	35.7	34.8
65 years and over, crude	74.3	78.7	79.0	54.2	63.3	64.5	40.1	44.2	44.2	31.7	35.7	34.8
65–74 years	60.2	71.4	72.3	42.2	60.2	59.6	32.6	41.9	40.2	24.9	33.8	29.3
75–84 years	69.6	76.4	76.1	54.2	61.8	63.4	38.9	44.9	43.9	30.1	34.7	33.5
85 years and over	83.1	81.9	82.6	58.2	65.0	66.4	43.5	44.3	45.4	35.5	36.9	37.1
Black												
65 years and over, age adjusted[2]	83.4	83.2	82.7	61.0	69.3	71.0	49.2	52.2	53.3	38.2	44.0	44.1
65 years and over, crude	81.1	82.1	82.0	59.9	69.1	69.2	47.9	51.7	53.3	37.7	43.7	43.2
65–74 years	70.9	79.6	75.9	48.6	68.3	55.8	43.1	51.2	53.2	33.8	43.1	38.4
75–84 years	82.5	77.8	84.1	70.1	68.9	72.4	47.9	49.5	52.9	40.6	42.3	42.0
85 years and over	87.4	88.0	83.5	57.9	69.8	74.0	51.7	54.3	53.6	37.6	45.5	47.2

[1]Nursing home residents who are dependent in mobility and eating require the assistance of a person or special equipment. Nursing home residents who are incontinent have difficulty in controlling bowels and/or bladder or have an ostomy or indwelling catheter.
[2]Age adjusted by the direct method to the 1995 National Nursing Home Survey population using the following 3 age groups: 65–74 years, 75–84 years, and 85 years and over.

NOTES: Age refers to age at time of interview. Excludes residents in personal care or domiciliary care homes.

SOURCES: Centers for Disease Control and Prevention: Hing E, Sekscenski E, Strahan G. The National Nursing Home Survey: 1985 summary for the United States. National Center for Health Statistics. Vital Health Stat 13(97). 1989; and unpublished data from the 1995 and 1997 National Nursing Home Surveys.

Table 99. Additions to selected inpatient psychiatric organizations according to sex, age, and race: United States, 1975, 1980, and 1986

[Data are based on a sample survey of patients]

Sex, age, and race	State and county mental hospitals			Private psychiatric hospitals			Non-Federal general hospitals[1]		
	1975	1980	1986	1975	1980	1986	1975	1980	1986
Both sexes				Additions in thousands					
Total	385	369	343	130	141	222	516	564	851
Under 18 years.	25	17	17	15	17	43	43	44	50
18–24 years	72	77	61	19	23	25	93	98	126
25–44 years	166	177	200	47	56	99	220	249	425
45–64 years	102	78	50	35	32	34	121	123	156
65 years and over	21	20	15	13	14	21	38	50	94
White	296	265	230	119	123	183	451	469	659
All other	89	104	113	10	18	39	65	95	192
Male									
Total	249	239	217	56	67	115	212	255	398
Under 18 years.	16	11	10	8	9	23	20	20	22
18–24 years	52	56	41	10	13	16	45	52	59
25–44 years	107	119	134	20	27	56	85	115	222
45–64 years	61	43	25	14	13	14	48	46	66
65 years and over	13	11	7	5	5	6	14	21	29
White.	191	171	145	51	58	89	184	213	292
All other	58	68	72	5	9	26	27	42	106
Female									
Total	136	130	126	74	74	107	304	309	453
Under 18 years.	9	5	7	8	7	20	23	23	28
18–24 years	20	22	20	9	10	8	48	45	67
25–44 years	59	58	66	28	29	44	135	135	203
45–64 years	41	35	24	21	18	20	74	77	90
65 years and over	8	9	8	3	9	15	24	29	65
White.	105	94	85	69	65	94	267	256	367
All other	31	36	41	5	9	13	37	53	86
Both sexes				Additions per 100,000 civilian population					
Total	182.2	163.6	143.4	61.4	62.6	92.5	243.8	250.0	355.4
Under 18 years.	38.1	26.1	26.9	23.3	26.3	67.5	64.4	68.5	78.7
18–24 years	271.8	264.6	225.6	73.7	79.6	91.6	352.8	334.2	467.0
25–44 years	314.1	282.9	267.0	89.3	89.1	132.7	416.8	399.0	566.8
45–64 years	233.5	175.7	110.9	80.1	71.0	75.2	278.5	276.4	346.2
65 years and over	91.8	78.0	52.5	57.7	54.1	71.4	170.3	195.4	323.6
White.	161.1	136.8	113.2	64.9	63.4	90.1	245.4	241.8	324.7
All other	321.9	328.0	311.4	37.9	57.5	106.1	233.3	300.0	526.2
Male									
Total	243.7	219.8	187.8	54.5	61.9	99.3	207.1	233.8	343.6
Under 18 years.	48.3	35.4	32.2	22.5	28.9	69.8	59.1	62.6	67.5
18–24 years	409.0	387.9	307.5	78.0	92.2	124.2	350.8	365.3	446.2
25–44 years	418.4	388.1	363.0	76.6	86.8	151.2	332.8	374.7	602.9
45–64 years	291.5	202.3	118.6	66.8	63.2	65.5	228.6	219.1	306.1
65 years and over	136.4	105.3	59.4	50.3	47.3	52.1	152.0	203.4	245.6
White.	214.2	182.2	147.2	57.0	61.7	90.3	206.9	226.3	296.4
All other	444.5	457.8	419.7	38.1	62.7	151.2	209.1	281.1	614.2
Female									
Total	124.7	111.1	101.8	67.8	63.3	86.2	278.1	265.1	366.4
Under 18 years.	27.5	16.4	21.4	24.1	23.6	65.0	70.0	74.6	90.3
18–24 years	143.1	145.8	146.6	69.6	67.4	60.2	354.6	304.4	487.1
25–44 years	215.9	182.3	174.1	101.2	91.2	114.9	495.8	422.2	531.9
45–64 years	180.5	151.7	103.8	92.3	78.1	84.0	324.3	328.2	382.8
65 years and over	60.8	59.6	47.8	62.8	58.8	84.6	182.9	190.0	376.7
White.	111.2	94.1	81.1	72.5	65.0	90.0	281.7	256.4	351.5
All other	212.0	212.6	214.2	37.7	52.8	65.5	254.9	316.7	447.0

[1]Non-Federal general hospitals include public and nonpublic facilities.

NOTES: An addition is a new admission, a readmission, a return from long-term leave, or a transfer. See Appendix II, Addition.

SOURCES: National Institute of Mental Health. Taube CA, Barrett SA. *Mental Health, United States, 1985*. DHHS. 1985; Manderscheid RW, Sonnenschein MA. *Mental Health, United States, 1992*. DHHS. 1992. Unpublished data.

Table 100. Additions to selected inpatient psychiatric organizations, according to selected primary diagnoses and age: United States, 1975, 1980, and 1986

[Data are based on a sample survey of patients]

Primary diagnosis and age	State and county mental hospitals			Private psychiatric hospitals			Non-Federal general hospitals[1]		
	1975	1980	1986	1975	1980	1986	1975	1980	1986
All diagnoses[2]	Additions per 100,000 civilian population								
All ages	182.2	163.6	143.4	61.4	62.6	92.5	243.3	250.0	355.4
Under 25 years	104.8	101.2	86.3		43.1	74.	146.7	152.2	194.7
25–44 years	314.1	282.9	267.0	...3	89.1	132.7	416.8	399.0	566.8
45–64 years	233.5	175.7	110.9	80.1	71.0	75.2	278.5	276.4	346.2
65 years and over	91.8	78.0	52.5	57.7	54.1	71.4	170.3	195.4	323.6
Alcohol related									
All ages	50.4	35.5	23.8	5.1	5.8	6.6	17.0	18.8	42.4
Under 25 years	10.7	12.4	16.8	0.4	1.4	2.2	2.4	4.4	13.7
25–44 years	86.2	64.0	45.4	7.6	9.3	10.0	31.0	34.3	94.8
45–64 years	110.0	57.7	15.3	12.5	10.9	11.0	34.5	30.6	32.9
65 years and over	14.8	11.5	*3.2	4.3	4.4	4.5	10.2	12.8	11.3
Drug related									
All ages	6.8	7.8	9.1	1.5	1.8	6.1	8.4	7.4	20.8
Under 25 years	7.2	9.4	6.3	1.5	1.8	7.5	7.7	7.8	18.8
25–44 years	12.6	12.9	14.8	2.3	3.0	9.3	13.8	9.3	42.0
45–64 years	*0.6	1.4	10.5	0.1	1.0	*1.8	6.5	7.1	*2.2
65 years and over	*3.5	*0.7	*0.8	0.4	0.6	- - -	*2.6	*2.0	*1.2
Organic disorders[3]									
All ages	9.6	6.8	4.5	2.5	2.2	2.0	9.0	7.4	10.7
Under 25 years	2.2	1.2	*0.2	0.7	0.5	*0.5	1.1	*0.8	1.7
25–44 years	6.4	4.7	3.0	1.1	0.9	*0.3	5.4	5.6	6.9
45–64 years	12.2	8.1	7.3	1.7	2.7	*1.5	9.3	6.9	6.8
65 years and over	43.3	30.0	17.2	14.5	10.8	11.7	49.3	36.4	54.5
Affective disorders									
All ages	21.3	22.0	23.6	26.0	26.8	45.4	91.9	79.2	135.9
Under 25 years	7.5	9.1	9.9	9.5	13.5	31.6	35.3	32.2	55.9
25–44 years	40.6	36.9	45.2	39.4	38.9	67.1	160.9	123.7	190.4
45–64 years	29.4	32.4	25.5	43.3	36.3	38.5	135.6	113.8	165.7
65 years and over	16.8	14.3	7.9	29.6	29.2	42.9	78.5	81.0	197.4
Schizophrenia									
All ages	61.2	62.1	53.2	13.4	13.3	11.0	58.9	59.9	66.2
Under 25 years	35.9	36.6	19.6	11.1	10.6	5.7	42.0	38.3	30.8
25–44 years	125.8	125.0	115.3	23.8	22.5	22.6	118.0	114.5	124.2
45–64 years	63.5	54.8	38.8	11.3	11.6	8.5	50.3	53.6	73.7
65 years and over	9.3	13.9	19.9	2.7	3.6	*1.8	5.6	16.3	15.3

* Based on 5 or fewer sample additions.
- - - Data not available.
[1]Non-Federal general hospitals include public and nonpublic facilities.
[2]Includes all other diagnoses not listed separately.
[3]Excludes alcohol- and drug-related diagnoses.

NOTES: An addition is a new admission, a readmission, a return from long-term leave, or a transfer. See Appendix II, Addition. Primary diagnosis categories are based on the then current *International Classification of Diseases* and *Diagnostic and Statistical Manual of Mental Disorders*. For a listing of the code numbers, see Appendix II, table IX.

SOURCES: National Institute of Mental Health. Taube CA, Barrett SA. *Mental Health, United States, 1985.* DHHS. 1985; Manderscheid RW, Sonnenschein MA. *Mental Health, United States, 1992.* DHHS. 1992. Unpublished data.

Table 101. Persons employed in health service sites: United States, selected years 1970-98

[Data are based on household interviews of a sample of the civilian noninstitutionalized population]

Site	1970	1975	1980	1985	1990	1992	1993	1994[1]	1995[1]	1996[1]	1997[1]	1998[1]
					Number of persons in thousands							
All employed civilians	76,805	85,846	99,303	107,150	117,914	117,598	119,306	123,060	124,900	126,708	129,558	131,463
All health service sites	4,246	5,945	7,339	7,910	9,447	10,271	10,553	10,587	10,928	11,199	11,525	11,504
Offices and clinics of physicians	477	618	777	894	1,098	1,434	1,450	1,404	1,512	1,501	1,559	1,581
Offices and clinics of dentists	222	331	415	480	580	583	567	596	644	614	662	666
Offices and clinics of chiropractors[2]	19	30	40	59	90	122	116	105	99	99	118	127
Hospitals	2,690	3,441	4,036	4,269	4,690	4,915	5,032	5,009	4,961	5,041	5,130	5,116
Nursing and personal care facilities	509	891	1,199	1,309	1,543	1,750	1,752	1,692	1,718	1,765	1,755	1,801
Other health service sites	330	634	872	899	1,446	1,467	1,635	1,781	1,995	2,178	2,301	2,213
					Percent of employed civilians							
All health service sites	5.[ ]	6.9	7.4	7.4	8.0	8.7	8.8	8.6	8.7	8.8	8.9	8.8
					Percent distribution							
All health service sites	100.0	100.0	100.0	100.0	100.0	100.0	100.0	100.0	100.0	100.0	100.0	100.0
Offices and clinics of physicians	11.2	10.4	10.6	11.3	11.6	14.0	13.7	13.3	13.8	13.4	13.5	13.7
Offices and clinics of dentists	5.2	5.6	5.7	6.1	6.1	5.7	5.4	5.6	5.9	5.5	5.7	5.8
Offices and clinics of chiropractors[2]	0.4	0.5	0.5	0.7	1.0	1.2	1.1	1.0	0.9	0.9	1.0	1.1
Hospitals	63.4	57.9	55.0	54.0	49.6	47.9	47.7	47.3	45.4	45.0	44.5	44.5
Nursing and personal care facilities	12.0	15.0	16.3	16.5	16.3	17.0	16.6	16.0	15.7	15.8	15.2	15.7
Other health service sites	7.8	10.7	11.9	11.4	15.3	14.3	15.5	16.8	18.3	19.4	20.0	19.2

[1]Data for 1994 and later years are not strictly comparable with data from previous years due to a redesign of the Current Population Survey. See Appendix I, Department of Commerce.

[2]Data for 1980 are from the American Chiropractic Association; data for all other years are from the U.S. Bureau of Labor Statistics.

NOTES: Employment is full- or part-time work. Totals exclude persons in health-related occupations who are working in nonhealth industries, as classified by the U.S. Bureau of the Census, such as pharmacists employed in drugstores, school nurses, and nurses working in private households. Totals include Federal, State, and county health workers. In 1970-82, employed persons were classified according to the industry groups used in the 1970 Census of Population. In 1983-91, persons were classified according to the system used in the 1980 Census of Population. Beginning in 1992 persons were classified according to the system used in the 1990 Census of Population. Data for additional years are available (see Appendix III).

SOURCES: U.S. Bureau of the Census: 1970 Census of Population, occupation by industry. Subject Reports. Final Report PC(2)-7C. Washington. U.S. Government Printing Office, Oct. 1972; U.S. Bureau of Labor Statistics: Labor Force Statistics Derived from the Current Population Survey: A Databook, Vol. I. Washington. U.S. Government Printing Office, Sept. 1982; Employment and Earnings, January issue 1986, 1991-99. U.S. Government Printing Office, Jan. 1986, 1991-99; American Chiropractic Association: Unpublished data.

Table 102 (page 1 of 2). Active non-Federal physicians and doctors of medicine in patient care, according to geographic division and State: United States, 1975, 1985, 1995, and 1997

[Data based on reporting by physicians]

Geographic division and State	Total physicians[1]				Doctors of medicine in patient care[2]			
	1975	1985	1995[3]	1997[4]	1975	1985	1995	1997
	Number per 10,000 civilian population							
United States	15.3	20.7	24.2	25.3	13.5	18.0	21.3	22.4
New England	19.1	26.7	32.5	34.2	16.9	22.9	28.8	30.4
Maine	12.8	18.7	22.3	23.9	10.7	15.6	18.2	19.7
New Hampshire	14.3	18.1	21.5	23.4	13.1	16.7	19.8	21.4
Vermont	18.2	23.8	26.9	28.8	15.5	20.3	24.2	26.0
Massachusetts	20.8	30.2	37.5	39.1	18.3	25.4	33.2	34.8
Rhode Island	17.8	23.3	30.4	33.3	16.1	20.2	26.7	29.4
Connecticut	19.8	27.6	32.8	34.0	17.7	24.3	29.5	30.6
Middle Atlantic	19.5	26.1	32.4	33.9	17.0	22.2	28.0	29.3
New York	22.7	29.0	35.3	37.1	20.2	25.2	31.6	33.2
New Jersey	16.2	23.4	29.3	30.6	14.0	19.8	24.9	26.0
Pennsylvania	16.6	23.6	30.1	31.3	13.9	19.2	24.6	25.5
East North Central	13.9	19.3	23.3	24.6	12.0	16.4	19.8	21.0
Ohio	14.1	19.9	23.8	25.1	12.2	16.8	20.0	21.1
Indiana	10.6	14.7	18.4	19.7	9.6	13.2	16.6	17.8
Illinois	14.5	20.5	24.8	26.2	13.1	18.2	22.1	23.4
Michigan	15.4	20.8	24.8	25.9	12.0	16.0	19.0	19.9
Wisconsin	12.5	17.7	21.5	22.8	11.4	15.9	19.6	20.8
West North Central	13.3	18.3	21.8	22.9	11.4	15.6	18.9	19.8
Minnesota	14.9	20.5	23.4	24.5	13.7	18.5	21.5	22.6
Iowa	11.4	15.6	19.2	19.8	9.4	12.4	15.1	15.6
Missouri	15.0	20.5	23.9	24.8	11.6	16.3	19.7	20.5
North Dakota	9.7	15.8	20.5	22.4	9.2	14.9	18.9	20.6
South Dakota	8.2	13.4	16.7	18.2	7.7	12.3	15.7	17.0
Nebraska	12.1	15.7	19.8	21.3	10.9	14.4	18.3	19.8
Kansas	12.8	17.3	20.8	21.9	11.2	15.1	18.0	18.9
South Atlantic	14.0	19.7	23.4	24.8	12.6	17.6	21.0	22.3
Delaware	14.3	19.7	23.4	24.9	12.7	17.1	19.7	21.4
Maryland	18.6	30.4	34.1	35.9	16.5	24.9	29.9	31.2
District of Columbia	39.6	55.3	63.6	69.2	34.6	45.6	53.6	58.6
Virginia	12.9	19.5	22.5	23.7	11.9	17.8	20.8	21.9
West Virginia	11.0	16.3	21.0	22.8	10.0	14.6	17.9	19.3
North Carolina	11.7	16.9	21.1	22.6	10.6	15.0	19.4	20.8
South Carolina	10.0	14.7	18.9	20.5	9.3	13.6	17.6	19.0
Georgia	11.5	16.2	19.7	20.8	10.6	14.7	18.0	19.0
Florida	15.2	20.2	22.9	24.4	13.4	17.8	20.3	21.6
East South Central	10.5	15.0	19.2	20.8	9.7	14.0	17.8	19.3
Kentucky	10.9	15.1	19.2	20.7	10.1	13.9	18.0	19.3
Tennessee	12.4	17.7	22.5	24.3	11.3	16.2	20.8	22.4
Alabama	9.2	14.2	18.4	19.7	8.6	13.1	17.0	18.2
Mississippi	8.4	11.8	13.9	16.0	8.0	11.1	13.0	14.8
West South Central	11.9	16.4	19.5	20.6	10.5	14.5	17.3	18.3
Arkansas	9.1	13.8	17.3	18.8	8.5	12.8	16.0	17.5
Louisiana	11.4	17.3	21.7	23.5	10.5	16.1	20.3	22.1
Oklahoma	11.6	16.1	18.8	19.6	9.4	12.9	14.7	15.5
Texas	12.5	16.8	19.4	20.3	11.0	14.7	17.3	18.1
Mountain	14.3	17.8	20.2	21.0	12.6	15.7	17.8	18.5
Montana	10.6	14.0	18.4	19.2	10.1	13.2	17.1	17.9
Idaho	9.5	12.1	13.9	15.5	8.9	11.4	13.1	14.4
Wyoming	9.5	12.9	15.3	17.1	8.9	12.0	13.9	15.6
Colorado	17.3	20.7	23.7	24.7	15.0	17.7	20.6	21.5
New Mexico	12.2	17.0	20.2	21.3	10.1	14.7	18.0	19.0
Arizona	16.7	20.2	21.4	21.7	14.1	17.1	18.2	18.5
Utah	14.1	17.2	19.2	19.7	13.0	15.5	17.6	18.0
Nevada	11.9	16.0	16.7	18.1	10.9	14.5	14.6	16.0

See footnotes at end of table.

Table 102 (page 2 of 2). Active non-Federal physicians and doctors of medicine in patient care, according to geographic division and State: United States, 1975, 1985, 1995, and 1997

[Data based on reporting by physicians]

Geographic division and State	Total physicians[1]				Doctors of medicine in patient care[2]			
	1975	1985	1995[3]	1997[4]	1975	1985	1995	1997
	Number per 10,000 civilian population							
Pacific	17.9	22.5	23.3	23.8	16.3	20.5	21.2	21.7
Washington...............	15.3	20.2	22.5	23.4	13.6	17.9	20.2	21.1
Oregon.................	15.6	19.7	21.6	22.6	13.8	17.6	19.5	20.4
California	18.8	23.7	23.7	24.1	17.3	21.5	21.7	22.0
Alaska	8.4	13.0	15.7	17.2	7.8	12.1	14.2	15.4
Hawaii	16.2	21.5	24.8	26.4	14.7	19.8	22.8	24.1

[1]Includes active non-Federal doctors of medicine and active doctors of osteopathy.
[2]Excludes doctors of osteopathy; States with large numbers are Florida, Michigan, Missouri, New Jersey, Ohio, Pennsylvania, and Texas. Excludes doctors of medicine in medical teaching, administration, research, and other nonpatient care activities.
[3]Data for doctors of osteopathy are as of July 1996.
[4]Data for doctors of osteopathy are as of November 1997.

NOTES: Data for doctors of medicine are as of December 31. See Appendix II for physician definitions.

SOURCES: American Medical Association (AMA). Physician distribution and medical licensure in the U.S., 1975; Physician characteristics and distribution in the U.S., 1986 edition; 1996–97 edition; 1999 edition. Department of Data Survey and Planning, Division of Survey and Data Resources, AMA. (Copyrights 1976, 1986, 1997, 1999: Used with the permission of the AMA); American Osteopathic Association: 1975–76 Yearbook and Directory of Osteopathic Physicians, 1985–86 Yearbook and Directory of Osteopathic Physicians; Rockville, Md. American Association of Colleges of Osteopathic Medicine: Annual Statistical Report, 1996 and 1998.

Table 103. Physicians, according to activity and place of medical education: United States and outlying U.S. areas, selected years 1975–97

[Data are based on reporting by physicians]

Activity and place of medical education	1975	1980	1985	1990	1995	1996	1997
				Number of physicians			
Doctors of medicine	393,742	467,679	552,716	615,421	720,325	737,764	756,710
Professionally active[1]	340,280	414,916	497,140	547,310	625,443	643,955	664,556
Place of medical education:							
U.S. medical graduates	- - -	333,325	392,007	432,884	481,137	495,463	509,942
International medical graduates[2]	- - -	81,591	105,133	114,426	144,306	148,492	154,614
Activity:[3]							
Non-Federal	312,089	397,129	475,573	526,835	604,364	623,526	645,203
Patient care	287,837	361,915	431,527	479,547	564,074	580,706	603,684
Office-based practice	213,334	271,268	329,041	359,932	427,275	445,765	458,209
General and family practice	46,347	47,772	53,862	57,571	59,932	61,760	62,022
Cardiovascular diseases	5,046	6,725	9,054	10,670	13,739	14,304	15,026
Dermatology	3,442	4,372	5,325	5,996	6,959	7,234	7,353
Gastroenterology	1,696	2,735	4,135	5,200	7,300	7,580	7,938
Internal medicine	28,188	40,514	52,712	57,799	72,612	77,929	81,352
Pediatrics	12,687	17,436	22,392	26,494	33,890	35,453	36,846
Pulmonary diseases	1,166	2,040	3,035	3,659	4,964	4,892	4,965
General surgery	19,710	22,409	24,708	24,498	24,086	25,425	27,865
Obstetrics and gynecology	15,613	19,503	23,525	25,475	29,111	29,872	30,063
Ophthalmology	8,795	10,598	12,212	13,055	14,596	14,931	15,118
Orthopedic surgery	8,148	10,719	13,033	14,187	17,136	17,637	18,482
Otolaryngology	4,297	5,262	5,751	6,360	7,139	7,152	7,378
Plastic surgery	1,706	2,437	3,299	3,835	4,612	5,012	5,257
Urological surgery	5,025	6,222	7,081	7,392	7,991	8,229	8,383
Anesthesiology	8,970	11,336	15,285	17,789	23,770	24,929	25,569
Diagnostic radiology	1,978	4,190	7,735	9,806	12,751	13,313	14,142
Emergency medicine	- - -	- - -	- - -	8,402	11,700	12,348	12,450
Neurology	1,862	3,245	4,691	5,587	7,623	7,898	8,199
Pathology, anatomical/clinical	4,195	5,952	6,877	7,269	9,031	9,661	10,229
Psychiatry	12,173	15,946	18,521	20,048	23,334	24,400	24,541
Radiology	6,970	7,791	7,355	6,056	5,994	6,276	6,297
Other specialty	15,320	24,064	28,453	22,784	29,005	29,530	28,734
Hospital-based practice	74,503	90,647	102,486	127,864	136,799	134,941	145,318
Residents and interns[4]	53,527	59,615	72,159	81,664	93,650	90,592	95,808
Full-time hospital staff	20,976	31,032	30,327	37,951	43,149	44,349	49,510
Other professional activity[5]	24,252	35,214	44,046	39,039	40,290	42,820	41,519
Federal[6]	28,191	17,787	21,567	20,475	21,079	20,429	19,353
Patient care	24,100	14,597	17,293	15,632	18,057	18,218	16,947
Office-based practice	2,095	732	1,156	1,063	. . .	. . .	. . .
Hospital-based practice	22,005	13,865	16,137	14,569	18,057	18,218	16,945
Residents and interns	4,275	2,427	3,252	1,725	2,702	5,749	4,068
Full-time hospital staff	17,730	11,438	12,885	12,844	15,355	12,469	12,877
Other professional activity[5]	4,091	3,190	4,274	4,843	3,022	2,211	2,406
Inactive	21,449	25,744	38,646	52,653	72,326	72,510	71,106
Not classified	26,145	20,629	13,950	12,678	20,579	19,998	20,049
Unknown address	5,868	6,390	2,980	2,780	1,977	1,311	999

- - - Data not available.
. . . Category not applicable.
[1]Excludes inactive, not classified, and address unknown.
[2]International medical graduates received their medical education in schools outside the United States and Canada.
[3]Specialty information based on the physician's self-designated primary area of practice. Categories include generalists and specialists.
[4]Beginning in 1990 clinical fellows are included in this category. In prior years clinical fellows were included in other professional activity.
[5]Includes medical teaching, administration, research, and other. Prior to 1990 this category included clinical fellows, also.
[6]Beginning in 1993 data collection for Federal physicians was revised.

NOTES: Data for doctors of medicine are as of December 31, except for 1990–94 data, which are as of January 1. See Appendix II for discussion of physician specialties. Outlying areas include Puerto Rico, Virgin Islands, and the Pacific islands of Canton, Caroline, Guam, Mariana, Marshall, American Samoa, and Wake. Data for additional years are available (see Appendix III).

SOURCES: American Medical Association (AMA). Distribution of physicians in the United States, 1970; Physician distribution and medical licensure in the U.S., 1975; Physician characteristics and distribution in the U.S., 1981 edition; 1986 edition; 1989 edition; 1990 edition; 1992 edition; 1993 edition; 1994 edition; 1995–96 edition; 1996–97 edition; 1997–98 edition; 1999 edition. Department of Data Survey and Planning, Division of Survey and Data Resources, AMA. (Copyrights 1971, 1976, 1982, 1986, 1989, 1990, 1992, 1993, 1994, 1996, 1997, 1997, 1999: Used with the permission of the AMA).

Table 104. Primary care doctors of medicine, according to specialty: United States and outlying U.S. areas, selected years 1949–97

[Data are based on reporting by physicians]

Specialty	1949[1]	1960[1]	1970	1980	1990	1994	1995	1996	1997
					Number				
Total[2]	201,277	260,484	334,028	467,679	615,421	684,414	720,325	737,764	756,710
Active doctors of medicine[3]	191,577	247,257	310,845	414,916	547,310	605,468	625,443	643,955	664,556
Primary care generalists	113,222	125,359	115,822	146,093	183,294	200,020	207,810	216,446	216,598
General/family practice	95,980	88,023	57,948	60,049	70,480	73,163	75,976	78,910	78,258
Internal medicine.	12,453	26,209	39,924	58,462	76,295	84,951	88,240	92,321	93,797
Pediatrics	4,789	11,127	17,950	27,582	36,519	41,906	43,594	45,215	44,543
Primary care specialists	- - -	- - -	2,817	14,949	27,434	33,927	35,290	39,315	32,918
Internal medicine.	- - -	- - -	1,948	13,069	22,054	26,476	26,928	29,804	24,582
Pediatrics	- - -	- - -	869	1,880	5,380	7,451	8,362	9,511	8,336
					Percent active doctors of medicine				
Primary care generalists	59.1	50.7	37.3	35.2	33.5	33.0	33.2	33.6	32.6
General/family practice	50.1	35.6	18.6	14.5	12.9	12.1	12.1	12.3	11.8
Internal medicine.	6.5	10.6	12.8	14.1	13.9	14.0	14.1	14.3	14.1
Pediatrics	2.5	4.5	5.8	6.6	6.7	6.9	7.0	7.0	6.7
Primary care specialists	- - -	- - -	0.9	3.6	5.0	5.6	5.6	6.1	5.0
Internal medicine.	- - -	- - -	0.6	3.1	4.0	4.4	4.3	4.6	3.7
Pediatrics	- - -	- - -	0.3	0.5	1.0	1.2	1.3	1.5	1.3

- - - Data not available.

[1]Estimated by the Bureau of Health Professions, Health Resources Administration. Active doctors of medicine (M.D.'s) include those with address unknown and primary specialty not classified.

[2]Includes M.D.'s engaged in Federal and non-Federal patient care (office-based or hospital-based) and other professional activities.

[3]Beginning in 1970, M.D.'s who are inactive, have unknown address, or primary specialty not classified are excluded.

NOTES: See Appendix II for definitions of physician specialties. Data are as of December 31 except for 1990–94 data, which are as of January 1, and 1949 data, which are as of midyear. Outlying areas include Puerto Rico, Virgin Islands, and the Pacific islands of Canton, Caroline, Guam, Mariana, Marshall, American Samoa, and Wake.

SOURCES: Health Manpower Source Book: Medical Specialists, USDHEW, 1962; American Medical Association (AMA). Distribution of physicians in the United States, 1970; Physician characteristics and distribution in the U.S., 1981 edition; 1992 edition; 1995–96 edition; 1996–97 edition; 1997–98 edition; 1999 edition. Department of Data Survey and Planning, Division of Survey and Data Resources, AMA. (Copyrights 1971, 1982, 1992, 1996, 1997, 1997, 1999: Used with the permission of the AMA).

Table 105. Active health personnel according to occupation and geographic region: United States, 1980, 1990, and 1996

[Data are compiled by the Bureau of Health Professions]

Year and occupation	Number of active health personnel	United States	Geographic region			
			Northeast	Midwest	South	West
1980		Number per 100,000 population[1]				
Physicians	427,122	189.8	- - -	- - -	- - -	- - -
Federal	17,642	7.8	- - -	- - -	- - -	- - -
Doctors of medicine[2]	16,585	7.4	- - -	- - -	- - -	- - -
Doctors of osteopathy	1,057	0.5	- - -	- - -	- - -	- - -
Non-Federal	409,480	182.0	224.5	165.2	157.0	200.0
Doctors of medicine[2]	393,407	174.9	216.1	153.3	152.8	195.8
Doctors of osteopathy	16,073	7.1	8.4	11.9	4.2	4.2
Dentists[3]	121,240	53.5	66.2	52.7	42.6	59.2
Optometrists	22,330	9.8	9.9	10.9	7.7	11.6
Pharmacists	142,780	62.5	66.5	67.8	62.1	51.8
Podiatrists[4]	7,000	3.0	- - -	- - -	- - -	- - -
Registered nurses	1,272,900	560.0	736.0	583.6	443.4	533.7
Associate and diploma	908,300	399.9	536.0	429.2	316.5	351.1
Baccalaureate	297,300	130.9	161.0	127.8	103.8	148.1
Masters and doctorate	67,300	29.6	39.0	26.7	23.0	34.6
1990						
Physicians	567,611	230.2	- - -	- - -	- - -	- - -
Federal[2]	20,784	8.4	- - -	- - -	- - -	- - -
Doctors of medicine[2]	19,166	7.7	- - -	- - -	- - -	- - -
Doctors of osteopathy	1,618	0.7	- - -	- - -	- - -	- - -
Non-Federal	546,826	221.8	285.5	203.9	195.5	223.3
Doctors of medicine[2]	520,450	211.1	271.6	186.8	188.6	216.9
Doctors of osteopathy	26,376	10.7	13.9	17.1	6.9	6.3
Dentists[3]	146,600	58.8	- - -	- - -	- - -	- - -
Optometrists	26,000	10.4	- - -	- - -	- - -	- - -
Pharmacists	161,900	64.4	- - -	- - -	- - -	- - -
Podiatrists[4]	10,600	4.2	- - -	- - -	- - -	- - -
Registered nurses	1,789,600	713.7	- - -	- - -	- - -	- - -
Associate and diploma	1,107,300	441.6	- - -	- - -	- - -	- - -
Baccalaureate	549,000	218.9	- - -	- - -	- - -	- - -
Masters and doctorate	133,300	53.2	- - -	- - -	- - -	- - -
1996						
Physicians	701,195	264.3	- - -	- - -	- - -	- - -
Federal	21,725	8.2	- - -	- - -	- - -	- - -
Doctors of medicine[2]	20,429	7.7	- - -	- - -	- - -	- - -
Doctors of osteopathy	1,296	0.5	- - -	- - -	- - -	- - -
Non-Federal	679,470	256.1	342.2	240.3	224.7	232.2
Doctors of medicine[2]	643,514	242.6	323.1	219.2	215.7	224.2
Doctors of osteopathy	35,956	13.6	19.1	21.1	9.0	8.0
Dentists[3]	159,500	58.2	- - -	- - -	- - -	- - -
Optometrists	29,500	11.1	- - -	- - -	- - -	- - -
Pharmacists	185,000	69.4	- - -	- - -	- - -	- - -
Podiatrists[4]	10,300	3.9	- - -	- - -	- - -	- - -
Registered nurses	2,161,700	814.9	- - -	- - -	- - -	- - -
Associate and diploma	1,252,600	472.2	- - -	- - -	- - -	- - -
Baccalaureate	693,200	261.3	- - -	- - -	- - -	- - -
Masters and doctorate	215,900	81.4	- - -	- - -	- - -	- - -

- - - Data not available.

[1]Ratios for physicians and dentists are based on civilian population; ratios for all other health occupations are based on resident population.

[2]Excludes physicians with unknown addresses and inactive from the number of active health personnel.

[3]Excludes dentists in military service, U.S. Public Health Service, and Department of Veterans Affairs.

[4]Podiatrists in patient care. Podiatric data shown in the bottom panel are from 1995.

NOTES: From 1989 to 1994 data for doctors of medicine are as of January 1; in other years these data are as of December 31. See Appendix II for physician definitions.

SOURCES: Division of Health Professions Analysis, Bureau of Health Professions: Supply and Characteristics of Selected Health Personnel. DHHS Pub. No. (HRA) 81–20. Health Resources Administration. Hyattsville, Md., June 1981; unpublished data; American Medical Association. Physician characteristics and distribution in the U.S., 1981, 1992, and 1997/98 editions. Chicago, 1982, 1992, and 1997; American Osteopathic Association. 1980–81 Yearbook and Directory of Osteopathic Physicians. Chicago, 1980. American Association of Colleges of Osteopathic Medicine. Annual statistical report, 1990 and 1997 editions. Rockville, Md., 1990 and 1997; unpublished data.

Table 106 (page 1 of 2). Full-time equivalent patient care staff in mental health organizations, according to type of organization and staff discipline: United States, selected years 1984–94

[Data are based on inventories of mental health organizations]

Organization and discipline	1984	1990	1992	1994	1984	1990	1992	1994
All organizations		Number				Percent distribution		
All patient care staff	313,243	416,282	434,620	457,503	100.0	100.0	100.0	100.0
Professional patient care staff	202,474	273,758	306,688	326,952	64.6	65.8	70.6	71.5
Psychiatrists	18,482	18,846	22,821	24,069	5.9	4.5	5.3	5.3
Psychologists	21,052	22,888	25,021	21,798	6.7	5.5	5.8	4.8
Social workers	36,397	53,487	57,201	55,493	11.6	12.8	13.2	12.1
Registered nurses	54,406	77,686	78,625	105,410	17.4	18.7	18.1	23.0
Other professional staff[1]	72,137	100,851	123,020	120,182	23.0	24.2	28.3	26.3
Other mental health workers	110,769	142,524	127,932	130,551	35.4	34.2	29.4	28.5
State and county mental hospitals								
All patient care staff	117,630	114,198	110,874	102,153	100.0	100.0	100.0	100.0
Professional patient care staff	51,290	50,035	56,953	41,359	43.6	43.8	51.4	40.5
Psychiatrists	4,108	3,849	4,457	3,177	3.5	3.4	4.0	3.1
Psychologists	3,239	3,324	3,620	2,697	2.8	2.9	3.3	2.6
Social workers	6,175	7,013	7,378	5,450	5.2	6.1	6.7	5.3
Registered nurses	16,051	20,848	21,119	17,685	13.6	18.3	19.0	17.3
Other professional staff[1]	21,717	15,001	20,379	12,350	18.5	13.1	18.4	12.1
Other mental health workers	66,340	64,163	53,921	60,794	56.4	56.2	48.6	59.5
Private psychiatric hospitals								
All patient care staff	26,359	57,200	56,877	58,262	100.0	100.0	100.0	100.0
Professional patient care staff	19,524	45,669	44,206	45,669	74.1	79.8	77.7	78.4
Psychiatrists	1,447	1,582	2,081	2,183	5.5	2.8	3.7	3.7
Psychologists	1,461	1,977	1,656	2,003	5.5	3.5	2.9	3.4
Social workers	2,179	4,044	4,587	5,473	8.3	7.1	8.1	9.4
Registered nurses	6,818	14,819	15,086	15,939	25.9	25.9	26.5	27.4
Other professional staff[1]	7,619	23,247	20,796	20,071	28.9	40.6	36.6	34.4
Other mental health workers	6,835	11,531	12,671	12,593	25.9	20.2	22.3	21.6
Non-Federal general hospitals' psychiatric services								
All patient care staff	59,848	72,214	72,880	87,304	100.0	100.0	100.0	100.0
Professional patient care staff	46,335	57,019	58,544	76,558	77.4	79.0	80.3	87.7
Psychiatrists	6,679	6,500	6,160	4,336	11.2	9.0	8.5	5.0
Psychologists	3,283	3,951	4,182	2,441	5.5	5.5	5.7	2.8
Social workers	4,898	7,241	7,985	5,355	8.2	10.0	11.0	6.1
Registered nurses	20,454	28,473	28,355	54,647	34.2	39.4	38.9	62.6
Other professional staff[1]	11,021	10,854	11,862	9,779	18.4	15.0	16.3	11.2
Other mental health workers	13,513	15,195	14,336	10,746	22.6	21.0	19.7	12.3
Department of Veterans Affairs psychiatric services								
All patient care staff	22,948	22,080	20,834	21,671	100.0	100.0	100.0	100.0
Professional patient care staff	16,265	14,619	16,274	18,393	70.9	66.2	78.1	84.9
Psychiatrists	2,463	2,103	3,403	6,272	10.7	9.5	16.3	28.9
Psychologists	1,247	1,476	2,479	587	5.4	6.7	11.9	2.7
Social workers	1,545	1,855	2,244	1,773	6.7	8.4	10.8	8.2
Registered nurses	5,699	5,888	5,485	8,475	24.8	26.7	26.3	39.1
Other professional staff[1]	5,311	3,297	2,663	1,286	23.1	14.9	12.8	5.9
Other mental health workers	6,683	7,461	4,560	3,278	29.1	33.8	21.9	15.1
Residential treatment centers for emotionally disturbed children								
All patient care staff	15,297	40,969	42,801	44,146	100.0	100.0	100.0	100.0
Professional patient care staff	10,551	26,032	30,207	31,079	69.0	63.5	70.6	70.4
Psychiatrists	240	498	748	840	1.6	1.2	1.7	1.9
Psychologists	820	1,492	1,641	1,707	5.4	3.6	3.8	3.9
Social workers	2,283	5,636	6,506	6,635	14.9	13.8	15.2	15.0
Registered nurses	485	1,238	1,367	1,468	3.2	3.0	3.2	3.3
Other professional staff[1]	6,723	17,168	19,945	20,429	43.9	41.9	46.6	46.3
Other mental health workers	4,746	14,937	12,594	13,067	31.0	36.5	29.4	29.6

See footnotes at end of table.

Table 106 (page 2 of 2). Full-time equivalent patient care staff in mental health organizations, according to type of organization and staff discipline: United States, selected years 1984–94

[Data are based on inventories of mental health organizations]

Organization and discipline	1984	1990	1992	1994	1984	1990	1992	1994
All other organizations[2]	Number				Percent distribution			
All patient care staff	71,161	109,621	130,354	143,967	100.0	100.0	100.0	100.0
Professional patient care staff	58,509	80,384	100,504	113,894	82.2	73.3	77.1	79.1
Psychiatrists	3,545	4,314	5,972	7,261	5.0	3.9	4.6	5.0
Psychologists	11,002	10,668	11,443	12,363	15.5	9.7	8.8	8.6
Social workers	19,317	27,698	28,501	30,807	27.1	25.3	21.9	21.4
Registered nurses	4,899	6,420	7,213	7,196	6.9	5.9	5.5	5.0
Other professional staff[1]	19,746	31,284	47,375	56,267	27.7	28.5	36.3	39.1
Other mental health workers	12,652	29,237	29,850	30,073	17.8	26.7	22.9	20.9

[1]Includes occupational therapists, recreation therapists, vocational rehabilitation counselors, and teachers.
[2]Includes freestanding outpatient clinics, freestanding day–night organizations, multiservice organizations, and other residential organizations.

NOTES: Full-time equivalent figures presented in this table combine staffing data for inpatient, residential, outpatient, and partial care treatment programs. Some mental health organizations provide a mixture of inpatient and outpatient care (for example Private psychiatric hospitals and Department of Veterans Affairs), while others provide predominantly inpatient (State and county mental hospitals) or outpatient (All other organizations) care. Caution should be exercised in comparing levels of FTE staff between different types of mental health organizations due to the different types of care provided. Figures for nonpatient care staff (administrative, clerical, and maintenance staff) are not shown. Data for additional years are available (see Appendix III).

SOURCES: Survey and Analysis Branch, Division of State and Community Systems Development, Center for Mental Health Services. Manderscheid RW, Sonnenschein MA. *Mental health, United States, 1996*. DHHS. 1996; Unpublished data.

Table 107. First-year enrollment and graduates of health professions schools and number of schools, according to profession: United States, selected years 1980–98

[Data are based on reporting by health professions schools]

Profession	1980	1985	1990	1995	1996	1997	1998
First-year enrollment							
Medicine	16,930	16,997	16,756	17,085	17,058	16,935	16,867
Osteopathy	1,426	1,750	1,844	2,217	2,274	2,535	2,692
Registered nursing, total	105,952	118,224	108,580	127,184	119,205	- - -	- - -
Baccalaureate	35,414	39,573	29,858	43,451	40,048	- - -	- - -
Associate degree	53,633	63,776	68,634	76,016	72,930	- - -	- - -
Diploma	16,905	14,875	10,088	7,717	6,227	- - -	- - -
Licensed practical nursing	56,316	47,034	52,969	57,906	- - -	- - -	- - -
Dentistry	6,066	4,983	3,938	4,078	4,190	4,204	- - -
Optometry	1,185	1,177	1,258	1,354	1,396	1,323	- - -
Pharmacy	7,905	6,749	8,009	9,091	8,662	8,719	8,487
Chiropractic[1]	- - -	1,383	1,485	- - -	- - -	- - -	- - -
Schools of Public Health[2]	3,348	3,836	4,087	5,332	5,275	5,083	- - -
Graduates							
Medicine	15,135	16,319	15,336	15,911	16,029	15,904	- - -
Osteopathy	1,059	1,474	1,529	1,843	1,932	2,009	- - -
Registered nursing, total	75,523	82,075	66,088	97,052	94,757	- - -	- - -
Baccalaureate	24,994	24,975	18,571	31,254	32,413	- - -	- - -
Associate degree	36,034	45,208	42,318	58,749	56,641	- - -	- - -
Diploma	14,495	11,892	5,199	7,049	5,703	- - -	- - -
Licensed practical nursing	41,892	36,955	35,417	44,234	- - -	- - -	- - -
Dentistry	5,256	5,353	4,233	3,840	3,768	3,930	- - -
Optometry	1,073	1,114	1,115	1,219	1,174	- - -	- - -
Pharmacy	7,432	5,724	6,956	7,837	8,003	7,772	- - -
Chiropractic	2,049	- - -	1,661	- - -	- - -	- - -	- - -
Schools of Public Health	3,326	3,047	3,549	4,636	5,350	5,100	- - -
Schools[3]							
Medicine	126	127	126	125	125	125	125
Osteopathy	14	15	15	16	17	17	19
Registered nursing, total	1,385	1,473	1,470	1,516	1,508	- - -	- - -
Baccalaureate	377	441	489	521	523	- - -	- - -
Associate degree	697	776	829	876	876	- - -	- - -
Diploma	311	256	152	119	109	- - -	- - -
Licensed practical nursing	1,299	1,165	1,154	1,210	- - -	- - -	- - -
Dentistry	60	60	56	53	53	53	53
Optometry	15	16	16	16	16	16	16
Pharmacy	72	72	74	75	75	75	78
Chiropractic	14	17	17	- - -	- - -	- - -	- - -
Schools of Public Health	21	23	25	27	28	28	- - -

- - - Data not available.

[1]Chiropractic first-year enrollment data are partial data from eight reporting schools.

[2]These are students entering Schools of Public Health for the first time.

[3]Some nursing schools offer more than one type of program. Numbers shown for nursing are number of nursing programs.

NOTE: Data on the number of schools are reported as of the beginning of the academic year while data on first-year enrollment and number of graduates are reported as of the end of the academic year.

SOURCES: Association of American Medical Colleges: AAMC Data Book, Statistical Information Related to Medical Education. Washington, DC. 1999; Bureau of Health Professions: Health Personnel in the United States, Eighth Report to Congress, 1991. Health Resources and Services Administration. DHHS Pub. No. HRS-P-OD–92–1, Rockville, Maryland. 1992 and unpublished data; National League for Nursing: Nursing data source, 1997 and unpublished data; American Nurses Association: Facts About Nursing, 1951 and 1961; American Dental Association 1996/97 Survey of predoctoral dental educational institutions, Chicago. 1996; American Medical Association: Medical education in the United States. *JAMA* 278(9). September 3, 1997; American Association of Colleges of Osteopathic Medicine. Annual statistical report 1998. Rockville, Maryland. 1998; American Chiropractic Association: Unpublished data; Association of Schools of Public Health: Unpublished data.

Table 108 (page 1 of 2). Total enrollment of minorities in schools for selected health occupations, according to detailed race and Hispanic origin: United States, academic years 1970–71, 1980–81, 1990–91, and 1996–97

[Data are based on reporting by health professions associations]

Occupation, detailed race, and Hispanic origin	1970–71[1]	1980–81	1990–91	1996–97[2]	1970–71[1]	1980–81	1990–91	1996–97[2]
Allopathic medicine	Number of students				Percent of students			
All races[3]	40,238	65,189	65,163	67,276	100.0	100.0	100.0	100.0
White, non-Hispanic	37,944	55,434	47,893	44,283	94.3	85.0	73.5	65.8
Black, non-Hispanic	1,509	3,708	4,241	5,400	3.8	5.7	6.5	8.0
Hispanic	196	2,761	3,538	4,424	0.5	4.2	5.4	6.6
Mexican	- - -	951	1,109	1,818	- - -	1.5	1.7	2.7
Mainland Puerto Rican	- - -	329	457	488	- - -	0.5	0.7	0.7
Other Hispanic[4]	- - -	1,481	1,972	2,118	- - -	2.3	3.0	3.1
American Indian	18	221	277	528	0.0	0.3	0.4	0.8
Asian	571	1,924	8,436	11,808	1.4	3.0	12.9	17.6
Osteopathic medicine								
All races	2,304	4,940	6,792	8,961	100.0	100.0	100.0	100.0
White, non-Hispanic[3]	2,241	4,688	5,680	7,148	97.3	94.9	83.6	79.8
Black, non-Hispanic	27	94	217	369	1.2	1.9	3.2	4.1
Hispanic	19	52	277	339	0.8	1.1	4.1	3.8
American Indian	6	19	36	83	0.3	0.4	0.5	0.9
Asian	11	87	582	1,022	0.5	1.8	8.6	11.4
Podiatry								
All races	1,268	2,577	2,226	2,175	100.0	100.0	100.0	100.0
White, non-Hispanic[3]	1,228	2,353	1,671	1,705	96.8	91.3	75.1	78.4
Black, non-Hispanic	27	110	237	80	2.1	4.3	10.6	3.7
Hispanic	5	39	148	73	0.4	1.5	6.6	3.4
American Indian	1	6	7	12	0.1	0.2	0.3	0.6
Asian	7	69	163	305	0.6	2.7	7.3	14.0
Dentistry[5]								
All races	19,187	22,842	15,770	16,400	100.0	100.0	100.0	100.0
White, non-Hispanic[3]	17,531	20,208	11,185	11,100	91.4	88.5	70.9	67.7
Black, non-Hispanic	872	1,022	940	891	4.5	4.5	6.0	5.4
Hispanic	185	519	1,073	654	1.0	2.3	6.8	4.0
American Indian	28	53	53	83	0.1	0.2	0.3	0.5
Asian	490	1,040	2,519	3,672	2.6	4.6	16.0	22.4
Optometry[5]								
All races	3,094	4,540	4,650	5,075	100.0	100.0	100.0	100.0
White, non-Hispanic[3]	2,913	4,148	3,706	3,705	94.1	91.4	79.7	73.0
Black, non-Hispanic	32	57	134	120	1.0	1.3	2.9	2.4
Hispanic	30	80	186	200	1.0	1.8	4.0	3.9
American Indian	2	12	21	23	0.1	0.3	0.5	0.5
Asian	117	243	603	1,027	3.8	5.4	13.0	20.2
Pharmacy[5,6]								
All races	17,909	21,628	22,764	32,853	100.0	100.0	100.0	100.0
White, non-Hispanic[3]	16,222	19,153	18,325	23,091	90.6	88.6	80.5	70.3
Black, non-Hispanic	659	945	1,301	2,529	3.7	4.4	5.7	7.7
Hispanic	254	459	945	934	1.4	2.1	4.2	2.8
American Indian	29	36	63	147	0.2	0.2	0.3	0.4
Asian	672	1,035	2,130	6,152	3.8	4.8	9.4	18.7

See footnotes at end of table.

Table 108 (page 2 of 2). Total enrollment of minorities in schools for selected health occupations, according to detailed race and Hispanic origin: United States, academic years 1970–71, 1980–81, 1990–91, and 1996–97

[Data are based on reporting by health professions associations]

Occupation, detailed race, and Hispanic origin	1970–71[1]	1980–81	1990–91	1996–97[2]	1970–71[1]	1980–81	1990–91	1996–97[2]
Registered nurses[5,7]		Number of students				Percent of students		
All races	211,239	230,966	221,170	238,244	100.0	100.0	100.0	100.0
White, non-Hispanic[3]	- - -	- - -	183,102	193,061	- - -	- - -	82.8	81.0
Black, non-Hispanic	- - -	- - -	23,094	23,611	- - -	- - -	10.4	9.9
Hispanic	- - -	- - -	6,580	9,227	- - -	- - -	3.0	3.9
American Indian	- - -	- - -	1,803	1,816	- - -	- - -	0.8	0.8
Asian	- - -	- - -	6,591	10,529	- - -	- - -	3.0	4.4

- - - Data not available.

[1]Data for osteopathic medicine, podiatry, and optometry are for 1971–72. Data for pharmacy and registered nurses are for 1972–73.
[2]Data for podiatry exclude New York College of Podiatric Medicine.
[3]Includes race and ethnicity unspecified.
[4]Includes Puerto Rican Commonwealth students.
[5]Excludes Puerto Rican schools.
[6]Prior to 1992–93 pharmacy total enrollment data are for students in the final 3 years of pharmacy education. Beginning in 1992–93 pharmacy data are for all students.
[7]In 1990 the National League for Nursing developed a new system for analyzing minority data. In evaluating the former system, much underreporting was noted. Therefore, race-specific data before 1990 would not be comparable and are not shown. Additional changes in the minority data question were introduced for academic years 1992–93 and 1993–94 resulting in a discontinuity in the trend.

NOTE: Total enrollment data are collected at the beginning of the academic year.

SOURCES: Association of American Medical Colleges: AAMC Data Book: Statistical Information Related to Medical Education. Washington, DC. 1998; American Association of Colleges of Osteopathic Medicine: 1997 Annual statistical report. Rockville, Maryland. 1997; Bureau of Health Professions: Minorities and women in the health fields, 1990 Edition; American Dental Association 1996/97 Survey of predoctoral dental educational institutions, Chicago. 1997; Association of Schools and Colleges of Optometry: Unpublished data; American Association of Colleges of Pharmacy: Profile of pharmacy students 1996, and unpublished data; American Association of Colleges of Podiatric Medicine: Unpublished data; National League for Nursing: Nursing datasource, 1997; Nursing data book. New York. 1982.

Table 109. First-year and total enrollment of women in schools for selected health occupations, according to detailed race and Hispanic origin: United States, academic years 1971–72, 1980–81, 1990–91, and 1996–97

[Data are based on reporting by health professions associations]

Enrollment, occupation, detailed race, and Hispanic origin	Both sexes				Women			
	1971–72[1]	1980–81	1990–91	1996–97[2]	1971–72[1]	1980–81	1990–91	1996–97[2]
First-year enrollment	Number of students				Percent of students			
Allopathic medicine[3]	12,361	17,186	16,876	16,935	13.7	28.9	38.8	42.9
White, non-Hispanic	- - -	14,262	11,830	10,916	- - -	27.4	37.7	40.4
Black, non-Hispanic	881	1,128	1,263	1,423	22.7	45.5	55.3	60.5
Hispanic	- - -	818	933	1,207	- - -	31.5	42.0	44.9
Mexican	118	258	285	501	8.5	30.6	39.3	44.3
Mainland Puerto Rican	40	95	120	150	15.0	43.2	43.3	50.7
Other Hispanic[4]	- - -	465	528	556	- - -	29.7	43.3	43.9
American Indian	23	67	76	149	34.8	35.8	40.8	50.3
Asian	217	572	2,527	3,039	19.4	31.5	40.3	42.3
Dentistry[5]	4,705	5,964	3,961	4,204	3.1	19.8	37.9	37.6
Osteopathic medicine	670	1,496	1,950	2,535	4.3	22.0	34.2	37.8
Podiatry[6]	399	695	622	616	- - -	- - -	- - -	31.0
Optometry[5]	906	1,174	1,207	1,323	5.3	25.3	50.6	53.4
Pharmacy[5,7]	6,532	7,442	8,009	8,719	25.8	48.4	- - -	63.1
Registered nurses[5]	93,344	110,201	113,526	119,205	94.5	92.7	89.3	87.5
Total enrollment								
Allopathic medicine[3]	43,650	65,189	65,163	67,276	10.9	26.5	37.3	42.2
White, non-Hispanic	- - -	55,434	47,893	44,283	- - -	25.0	35.4	39.9
Black, non-Hispanic	2,055	3,708	4,241	5,400	20.4	44.3	55.8	60.4
Hispanic	- - -	2,761	3,538	4,424	- - -	30.1	39.0	43.6
Mexican	252	951	1,109	1,818	9.5	26.4	38.5	42.1
Mainland Puerto Rican	76	329	457	488	17.1	35.9	43.1	47.1
Other Hispanic[4]	- - -	1,481	1,972	2,118	- - -	31.1	38.4	44.2
American Indian	42	221	277	528	23.8	28.5	42.6	45.8
Asian	647	1,924	8,436	11,808	17.9	30.4	37.7	42.0
Dentistry[5]	16,553	22,842	15,770	16,400	- - -	17.0	34.2	36.7
Osteopathic medicine	2,304	4,940	6,792	8,961	3.4	19.7	32.7	36.9
Podiatry[6]	1,268	2,577	2,226	2,175	1.2	11.9	- - -	30.2
Optometry[5]	3,094	4,540	4,650	5,075	- - -	- - -	47.3	52.9
Registered nurses[5]	211,239	230,966	221,170	238,244	95.5	94.3	- - -	87.9

- - - Data not available.

[1]Total enrollments for registered nurse students are for 1972–73.
[2]First-year enrollments for registered nurse students are for 1995–96.
[3]Includes race and ethnicity unspecified.
[4]Includes Puerto Rican Commonwealth students.
[5]Excludes Puerto Rican schools.
[6]Podiatry data for 1996–97 exclude New York College of Podiatric Medicine.
[7]Pharmacy first-year enrollment data are for students in the first year of the final 3 years of pharmacy education.

NOTES: Data not available on total enrollment of women in schools of pharmacy. Total enrollment data are collected at the beginning of the academic year while first-year enrollment data are collected during the academic year.

SOURCES: Association of American Medical Colleges: AAMC Data Book: Statistical Information Related to Medical Education. Washington, DC. 1998 and unpublished data; American Association of Colleges of Osteopathic Medicine: 1997 Annual Statistical Report. Rockville, Maryland. 1997; Bureau of Health Professions: Minorities and women in the health fields, 1990 edition; American Dental Association 1996/97 Survey of predoctoral dental educational institutions, Chicago. 1997; Association of Schools and Colleges of Optometry: Unpublished data; American Association of Colleges of Pharmacy: Unpublished data; American Association of Colleges of Podiatric Medicine: Unpublished data; National League for Nursing: Nursing datasource. New York. 1997; Nursing data book. New York. 1982; State-Approved Schools of Nursing-RN. New York. 1973.

Table 110. Hospitals, beds, and occupancy rates, according to type of ownership and size of hospital: United States, selected years 1975–97

[Data are based on reporting by a census of hospitals]

Type of ownership and size of hospital	1975	1980	1985	1990	1994	1995	1996	1997
Hospitals				Number				
All hospitals	7,156	6,965	6,872	6,649	6,374	6,291	6,201	6,097
Federal	382	359	343	337	307	299	290	285
Non-Federal[1]	6,774	6,606	6,529	6,312	6,067	5,992	5,911	5,812
Community[2]	5,875	5,830	5,732	5,384	5,229	5,194	5,134	5,057
Nonprofit	3,339	3,322	3,349	3,191	3,139	3,092	3,045	3,000
For profit	775	730	805	749	719	752	759	797
State-local government	1,761	1,778	1,578	1,444	1,371	1,350	1,330	1,260
6–24 beds	299	259	208	226	235	278	262	281
25–49 beds	1,155	1,029	982	935	900	922	906	890
50–99 beds	1,481	1,462	1,399	1,263	1,157	1,139	1,128	1,111
100–199 beds	1,363	1,370	1,407	1,306	1,331	1,324	1,338	1,289
200–299 beds	678	715	739	739	746	718	692	679
300–399 beds	378	412	439	408	377	354	361	367
400–499 beds	230	266	239	222	210	195	196	185
500 beds or more	291	317	319	285	273	264	251	255
Beds								
All hospitals	1,465,828	1,364,516	1,317,630	1,213,327	1,128,066	1,080,601	1,061,688	1,035,390
Federal	131,946	117,328	112,023	98,255	83,823	77,079	73,171	61,937
Non-Federal[1]	1,333,882	1,247,188	1,205,607	1,115,072	1,044,243	1,003,522	988,517	973,453
Community[2]	941,844	988,387	1,000,678	927,360	902,061	872,736	862,352	853,287
Nonprofit	658,195	692,459	707,451	656,755	636,949	609,729	598,162	590,636
For profit	73,495	87,033	103,921	101,377	100,667	105,737	109,197	115,074
State-local government	210,154	208,895	189,306	169,228	164,445	157,270	154,993	147,577
6–24 beds	5,615	4,932	4,031	4,427	4,388	5,085	4,770	5,128
25–49 beds	41,783	37,478	36,833	35,420	33,635	34,352	33,814	33,138
50–99 beds	106,776	105,278	101,680	90,394	83,018	82,024	81,185	79,837
100–199 beds	192,438	192,892	199,690	183,867	187,369	187,381	189,630	182,284
200–299 beds	164,405	172,390	180,165	179,670	182,111	175,240	168,977	165,197
300–399 beds	127,728	139,434	151,919	138,938	129,300	121,136	123,822	126,307
400–499 beds	101,278	117,724	106,653	98,833	93,415	86,459	86,913	82,250
500 beds or more	201,821	218,259	219,707	195,811	188,825	181,059	173,241	179,146
Occupancy rate				Percent of beds occupied				
All hospitals	76.7	77.7	69.0	69.5	66.0	65.7	64.5	65.0
Federal	80.7	80.1	76.3	72.9	74.9	72.6	71.4	79.1
Non-Federal[1]	76.3	77.4	68.4	69.2	65.3	65.1	64.0	64.1
Community[2]	75.0	75.6	64.8	66.8	62.9	62.8	61.5	61.8
Nonprofit	77.5	78.2	67.2	69.3	64.8	64.5	63.3	63.6
For profit	65.9	65.2	52.1	52.8	50.1	51.8	51.6	52.0
State-local government	70.4	71.1	62.9	65.3	63.5	63.7	61.7	62.3
6–24 beds	48.0	46.8	34.7	32.3	31.7	36.9	33.2	35.4
25–49 beds	56.7	52.8	40.0	41.3	40.9	42.6	40.0	40.3
50–99 beds	64.7	64.2	51.8	53.8	53.1	54.1	53.1	54.2
100–199 beds	71.2	71.4	59.7	61.5	58.2	58.8	57.8	58.2
200–299 beds	77.1	77.4	65.7	67.1	62.9	63.1	62.0	61.8
300–399 beds	79.7	79.7	68.4	70.0	65.5	64.8	63.6	63.2
400–499 beds	81.1	81.2	70.1	73.5	68.9	68.1	67.4	68.0
500 beds or more	80.9	82.1	74.6	77.3	71.8	71.4	69.7	69.8

[1]The category of non-Federal hospitals is comprised of psychiatric, tuberculosis and other respiratory disease hospitals, and long-term and short-term hospitals.
[2]Community hospitals are short-term hospitals excluding hospital units in institutions such as prison and college infirmaries, facilities for the mentally retarded, and alcoholism and chemical dependency hospitals.

NOTE: Data for additional years are available (see Appendix III).

SOURCES: American Hospital Association: Hospital Statistics, 1976, 1981, 1986, 1991–99 Editions. Chicago, 1976, 1981, 1986, 1991–99. (Copyrights 1976, 1981, 1986, 1991–99: Used with the permission of the American Hospital Association (AHA) and Health Forum, an AHA company.)

Table 111. Inpatient and residential mental health organizations and beds, according to type of organization: United States, selected years 1984–94

[Data are based on inventories of mental health organizations]

Type of organization	1984	1986	1988	1990	1992	1994
	Number of mental health organizations					
All organizations.	2,849	3,039	3,231	3,430	3,415	3,319
State and county mental hospitals	277	285	285	273	273	256
Private psychiatric hospitals.	220	314	444	462	475	430
Non-Federal general hospital psychiatric services . . .	1,259	1,287	1,425	1,571	1,517	1,531
Department of Veterans Affairs psychiatric services[1]	124	124	125	130	133	135
Residential treatment centers for emotionally disturbed children	322	437	440	501	497	459
All other[2]	647	592	512	493	520	508
	Number of beds					
All organizations.	262,673	267,613	271,923	272,253	270,867	252,333
State and county mental hospitals	130,411	119,033	107,109	98,789	93,058	79,294
Private psychiatric hospitals.	21,474	30,201	42,255	44,871	43,684	41,195
Non-Federal general hospital psychiatric services . . .	46,045	45,808	48,421	53,479	52,059	52,984
Department of Veterans Affairs psychiatric services[1]	23,546	26,874	25,742	21,712	22,466	21,146
Residential treatment centers for emotionally disturbed children	16,745	24,547	25,173	29,756	30,089	32,110
All other[2]	24,452	21,150	23,223	23,646	29,511	25,604
	Beds per 100,000 civilian population					
All organizations.	112.9	111.7	111.4	111.6	107.4	97.5
State and county mental hospitals	56.1	49.7	44.0	40.5	36.9	30.6
Private psychiatric hospitals.	9.2	12.6	17.3	18.4	17.3	15.9
Non-Federal general hospital psychiatric services . . .	19.8	19.1	19.8	21.9	20.7	20.5
Department of Veterans Affairs psychiatric services[1]	10.1	11.2	10.5	8.9	8.9	8.2
Residential treatment centers for emotionally disturbed children	7.2	10.3	10.3	12.2	11.9	12.4
All other[2]	10.5	8.8	9.5	9.7	11.7	9.9

[1]Includes Department of Veterans Affairs neuropsychiatric hospitals and general hospital psychiatric services.
[2]Includes other multiservice mental health organizations with inpatient and residential treatment services that are not elsewhere classified. See Appendix I.

SOURCES: Survey and Analysis Branch, Division of State and Community Systems Development, Center for Mental Health Services. Manderscheid RW, Sonnenschein MA. *Mental health, United States, 1996*. DHHS. 1996.

Table 112. Community hospital beds and average annual percent change, according to geographic division and State: United States, selected years 1940–97

[Data are based on reporting by facilities]

Geographic division and State	Beds per 1,000 civilian population							Average annual percent change				
	1940[1,2]	1950[1,2]	1960[2,3]	1970[2]	1980[2]	1990[4]	1997[4]	1940–60[1,2,3]	1960–70[2,3]	1970–80[2]	1980–90[5]	1990–97[4]
United States	3.2	3.3	3.6	4.3	4.5	3.7	3.2	0.6	1.8	0.5	−1.9	−2.1
New England	4.4	4.2	3.9	4.1	4.1	3.4	2.6	−0.6	0.5	0.0	−1.9	−3.8
Maine	3.0	3.2	3.4	4.7	4.7	3.7	3.0	0.6	3.3	0.0	−2.4	−3.0
New Hampshire	4.2	4.2	4.4	4.0	3.9	3.1	2.5	0.2	−0.9	−0.3	−2.3	−3.0
Vermont	3.3	4.0	4.5	4.5	4.4	3.0	2.7	1.6	0.0	−0.2	−3.8	−1.5
Massachusetts	5.1	4.8	4.2	4.4	4.4	3.6	2.8	−1.0	0.5	0.0	−2.0	−3.5
Rhode Island	3.9	3.8	3.7	4.0	3.8	3.2	2.6	−0.3	0.8	−0.5	−1.7	−2.9
Connecticut	3.7	3.6	3.4	3.4	3.5	2.9	2.2	−0.4	0.0	0.3	−1.9	−3.9
Middle Atlantic	3.9	3.8	4.0	4.4	4.6	4.1	3.8	0.1	1.0	0.4	−1.1	−1.1
New York	4.3	4.1	4.3	4.6	4.5	4.1	3.9	0.0	0.7	−0.2	−0.9	−0.7
New Jersey	3.5	3.2	3.1	3.6	4.2	3.7	3.5	−0.6	1.5	1.6	−1.3	−0.8
Pennsylvania	3.5	3.8	4.1	4.7	4.8	4.4	3.8	0.8	1.4	0.2	−0.9	−2.1
East North Central	3.2	3.2	3.6	4.4	4.7	3.9	3.2	0.6	2.0	0.7	−1.8	−2.8
Ohio	2.7	2.9	3.4	4.2	4.7	4.0	3.2	1.2	2.1	1.1	−1.6	−3.1
Indiana	2.3	2.6	3.1	4.0	4.5	3.9	3.3	1.5	2.6	1.2	−1.4	−2.4
Illinois	3.4	3.6	4.0	4.7	5.1	4.0	3.4	0.8	1.6	0.8	−2.4	−2.3
Michigan	4.0	3.3	3.3	4.3	4.4	3.7	2.9	−1.0	2.7	0.2	−1.7	−3.4
Wisconsin	3.4	3.7	4.3	5.2	4.9	3.8	3.2	1.2	1.9	−0.6	−2.5	−2.4
West North Central	3.1	3.7	4.3	5.7	5.8	4.9	4.2	1.6	2.9	0.2	−1.7	−2.2
Minnesota	3.9	4.4	4.8	6.1	5.7	4.4	3.6	1.0	2.4	−0.7	−2.6	−2.8
Iowa	2.7	3.2	3.9	5.6	5.7	5.1	4.3	1.9	3.7	0.2	−1.1	−2.4
Missouri	2.9	3.3	3.9	5.1	5.7	4.8	3.9	1.5	2.7	1.1	−1.7	−2.9
North Dakota	3.5	4.3	5.2	6.8	7.4	7.0	6.1	2.0	2.7	0.8	−0.6	−1.9
South Dakota	2.8	4.4	4.5	5.6	5.5	6.1	6.0	2.4	2.2	−0.2	1.0	−0.2
Nebraska	3.4	4.2	4.4	6.2	6.0	5.5	4.7	1.3	3.5	−0.3	−0.9	−2.2
Kansas	2.8	3.4	4.2	5.4	5.8	4.8	4.2	2.0	2.5	0.7	−1.9	−1.9
South Atlantic	2.5	2.8	3.3	4.0	4.5	3.7	3.2	1.4	1.9	1.2	−1.9	−2.1
Delaware	4.4	3.9	3.7	3.7	3.6	3.0	2.6	−0.9	0.0	−0.3	−1.8	−2.0
Maryland	3.9	3.6	3.3	3.1	3.6	2.8	2.5	−0.8	−0.6	1.5	−2.5	−1.6
District of Columbia	5.5	5.5	5.9	7.4	7.3	7.6	6.8	0.4	2.3	−0.1	0.4	−1.6
Virginia	2.2	2.5	3.0	3.7	4.1	3.3	2.7	1.6	2.1	1.0	−2.1	−2.8
West Virginia	2.7	3.1	4.1	5.4	5.5	4.7	4.5	2.1	2.8	0.2	−1.6	−0.6
North Carolina	2.2	2.6	3.4	3.8	4.2	3.3	3.1	2.2	1.1	1.0	−2.4	−0.9
South Carolina	1.8	2.4	2.9	3.7	3.9	3.3	3.2	2.4	2.5	0.5	−1.7	−0.4
Georgia	1.7	2.0	2.8	3.8	4.6	4.0	3.4	2.5	3.1	1.9	−1.4	−2.3
Florida	2.8	2.9	3.1	4.4	5.1	3.9	3.4	0.5	3.6	1.5	−2.6	−1.9
East South Central	1.7	2.1	3.0	4.4	5.1	4.7	4.2	2.9	3.9	1.5	−0.8	−1.6
Kentucky	1.8	2.2	3.0	4.0	4.5	4.3	3.9	2.6	2.9	1.2	−0.5	−1.4
Tennessee	1.9	2.3	3.4	4.7	5.5	4.8	3.9	3.0	3.3	1.6	−1.4	−2.9
Alabama	1.5	2.0	2.8	4.3	5.1	4.6	4.3	3.2	4.4	1.7	−1.0	−1.0
Mississippi	1.4	1.7	2.9	4.4	5.3	5.0	4.7	3.7	4.3	1.9	−0.6	−0.9
West South Central	2.1	2.7	3.3	4.3	4.7	3.8	3.2	2.3	2.7	0.9	−2.1	−2.4
Arkansas	1.4	1.6	2.9	4.2	5.0	4.6	4.0	3.7	3.8	1.8	−0.8	−2.0
Louisiana	3.1	3.8	3.9	4.2	4.8	4.6	4.3	1.2	0.7	1.3	−0.4	−1.0
Oklahoma	1.9	2.5	3.2	4.5	4.6	4.0	3.3	2.6	3.5	0.2	−1.4	−2.7
Texas	2.0	2.7	3.3	4.3	4.7	3.5	2.9	2.5	2.7	0.9	−2.9	−2.7
Mountain	3.6	3.8	3.5	4.3	3.8	3.1	2.5	−0.1	2.1	−1.2	−2.0	−3.0
Montana	4.9	5.3	5.1	5.8	5.9	5.8	5.1	0.2	1.3	0.2	−0.2	−1.8
Idaho	2.6	3.4	3.2	4.0	3.7	3.2	2.9	1.0	2.3	−0.8	−1.4	−1.4
Wyoming	3.5	3.9	4.6	5.5	3.6	4.8	4.1	1.4	1.8	−4.1	2.9	−2.2
Colorado	3.9	4.2	3.8	4.6	4.2	3.2	2.3	−0.1	1.9	−0.9	−2.7	−4.6
New Mexico	2.7	2.2	2.9	3.5	3.1	2.8	2.1	0.4	1.9	−1.2	−1.0	−4.0
Arizona	3.4	4.0	3.0	4.1	3.6	2.7	2.3	−0.6	3.2	−1.3	−2.8	−2.3
Utah	3.2	2.9	2.8	3.6	3.1	2.6	2.0	−0.7	2.5	−1.5	−1.7	−3.7
Nevada	5.0	4.4	3.9	4.2	4.2	2.8	2.1	−1.2	0.7	0.0	−4.0	−4.0
Pacific	4.1	3.2	3.1	3.7	3.5	2.7	2.2	−1.4	1.8	−0.6	−2.6	−2.9
Washington	3.4	3.6	3.3	3.5	3.1	2.5	1.9	−0.1	0.6	−1.2	−2.1	−3.8
Oregon	3.5	3.1	3.5	4.0	3.5	2.8	2.2	0.0	1.3	−1.3	−2.2	−3.4
California	4.4	3.3	3.0	3.8	3.6	2.7	2.3	−1.9	2.4	−0.5	−2.8	−2.3
Alaska	. . .	. . .	2.4	2.3	2.7	2.3	2.4	. . .	−0.4	1.6	−1.6	0.6
Hawaii	. . .	. . .	3.7	3.4	3.1	2.7	2.3	. . .	−0.8	−0.9	−1.4	−2.3

0.0 Quantity more than zero but less than 0.05.   . . . Category not applicable.   [1]1940 and 1950 data are estimated based on published figures.
[2]Data exclude facilities for the mentally retarded. See Appendix II, Hospital.   [3]1960 data include hospital units of institutions.
[4]Starting with 1990, data exclude hospital units of institutions, facilities for the mentally retarded, and alcoholism and chemical dependency hospitals. See Appendix II.
[5]1990 data used in this calculation (not shown in table) exclude only facilities for the mentally retarded, consistent with exclusions from 1980 data.
NOTE: Data for additional years are available (see Appendix III).
SOURCES: American Medical Association (AMA): Hospital service in United States. JAMA 116(11):1055–1144, 1941 and 146(2):109–184, 1951 (Copyright 1941, 1951: Used with permission of AMA); American Hospital Association (AHA): Hospitals. JAHA 35(15):383–430, 1961 (Copyright 1961: Used with permission of AHA); data computed by National Center for Health Statistics, Division of Health and Utilization Analysis from data compiled by Division of Health Care Statistics and AHA annual surveys for 1970, 1980; Hospital Statistics 1991–92, 1999 Editions. Chicago (Copyrights 1971, 1981, 1991, 1999: Used with permission of AHA and Health Forum, an AHA company).

Table 113. Occupancy rates in community hospitals and average annual percent change, according to geographic division and State: United States, selected years 1940–97

[Data are based on reporting by facilities]

Geographic division and State	Percent of beds occupied						Average annual percent change				
	1940[1,2]	1960[2,3]	1970[2]	1980[2]	1990[4]	1997[4]	1940–60[1,2,3]	1960–70[2,3]	1970–80[2]	1980–90[5]	1990–97[4]
United States	69.9	74.7	77.3	75.2	66.8	61.8	0.3	0.3	−0.3	−1.2	−1.1
New England	72.5	75.2	79.7	80.1	74.0	67.3	0.2	0.6	0.1	−0.8	−1.3
Maine	72.4	73.2	73.0	74.5	71.5	63.6	0.1	−0.0	0.2	−0.4	−1.7
New Hampshire	65.3	66.5	73.4	73.2	66.8	63.4	0.1	1.0	−0.0	−0.9	−0.7
Vermont	68.8	68.5	76.3	73.7	67.3	71.2	−0.0	1.1	−0.3	−0.9	0.8
Massachusetts	71.8	75.8	80.3	81.7	74.2	67.3	0.3	0.6	0.2	−1.0	−1.4
Rhode Island	77.7	75.7	82.9	85.9	79.4	70.9	−0.1	0.9	0.4	−0.8	−1.6
Connecticut	75.9	78.2	82.6	80.4	77.0	68.7	0.1	0.5	−0.3	−0.4	−1.6
Middle Atlantic	75.5	78.1	82.4	83.2	80.5	71.5	0.2	0.5	0.1	−0.3	−1.7
New York	78.9	79.4	82.9	85.9	36.0	75.9	0.0	0.4	0.4	−0.0	−1.8
New Jersey	72.4	78.4	82.5	82.8	80.2	68.0	0.4	0.5	0.0	−0.3	−2.3
Pennsylvania	71.3	76.0	81.5	79.5	72.9	66.9	0.3	0.7	−0.2	−0.9	−1.2
East North Central	71.0	78.4	79.5	76.9	64.6	59.3	0.5	0.1	−0.3	−1.7	−1.2
Ohio	72.1	81.3	81.8	79.2	64.7	58.3	0.6	0.1	−0.3	−2.0	−1.5
Indiana	68.5	79.6	80.3	77.6	60.6	57.6	0.8	0.1	−0.3	−2.4	−0.7
Illinois	73.1	76.0	79.3	74.9	65.7	58.1	0.2	0.4	−0.6	−1.3	−1.7
Michigan	71.5	80.5	80.6	78.2	65.5	64.7	0.6	0.0	−0.3	−1.8	−0.2
Wisconsin	65.2	73.9	73.2	73.6	64.6	57.0	0.6	−0.1	0.1	−1.3	−1.8
West North Central	65.7	71.8	73.6	71.2	61.8	59.6	0.4	0.2	−0.3	−1.4	−0.5
Minnesota	71.0	72.3	73.9	73.7	66.8	68.3	0.1	0.2	−0.0	−1.0	0.3
Iowa	63.6	72.6	71.9	68.7	61.7	56.1	0.7	−0.1	−0.5	−1.1	−1.4
Missouri	68.6	75.8	79.3	75.1	61.8	56.6	0.5	0.5	−0.5	−1.9	−1.2
North Dakota	61.9	71.3	67.1	68.6	64.2	61.6	0.7	−0.6	0.2	−0.7	−0.6
South Dakota	59.1	66.0	66.3	60.6	62.1	65.0	0.6	0.0	−0.9	0.2	0.7
Nebraska	59.0	65.6	69.9	67.4	57.6	59.5	0.5	0.6	−0.4	−1.6	0.5
Kansas	60.4	69.1	71.4	68.8	55.6	53.0	0.7	0.3	−0.4	−2.1	−0.7
South Atlantic	66.7	74.8	77.9	75.5	67.4	62.3	0.6	0.4	−0.3	−1.1	−1.1
Delaware	59.2	70.2	78.8	81.8	76.5	70.9	0.9	1.2	0.4	−0.7	−1.1
Maryland	74.6	73.9	79.3	84.0	78.6	67.6	−0.0	0.7	0.6	−0.7	−2.1
District of Columbia	76.2	80.8	77.7	83.0	75.3	71.1	0.3	−0.4	0.7	−1.0	−0.8
Virginia	70.0	78.0	81.1	77.8	67.4	63.6	0.5	0.4	−0.4	−1.4	−0.8
West Virginia	62.1	74.5	79.3	75.6	62.7	58.6	0.9	0.6	−0.5	−1.9	−1.0
North Carolina	64.6	73.9	78.5	77.8	73.2	68.2	0.7	0.6	−0.1	−0.6	−1.0
South Carolina	69.1	76.9	76.4	77.0	70.9	64.1	0.5	−0.1	0.1	−0.8	−1.4
Georgia	62.7	71.7	76.5	70.4	65.8	58.9	0.7	0.7	−0.8	−0.7	−1.6
Florida	57.5	73.9	76.2	71.7	61.8	58.7	1.3	0.3	−0.6	−1.5	−0.7
East South Central	62.6	71.8	78.2	74.6	62.6	58.8	0.7	0.9	−0.5	−1.7	−0.9
Kentucky	61.6	73.4	79.6	77.4	62.4	56.9	0.9	0.8	−0.3	−2.1	−1.3
Tennessee	65.5	75.9	78.2	75.9	64.4	58.8	0.7	0.3	−0.3	−1.6	−1.3
Alabama	59.0	70.8	80.0	73.3	62.5	57.8	0.9	1.2	−0.9	−1.6	−1.1
Mississippi	63.8	62.8	73.6	70.5	59.4	62.6	−0.1	1.6	−0.4	−1.7	0.8
West South Central	62.5	68.7	73.2	69.7	57.8	55.5	0.5	0.6	−0.5	−1.9	−0.6
Arkansas	55.6	70.0	74.4	69.6	62.0	57.6	1.2	0.6	−0.7	−1.1	−1.0
Louisiana	75.0	67.9	73.6	69.7	57.4	54.2	−0.5	0.8	−0.5	−1.9	−0.8
Oklahoma	54.5	71.0	72.5	68.1	57.7	54.1	1.3	0.2	−0.6	−1.6	−0.9
Texas	59.6	68.2	73.0	70.1	57.2	55.8	0.7	0.7	−0.4	−2.0	−0.4
Mountain	60.9	69.9	71.2	69.6	60.5	58.6	0.7	0.2	−0.2	−1.4	−0.5
Montana	62.8	60.3	65.9	66.1	61.2	62.0	−0.2	0.9	0.0	−0.8	0.2
Idaho	65.4	55.9	66.1	65.2	55.7	53.7	−0.8	1.7	−0.1	−1.6	−0.5
Wyoming	47.5	61.1	63.1	57.2	53.8	52.4	1.3	0.3	−1.0	−0.6	−0.4
Colorado	62.1	80.6	74.0	71.6	64.0	55.0	1.3	−0.9	−0.3	−1.1	−2.1
New Mexico	47.8	65.1	69.8	66.2	57.5	57.9	1.6	0.7	−0.5	−1.4	0.1
Arizona	61.2	74.2	73.3	74.2	61.8	61.9	1.0	−0.1	0.1	−1.8	0.0
Utah	65.8	70.0	73.7	70.0	58.7	54.4	0.3	0.5	−0.5	−1.7	−1.1
Nevada	67.9	70.7	72.7	68.8	60.2	67.3	0.2	0.3	−0.5	−1.3	1.6
Pacific	69.7	71.4	71.0	69.0	63.8	59.6	0.1	−0.1	−0.3	−0.8	−1.0
Washington	67.5	63.4	69.7	71.7	62.7	56.9	−0.3	1.0	0.3	−1.3	−1.4
Oregon	71.2	65.8	69.3	69.3	56.7	52.9	−0.4	0.5	0.0	−2.0	−1.0
California	69.9	74.3	71.3	68.5	64.1	59.6	0.3	−0.4	−0.4	−0.7	−1.0
Alaska	...	53.8	59.1	58.3	49.5	73.0	...	0.9	−0.1	−1.6	5.7
Hawaii	...	61.5	75.7	74.7	85.1	81.7	...	2.1	−0.1	1.3	−0.6

0.0 Quantity more than zero but less than 0.05.   ... Category not applicable.
[1]1940 data are estimated based on published figures.
[2]Data exclude facilities for the mentally retarded. See Appendix II, Hospital.   [3]1960 data include hospital units of institutions.
[4]Starting with 1990, data exclude hospital units of institutions, facilities for the mentally retarded, and alcoholism and chemical dependency hospitals. See Appendix II.
[5]1990 data used in this calculation (not shown in table) exclude only facilities for the mentally retarded, consistent with exclusions from 1980 data.

NOTES: Occupancy rates exclude data for newborns from the numerator. Data for additional years are available (see Appendix III).

SOURCES: American Medical Association (AMA): Hospital service in United States. JAMA 116(11):1055–1144, 1941. (Copyright 1941: Used with permission of AMA); American Hospital Association (AHA): Hospitals. JAHA 35(15):383–430, Aug. 1, 1961. (Copyright 1961: Used with permission of AHA); data computed by National Center for Health Statistics, Division of Health and Utilization Analysis from data compiled by Division of Health Care Statistics, and AHA annual surveys for 1970 and 1980; Hospital Statistics 1991–92, 1999 Editions. Chicago (Copyrights 1971, 1981, 1991, 1999: Used with permission of AHA and Health Forum, an AHA company).

Table 114 (page 1 of 2). Nursing homes, beds, occupancy, and residents, according to geographic division and State: United States, selected years 1993–97

[Data are based on a census of certified nursing facilities]

Geographic division and State	Nursing homes				Beds			
	1993	1995	1996	1997	1993	1995	1996	1997
United States	15,535	15,647	16,197	16,052	1,665,459	1,666,942	1,727,016	1,714,756
New England	1,111	1,063	1,104	1,122	110,446	106,924	112,192	116,144
Maine	136	121	128	128	9,052	8,332	9,230	8,874
New Hampshire	69	78	78	78	6,531	7,417	7,794	7,591
Vermont	43	43	38	39	3,592	3,654	3,121	3,310
Massachusetts	521	483	522	532	52,051	47,605	51,920	55,029
Rhode Island	84	83	92	93	8,363	8,672	9,400	9,442
Connecticut	258	255	246	252	30,857	31,244	30,727	31,898
Middle Atlantic	1,552	1,607	1,657	1,669	231,795	237,304	241,974	240,966
New York	588	596	589	561	100,875	102,907	102,924	99,159
New Jersey	276	311	316	314	41,492	45,659	46,697	45,935
Pennsylvania	688	700	752	794	89,428	88,738	92,353	95,872
East North Central	3,045	3,045	3,205	3,140	347,526	350,701	376,421	368,442
Ohio	934	894	996	931	100,362	99,358	117,892	111,145
Indiana	522	529	545	549	55,940	56,455	57,988	59,152
Illinois	795	823	841	841	97,750	102,200	105,512	104,873
Michigan	390	396	418	417	45,194	45,477	48,446	47,960
Wisconsin	404	403	405	402	48,280	47,211	46,583	45,312
West North Central	2,242	2,165	2,185	2,186	201,397	193,866	196,080	195,064
Minnesota	443	381	383	396	45,796	38,660	38,753	39,804
Iowa . . . . :	461	428	442	424	44,800	42,832	44,080	41,506
Missouri	484	532	536	549	47,086	51,195	52,332	53,855
North Dakota	83	85	87	80	7,020	6,776	7,128	6,517
South Dakota	113	111	101	100	8,340	8,140	7,283	7,016
Nebraska	233	228	233	234	18,284	17,910	18,000	17,923
Kansas	425	400	403	403	30,071	28,353	28,504	28,443
South Atlantic	2,057	2,106	2,173	2,161	228,161	229,291	232,781	236,958
Delaware	40	38	37	43	4,558	4,332	3,869	4,985
Maryland	197	205	221	228	25,570	26,299	27,394	29,174
District of Columbia	16	14	18	22	3,023	2,156	2,451	3,124
Virginia	263	259	264	245	29,708	29,070	29,593	27,229
West Virginia	94	85	111	79	7,756	6,956	8,924	8,000
North Carolina	356	391	382	384	34,854	38,250	37,717	37,763
South Carolina	138	155	171	176	14,246	15,718	17,002	17,604
Georgia	344	357	358	346	37,318	38,279	38,330	38,652
Florida	609	602	611	638	71,128	68,231	67,501	70,427
East South Central	941	943	1,038	1,007	94,778	92,268	100,336	97,292
Kentucky	271	235	302	266	22,437	19,268	24,180	21,512
Tennessee	298	300	332	341	34,946	34,013	37,394	37,500
Alabama	204	212	209	198	21,703	22,345	22,530	21,677
Mississippi	168	196	195	202	15,692	16,642	16,232	16,603
West South Central	2,136	2,236	2,250	2,210	214,314	221,770	224,665	221,099
Arkansas	249	262	261	256	28,311	30,821	31,461	31,465
Louisiana	321	343	341	333	36,137	39,008	38,183	37,627
Oklahoma	395	388	395	400	33,369	32,519	33,466	33,216
Texas	1,171	1,243	1,253	1,221	116,497	119,422	121,555	118,791
Mountain	721	733	768	762	64,832	63,080	66,458	66,314
Montana	98	102	93	96	6,961	7,331	6,498	6,844
Idaho	68	80	80	78	5,386	5,868	5,860	5,794
Wyoming	28	38	38	37	2,169	3,125	3,125	3,054
Colorado	202	205	205	222	19,017	18,623	18,010	19,457
New Mexico	70	77	79	77	6,493	6,451	6,911	6,518
Arizona	127	114	143	118	14,125	12,097	15,252	12,955
Utah	91	79	88	92	6,983	5,854	6,997	7,403
Nevada	37	38	42	42	3,698	3,731	3,805	4,289
Pacific	1,730	1,749	1,817	1,795	172,210	171,738	176,109	172,477
Washington	275	270	272	275	27,622	26,354	26,423	25,905
Oregon	165	153	159	152	14,346	13,335	13,598	13,207
California	1,248	1,270	1,329	1,311	127,434	127,790	131,726	128,913
Alaska	13	14	16	15	847	724	829	738
Hawaii	29	42	41	42	1,961	3,535	3,533	3,714

See footnotes at end of table.

[Data are based on a census of certified nursing facilities]

Geographic division and State	Occupancy rate[1]				Resident rate[2]			
	1993	1995	1996	1997	1993	1995	1996	1997
United States	85.5	84.2	82.7	82.0	414.8	383.5	379.7	363.2
New England	92.8	91.9	91.4	90.5	484.4	440.6	447.8	447.0
Maine	95.7	90.5	87.4	87.9	438.2	366.9	385.4	365.0
New Hampshire	93.1	93.4	91.6	92.8	403.5	437.2	439.0	424.4
Vermont	94.3	96.7	94.2	94.0	414.1	408.0	332.4	344.4
Massachusetts	93.2	91.1	90.5	89.3	486.1	416.0	440.0	449.3
Rhode Island	95.0	91.2	93.0	91.3	457.2	427.6	457.0	436.1
Connecticut	90.6	92.8	93.4	92.2	542.9	524.6	502.3	498.2
Middle Atlantic	93.3	93.3	93.0	92.5	384.8	371.7	368.5	355.3
New York	95.6	95.5	96.1	95.2	364.1	353.2	348.5	325.1
New Jersey	92.2	91.8	91.9	91.9	359.8	364.9	360.0	341.0
Pennsylvania	91.2	91.5	90.1	90.1	427.5	401.2	400.8	404.7
East North Central	81.8	79.9	77.2	76.8	481.6	453.3	459.9	437.6
Ohio	77.5	74.0	69.2	69.1	513.4	464.5	505.3	466.2
Indiana	75.4	74.1	73.3	71.9	542.4	517.8	515.1	504.4
Illinois	82.3	80.5	78.7	78.2	499.5	486.6	480.6	463.8
Michigan	88.2	87.8	86.0	86.4	335.1	318.4	323.0	312.9
Wisconsin	91.2	90.5	90.0	88.3	543.1	504.1	485.6	454.5
West North Central	82.9	80.6	79.3	79.4	515.1	464.9	456.5	447.9
Minnesota	93.7	93.7	91.6	92.6	584.3	472.9	456.1	465.5
Iowa	68.8	66.3	65.5	66.4	530.3	473.2	475.9	449.7
Missouri	77.4	74.0	73.7	73.3	409.5	410.8	412.9	416.1
North Dakota	96.7	96.4	95.2	93.9	546.3	496.6	503.6	443.7
South Dakota	95.2	94.4	94.1	94.2	563.8	526.8	464.2	441.6
Nebraska	87.9	88.0	87.2	85.4	516.9	488.8	482.2	464.8
Kansas	86.3	84.2	81.7	80.6	565.5	502.1	484.0	470.8
South Atlantic	90.5	90.0	88.8	87.0	347.2	318.6	308.1	296.7
Delaware	77.8	83.3	84.6	75.0	450.2	423.8	369.7	406.3
Maryland	89.4	87.7	85.4	82.1	429.7	403.9	394.7	389.9
District of Columbia	90.5	97.1	87.1	94.9	326.1	241.8	245.3	338.2
Virginia	93.1	93.8	91.4	90.8	408.6	373.3	358.9	317.7
West Virginia	94.6	94.9	93.0	69.5	266.4	229.4	282.2	184.8
North Carolina	91.9	93.1	93.5	93.7	397.4	402.2	385.8	375.0
South Carolina	87.6	87.4	87.8	86.6	347.0	345.0	361.3	355.8
Georgia	93.6	93.9	93.5	92.5	528.8	495.9	479.1	462.0
Florida	88.5	85.8	83.8	83.5	254.4	216.0	200.6	200.8
East South Central	93.5	91.3	90.9	90.9	428.7	383.3	405.3	383.6
Kentucky	90.1	88.6	89.2	88.7	400.1	323.3	398.7	343.9
Tennessee	93.8	90.1	90.4	90.3	495.0	433.3	465.6	454.6
Alabama	93.8	93.5	91.9	93.0	373.9	356.3	345.5	328.8
Mississippi	97.0	93.9	93.5	92.6	429.7	415.6	394.3	390.6
West South Central	77.0	74.8	72.4	71.2	503.1	476.9	455.7	429.9
Arkansas	72.8	68.1	64.8	63.5	531.3	512.7	489.9	472.2
Louisiana	86.1	85.3	82.2	81.1	647.5	654.9	604.3	573.9
Oklahoma	79.5	78.3	74.9	72.4	525.0	481.7	466.4	439.6
Texas	74.5	72.1	70.6	69.8	455.1	423.9	409.3	383.7
Mountain	84.3	84.3	84.2	79.8	346.5	304.2	305.0	275.4
Montana	90.5	88.4	86.6	83.1	525.6	496.2	412.1	398.3
Idaho	81.7	83.3	78.6	74.0	332.0	334.8	302.8	270.4
Wyoming	79.9	87.2	83.5	84.0	337.4	479.3	447.5	428.0
Colorado	85.6	86.3	87.8	83.1	433.1	396.4	375.5	369.9
New Mexico	87.9	86.6	84.2	84.0	345.3	306.7	306.6	276.5
Arizona	80.2	76.9	80.9	75.3	240.5	175.2	220.5	165.6
Utah	80.8	82.3	82.0	78.3	347.0	267.2	303.7	292.8
Nevada	87.7	89.3	89.1	74.4	330.3	285.2	265.3	230.2
Pacific	80.5	79.7	78.4	78.4	303.8	276.8	269.0	253.8
Washington	88.8	86.3	84.3	82.3	388.0	330.5	310.2	284.7
Oregon	84.0	82.8	91.1	79.7	274.0	231.7	223.6	206.1
California	78.2	77.7		77.1	296.9	273.9	268.6	255.4
Alaska	68.8	75.3	76.1	73.6	374.2	299.1	324.1	261.2
Hawaii	93.6	90.9	90.7	91.4	152.5	237.8	221.2	220.1

[1]Percent of beds occupied.

[2]Number of nursing home residents (all ages) per 1,000 resident population 85 years of age and over.

NOTE: Data are not comparable to OSCAR data shown in previous editions of *Health, United States* due to the use of different methodology for editing nursing home information.

SOURCE: Health Care Financing Administration. Division of Payment Systems. Data from the Online Survey Certification and Reporting (OSCAR) database and Cowles Research Group tabulation of OSCAR data.

Table 115. Total health expenditures as a percent of gross domestic product and per capita health expenditures in dollars: Selected countries and years 1960–97

[Data compiled by the Organization for Economic Cooperation and Development]

Country	1960	1965	1970	1975	1980	1985	1990	1994	1995	1996	1997[1]
Health expenditures as a percent of gross domestic product											
Australia	4.9	5.1	5.7	7.5	7.3	7.7	8.2	8.4	8.4	8.5	8.4
Austria	4.4	4.7	5.4	7.3	7.9	6.7	7.1	7.8	8.0	8.0	7.9
Belgium	3.4	3.9	4.1	5.9	6.6	7.4	7.6	8.1	7.9	7.8	7.6
Canada	5.5	6.0	7.1	7.2	7.3	8.4	9.2	9.9	9.7	9.6	9.0
Czechoslovakia	- - -	- - -	- - -	- - -	- - -	- - -	5.5	8.3	7.5	7.2	7.0
Denmark	3.6	4.8	6.1	6.5	6.8	6.3	6.5	6.6	8.0	8.0	7.4
Finland	3.9	4.9	5.7	6.4	6.5	7.3	8.0	7.9	7.6	7.4	7.2
France	4.2	5.2	5.8	7.0	7.6	8.5	8.9	9.7	9.9	9.7	9.6
Germany	4.3	4.6	5.7	8.0	8.1	8.5	8.2	10.3	10.4	10.5	10.4
Greece	2.4	2.6	3.3	3.4	3.6	4.0	4.2	5.5	5.8	6.8	7.1
Hungary	- - -	- - -	- - -	- - -	- - -	- - -	6.6	7.3	7.1	6.7	6.5
Iceland	3.3	3.9	5.0	5.8	6.2	7.3	8.0	8.1	8.2	8.2	8.0
Ireland	3.8	4.2	5.3	7.7	8.8	7.8	6.6	7.6	7.0	7.0	7.0
Italy	3.6	4.3	5.2	6.2	7.0	7.1	8.1	8.4	7.7	7.8	7.6
Japan	- - -	- - -	4.4	5.5	6.4	6.7	6.0	6.9	7.2	7.2	7.3
Korea	- - -	- - -	2.1	2.5	2.9	3.9	3.9	4.6	3.9	4.0	4.0
Luxembourg	- - -	- - -	3.7	5.1	6.2	6.1	6.6	6.5	6.7	6.8	7.1
Mexico	- - -	- - -	- - -	- - -	- - -	- - -	- - -	4.7	4.9	4.6	4.7
Netherlands	3.8	4.3	5.9	7.5	7.9	7.9	8.3	8.8	8.8	8.6	8.6
New Zealand	4.3	- - -	5.2	6.7	6.0	5.3	7.0	7.1	7.3	7.3	7.7
Norway	3.0	3.6	4.6	6.1	7.0	6.6	7.8	8.0	8.0	7.9	7.5
Poland	- - -	- - -	- - -	- - -	- - -	- - -	4.4	4.4	4.5	5.0	5.2
Portugal	- - -	- - -	2.8	5.6	5.8	6.3	6.5	7.8	8.2	8.3	7.8
Spain	1.5	2.6	3.7	4.9	5.7	5.7	6.9	7.3	7.3	7.4	7.4
Sweden	4.7	5.5	7.1	7.9	9.4	9.0	8.8	7.6	8.5	8.6	8.6
Switzerland	3.3	3.8	5.2	7.0	7.3	8.1	8.4	9.5	9.6	10.2	10.1
Turkey	- - -	- - -	2.4	2.7	3.3	2.2	2.5	5.2	3.3	3.8	4.0
United Kingdom	3.9	4.1	4.5	5.5	5.6	5.9	6.0	6.9	6.9	6.9	6.7
United States	5.1	5.7	7.1	8.0	8.9	10.3	12.2	13.6	13.7	13.6	13.5
Per capita health expenditures[2]											
Australia	$ 98	$125	$212	$443	$ 669	$ 989	$1,316	$1,609	$1,699	$1,775	$1,805
Austria	67	92	166	377	697	815	1,180	1,573	1,641	1,748	1,793
Belgium	53	82	131	311	588	890	1,247	1,653	1,664	1,708	1,747
Canada	105	151	255	433	729	1,206	1,691	2,005	2,029	2,065	2,095
Czechoslovakia	- - -	- - -	- - -	- - -	- - -	- - -	538	735	- - -	904	904
Denmark	67	120	215	348	535	816	1,069	1,344	1,708	1,802	1,848
Finland	55	92	165	312	521	852	1,292	1,289	1,370	1,380	1,447
France	73	121	208	398	716	1,088	1,539	1,868	1,971	1,983	2,051
Germany	91	127	230	498	860	1,274	1,642	2,020	2,128	2,278	2,339
Greece	16	27	60	106	190	288	389	634	703	888	974
Hungary	- - -	- - -	- - -	- - -	- - -	- - -	- - -	459	- - -	602	602
Iceland	50	85	139	295	637	929	1,375	1,571	1,789	1,893	2,005
Ireland	37	52	98	240	468	586	748	1,201	1,204	1,276	1,324
Italy	50	81	157	295	591	834	1,322	1,559	1,503	1,584	1,589
Japan	27	64	132	269	535	823	1,082	1,454	1,576	1,677	1,741
Korea	- - -	- - -	14	32	71	171	310	525	483	537	587
Luxembourg	- - -	- - -	150	315	617	895	1,499	1,962	2,077	2,139	2,340
Mexico	- - -	- - -	- - -	- - -	- - - -	- - -	- - -	379	361	358	391
Netherlands	68	99	205	408	693	932	1,325	1,643	1,743	1,766	1,838
New Zealand	92	- - -	177	358	463	592	937	1,151	1,238	1,270	1,352
Norway	47	74	135	308	639	910	1,365	1,754	1,809	1,928	1,814
Poland	- - -	- - -	- - -	- - -	- - -	- - -	- - -	219	- - -	371	371
Portugal	- - -	- - -	45	154	264	387	616	939	1,025	1,071	1,125
Spain	14	37	83	190	332	455	813	992	1,042	1,115	1,168
Sweden	90	146	274	476	867	1,174	1,492	1,339	1,590	1,675	1,728
Switzerland	93	137	270	523	850	1,297	1,782	2,280	2,403	2,499	2,547
Turkey	- - -	- - -	23	41	77	73	119	272	190	232	260
United Kingdom	77	98	149	278	453	670	957	1,213	1,234	1,317	1,347
United States	141	202	341	582	1,052	1,735	2,690	3,500	3,637	3,781	3,925

- - - Data not available.

[1]Preliminary figures.

[2]Per capita health expenditures for each country have been adjusted to U.S. dollars using gross domestic product purchasing power parities for each year.

NOTE: Some numbers in this table have been revised and differ from previous editions of *Health, United States*.

SOURCES: Schieber GJ, Poullier JP, and Greenwald LG. U.S. health expenditure performance: An international comparison and data update. Health Care Financing Review vol 13 no 4. Washington: Health Care Financing Administration. September 1992; Anderson GF and Poullier JP. Health spending, access, and outcomes: Trends in industrialized countries. Health Affairs vol 18 no 3. May/June 1999; Office of National Health Statistics, Office of the Actuary. National health expenditures, 1997. Health Care Financing Review vol 20 no 1. HCFA pub no 03412. Washington: Health Care Financing Administration. March 1999; Organization for Economic Cooperation and Development Health Data File: Unpublished data.

Table 116. Gross domestic product, national health expenditures, Federal and State and local government expenditures, and average annual percent change: United States, selected years 1960–97

[Data are compiled by the Health Care Financing Administration]

Gross domestic product, national health expenditures, and government health expenditures	1960	1965	1970	1975	1980	1985	1990	1994	1995	1996	1997
					Amount in billions						
Gross domestic product (GDP)	$ 527	$ 719	$1,036	$1,631	$2,784	$4,181	$ 5,744	$ 6,947	$ 7,270	$ 7,662	$ 8,111
					Percent						
National health expenditures as percent of GDP	5.1	5.7	7.1	8.0	8.9	10.3	12.2	13.6	13.7	13.6	13.5
Source of funds for national health expenditures					Amount in billions						
National health expenditures	$ 26.9	$ 41.1	$ 73.2	$130.7	$247.3	$428.7	$ 699.4	$ 947.7	$ 993.7	$1,042.5	$1,092.4
Private funds	20.2	30.9	45.5	75.7	142.5	254.5	416.2	524.9	538.5	561.1	585.3
Public funds	6.6	10.3	27.7	55.0	104.8	174.2	283.2	422.8	455.2	481.4	507.1
					Percent distribution						
National health expenditures	100.0	100.0	100.0	100.0	100.0	100.0	100.0	100.0	100.0	100.0	100.0
Private funds	75.2	75.0	62.2	57.9	57.6	59.4	59.5	55.4	54.2	53.8	53.6
Public funds	24.8	25.0	37.8	42.1	42.4	40.6	40.5	44.6	45.8	46.2	46.4
Per capita health expenditures					Amount						
National health expenditures	$ 141	$ 202	$ 341	$ 582	$1,052	$1,735	$ 2,690	$ 3,500	$ 3,637	$ 3,781	$ 3,925
Private health expenditures	106	151	212	337	606	1,030	1,601	1,939	1,971	2,035	2,103
Public health expenditures	35	50	129	245	446	705	1,089	1,561	1,666	1,746	1,822
Federal government expenditures					Amount in billions						
Total	$ 89.6	$122.4	$209.1	$371.3	$622.5	$974.2	$1,284.5	$1,561.4	$1,634.7	$1,695.0	$1,741.0
Health	2.9	4.8	17.8	36.4	72.0	123.2	195.2	301.2	326.0	348.0	367.0
State and local government expenditures											
Total	$ 38.4	$ 57.2	$108.2	$198.0	$307.0	$437.8	$ 648.8	$ 852.3	$ 886.0	$ 922.6	$ 960.1
Health	3.7	5.5	9.9	18.6	32.8	51.0	88.0	121.6	129.2	133.4	140.0
Health as a percent of total					Percent						
Federal government expenditures	3.3	3.9	8.5	9.8	11.6	12.6	15.2	19.3	19.9	20.5	21.1
State and local government expenditures	9.7	9.5	9.1	9.4	10.7	11.7	13.6	14.3	14.6	14.5	14.6
Growth					Average annual percent change from previous year shown						
Gross domestic product	...	6.4	7.6	9.5	11.3	8.5	6.6	4.9	4.6	5.4	5.9
National health expenditures											
Total	...	8.9	12.2	12.3	13.6	11.6	10.2	7.9	4.9	4.9	4.8
Per capita	...	7.4	11.1	11.3	12.6	10.5	9.2	6.8	3.9	4.0	3.8
Private health expenditures											
Total	...	8.8	12.2	12.3	13.6	12.3	10.3	6.0	2.6	4.2	4.3
Per capita	...	7.3	12.2	12.3	13.6	11.2	9.2	4.9	1.7	3.3	3.4
Public health expenditures											
Total	...	9.1	12.2	12.3	-13.6	10.7	10.2	10.5	7.7	5.7	5.3
Per capita	...	7.6	12.2	12.3	13.6	9.6	9.1	9.4	6.7	4.8	4.4
Federal government expenditures											
Total	...	6.4	11.3	12.2	10.9	9.4	5.7	5.0	4.7	3.7	2.7
Health	...	10.6	29.9	15.4	14.6	11.3	9.6	11.5	8.2	6.8	5.5
State and local government expenditures											
Total	...	8.3	13.6	12.8	9.2	7.4	8.2	7.1	4.0	4.1	4.1
Health	...	7.9	12.6	13.5	12.0	9.2	11.5	8.4	6.2	3.2	5.0

... Category not applicable.

NOTES: These data include revisions in health expenditures and differ from previous editions of *Health, United States*. They reflect Social Security Administration population revisions as of July 1998.

SOURCE: National Health Statistics Group, Office of the Actuary. National health expenditures, 1997. Health Care Financing Review vol 20 no 1. HCFA pub no 03412. Health Care Financing Administration. Washington: U.S. Government Printing Office, March 1999.

Table 117. Consumer Price Index and average annual percent change for all items, selected items, and medical care components: United States, selected years 1960–98

[Data are based on reporting by samples of providers and other retail outlets]

Items and medical care components	1960	1970	1980	1985	1990	1995	1996	1997	1998
	Consumer Price Index (CPI)								
All items	29.6	38.8	82.4	107.6	130.7	152.4	156.9	160.5	163.0
All items excluding medical care	30.2	39.2	82.8	107.2	128.8	148.6	152.8	156.3	158.6
All services	24.1	35.0	77.9	109.9	139.2	168.7	174.1	179.4	184.2
Selected items									
Food	30.0	39.2	86.8	105.6	132.4	148.4	153.3	157.3	160.7
Apparel	45.7	59.2	90.9	105.0	124.1	132.0	131.7	132.9	133.0
Housing	- - -	36.4	81.1	107.7	128.5	148.5	152.8	156.8	160.4
Energy	22.4	25.5	86.0	101.6	102.1	105.2	110.1	111.5	102.9
Medical care	22.3	34.0	74.9	113.5	162.8	220.5	228.2	234.6	242.1
Components of medical care									
Medical care services	19.5	32.3	74.8	113.2	162.7	224.2	232.4	239.1	246.8
Professional medical services	- - -	37.0	77.9	113.5	156.1	201.0	208.3	215.4	222.2
Physicians' services	21.9	34.5	76.5	113.3	160.8	208.8	216.4	222.9	229.5
Dental services	27.0	39.2	78.9	114.2	155.8	206.8	216.5	226.6	236.2
Eye care[1]	- - -	- - -	- - -	- - -	117.3	137.0	139.3	141.5	144.1
Services by other medical professionals[1]	- - -	- - -	- - -	- - -	120.2	143.9	146.6	151.8	155.4
Hospital and related services	- - -	- - -	69.2	116.1	178.0	257.8	269.5	278.4	287.5
Hospital services[2]	- - -	- - -	- - -	- - -	- - -	- - -	- - -	101.7	105.0
Inpatient services[2]	- - -	- - -	- - -	- - -	- - -	- - -	- - -	101.3	104.0
Outpatient services[1]	- - -	- - -	- - -	- - -	138.7	204.6	215.1	224.9	233.2
Hospital rooms	9.3	23.6	68.0	115.4	175.4	251.2	261.0	- - -	- - -
Other inpatient services[1]	- - -	- - -	- - -	- - -	142.7	206.8	216.9	- - -	- - -
Nursing home services[2]	- - -	- - -	- - -	- - -	- - -	- - -	- - -	102.3	107.1
Medical care commodities	46.9	46.5	75.4	115.2	163.4	204.5	210.4	215.3	221.8
Prescription drugs	54.0	47.4	72.5	120.1	181.7	235.0	242.9	249.3	258.6
Nonprescription drugs and medical supplies[1]	- - -	- - -	- - -	- - -	120.6	140.5	143.1	145.4	147.7
Internal and respiratory over-the-counter drugs	- - -	42.3	74.9	112.2	145.9	167.0	170.2	173.1	175.4
Nonprescription medical equipment and supplies	- - -	- - -	79.2	109.6	138.0	166.3	169.1	171.5	174.9
	Average annual percent change from previous year shown								
All items	...	4.3	8.9	5.5	4.0	3.1	3.0	2.3	1.6
All items excluding medical care	...	4.1	8.8	5.3	3.7	2.9	2.8	2.3	1.5
All services	...	5.6	10.2	7.1	4.8	3.9	3.2	3.0	2.7
Selected items									
Food	...	4.0	7.7	4.0	4.6	2.3	3.3	2.6	2.2
Apparel	...	4.4	4.6	2.9	3.4	1.2	−0.2	0.9	0.1
Housing	...	- - -	9.9	5.8	3.6	2.9	2.9	2.6	2.3
Energy	...	2.2	15.4	3.4	0.1	0.6	4.7	1.3	−7.7
Medical care	...	6.2	9.5	8.7	7.5	6.3	3.5	2.8	3.2
Components of medical care									
Medical care services	...	7.3	9.9	8.6	7.5	6.6	3.7	2.9	3.2
Professional medical services	...	- - -	8.9	7.8	6.6	5.2	3.6	3.4	3.2
Physicians' services	...	6.6	9.7	8.2	7.3	5.4	3.6	3.0	3.0
Dental services	...	5.3	8.2	7.7	6.4	5.8	4.7	4.7	4.2
Eye care[1]	...	- - -	- - -	- - -	- - -	3.2	1.7	1.6	1.8
Services by other medical professionals[1]	...	- - -	- - -	- - -	- - -	3.7	1.9	3.5	2.4
Hospital and related services	...	- - -	- - -	10.9	8.9	7.7	4.5	3.3	3.3
Hospital services[2]	...	- - -	- - -	- - -	- - -	- - -	- - -	- - -	3.2
Inpatient services[2]	...	- - -	- - -	- - -	- - -	- - -	- - -	- - -	2.7
Outpatient services[1]	...	- - -	- - -	- - -	- - -	8.1	5.1	4.6	3.7
Hospital rooms	...	13.9	12.2	11.2	8.7	7.4	3.9	- - -	- - -
Other inpatient services[1]	...	- - -	- - -	- - -	- - -	7.7	4.9	- - -	- - -
Nursing home services[2]	...	- - -	- - -	- - -	- - -	- - -	- - -	- - -	4.7
Medical care commodities	...	0.7	7.2	8.8	7.2	4.6	2.9	2.3	3.0
Prescription drugs	...	−0.2	7.2	10.6	8.6	5.3	3.4	2.6	3.7
Nonprescription drugs and medical supplies[1]	...	- - -	- - -	- - -	- - -	3.1	1.9	1.6	1.6
Internal and respiratory over-the-counter drugs	...	1.6	7.7	8.4	5.4	2.7	1.9	1.7	1.3
Nonprescription medical equipment and supplies	...	- - -	- - -	6.7	4.7	3.8	1.7	1.4	2.0

- - - Data not available. . . . Category not applicable.
[1]Dec. 1986 = 100. [2]Dec. 1996 = 100.

NOTES: 1982–84 = 100, except where noted. Data for additional years are available (see Appendix III).

SOURCE: U.S. Department of Labor, Bureau of Labor Statistics. Consumer Price Index. Various releases.

Table 118. Growth in personal health care expenditures and percent distribution of factors affecting growth: United States, 1960–97

[Data are compiled by the Health Care Financing Administration]

Period	Average annual percent increase	All factors	Inflation[1] Economy-wide	Inflation[1] Medical	Population	Intensity[2]
			Percent distribution			
1960–97	10.6	100	42	15	10	32
1960–61	6.1	100	20	6	27	47
1961–62	7.6	100	17	11	21	51
1962–63	9.3	100	13	7	16	64
1963–64	9.9	100	15	15	14	56
1964–65	8.6	100	23	9	15	53
1965–66	10.4	100	29	21	11	39
1966–67	13.7	100	25	13	8	54
1967–68	12.9	100	35	11	8	46
1968–69	12.8	100	38	10	8	44
1969–70	13.5	100	40	8	8	43
1970–71	9.8	100	54	11	11	24
1971–72	11.4	100	39	−3	9	55
1972–73	11.6	100	50	−15	8	57
1973–74	14.7	100	62	1	6	30
1974–75	14.7	100	66	9	6	19
1975–76	14.0	100	44	21	6	29
1976–77	13.2	100	50	11	7	32
1977–78	11.6	100	64	5	9	22
1978–79	13.7	100	64	4	7	25
1979–80	15.8	100	60	13	7	20
1980–81	16.1	100	60	17	7	16
1981–82	12.4	100	52	35	9	4
1982–83	10.0	100	44	32	11	13
1983–84	9.6	100	39	40	11	10
1984–85	10.2	100	36	36	10	18
1985–86	9.0	100	29	26	11	34
1986–87	9.6	100	33	19	11	37
1987–88	11.0	100	34	24	10	32
1988–89	10.2	100	42	27	11	20
1989–90	11.7	100	38	21	9	31
1990–91	10.6	100	39	16	10	35
1991–92	9.0	100	32	28	12	28
1992–93	6.7	100	39	32	16	13
1993–94	5.5	100	41	29	18	12
1994–95	5.4	100	48	20	17	15
1995–96	5.1	100	48	11	18	22
1996–97	4.9	100	42	3	19	35

[1]Total inflation is economy-wide and medical inflation is the medical inflation above economy-wide inflation.
[2]The residual percent of growth which cannot be attributed to price increases or population growth and represents changes in use or kinds of services and supplies.

NOTE: These data include revisions in health expenditures and in population back to 1990 and differ from previous editions of Health, United States.

SOURCE: National Health Statistics Group, Office of the Actuary. National health expenditures, 1997. Health Care Financing Review vol 20 no 1. HCFA pub no 03412. Washington: Health Care Financing Administration. March 1999.

Table 119 (page 1 of 2). National health expenditures, average annual percent change, and percent distribution, according to type of expenditure: United States, selected years 1960–97

[Data are compiled by the Health Care Financing Administration]

Type of expenditure	1960	1965	1970	1975	1980	1985	1990	1994	1995	1996	1997
					Amount in billions						
All expenditures	$26.9	$41.1	$73.2	$130.7	$247.3	$428.7	$699.4	$947.7	$993.7	$1,042.5	$1,092.4
Health services and supplies	25.2	37.7	67.9	122.3	235.6	412.3	674.8	917.2	963.1	1,010.6	1,057.5
Personal health care	23.6	35.2	63.8	114.5	217.0	376.4	614.7	834.0	879.3	924.0	969.0
Hospital care	9.3	14.0	28.0	52.6	102.7	168.3	256.4	335.7	347.2	360.8	371.1
Physician services	5.3	8.2	13.6	23.9	45.2	83.6	146.3	193.0	201.9	208.5	217.6
Dentist services	2.0	2.8	4.7	8.0	13.3	21.7	31.6	42.4	45.0	47.5	50.6
Nursing home care	0.8	1.5	4.2	8.7	17.6	30.7	50.9	71.1	75.5	79.4	82.8
Other professional services	0.6	0.9	1.4	2.7	6.4	16.6	34.7	49.6	53.6	57.5	61.9
Home health care	0.1	0.1	0.2	0.6	2.4	5.6	13.1	26.2	29.1	31.2	32.3
Drugs and other medical nondurables	4.2	5.9	8.8	13.0	21.6	37.1	59.9	81.6	88.9	98.3	108.9
Vision products and other medical durables	0.6	1.0	1.6	2.5	3.8	6.7	10.5	12.5	13.1	13.4	13.9
Other personal health care	0.7	0.8	1.3	2.5	4.0	6.1	11.2	21.9	25.1	27.4	29.9
Program administration and net cost of health insurance	1.2	1.9	2.7	4.9	11.9	24.3	40.5	55.1	53.3	52.5	50.0
Government public health activities[1]	0.4	0.6	1.3	2.9	6.7	11.6	19.6	28.2	30.4	34.0	38.5
Research and construction	1.7	3.4	5.3	8.4	11.6	16.4	24.5	30.5	30.6	32.0	34.9
Noncommercial research	0.7	1.5	2.0	3.3	5.5	7.8	12.2	15.9	16.7	17.2	18.0
Construction	1.0	1.9	3.4	5.1	6.2	8.5	12.3	14.6	13.9	14.8	16.9
				Average annual percent change from previous year shown							
All expenditures	...	8.9	12.2	12.3	13.6	11.6	10.3	7.9	4.9	4.9	4.8
Health services and supplies	...	8.4	12.5	12.5	14.0	11.8	10.4	8.0	5.0	4.9	4.6
Personal health care	...	8.3	12.7	12.4	13.6	11.6	10.3	7.9	5.4	5.1	4.9
Hospital care	...	8.6	14.8	13.4	14.3	10.4	8.8	7.0	3.4	3.9	2.9
Physician services	...	9.2	10.6	12.0	13.6	13.1	11.8	7.2	4.6	3.3	4.4
Dentist services	...	7.3	10.8	11.2	10.9	10.2	7.8	7.7	6.1	5.6	6.5
Nursing home care	...	11.6	23.4	15.5	15.3	11.7	10.7	8.7	6.2	5.2	4.3
Other professional services	...	7.4	10.2	14.2	18.4	21.2	15.8	9.4	8.1	7.2	7.7
Home health care	...	9.6	19.7	23.2	30.7	18.9	18.4	18.9	11.0	7.1	3.7
Drugs and other medical nondurables	...	6.8	8.4	8.1	10.7	11.4	10.1	8.0	9.0	10.6	10.7
Vision products and other medical durables	...	9.1	10.2	9.5	8.1	12.4	9.2	4.5	4.9	2.3	3.6
Other personal health care	...	3.5	9.5	13.8	10.2	8.8	12.9	18.2	14.5	9.5	9.0
Program administration and net cost of health insurance	...	10.6	7.1	12.5	19.3	15.4	10.8	8.0	-3.2	-1.5	-4.8
Government public health activities[1]	...	10.8	17.0	16.8	18.1	11.5	11.0	9.5	8.0	11.9	13.1
Research and construction	...	15.1	9.2	9.4	6.8	7.1	8.4	5.6	0.5	4.3	9.2
Noncommercial research	...	17.1	5.1	11.2	10.4	7.5	9.3	6.8	5.2	2.6	4.7
Construction	...	13.7	12.1	8.3	4.1	6.7	7.6	4.4	-4.6	6.3	14.3

See footnotes at end of table.

Table 119 (page 2 of 2). National health expenditures, average annual percent change, and percent distribution, according to type of expenditure: United States, selected years 1960–97

[Data are compiled by the Health Care Financing Administration]

Type of expenditure	1960	1965	1970	1975	1980	1985	1990	1994	1995	1996	1997
					Percent distribution						
All expenditures	100.0	100.0	100.0	100.0	100.0	100.0	100.0	100.0	100.0	100.0	100.0
Health services and supplies	93.7	91.6	92.7	93.6	95.3	96.2	96.5	96.8	96.9	96.9	96.8
Personal health care	88.0	85.5	87.1	87.6	87.8	87.8	87.9	88.0	88.5	88.6	88.7
Hospital care	34.5	34.1	38.2	40.2	41.5	39.3	36.7	35.4	34.9	34.6	34.0
Physician services	19.7	19.9	18.5	18.3	18.3	19.5	20.9	20.4	20.3	20.0	19.9
Dentist services	7.3	6.8	6.4	6.1	5.4	5.0	4.5	4.5	4.5	4.6	4.6
Nursing home care	3.2	3.6	5.8	6.6	7.1	7.2	7.3	7.5	7.6	7.6	7.6
Other professional services	2.3	2.1	1.9	2.1	2.6	3.9	5.0	5.2	5.4	5.5	5.7
Home health care	0.2	0.2	0.3	0.5	1.0	1.3	1.9	2.8	2.9	3.0	3.0
Drugs and other medical nondurables	15.8	14.3	12.0	10.0	8.7	8.6	8.6	8.6	8.9	9.4	10.0
Vision products and other medical durables	2.4	2.4	2.2	2.0	1.5	1.6	1.5	1.3	1.3	1.3	1.3
Other personal health care	2.6	2.0	1.8	1.9	1.6	1.4	1.6	2.3	2.5	2.6	2.7
Program administration and net cost of health insurance	4.3	4.7	3.7	3.8	4.8	5.7	5.8	5.8	5.4	5.0	4.6
Government public health activities[1]	1.4	1.5	1.8	2.2	2.7	2.7	2.8	3.0	3.1	3.3	3.5
Research and construction	6.3	8.4	7.3	6.4	4.7	3.8	3.5	3.2	3.1	3.1	3.2
Noncommercial research	2.6	3.7	2.7	2.5	2.2	1.8	1.7	1.7	1.7	1.6	1.6
Construction	3.7	4.7	4.6	3.9	2.5	2.0	1.8	1.5	1.4	1.4	1.6

. . . Category not applicable.

[1]Includes personal care services delivered by government public health agencies.

NOTE: These data include revisions in health expenditures and differ from previous editions of *Health, United States*.

SOURCE: National Health Statistics Group, Office of the Actuary. National health expenditures, 1997. Health Care Financing Review vol 20 no 1. HCFA pub no 03412. Health Care Financing Administration. Washington: U.S. Government Printing Office, March 1999.

Table 120. Personal health care expenditures, according to type of expenditure and source of funds: United States, selected years 1960–97

[Data are compiled by the Health Care Financing Administration]

Type of personal health care expenditures and source of funds	1960	1965	1970	1975	1980	1985	1990	1994	1995	1996	1997
					Amount in billions						
Total[1]	$ 23.6	$ 35.2	$ 63.8	$114.5	$217.0	$376.4	$614.7	$834.0	$879.3	$924.0	$969.0
					Amount						
Per capita	$ 124	$ 172	$ 297	$ 510	$ 923	$1,523	$2,364	$3,080	$3,218	$3,351	$3,482
Source of funds					Percent distribution						
All sources	100.0	100.0	100.0	100.0	100.0	100.0	100.0	100.0	100.0	100.0	100.0
Out-of-pocket payments	55.3	52.7	39.0	33.3	27.8	26.7	23.6	20.2	19.4	19.3	19.4
Private health insurance	21.2	24.7	23.2	24.8	28.6	30.3	33.8	32.9	32.6	32.4	32.3
Other private funds	1.8	2.0	2.6	2.4	3.6	3.7	3.4	3.5	3.6	3.6	3.7
Government	21.7	20.6	35.3	39.6	40.1	39.2	39.2	43.4	44.4	44.7	44.6
Federal	9.0	8.4	23.0	27.0	29.2	29.5	28.8	33.1	34.0	34.6	34.8
State and local	12.6	12.2	12.2	12.5	10.9	9.7	10.4	10.3	10.4	10.0	9.8
					Amount in billions						
Hospital care expenditures[2]	$ 9.3	$ 14.0	$ 28.0	$ 52.6	$102.7	$168.3	$256.4	$335.7	$347.2	$360.8	$371.1
					Percent distribution						
All sources	100.0	100.0	100.0	100.0	100.0	100.0	100.0	100.0	100.0	100.0	100.0
Out-of-pocket payments	20.7	19.6	9.0	8.3	5.2	5.2	4.3	3.8	3.3	3.3	3.3
Private health insurance	35.6	40.9	32.4	32.9	35.5	35.0	37.3	32.3	30.9	30.5	30.5
Other private funds	1.2	1.9	3.2	2.7	4.9	4.9	4.0	4.1	4.3	4.5	4.6
Government[3]	42.5	37.6	55.4	56.0	54.4	54.8	54.5	59.8	61.5	61.8	61.6
Medicaid	...	...	9.5	10.0	10.3	9.3	11.5	15.7	16.3	16.4	15.5
Medicare	...	...	19.2	22.0	25.7	29.1	26.8	29.7	31.4	32.2	33.3
					Amount in billions						
Nursing home care expenditures[4]	$ 0.8	$ 1.5	$ 4.2	$ 8.7	$ 17.6	$ 30.7	$ 50.9	$ 71.1	$ 75.5	$ 79.4	$ 82.8
					Percent distribution						
All sources	100.0	100.0	100.0	100.0	100.0	100.0	100.0	100.0	100.0	100.0	100.0
Out-of-pocket payments	77.9	60.1	53.5	42.6	41.8	44.3	43.1	35.6	35.3	33.6	31.1
Private health insurance	0.0	0.1	0.4	0.8	1.2	2.7	4.1	4.3	4.5	4.7	4.9
Other private funds	6.3	5.7	4.9	4.8	3.0	1.8	1.8	1.9	1.9	1.9	1.9
Government[3]	15.7	34.1	41.2	51.9	54.0	51.2	51.0	58.3	58.3	59.8	62.2
Medicaid	...	...	22.3	47.1	50.0	47.2	45.4	48.2	47.1	47.4	47.6
Medicare	...	...	3.4	2.5	1.7	1.5	3.4	7.8	8.9	10.1	12.3
					Amount in billions						
Physician services expenditures	$ 5.3	$ 8.2	$ 13.6	$ 23.9	$ 45.2	$ 83.6	$146.3	$193.0	$201.9	$208.5	$217.6
					Percent distribution						
All sources	100.0	100.0	100.0	100.0	100.0	100.0	100.0	100.0	100.0	100.0	100.0
Out-of-pocket payments	62.7	60.6	42.2	36.7	32.4	29.2	22.0	16.3	14.9	14.9	15.7
Private health insurance	30.2	32.5	35.2	35.3	37.9	40.1	45.7	51.3	51.7	51.3	50.2
Other private funds	0.1	0.1	0.1	0.2	0.8	1.6	1.8	1.9	2.1	2.0	2.0
Government[3]	7.1	6.8	22.5	27.7	28.9	29.1	30.5	30.6	31.3	31.8	32.2
Medicaid	...	...	4.8	7.5	5.5	4.2	4.8	7.0	7.2	7.3	7.2
Medicare	...	...	12.2	14.1	17.6	19.5	20.0	18.8	19.8	20.5	21.3
					Amount in billions						
All other personal health care expenditures[5]	$ 8.2	$ 11.5	$ 18.0	$ 29.4	$ 51.5	$ 93.9	$161.0	$234.2	$254.8	$275.3	$297.5
					Percent distribution						
All sources	100.0	100.0	100.0	100.0	100.0	100.0	100.0	100.0	100.0	100.0	100.0
Out-of-pocket payments	87.4	86.7	79.9	72.4	63.9	57.3	49.6	42.4	40.4	39.4	38.8
Private health insurance	1.5	2.4	5.0	8.7	15.9	22.2	26.9	27.3	28.1	28.7	29.3
Other private funds	3.0	2.9	2.8	2.9	3.6	4.1	4.3	4.4	4.4	4.2	4.2
Government[3]	8.1	8.0	12.3	16.1	16.5	16.4	19.2	25.9	27.2	27.6	27.7
Medicaid	...	...	4.5	6.0	5.5	5.7	7.3	11.2	12.0	12.5	13.3
Medicare	...	...	0.7	1.8	3.2	4.6	5.5	9.0	9.9	10.1	9.6

... Category not applicable.

[1]Includes all expenditures for health services and supplies other than expenses for program administration, net cost of private health insurance, and government public health activities.

[2]Includes expenditures for hospital-based nursing home care and home health agency care.

[3]Includes other government expenditures for these health care services, for example, care funded by the Department of Veterans Affairs and State and locally financed subsidies to hospitals.

[4]Includes expenditures for care in freestanding nursing homes. Expenditures for care in facility-based nursing homes are included with hospital care.

[5]Includes expenditures for dental services, other professional services, home health care, drugs and other medical nondurables, vision products and other medical durables, and other personal health care.

NOTE: These data include revisions in health expenditures and differ from previous editions of *Health, United States*.

SOURCE: National Health Statistics Group, Office of the Actuary. National health expenditures, 1997. Health Care Financing Review vol 20 no 1. HCFA pub no 03412. Health Care Financing Administration. Washington: U.S. Government Printing Office, March 1999.

Table 121 (page 1 of 2). Expenditures for health services and supplies and percent distribution, by type of payer: United States, selected calendar years 1965–95

[Data are compiled by the Health Care Financing Administration]

Type of payer	1965	1970	1975	1980	1985	1990	1991	1992	1993	1994	1995
					Amount in billions						
Total[1]	$ 37.7	$ 67.9	$122.3	$235.6	$411.8	$672.9	$736.8	$806.7	$863.1	$906.7	$957.8
Private	29.8	48.9	83.7	158.4	282.2	450.8	483.4	522.4	547.0	569.5	597.4
Private business	5.9	13.6	27.5	61.7	108.6	185.8	200.1	217.9	229.5	239.0	249.4
Employer contribution to private health insurance premiums	4.9	9.7	19.7	45.3	79.1	138.4	148.2	162.4	172.3	177.1	183.8
Private employer contribution to Medicare hospital insurance trust fund[2]	0.0	2.1	5.0	10.5	20.3	29.5	32.7	34.3	36.0	40.2	43.1
Workers compensation and temporary disability insurance	0.8	1.4	2.4	5.1	7.7	15.7	16.7	18.5	18.4	18.6	19.3
Industrial inplant health services	0.2	0.3	0.5	0.9	1.4	2.2	2.4	2.6	2.8	3.1	3.3
Household	23.2	33.8	53.8	89.5	160.5	245.3	261.8	282.2	293.7	306.7	323.3
Employee contribution to private health insurance premiums and individual policy premiums	4.7	5.6	8.2	14.6	30.7	51.3	56.8	62.6	66.4	66.0	68.5
Employee and self-employment contributions and voluntary premiums paid to Medicare hospital insurance trust fund[2]	0.0	2.4	5.7	12.0	24.1	35.5	39.7	41.7	43.8	50.3	55.9
Premiums paid by individuals to Medicare supplementary medical insurance trust fund	0.0	1.0	1.7	2.7	5.2	10.1	10.3	12.1	11.9	14.4	16.3
Out-of-pocket health spending	18.5	24.9	38.1	60.3	100.6	148.4	155.0	165.8	171.6	176.0	182.6
Nonpatient revenues	0.6	1.5	2.4	7.2	13.1	19.8	21.6	22.4	23.8	23.7	24.7
Public	7.9	19.0	38.6	77.3	129.6	222.1	253.3	284.2	316.1	337.3	360.4
Federal Government	3.4	10.4	21.2	42.4	68.4	115.1	135.7	159.1	179.5	189.1	203.4
Employer contributions to private health insurance premiums	0.2	0.3	1.2	2.2	4.3	9.2	9.8	10.7	11.5	11.9	11.3
Medicaid[3]	0.0	2.9	7.6	14.7	23.1	43.4	57.8	69.2	78.2	83.2	88.7
Other[4]	3.2	7.2	12.4	25.5	41.0	62.5	68.1	79.2	89.8	94.0	103.4
State and local government	4.5	8.6	17.4	34.8	61.2	107.0	117.6	125.2	136.6	148.1	157.0
Employer contributions to private health insurance premiums	0.3	0.7	2.2	7.6	18.2	33.5	37.5	41.2	45.2	47.7	47.1
Medicaid[3]	0.0	2.5	6.1	11.7	18.6	33.2	37.9	39.2	43.9	49.8	55.6
Other[5]	1.2	5.4	9.1	15.5	24.4	40.2	42.2	44.8	47.5	50.6	54.3
					Percent distribution						
Total	100.0	100.0	100.0	100.0	100.0	100.0	100.0	100.0	100.0	100.0	100.0
Private	79.0	72.0	68.4	67.2	68.5	67.0	65.6	64.8	63.4	62.8	62.4
Private business	15.6	20.0	22.5	26.2	26.4	27.6	27.2	27.0	26.6	26.4	26.0
Employer contribution to private health insurance premiums	13.0	14.3	16.1	19.2	19.2	20.6	20.1	20.1	20.0	19.5	19.2
Private employer contribution to Medicare hospital insurance trust fund[2]	0.0	3.1	4.1	4.5	4.9	4.4	4.4	4.3	4.2	4.4	4.5
Workers compensation and temporary disability insurance	2.1	2.1	2.0	2.2	1.9	2.3	2.3	2.3	2.1	2.1	2.0
Industrial inplant health services	0.5	0.4	0.4	0.4	0.3	0.3	0.3	0.3	0.3	0.3	0.3
Household	61.5	49.8	44.0	38.0	39.0	36.5	35.5	35.0	34.0	33.8	33.7
Employee contribution to private health insurance premiums and individual policy premiums	12.5	8.2	6.7	6.2	7.5	7.6	7.7	7.8	7.7	7.3	7.1
Employee and self-employment contributions and voluntary premiums paid to Medicare hospital insurance trust fund[2]	0.0	3.5	4.7	5.1	5.9	5.3	5.4	5.2	5.1	5.6	5.8
Premiums paid by individuals to Medicare supplementary medical insurance trust fund	0.0	1.5	1.4	1.1	1.3	1.5	1.4	1.5	1.4	1.6	1.7
Out-of-pocket health spending	49.1	36.7	31.2	25.6	24.4	22.1	21.0	20.5	19.9	19.4	19.1
Nonpatient revenues	1.6	2.2	2.0	3.1	3.2	2.9	2.9	2.8	2.8	2.6	2.6

See footnotes at end of table.

Table 121 (page 2 of 2). Expenditures for health services and supplies and percent distribution, by type of payer: United States, selected calendar years 1965–95

[Data are compiled by the Health Care Financing Administration]

Type of payer	1965	1970	1975	1980	1985	1990	1991	1992	1993	1994	1995
					Percent distribution						
Public	21.0	28.0	31.6	32.8	31.5	33.0	34.4	35.2	36.6	37.2	37.6
Federal Government	9.0	15.3	17.3	18.0	16.6	17.1	18.4	19.7	20.8	20.9	21.2
Employer contributions to private health insurance premiums	0.5	0.4	1.0	0.9	1.0	1.4	1.3	1.3	1.3	1.3	1.2
Medicaid[3]	0.0	4.3	6.2	6.2	5.6	6.4	7.8	8.6	9.1	9.2	9.3
Other[4]	8.5	10.6	10.1	10.8	10.0	9.3	9.2	9.8	10.4	10.4	10.8
State and local government	11.9	12.7	14.2	14.8	14.9	15.9	16.0	15.5	15.8	16.3	16.4
Employer contributions to private health insurance premiums	0.8	1.0	1.8	3.2	4.4	5.0	5.1	5.1	5.2	5.3	4.9
Medicaid[3]	0.0	3.7	5.0	5.0	4.5	4.9	5.1	4.9	5.1	5.5	5.8
Other[5]	11.1	8.0	7.4	6.6	5.9	6.0	5.7	5.6	5.5	5.6	5.7

[1]Excludes research and construction.
[2]Includes one-half of self-employment contribution to Medicare hospital insurance trust fund.
[3]Includes Medicaid buy-in premiums for Medicare.
[4]Includes expenditures for Medicare with adjustments for contributions by employers and individuals and premiums paid to the Medicare insurance trust fund and maternal and child health, vocational rehabilitation, Substance Abuse and Mental Health Services Administration, Indian Health Service, Federal workers' compensation, and other miscellaneous general hospital and medical programs, public health activities, Department of Defense, and Department of Veterans Affairs.
[5]Includes other public and general assistance, maternal and child health, vocational rehabilitation, public health activities, hospital subsidies, and employer contributions to Medicare hospital insurance trust fund.

NOTES: This table disaggregates health expenditures according to four classes of payers: businesses, households (individuals), Federal Government, and State and local governments. Where businesses or households pay dedicated funds into government health programs (for example, Medicare) or employers and employees share in the cost of health premiums, these costs are assigned to businesses or households accordingly. This results in a lower share of expenditures being assigned to the Federal Government than for tabulations of expenditures by source of funds. Estimates of national health expenditure by source of funds aim to track government-sponsored health programs over time and do not delineate the role of business employers in paying for health care. Figures may not sum to totals due to rounding. These data include revisions and differ from previous editions of *Health, United States*.

SOURCE: Office of National Health Statistics, Office of the Actuary. Business, households, and government: Health spending 1995. Health Care Financing Review vol 18, no 3. Washington: Health Care Financing Administration. Spring 1997.

Table 122. Employers' costs per employee hour worked for total compensation, wages and salaries, and health insurance, according to selected characteristics: United States, selected years 1991-98

[Data are based on surveys of employers]

Characteristic	Total compensation				Wages and salaries			
	1991	1994	1997	1998	1991	1994	1997	1998
	Amount per employee-hour worked							
State and local government............	$22.31	$25.27	$26.58	$27.28	$15.52	$17.57	$18.61	$19.19
Total private industry	15.40	17.08	17.97	18.50	11.14	12.14	13.04	13.47
Industry:								
Goods producing................	18.48	20.85	21.86	22.26	12.70	13.87	14.92	15.35
Service producing	14.31	15.82	16.73	17.31	10.58	11.56	12.44	12.88
Manufacturing	18.22	20.72	21.84	22.29	12.40	13.69	14.79	15.22
Nonmanufacturing	14.67	16.19	17.10	17.66	10.81	11.76	12.64	13.09
Occupation:								
White collar....................	18.15	20.26	21.60	22.38	13.40	14.72	15.94	16.54
Blue collar.....................	15.15	16.92	17.19	17.56	10.37	11.31	11.80	12.15
Service........................	7.82	8.38	9.04	9.37	5.96	6.33	6.94	7.25
Region:								
Northeast......................	17.56	20.03	20.27	20.38	12.65	14.13	14.52	14.70
Midwest	15.05	16.26	17.33	18.15	10.70	11.34	12.33	12.99
South.........................	13.68	15.05	15.79	16.45	10.03	10.85	11.61	12.15
West..........................	15.97	18.08	19.68	19.94	11.62	13.01	14.57	14.75
Union status:								
Union.........................	19.76	23.26	23.48	23.59	13.02	14.76	15.13	15.38
Nonunion......................	14.54	16.04	17.21	17.80	10.78	11.70	12.75	13.21
Establishment employment size:								
1-99 employees	13.38	14.58	15.37	15.92	10.00	10.72	11.54	12.01
100 or more	17.34	19.45	20.61	21.20	12.23	13.48	14.55	15.01
100-499...................	14.31	15.88	16.97	17.52	10.32	11.37	12.29	12.67
500 or more.................	20.60	23.35	24.75	25.56	14.28	15.79	17.12	17.78

Characteristic	Health insurance				Health insurance as a percent of total compensation			
	1991	1994	1997	1998	1991	1994	1997	1998
	Amount per employee-hour worked							
State and local government............	$1.54	$2.06	$1.99	$2.05	6.9	8.2	7.5	7.5
Total private industry	0.92	1.14	0.99	1.00	6.0	6.7	5.5	5.4
Industry:								
Goods producing................	1.28	1.70	1.49	1.48	6.9	8.1	6.8	6.6
Service producing	0.79	0.95	0.83	0.85	5.5	6.0	4.9	4.9
Manufacturing	1.37	1.79	1.55	1.54	7.5	8.6	7.1	6.9
Nonmanufacturing	0.80	0.98	0.86	0.88	5.5	6.0	5.0	5.0
Occupation:								
White collar....................	1.02	1.25	1.07	1.11	5.6	6.2	5.0	5.0
Blue collar.....................	1.06	1.35	1.19	1.17	7.0	8.0	6.9	6.7
Service........................	0.36	0.45	0.40	0.40	4.6	5.4	4.5	4.3
Region:								
Northeast......................	1.08	1.37	1.17	1.15	6.2	6.9	5.8	5.6
Midwest	0.95	1.19	1.02	1.04	6.3	7.3	5.9	5.7
South.........................	0.76	0.95	0.86	0.87	5.5	6.3	5.4	5.3
West..........................	0.92	1.10	0.95	0.97	5.8	6.1	4.8	4.9
Union status:								
Union.........................	1.63	2.28	2.01	1.97	8.2	9.8	8.5	8.4
Nonunion......................	0.78	0.94	0.85	0.86	5.4	5.9	4.9	4.8
Establishment employment size:								
1-99 employees	0.68	0.84	0.72	0.73	5.1	5.7	4.7	4.6
100 or more	1.14	1.42	1.26	1.28	6.6	7.3	6.1	6.0
100-499...................	0.90	1.03	0.98	1.01	6.3	6.5	5.8	5.8
500 or more.................	1.40	1.84	1.57	1.59	6.8	7.9	6.3	6.2

NOTES: Costs are calculated from March survey data each year. Data for additional years are available (see Appendix III).

SOURCES: U.S. Department of Labor, Bureau of Labor Statistics: Employment Cost Indexes and Levels, 1975-92. Bulletin 2413, Nov. 1992; U.S. Department of Labor: News pub nos 91-292, 94-290, 96-424, 97-371, and 98-285. June 19, 1991, June 16, 1994, Oct. 10, 1996, Oct. 21, 1997, and July 9, 1998. Washington.

Table 123. Hospital expenses, according to type of ownership and size of hospital: United States, selected years 1975–97

[Data are based on reporting by a census of hospitals]

Type of ownership and size of hospital	1975	1980	1985	1990	1993	1995	1996	1997	1985–93	1993–97
Total expenses				Amount in billions					Average annual percent change	
All hospitals	$ 48.7	$ 91.9	$153.3	$234.9	$301.5	$320.3	$330.5	$342.3	8.8	3.2
Federal	4.5	7.9	12.3	15.2	19.6	20.2	22.3	22.7	6.0	3.7
Non-Federal[1]	44.2	84.0	141.0	219.6	281.9	300.0	308.3	319.6	9.0	3.2
Community[2]	39.0	76.9	130.5	203.7	266.1	285.6	293.8	305.8	9.3	3.5
Nonprofit	27.9	55.8	96.1	150.7	197.2	209.6	216.0	225.3	9.4	3.4
For profit	2.6	5.8	11.5	18.8	23.1	26.7	28.4	31.2	9.1	7.8
State-local government	8.5	15.2	22.9	34.2	45.8	49.3	49.4	49.3	9.1	1.9
6–24 beds	0.1	0.2	0.3	0.5	0.7	1.1	1.1	1.3	11.2	16.7
25–49 beds	1.0	1.7	2.6	4.0	5.6	7.2	7.5	8.1	10.1	9.7
50–99 beds	2.9	5.4	8.6	12.6	15.8	17.8	18.4	19.5	7.9	5.4
100–199 beds	6.7	12.5	21.4	33.3	44.5	50.7	53.7	54.9	9.6	5.4
200–299 beds	6.8	13.4	23.3	38.7	50.6	55.8	56.5	57.1	10.2	3.1
300–399 beds	5.8	11.5	21.8	33.1	43.7	43.3	46.0	48.4	9.1	2.6
400–499 beds	4.8	10.5	15.7	25.3	30.4	33.7	35.5	35.0	8.6	3.6
500 beds or more	11.0	21.6	36.8	56.2	74.9	76.1	75.0	81.7	9.3	2.2
Employee expenses as percent of total expenses[3]				Percent						
Federal	64.5	68.4	68.1	67.1	65.6	65.8	63.0	63.1	...	...
Non-Federal[1]	54.8	58.1	56.6	54.8	53.7	54.5	53.9	53.2	...	...
Community[2]	53.0	56.3	55.2	53.6	52.7	53.6	53.0	52.4	...	...
Nonprofit	53.5	57.2	55.9	54.3	53.4	53.9	53.4	52.7	...	...
For profit	43.5	45.7	45.2	43.7	45.7	47.9	48.2	47.7	...	...
State-local government	54.3	57.3	57.1	55.8	53.6	55.2	54.2	54.2	...	...
6–24 beds	51.3	54.9	55.0	54.4	53.9	54.2	54.1	55.6	...	...
25–49 beds	50.2	54.0	54.1	53.0	52.8	53.9	53.8	53.0	...	...
50–99 beds	50.6	53.7	52.9	51.8	52.4	53.7	53.0	53.0	...	...
100–199 beds	51.0	54.2	52.6	51.7	52.2	52.9	52.9	52.2	...	...
200–299 beds	52.8	55.6	54.6	53.0	52.6	53.3	52.8	52.0	...	...
300–399 beds	53.8	56.9	55.7	54.1	53.1	53.4	52.5	52.1	...	...
400–499 beds	54.2	57.8	56.2	55.1	53.2	54.1	53.9	52.7	...	...
500 beds or more	54.3	57.9	56.9	54.5	52.9	54.1	53.1	52.6	...	...
Expenses per inpatient day				Amount						
Community[2]	$ 151	$ 245	$ 460	$ 687	$ 881	$ 968	$1,006	$1,033	8.5	4.1
Nonprofit	150	246	463	692	898	994	1,042	1,074	8.6	4.6
For profit	146	257	500	752	914	947	945	962	7.8	1.3
State-local government	157	239	433	634	800	878	903	914	8.0	3.4
6–24 beds	121	203	380	526	664	678	757	731	7.2	2.4
25–49 beds	111	197	379	489	635	696	749	775	6.7	5.1
50–99 beds	115	191	363	493	598	647	664	686	6.4	3.5
100–199 beds	134	215	402	585	729	796	827	853	7.7	4.0
200–299 beds	146	239	449	665	854	943	993	1,011	8.4	4.3
300–399 beds	156	248	484	731	956	1,070	1,109	1,129	8.9	4.2
400–499 beds	159	215	489	756	977	1,135	1,175	1,195	9.0	5.2
500 beds or more	184	239	527	825	1,087	1,212	1,267	1,304	9.5	4.7
Expenses per inpatient stay										
Community[2]	$1,165	$1,851	$3,245	$4,947	$6,132	$6,216	$6,225	$6,262	8.3	0.5
Nonprofit	1,178	1,902	3,307	5,001	6,178	6,279	6,344	6,393	8.1	0.9
For profit	968	1,676	3,033	4,727	5,643	5,425	5,207	5,219	8.1	-1.9
State-local government	1,197	1,750	3,106	4,838	6,206	6,445	6,419	6,475	9.0	1.1
6–24 beds	684	1,072	1,876	2,701	3,471	3,578	3,630	3,348	8.0	-0.9
25–49 beds	673	1,138	2,007	2,967	3,687	3,797	3,879	3,989	7.9	2.0
50–99 beds	785	1,271	2,342	3,461	4,312	4,427	4,474	4,598	7.9	1.6
100–199 beds	955	1,512	2,683	4,109	4,999	5,103	5,121	5,146	8.1	0.7
200–299 beds	1,096	1,767	3,044	4,618	5,713	5,851	5,917	5,948	8.2	1.0
300–399 beds	1,225	1,881	3,394	5,096	6,351	6,512	6,550	6,429	8.1	0.3
400–499 beds	1,290	2,090	3,571	5,500	6,706	7,164	7,253	7,279	8.2	2.1
500 beds or more	1,677	2,517	4,254	6,667	8,460	8,531	8,450	8,508	9.0	0.1

... Category not applicable.

[1]The category of non-Federal hospitals is comprised of psychiatric, tuberculosis and other respiratory diseases hospitals, and long-term and short-term hospitals.
[2]Community hospitals are short-term hospitals excluding hospital units in institutions such as prison and college infirmaries, facilities for the mentally retarded, and alcoholism and chemical dependency hospitals.
[3]Includes employee payroll and benefit expenses. Does not include contracted labor services.

NOTE: Data for additional years are available (see Appendix III).

SOURCES: American Hospital Association: Hospital Statistics, 1976, 1981, 1986, 1991–99 Editions. Chicago, 1976, 1981, 1986, 1991–99 (Copyrights 1976, 1981, 1986, 1991–99: Used with the permission of the American Hospital Association); and unpublished data.

Table 124. Nursing home average monthly charges per resident and percent of residents, according to selected facility and resident characteristics: United States, 1964, 1973–74, 1977, 1985, and 1995

[Data are based on reporting by a sample of nursing homes]

Facility and resident characteristic	Average monthly charge[1]					Percent of residents				
	1964	1973–74[2]	1977	1985	1995	1964	1973–74[2]	1977	1985	1995
Facility characteristic										
All facilities	$186	$479	$689	$1,456	$3,135	100.0	100.0	100.0	100.0	100.0
Ownership:										
Proprietary	205	489	670	1,379	3,047	60.2	69.8	68.2	68.7	63.6
Nonprofit and government	145	456	732	1,624	3,288	39.8	30.2	31.8	31.3	36.4
Certification:[3]										
Skilled nursing facility	. . .	566	880	1,905	- - -	. . .	39.8	20.7	18.5	- - -
Skilled nursing and intermediate facility	. . .	514	762	1,571	- - -	. . .	24.5	40.5	45.2	- - -
Intermediate facility	. . .	376	556	1,179	- - -	. . .	22.4	28.3	24.9	- - -
Not certified	. . .	329	390	875	- - -	. . .	13.3	10.6	11.4	- - -
Both Medicare and Medicaid	- - -	- - -	- - -	- - -	3,317	- - -	- - -	- - -	- - -	78.4
Medicare only	- - -	- - -	- - -	- - -	4,211	- - -	- - -	- - -	- - -	3.0
Medicaid only	- - -	- - -	- - -	- - -	2,169	- - -	- - -	- - -	- - -	15.8
Neither	- - -	- - -	- - -	- - -	2,323	- - -	- - -	- - -	- - -	2.8
Bed size:										
Less than 50 beds	- - -	397	546	1,036	4,978	- - -	15.2	12.9	8.9	4.5
50–99 beds	- - -	448	643	1,335	2,691	- - -	34.1	30.5	27.6	24.9
100–199 beds	- - -	502	706	1,478	3,028	- - -	35.6	38.8	43.2	51.1
200 beds or more	- - -	576	837	1,759	3,560	- - -	15.1	17.9	20.2	19.5
Geographic region:										
Northeast	213	651	918	1,781	3,904	28.6	22.0	22.4	23.6	22.8
Midwest	171	433	640	1,399	2,740	36.6	34.6	34.5	32.5	32.3
South	161	410	585	1,256	2,752	18.1	26.0	27.2	29.4	32.0
West	204	454	653	1,458	3,710	16.7	17.4	15.9	14.5	12.9
Resident characteristic										
All residents	186	479	689	1,456	3,135	100.0	100.0	100.0	100.0	100.0
Age:										
Under 65 years	155	434	585	1,379	3,662	12.0	10.6	13.6	11.6	8.0
65–74 years	184	473	669	1,372	3,409	18.9	15.0	16.2	14.2	12.0
75–84 years	191	488	710	1,468	3,138	41.7	35.5	35.7	34.1	32.5
85 years and over	194	485	719	1,497	2,974	27.5	38.8	34.5	40.0	47.5
Sex:										
Male	171	466	652	1,438	3,345	35.0	29.1	28.8	28.4	26.6
Female	194	484	705	1,463	3,059	65.0	70.9	71.2	71.6	73.4

. . . Category not applicable.

- - - Data not available.

[1]Includes life-care residents and no-charge residents.

[2]Data exclude residents of personal care homes.

[3]Medicare extended care facilities and Medicaid skilled nursing homes from the 1973–74 survey were considered to be equivalent to Medicare or Medicaid skilled nursing facilities in 1977 and 1985 for the purposes of this comparison. In the 1995 survey the certification categories were based on Medicare and Medicaid certification.

SOURCES: Centers for Disease Control and Prevention: Van Nostrand JF, Sutton JF. Charges for care and sources of payment for residents in nursing homes, United States, June–August 1969. National Center for Health Statistics. Vital Health Stat 12(21). 1973; Hing E. Charges for care and sources of payment for residents in nursing homes, United States, National Nursing Home Survey, August 1973–April 1974. National Center for Health Statistics. Vital Health Stat 13(32). 1977; Van Nostrand JF, Zappolo A, Hing E, et al. The National Nursing Home Survey, 1977 summary for the United States. National Center for Health Statistics. Vital Health Stat 13(43). 1979; and Hing E, Sekscenski E, Strahan G. The National Nursing Home Survey: 1985 summary for the United States. National Center for Health Statistics. Vital Health Stat 13(97). 1989; and unpublished data.

Table 125. Nursing home average monthly charges per resident and percent of residents, according to primary source of payments and selected facility characteristics: United States, 1977, 1985, and 1995

[Data are based on reporting by a sample of nursing homes]

Facility characteristic	All sources 1995	Own income or family support[1] 1977	Own income or family support[1] 1985	Own income or family support[1] 1995	Medicare 1977	Medicare 1985	Medicare 1995	Medicaid 1977	Medicaid 1985	Medicaid 1995
					Average monthly charge[2]					
All facilities	$3,135	$ 690	$1,450	$3,081	$ 1,167	$ 2,141	$ 5,546	$ 720	$1,504	$2,769
Ownership										
Proprietary	3,047	686	1,444	3,190	1,048	2,058	5,668	677	1,363	2,560
Nonprofit and government	3,288	698	1,462	2,967	1,325	*2,456	5,304	825	1,851	3,201
Certification[3]										
Skilled nursing facility	- - -	866	1,797	- - -	1,136	2,315	- - -	955	2,000	- - -
Skilled nursing and intermediate facility	- - -	800	1,643	- - -	1,195	2,156	- - -	739	1,509	- - -
Intermediate facility	- - -	567	1,222	- - -	. . .	. . .	- - -	563	1,150	- - -
Not certified	- - -	447	999	- - -	. . .	. . .	- - -	. . .	. . .	- - -
Both Medicare and Medicaid	3,317	- - -	- - -	3,364	- - -	- - -	5,472	- - -	- - -	2,910
Medicare only	4,211	- - -	- - -	3,344	- - -	- - -	4*10,074	- - -	- - -	- - -
Medicaid only	2,169	- - -	- - -	2,352	- - -	- - -	. . .	- - -	- - -	2,069
Neither	2,323	- - -	- - -	2,390	- - -	- - -	. . .	- - -	- - -	- - -
Bed size										
Less than 50 beds	4,978	516	886	3,377	*869	*1,348	4*17,224	663	1,335	2,990
50–99 beds	2,691	686	1,388	2,849	*1,141	1,760	4,929	634	1,323	2,335
100–199 beds	3,028	721	1,567	3,138	1,242	2,192	4,918	691	1,413	2,659
200 beds or more	3,560	823	1,701	3,316	*1,179	2,767	4,523	925	1,919	3,520
Geographic region										
Northeast	3,904	909	1,645	4,117	1,369	2,109	4,883	975	2,035	3,671
Midwest	2,740	652	1,398	2,650	*1,160	2,745	5,439	639	1,382	2,478
South	2,752	585	1,359	2,945	*1,096	2,033	4,889	619	1,200	2,333
West	3,710	663	1,498	3,666	*868	1,838	8,825	663	1,501	2,848
					Percent of residents					
All facilities	100.0	38.4	41.6	27.8	2.0	1.4	9.9	47.8	50.4	60.2
Ownership										
Proprietary	100.0	37.5	40.1	24.1	1.7	1.6	10.4	49.6	52.1	63.8
Nonprofit and government	100.0	40.4	44.9	34.3	2.7	*0.9	9.2	43.8	46.6	54.0
Certification[3]										
Skilled nursing facility	- - -	41.5	39.1	- - -	4.6	2.6	- - -	41.4	53.7	- - -
Skilled nursing and intermediate facility	- - -	31.6	36.8	- - -	2.6	1.9	- - -	58.3	57.8	- - -
Intermediate facility	- - -	36.3	41.4	- - -	. . .	. . .	- - -	55.3	55.9	- - -
Not certified	- - -	64.2	65.5	- - -	. . .	. . .	- - -	. . .	. . .	- - -
Both Medicare and Medicaid	100.0	- - -	- - -	23.1	- - -	- - -	11.6	- - -	- - -	63.9
Medicare only	100.0	- - -	- - -	71.2	- - -	- - -	16.2	- - -	- - -	- - -
Medicaid only	100.0	- - -	- - -	32.1	- - -	- - -	- - -	- - -	- - -	63.0
Neither	100.0	- - -	- - -	91.0	- - -	- - -	- - -	- - -	- - -	- - -
Bed size										
Less than 50 beds	100.0	49.6	53.1	35.3	*1.8	*1.2	13.1	32.7	33.8	49.9
50–99 beds	100.0	39.5	49.5	34.5	*1.2	*1.3	6.2	46.5	42.9	57.6
100–199 beds	100.0	38.4	39.6	26.2	2.6	1.5	10.6	50.4	55.2	61.5
200 beds or more	100.0	28.6	30.1	22.0	2.3	*1.5	12.1	55.5	57.7	62.4
Geographic region										
Northeast	100.0	34.6	34.8	18.2	3.3	1.7	14.0	53.3	52.9	64.9
Midwest	100.0	44.5	49.1	36.3	1.5	*0.8	6.7	42.1	45.9	55.8
South	100.0	32.2	39.4	26.1	*1.4	*1.2	10.1	52.5	53.8	62.2
West	100.0	41.3	40.4	27.9	2.5	*2.7	10.5	44.7	49.2	57.9

* Relative standard error greater than 30 percent.

- - - Data not available.

. . . Category not applicable.

[1]Includes private health insurance.

[2]Includes life-care residents and no-charge residents.

[3]In the 1995 survey the certification categories were based on Medicare and Medicaid certification.

[4]Likely to include a high proportion of patients in subacute units of hospitals.

SOURCES: Centers for Disease Control and Prevention: Van Nostrand JF, Zappolo A, Hing E, et al. The National Nursing Home Survey, 1977 summary for the United States. National Center for Health Statistics. Vital Health Stat 13(43). 1979; and Hing E, Sekscenski E, Strahan G. The National Nursing Home Survey: 1985 summary for the United States. National Center for Health Statistics. Vital Health Stat 13(97). 1985; and unpublished data.

Table 126. Mental health expenditures, percent distribution, and per capita expenditures, according to type of mental health organization: United States, selected years 1975–94

[Data are based on inventories of mental health organizations]

Type of organization	1975	1979	1983	1986	1988	1990	1992	1994
				Amount in millions				
All organizations	$6,564	$8,764	$14,432	$18,458	$23,028	$28,410	$29,765	$33,136
State and county mental hospitals	3,185	3,757	5,491	6,326	6,978	7,774	7,970	7,825
Private psychiatric hospitals	467	743	1,712	2,629	4,588	6,101	5,302	6,468
Non-Federal general hospitals with separate psychiatric services	621	723	2,176	2,878	3,610	4,662	5,193	5,344
Department of Veterans Affairs medical centers[1]	699	848	1,316	1,338	1,290	1,480	1,530	1,386
Residential treatment centers for emotionally disturbed children	279	436	573	978	1,305	1,969	2,167	2,360
Freestanding psychiatric outpatient clinics	422	589	430	518	657	671	821	878
All other organizations[2]	116	187	2,734	3,792	4,600	5,753	6,782	8,875
				Percent distribution				
All organizations	100.0	100.0	100.0	100.0	100.0	100.0	100.0	100.0
State and county mental hospitals	48.5	42.9	38.0	34.4	30.3	27.4	26.8	23.6
Private psychiatric hospitals	7.1	8.5	11.9	14.2	19.9	21.5	17.8	19.5
Non-Federal general hospitals with separate psychiatric services	9.5	8.2	15.1	15.6	15.7	16.4	17.4	16.1
Department of Veterans Affairs medical centers[1]	10.6	9.7	9.1	7.2	5.6	5.2	5.1	4.2
Residential treatment centers for emotionally disturbed children	4.3	5.0	4.0	5.3	5.7	6.9	7.3	7.1
Freestanding psychiatric outpatient clinics	6.4	6.7	3.0	2.8	2.8	2.4	2.8	2.7
All other organizations[2]	1.8	2.1	18.9	20.5	20.0	20.2	22.8	26.8
				Amount per capita[3]				
All organizations	$ 31	$ 40	$ 62	$ 77	$ 95	$ 117	$ 117	$ 128
State and county mental hospitals	15	17	24	26	29	32	31	30
Private psychiatric hospitals	2	3	7	11	19	25	21	25
Non-Federal general hospitals with separate psychiatric services	3	3	9	12	15	19	20	21
Department of Veterans Affairs medical centers[1]	3	4	6	6	5	6	6	5
Residential treatment centers for emotionally disturbed children	1	2	3	4	5	8	9	9
Freestanding psychiatric outpatient clinics	2	3	2	2	3	3	3	3
All other organizations[2]	1	1	12	16	19	24	27	35

[1]Includes Department of Veterans Affairs neuropsychiatric hospitals, general hospital psychiatric services, and psychiatric outpatient clinics.
[2]Includes freestanding outpatient clinics, freestanding day–night organizations, multiservice organizations, and other residential organizations. Multiservice mental health organizations were redefined in 1983; see Appendix I, Substance Abuse and Mental Health Services Administration.
[3]Civilian population.

NOTES: Comparisons of data from 1979 and 1983 with data from other years should be made with caution because changes in reporting procedures may affect the comparability of data. Mental health expenditures include salaries, other operating expenditures, and capital expenditures.

SOURCES: Survey and Analysis Branch, Division of State and Community Systems Development, Center for Mental Health Services. Manderscheid RW, Sonnenschein MA. *Mental Health, United States, 1996.* U.S. Government Printing Office, 1996; unpublished data from the 1994 inventory of mental health organizations and general hospital mental health services.

Table 127. Funding for health research and development, according to source of funds: United States, selected fiscal years 1970–97

[Data are compiled by the National Institutes of Health from Federal Government sources]

Source of funds	1970	1975	1980	1985	1990	1993[1]	1994	1995	1996	1997
	Amount in millions									
All funding	$2,847	$4,701	$7,967	$13,567	$23,095	$31,088	$33,399	$35,816	- - -	- - -
Industry[2]	795	1,319	2,459	5,360	10,719	15,711	17,106	18,645	- - -	- - -
Private nonprofit organizations	215	264	305	538	960	1,215	1,276	1,325	- - -	- - -
State and local governments	170	286	480	878	1,625	2,054	2,196	2,423	- - -	- - -
Federal government	1,667	2,832	4,723	6,791	9,791	12,108	12,821	13,423	- - -	- - -
National Institutes of Health	- - -	- - -	- - -	- - -	- - -	9,756	10,329	10,681	11,251	11,993
National Institute on Aging	- - -	- - -	- - -	- - -	- - -	382	405	419	441	470
National Institute of Allergy and Infectious Diseases	- - -	- - -	- - -	- - -	- - -	1,001	1,060	1,096	1,154	1,230
National Cancer Institute	- - -	- - -	- - -	- - -	- - -	1,903	2,015	2,084	2,195	2,340
National Institute of Child Health and Human Development	- - -	- - -	- - -	- - -	- - -	497	526	544	573	610
National Institute of Diabetes and Digestive and Kidney Diseases	- - -	- - -	- - -	- - -	- - -	637	675	698	735	783
National Institute on Drug Abuse	- - -	- - -	- - -	- - -	- - -	396	419	434	457	487
National Institute of General Medical Sciences	- - -	- - -	- - -	- - -	- - -	715	757	783	825	879
National Heart, Lung, and Blood Institute	- - -	- - -	- - -	- - -	- - -	1,123	1,189	1,229	1,295	1,380
National Institute of Mental Health	- - -	- - -	- - -	- - -	- - -	540	572	592	623	664
National Institute of Neurological Disorders and Stroke	- - -	- - -	- - -	- - -	- - -	578	613	633	667	711
Other National Institutes of Health[3]	- - -	- - -	- - -	- - -	- - -	1,984	2,098	2,169	2,286	2,439
	Average annual percent change from previous year shown									
All funding	...	10.6	11.1	11.2	11.2	6.3	7.4	7.2	- - -	- - -
Industry[2]	...	10.7	13.3	16.9	14.9	9.1	8.9	9.0	- - -	- - -
Private nonprofit organizations	...	4.2	2.9	12.0	12.3	2.7	5.0	3.8	- - -	- - -
State and local governments	...	11.0	10.9	12.8	13.1	6.3	6.9	10.3	- - -	- - -
Federal government	...	11.2	10.8	7.5	7.6	3.3	5.9	4.7	- - -	- - -
	Percent distribution of Federal funding									
All Federal agencies	100.0	100.0	100.0	100.0	100.0	100.0	100.0	100.0	- - -	- - -
Department of Health and Human Services	70.6	77.6	78.2	79.7	85.2	85.0	85.6	85.1	- - -	- - -
National Institutes of Health	52.4	66.4	67.4	71.1	72.9	80.7	80.6	79.6	- - -	- - -
Centers for Disease Control and Prevention	- - -	1.5	1.8	0.7	1.0	1.3	1.6	2.4	- - -	- - -
Other Public Health Service	16.2	8.3	7.9	7.3	10.8	2.4	2.7	2.5	- - -	- - -
Other Department of Health and Human Services	2.0	1.3	1.1	0.6	0.5	0.6	0.6	0.6	- - -	- - -
Other departments and agencies	29.4	22.4	21.8	20.3	14.8	15.0	14.4	14.9	- - -	- - -
Department of Defense	7.5	4.1	4.5	6.5	4.4	5.6	5.3	5.3	- - -	- - -
Department of Energy[4]	6.3	5.8	4.5	2.6	2.8	2.6	2.5	2.5	- - -	- - -
Department of Veterans Affairs	3.5	3.3	2.8	3.3	2.4	2.0	1.9	1.8	- - -	- - -
Environmental Protection Agency	...	1.3	1.7	0.8	0.3	0.4	0.3	0.2	- - -	- - -
National Aeronautics and Space Administration	5.2	2.6	1.5	1.7	1.5	1.7	1.5	2.6	- - -	- - -
All other departments and agencies	6.9	5.3	6.8	5.4	3.4	2.7	2.9	2.5	- - -	- - -

- - - Data not available.
... Category not applicable.

[1]In fiscal year 1993 the Alcohol, Drug Abuse, and Mental Health Administration was reorganized and renamed the Substance Abuse and Mental Health Services Administration and its three research institutes were transferred into the National Institutes of Health.
[2]Includes expenditures for drug research. These expenditures are included in the "drugs and sundries" component of the Health Care Financing Administration's National Health Expenditure Series, not under "research."
[3]Includes the National Institutes on Alcohol Abuse and Alcoholism, of Arthritis and Musculoskeletal and Skin Diseases, on Deafness and Other Communication Disorders, of Dental Research, of Environmental Health Sciences, of Nursing Research, and the National Eye Institute, the National Center for Human Genome Research, the National Library of Medicine, the Fogarty International Center, the Division of Research Resources, and the Office of the Director.
[4]Includes Atomic Energy Commission and Energy Research and Development Administration.

NOTES: Data for 1970 and 1975 fiscal years ending June 30; all other data for fiscal year ending September 30. Data on the National Institutes of Health are presented from 1993 onwards since there was frequent reorganization of the Institutes in prior years. Data for additional years are available (see Appendix III).

SOURCE: National Institutes of Health, Office of Reports and Analysis.

Table 128. Federal spending for human immunodeficiency virus (HIV)-related activities, according to agency and type of activity: United States, selected fiscal years 1985–98

[Data are compiled from Federal Government appropriations]

Agency and type of activity	1985	1990	1991	1992	1993	1994	1995	1996	1997	1998[1]
Agency					Amount in millions					
All Federal spending	$205	$3,064	$3,806	$4,498	$5,328	$6,329	$6,821	$7,522	$8,363	$8,931
Department of Health and Human Services, total	197	2,620	3,302	3,824	4,426	5,399	4,941	5,598	6,367	6,835
Department of Health and Human Services discretionary spending, total[2]	109	1,591	1,891	1,963	2,081	2,569	2,700	2,898	3,267	3,535
National Institutes of Health	66	907	1,014	1,047	1,073	1,296	1,334	1,411	1,501	1,604
Substance Abuse and Mental Health Services Administration	–	50	30	26	26	27	24	54	64	70
Centers for Disease Control and Prevention	33	443	497	480	498	543	590	584	617	625
Food and Drug Administration	9	57	63	72	73	72	73	73	73	73
Health Resources and Services Administration	–	113	266	317	390	608	661	762	1,001	1,155
Agency for Health Care Policy and Research	–	8	10	10	10	11	9	6	4	1
Office of the Assistant Secretary for Health	–	8	6	5	5	5	4	4	4	4
Indian Health Service	–	3	2	3	3	4	4	3	4	4
Other Department of Health and Human Services agencies	–	3	3	3	3	2	2	2	–	–
Health Care Financing Administration	75	780	1,050	1,360	1,675	1,990	2,240	2,700	3,100	3,300
Social Security Administration[3]	13	249	360	501	670	840	...	...	...	...
Social Security Administration[3]	...	...	...	...	...	...	940	976	1,001	1,061
Department of Veterans Affairs	8	220	258	279	325	312	317	331	332	343
Department of Defense	–	125	127	129	159	129	112	98	100	105
Agency for International Development	–	71	78	94	117	115	120	115	117	121
Department of Housing and Urban Development	–	–	–	107	196	258	171	171	196	204
Office of Personnel Management	–	21	34	58	98	108	212	226	241	253
Other departments	–	7	7	7	7	8	8	7	9	9
Activity										
Research	84	1,142	1,275	1,311	1,361	1,561	1,589	1,653	1,730	1,831
Department of Health and Human Services discretionary spending[2]	83	1,093	1,221	1,259	1,284	1,508	1,544	1,619	1,702	1,801
Department of Veterans Affairs	1	15	10	6	7	6	5	6	6	6
Department of Defense	–	34	44	46	70	47	40	28	22	24
Education and prevention	26	486	528	518	576	619	658	635	685	701
Department of Health and Human Services discretionary spending[2]	25	351	391	378	395	445	492	476	522	534
Department of Veterans Affairs	1	31	34	22	31	31	31	31	31	31
Department of Defense	–	28	19	18	27	22	12	11	12	13
Agency for International Development	–	71	78	94	117	115	120	115	117	121
Other	–	5	6	6	6	6	3	2	3	2
Medical care	81	1,187	1,642	2,061	2,523	3,051	3,462	4,087	4,752	5,134
Health Care Financing Administration:										
Medicaid (Federal share)	70	670	870	1,080	1,290	1,490	1,640	1,600	1,800	1,900
Medicare	5	110	180	280	385	500	600	1,100	1,300	1,400
Department of Health and Human Services discretionary spending[2]	–	144	274	323	397	613	664	803	1,044	1,200
Department of Veterans Affairs	6	174	214	251	287	275	281	294	295	306
Department of Defense	–	63	64	65	62	60	60	59	66	68
Office of Personnel Management	–	21	34	58	98	108	212	226	241	253
Other	–	5	4	4	4	5	5	5	6	7
Cash assistance	13	249	360	608	866	1,098	1,111	1,147	1,197	1,265
Social Security Administration:										
Disability Insurance	10	210	295	390	505	600	640	696	691	726
Supplemental Security Income	3	39	65	111	165	240	300	280	310	335
Department of Housing and Urban Development	–	–	–	107	196	258	171	171	196	204

– Quantity zero.

... Category not applicable.

[1] Preliminary figures.

[2] Department of Health and Human Services discretionary spending is spending that is not entitlement spending. Medicare and Medicaid are examples of entitlement spending.

[3] Prior to 1995 the Social Security Administration was part of the Department of Health and Human Services.

NOTES: These data include revisions and differ from the previous edition of Health, United States. Federal expenditures on HIV-related activities are estimated at about 35 to 40 percent of total HIV-related expenditures that include, for example, expenditures covered by private health insurance, out-of-pocket costs to patients, and the States' share of Medicaid, public hospital, and other local expenditures.

SOURCE: Budget Office, Public Health Service. Unpublished data.

Table 129 (page 1 of 2). Health care coverage for persons under 65 years of age, according to type of coverage and selected characteristics: United States, selected years 1984–97

[Data are based on household interviews of a sample of the civilian noninstitutionalized population]

Characteristic	Private insurance						Private insurance obtained through workplace[1]					
	1984	1989	1994[2]	1995	1996	1997[2,3]	1984	1989	1994[2]	1995	1996	1997[2,3]
	Number in millions											
Total[4]	157.5	162.7	160.7	165.0	165.9	165.8	141.8	146.3	146.7	151.4	151.4	152.5
	Percent of population											
Total, age adjusted[4]	76.6	75.7	69.9	71.2	71.1	70.4	68.9	68.1	63.8	65.4	64.8	64.7
Total, crude[4]	76.8	75.9	70.3	71.6	71.4	70.7	69.1	68.3	64.2	65.7	65.1	65.0
Age												
Under 18 years	72.6	71.8	63.8	65.7	66.4	66.1	66.5	65.8	59.0	60.9	61.1	61.3
Under 6 years	68.1	67.9	58.3	60.1	61.1	61.3	62.1	62.3	53.9	55.6	56.5	57.3
6–17 years	74.9	74.0	66.8	68.7	69.1	68.5	68.7	67.7	61.8	63.7	63.4	63.4
18–44 years	76.5	75.5	69.8	71.2	70.6	69.4	69.6	68.4	63.9	65.6	64.7	64.4
18–24 years	67.4	64.5	58.3	61.2	60.4	59.3	58.7	55.3	50.7	53.9	52.3	53.8
25–34 years	77.4	75.9	69.4	70.3	69.5	68.1	71.2	69.5	64.1	65.3	64.4	63.6
35–44 years	83.9	82.7	77.1	78.0	77.5	76.4	77.4	76.2	71.6	72.9	72.0	71.2
45–64 years	83.3	82.5	80.3	80.4	79.5	79.1	71.8	71.6	71.8	72.4	71.4	70.8
45–54 years	83.3	83.4	81.3	81.1	80.4	80.4	74.6	74.4	74.6	74.9	74.0	73.6
55–64 years	83.3	81.6	78.8	79.3	78.1	76.9	69.0	68.3	67.9	68.6	67.5	66.6
Sex[5]												
Male	77.1	76.0	70.4	71.6	71.4	70.7	69.7	68.6	64.3	65.9	65.2	65.0
Female	76.0	75.4	69.5	70.8	70.8	70.1	68.1	67.6	63.4	64.8	64.4	64.4
Race[5,6]												
White	79.7	79.0	73.5	74.4	74.2	74.1	71.9	71.1	67.0	68.4	67.6	67.9
Black	58.3	57.8	51.5	54.2	54.9	54.9	52.4	52.9	48.8	50.4	51.8	52.6
Asian or Pacific Islander	69.8	71.1	67.3	68.0	67.8	68.0	63.6	60.2	57.4	59.8	59.3	60.4
Hispanic origin and race[5,6]												
All Hispanic	56.3	52.6	48.6	47.3	47.5	47.3	52.3	48.0	44.5	44.0	43.8	44.0
Mexican	54.3	48.0	45.7	43.9	43.8	43.3	51.1	45.2	43.7	41.9	40.9	41.2
Puerto Rican	48.8	45.9	48.3	47.9	50.7	47.2	46.4	42.6	45.2	44.7	48.1	44.6
Cuban	71.7	69.0	63.9	62.4	65.4	70.5	57.7	55.8	46.5	53.1	54.4	56.0
Other Hispanic	61.6	61.9	52.3	52.2	52.6	50.7	57.4	55.4	46.2	47.1	47.6	47.1
White, non-Hispanic	82.3	82.4	77.3	78.6	78.5	77.9	74.0	74.1	70.4	72.1	71.5	71.4
Black, non-Hispanic	58.5	57.9	51.9	54.6	55.4	55.1	52.6	53.0	49.2	50.9	52.2	52.8
Age and percent of poverty level[6,7]												
All ages:[5]												
Below 100 percent	32.4	26.7	21.3	21.9	20.0	22.7	23.7	19.4	16.1	17.0	15.5	18.9
100–149 percent	62.4	54.9	46.8	47.8	47.1	42.1	51.9	45.8	40.9	41.9	40.8	37.0
150–199 percent	77.7	71.3	65.7	66.5	67.9	64.0	69.5	62.9	59.0	60.4	60.9	58.7
200 percent or more	91.7	91.2	88.9	89.3	89.5	87.7	85.2	84.2	83.0	83.7	83.2	82.0
Under 18 years:												
Below 100 percent	28.7	22.3	14.9	16.8	16.1	17.4	23.2	17.5	12.4	13.4	13.4	15.4
100–149 percent	66.2	59.6	47.8	48.5	49.5	42.5	58.3	52.5	43.2	43.6	43.7	38.5
150–199 percent	80.9	75.9	69.3	68.5	73.0	66.8	75.8	70.1	64.0	63.0	67.4	63.1
200 percent or more	92.3	92.7	89.7	90.4	90.7	88.9	86.9	86.7	84.5	85.5	84.6	83.7
Geographic region[5]												
Northeast	80.1	81.8	74.8	75.1	74.9	74.0	73.8	74.9	69.5	69.5	68.7	69.4
Midwest	80.4	81.4	77.2	77.2	78.4	76.9	71.9	73.3	71.0	71.1	72.3	71.1
South	74.0	71.1	65.0	66.7	65.9	66.8	65.9	63.3	59.1	61.7	60.4	61.0
West	71.8	71.3	65.2	67.9	67.1	65.3	64.5	63.9	58.1	60.7	59.6	58.9
Location of residence[5]												
Within MSA[8]	77.2	76.3	70.4	72.1	72.5	71.0	70.6	69.5	64.8	66.6	66.5	65.6
Outside MSA[8]	75.1	73.6	68.1	67.7	65.8	68.0	65.1	63.4	60.4	60.5	58.6	61.4

See footnotes at end of table.

Table 129 (page 2 of 2). Health care coverage for persons under 65 years of age, according to type of coverage and selected characteristics: United States, selected years 1984–97

[Data are based on household interviews of a sample of the civilian noninstitutionalized population]

Characteristic	Medicaid[9]						Not covered[10]					
	1984	1989	1994[2]	1995	1996	1997[2,3]	1984	1989	1994[2]	1995	1996	1997[2,3]
						Number in millions						
Total[4]	14.0	15.4	24.1	25.3	25.0	22.9	29.8	33.4	40.4	37.4	38.9	41.0
						Percent of population						
Total, age adjusted[4]	7.3	7.8	11.5	12.0	11.7	10.7	14.2	15.2	17.1	15.6	16.1	16.8
Total, crude[4]	6.8	7.2	10.6	11.0	10.8	9.7	14.5	15.6	17.7	16.2	16.7	17.5
Age												
Under 18 years	11.9	12.6	20.0	20.6	20.1	18.4	13.9	14.7	15.3	13.6	13.4	14.0
Under 6 years	15.5	15.7	27.2	28.3	27.4	24.7	14.9	15.1	13.7	11.9	11.9	12.5
6–17 years	10.1	10.9	16.2	16.6	16.4	15.2	13.4	14.5	16.2	14.5	14.1	14.7
18–44 years	5.1	5.2	7.3	7.4	7.3	6.6	17.1	18.4	21.9	20.5	21.2	22.4
18–24 years	6.4	6.8	9.6	9.7	9.2	8.8	25.0	27.1	31.1	28.2	29.6	30.1
25–34 years	5.3	5.2	7.7	7.7	7.5	6.8	16.2	18.3	22.1	21.3	22.5	23.8
35–44 years	3.5	4.0	5.4	5.6	6.0	5.2	11.2	12.3	16.0	15.2	15.2	16.7
45–64 years	3.4	4.3	4.5	5.3	5.2	4.6	9.6	10.5	12.0	11.0	12.1	12.4
45–54 years	3.2	3.8	3.8	4.9	4.8	4.0	10.5	11.0	12.6	11.7	12.5	12.8
55–64 years	3.6	4.9	5.5	6.0	5.7	5.6	8.7	10.0	11.2	10.0	11.6	11.8
Sex[5]												
Male	6.1	6.5	9.8	10.3	10.1	9.4	14.8	16.1	18.1	16.7	17.2	17.8
Female	8.5	9.1	13.2	13.6	13.3	11.9	13.6	14.3	16.1	14.6	15.1	15.9
Race[5,6]												
White	5.0	5.6	8.7	9.4	9.3	8.2	13.3	14.1	16.4	15.0	15.4	15.8
Black	20.5	19.3	27.0	27.0	24.5	22.7	19.5	21.0	19.5	17.9	19.0	19.3
Asian or Pacific Islander	10.1	11.8	10.2	11.4	12.4	10.3	17.8	18.2	19.9	17.8	18.6	18.8
Hispanic origin and race[5,6]												
All Hispanic	13.1	13.5	19.6	21.2	20.1	17.8	29.0	32.4	31.4	30.8	31.6	33.2
Mexican	11.8	12.3	18.3	20.1	19.0	17.1	33.1	38.6	35.7	35.4	36.7	38.1
Puerto Rican	31.1	28.0	36.2	32.7	33.8	30.9	17.9	23.3	15.4	17.8	14.4	18.5
Cuban	5.0	8.0	9.8	15.3	13.9	9.2	21.6	21.8	26.1	21.6	17.6	19.8
Other Hispanic	8.0	11.2	16.2	18.4	16.3	15.6	27.1	24.8	30.2	29.0	29.8	31.8
White, non-Hispanic	4.0	4.6	7.1	7.5	7.5	6.8	11.6	11.7	14.2	12.7	12.9	13.3
Black, non-Hispanic	20.8	19.4	27.0	26.7	24.2	22.5	19.2	20.8	19.1	17.8	18.9	19.3
Age and percent of poverty level[6,7]												
All ages:[5]												
Below 100 percent	32.1	37.0	45.0	46.9	46.8	41.6	34.0	35.2	32.7	30.9	32.7	32.8
100–149 percent	7.7	11.2	16.0	18.4	17.2	19.1	26.4	30.6	34.0	31.2	32.8	34.8
150–199 percent	3.3	5.1	5.9	7.7	7.7	8.0	16.7	21.0	24.9	22.8	22.5	25.1
200 percent or more	0.6	1.1	1.4	1.6	1.6	1.9	5.6	6.5	8.4	7.8	7.4	8.5
Under 18 years:												
Below 100 percent	43.1	47.8	63.6	65.6	65.9	59.9	28.9	31.6	23.3	20.6	21.3	22.4
100–149 percent	9.0	12.3	22.9	26.3	24.8	30.2	28.2	26.1	27.7	25.5	25.2	26.1
150–199 percent	4.4	6.1	8.6	11.7	10.8	12.2	12.7	15.8	19.0	17.7	16.1	19.7
200 percent or more	0.8	1.6	2.2	2.7	2.6	2.9	4.2	4.4	6.8	6.0	5.3	6.1
Geographic region[5]												
Northeast	9.4	7.4	12.0	12.5	12.3	12.4	9.8	10.5	13.3	12.7	13.2	12.8
Midwest	7.9	8.2	10.4	11.0	9.4	9.2	10.9	10.2	11.9	11.8	11.9	12.6
South	5.5	7.0	11.3	11.6	12.0	9.8	17.4	19.4	20.9	19.1	19.7	20.3
West	7.5	9.1	12.6	13.2	13.4	12.5	17.6	18.1	20.2	17.3	18.1	19.8
Location of residence[5]												
Within MSA[8]	7.8	7.7	11.7	11.8	11.1	10.6	13.2	14.7	16.6	14.9	15.3	16.2
Outside MSA[8]	6.4	8.3	11.1	12.8	13.9	11.0	16.3	16.7	18.8	18.4	19.2	19.4

[1]Private insurance originally obtained through a present or former employer or union.
[2]The questionnaire changed compared with previous years. See Appendix II, Health insurance coverage.
[3]Preliminary data.   [4]Includes all other races not shown separately and unknown poverty level.
[5]Age adjusted. See Appendix II for age-adjustment procedure.
[6]The race groups white, black, and Asian or Pacific Islander include persons of Hispanic and non-Hispanic origin; persons of Hispanic origin may be of any race.
[7]Poverty level is based on family income and family size using Bureau of the Census poverty thresholds. See Appendix II.
[8]Metropolitan statistical area.
[9]Includes other public assistance through 1996. In 1997 includes state-sponsored health plans. In 1997 the age-adjusted percent of the population under 65 years of age covered by Medicaid was 9.5 percent, and 1.2 percent were covered by state-sponsored health plans.
[10]Includes persons not covered by private insurance, Medicaid, public assistance (through 1996), state-sponsored or other government-sponsored health plans (1997), Medicare, or military plans. Estimates of the percentage of persons lacking health care coverage based on the National Health Interview Survey (NHIS) are slightly higher than those based on the March Current Population Survey (CPS) (table 146). See Appendix II, Health insurance coverage.

NOTE: Percents do not add to 100 because the percent with other types of health insurance (for example, Medicare, military) is not shown, and because persons with both private insurance and Medicaid appear in both columns.

SOURCE: Centers for Disease Control and Prevention, National Center for Health Statistics. Data computed by the Division of Health and Utilization Analysis from the National Health Interview Survey.

Table 130 (page 1 of 2). Health care coverage for persons 65 years of age and over, according to type of coverage and selected characteristics: United States, selected years 1984–97

[Data are based on household interviews of a sample of the civilian noninstitutionalized population]

Characteristic	Private insurance[1]						Private insurance obtained through workplace[1,2]					
	1984	1989	1994[3]	1995	1996	1997[3,4]	1984	1989	1994[3]	1995	1996	1997[3,4]
	Number in millions											
Total[5]	19.4	22.4	24.0	23.5	22.9	22.3	10.2	11.2	12.5	12.5	12.1	12.0
	Percent of population											
Total, age adjusted[5]	73.5	76.6	77.5	74.9	72.0	69.6	39.1	38.8	41.0	40.1	38.6	38.2
Total, crude[5]	73.3	76.5	77.3	74.8	72.0	69.5	38.8	38.4	40.4	39.6	38.1	37.5
Age												
65–74 years	76.5	78.2	78.4	75.3	72.4	69.9	45.1	43.7	45.6	43.3	41.5	42.0
75 years and over	68.1	73.9	75.8	74.2	71.3	69.1	28.6	30.2	33.0	34.3	33.3	31.6
75–84 years	70.8	75.9	77.9	76.0	73.3	70.2	30.8	32.0	35.0	36.1	35.5	33.2
85 years and over	56.8	65.5	67.9	67.8	63.9	64.7	18.9	22.8	25.1	27.5	25.3	25.6
Sex[6]												
Male	74.3	77.5	78.9	76.5	73.6	72.0	44.2	43.4	45.1	44.3	42.7	42.9
Female	72.9	76.2	76.5	73.9	71.0	67.8	35.7	35.6	38.1	37.0	35.5	34.9
Race[6,7]												
White	76.8	80.3	81.2	78.6	75.3	72.9	40.9	40.3	42.7	41.6	39.8	39.1
Black	42.3	43.0	44.7	41.9	44.0	43.5	24.0	24.9	26.5	26.4	30.1	32.1
Hispanic origin and race[6,7]												
All Hispanic	40.5	44.6	51.2	40.9	38.6	31.9	25.4	24.3	22.1	20.1	19.4	19.0
Mexican	41.4	36.6	44.6	33.0	35.6	32.4	25.5	22.4	23.1	17.4	18.7	19.0
White, non-Hispanic	77.9	81.5	82.6	80.7	77.2	75.0	41.4	40.9	43.8	42.9	40.8	40.2
Black, non-Hispanic	42.0	43.1	45.2	41.7	44.8	43.7	23.8	24.9	26.8	26.1	30.7	32.1
Percent of poverty level[6,8]												
Below 100 percent	43.0	45.3	40.1	36.8	32.7	31.0	13.4	11.5	10.6	11.3	10.2	7.3
100–149 percent	67.3	66.7	68.0	67.4	58.8	53.2	27.8	22.4	25.2	25.3	22.3	17.2
150–199 percent	78.6	81.1	81.3	77.4	75.0	69.0	41.4	39.8	37.3	39.9	37.3	32.9
200 percent or more	85.7	86.2	88.9	86.6	84.0	81.4	52.8	51.5	54.0	51.7	49.9	49.4
Geographic region[6]												
Northeast	76.8	76.7	78.3	76.0	72.9	73.0	43.9	44.2	45.2	45.3	42.5	43.8
Midwest	79.6	82.3	84.6	82.5	80.8	78.5	40.6	41.4	43.6	46.0	42.3	41.9
South	68.0	73.5	71.2	71.6	67.2	66.3	35.3	33.5	36.8	35.1	34.7	34.2
West	70.8	75.1	78.2	69.3	69.0	59.5	38.2	38.5	40.1	34.9	36.2	34.4
Location of residence[6]												
Within MSA[9]	74.5	77.2	78.0	75.1	72.2	68.4	42.3	41.6	42.6	42.0	40.5	39.8
Outside MSA[9]	71.8	75.1	76.0	74.4	71.3	73.6	33.7	31.3	36.5	33.5	32.2	33.0

See footnotes at end of table.

Table 130 (page 2 of 2). Health care coverage for persons 65 years of age and over, according to type of coverage and selected characteristics: United States, selected years 1984–97

[Data are based on household interviews of a sample of the civilian noninstitutionalized population]

Characteristic	Medicaid[1,10]						Medicare only[11]					
	1984	1989	1994[3]	1995	1996	1997[3,4]	1984	1989	1994[3]	1995	1996	1997[3,4]
	Number in millions											
Total[5]	1.8	2.0	2.5	2.9	2.7	2.5	4.7	4.5	4.1	4.6	5.7	6.7
	Percent of population											
Total, age adjusted[5]	6.9	7.0	7.8	9.0	8.3	7.8	17.7	15.3	13.1	14.7	18.1	20.7
Total, crude[5]	7.0	7.0	7.9	9.2	8.5	7.9	17.9	15.4	13.2	14.8	18.1	20.8
Age												
65–74 years	6.0	6.3	6.8	8.3	7.5	7.5	15.2	13.8	12.3	14.4	18.0	20.3
75 years and over	8.5	8.2	9.6	10.4	9.9	8.4	22.3	17.8	14.5	15.2	18.2	21.5
75–84 years.	7.7	7.9	8.4	9.5	9.0	7.9	20.6	16.2	13.3	14.1	16.8	20.5
85 years and over	11.7	9.7	14.2	13.7	13.0	10.2	29.8	24.9	19.1	19.3	23.4	25.2
Sex[6]												
Male.	4.5	5.0	4.7	5.6	5.5	5.2	17.4	14.6	12.9	14.4	17.1	19.6
Female	8.6	8.4	10.0	11.5	10.4	9.7	18.1	15.6	13.3	14.9	18.7	21.5
Race[6,7]												
White	5.0	5.4	6.0	6.9	6.6	6.4	16.5	13.4	11.6	13.4	16.9	19.2
Black	24.9	20.4	21.7	26.8	21.8	19.3	30.7	34.5	28.7	28.6	30.1	33.9
Hispanic origin and race[6,7]												
All Hispanic.	24.9	25.6	26.5	31.1	28.9	27.6	28.5	21.6	18.7	24.5	29.0	34.9
White, non-Hispanic.	4.4	4.7	5.1	5.6	5.4	5.4	16.1	13.1	11.3	12.8	16.3	18.3
Black, non-Hispanic	25.2	20.4	21.2	27.0	21.7	19.0	30.8	34.5	28.8	28.7	29.3	34.0
Percent of poverty level[6,8]												
Below 100 percent.	28.0	29.0	37.4	40.6	39.9	41.0	27.5	26.0	23.0	22.1	25.6	26.9
100–149 percent	6.9	9.2	10.8	13.3	12.5	14.6	22.5	21.1	19.0	18.3	26.6	28.6
150–199 percent	3.3	4.7	3.8	5.2	4.6	5.1	16.2	13.5	12.8	16.2	19.6	23.1
200 percent or more	1.8	2.3	1.8	1.8	1.9	2.5	11.0	10.4	7.8	9.9	12.4	15.0
Geographic region[6]												
Northeast	5.3	5.4	7.3	8.9	7.3	6.4	17.1	16.8	14.0	15.4	20.3	19.5
Midwest	4.2	3.6	3.7	5.6	5.1	5.0	15.2	13.4	10.7	10.9	12.8	15.2
South	9.5	9.1	10.3	10.8	9.9	9.7	19.8	16.3	16.0	15.8	19.7	21.3
West	7.9	9.3	9.4	10.8	10.8	9.9	18.4	13.8	10.3	17.3	18.6	28.5
Location of residence[6]												
Within MSA[9]	6.2	6.4	7.3	8.4	7.7	7.4	17.6	15.3	12.9	14.9	18.7	22.2
Outside MSA[9]	8.1	8.4	9.2	11.1	10.4	9.2	17.9	15.2	13.9	14.1	15.9	15.6

[1]Almost all persons 65 years of age and over are covered by Medicare also. In 1997, 92 percent of older persons with private insurance also had Medicare.
[2]Private insurance originally obtained through a present or former employer or union.
[3]The questionnaire changed compared with previous years. See Appendix II, Health insurance coverage.
[4]Preliminary data.
[5]Includes all other races not shown separately and unknown poverty level.
[6]Age adjusted. See Appendix II for age-adjustment procedure.
[7]The race groups white and black include persons of Hispanic and non-Hispanic origin; persons of Hispanic origin may be of any race.
[8]Poverty level is based on family income and family size using Bureau of the Census poverty thresholds. See Appendix II.
[9]Metropolitan statistical area.
[10]Includes public assistance through 1996. In 1997 includes state-sponsored health plans. In 1997 the age-adjusted percent of the population 65 years of age and over covered by Medicaid was 7.4 percent, and 0.4 percent were covered by state-sponsored health plans.
[11]Persons covered by Medicare but not covered by private health insurance, Medicaid, public assistance (through 1996), state-sponsored or other government-sponsored health plans (1997), or military plans. See Appendix II, Health insurance coverage.

NOTE: Percents do not add to 100 because persons with both private health insurance and Medicaid appear in more than one column, and because the percent of persons without health insurance (1.1 percent in 1997) is not shown.

SOURCE: Centers for Disease Control and Prevention, National Center for Health Statistics. Data computed by the Division of Health and Utilization Analysis from the National Health Interview Survey.

Table 131. Private health insurance by health maintenance organization (HMO) and other types of coverage according to selected characteristics: United States, selected years 1989–97

[Data are based on household interviews of a sample of the civilian noninstitutionalized population]

	Private health insurance									
	Health maintenance organization[1]					Other				
Characteristic	1989	1994	1995	1996	1997[2]	1989	1994	1995	1996	1997[2]
	Number of persons in millions									
Total[3]	45.0	61.3	68.4	76.4	76.5	140.3	123.3	120.2	112.6	111.5
	Percent of population									
Total, age adjusted[3,4]	18.7	23.8	25.4	29.3	29.1	57.2	46.8	45.1	41.9	41.2
Total, crude[3]	18.5	23.6	26.1	28.9	28.7	57.6	47.5	45.9	42.6	41.8
Age										
Under 18 years	20.1	24.0	27.4	30.2	29.9	51.7	39.8	38.3	36.2	36.2
Under 6 years	20.1	22.7	26.8	28.9	29.8	47.8	35.5	33.2	32.2	31.5
6–17 years	20.2	24.6	27.6	30.9	30.0	53.8	42.2	41.0	38.2	38.5
18–44 years	20.3	25.6	28.7	31.6	31.4	55.2	44.1	42.5	39.0	38.1
18–24 years	16.6	20.0	22.0	24.6	24.9	47.8	38.2	39.1	35.8	34.4
25–34 years	21.2	26.8	29.3	32.0	32.4	54.7	42.5	41.0	37.5	35.7
35–44 years	21.7	27.8	32.0	35.3	34.1	61.0	49.3	46.0	42.2	42.3
45–64 years	17.6	25.5	27.7	31.5	31.3	65.0	54.8	52.6	48.0	47.7
45–54 years	19.6	27.8	29.5	34.3	33.6	63.9	53.4	51.5	46.2	46.9
55–64 years	15.3	22.1	24.9	27.2	27.9	66.4	56.7	54.3	50.9	49.0
65 years or more	10.4	13.1	12.2	12.3	12.5	67.0	64.3	62.6	59.6	57.0
65–74 years	11.4	14.8	13.9	14.0	14.4	67.7	63.6	61.3	58.4	55.5
75 years or more	8.9	10.6	9.8	10.0	10.0	65.9	65.2	64.4	61.4	59.0
Sex[4]										
Male	18.9	23.7	26.6	29.2	29.0	57.4	47.4	45.4	42.3	41.8
Female	18.6	23.9	26.3	29.3	29.1	57.0	46.2	44.7	41.4	40.7
Race[4,5]										
White	18.2	23.6	26.1	29.7	29.3	61.2	51.2	49.1	44.6	44.7
Black	20.3	22.6	24.4	26.6	27.9	36.5	27.9	28.4	27.3	25.8
Asian or Pacific Islander	24.6	30.5	32.4	34.1	35.2	44.8	35.0	33.4	30.2	30.5
Hispanic origin and race[4,5]										
All Hispanic	18.8	23.1	23.2	25.8	25.4	33.1	25.5	23.4	20.8	20.4
Mexican	16.8	23.9	21.6	24.5	23.6	30.2	21.6	21.1	18.4	18.7
Puerto Rican	16.1	22.9	22.1	24.1	23.9	28.5	25.3	24.9	25.5	20.9
Cuban	25.6	24.9	31.1	34.9	37.7	41.9	38.3	29.3	28.9	28.7
Other Hispanic	22.2	21.3	25.6	28.3	27.4	39.5	31.5	26.4	22.7	21.9
White, non-Hispanic	18.6	24.2	27.3	30.5	30.0	63.8	53.6	51.5	47.9	47.7
Black, non-Hispanic	20.0	22.4	24.3	26.7	27.9	36.8	28.8	29.0	27.7	26.1
Percent of poverty level[4,6]										
Below 100 percent	5.4	6.3	6.7	6.5	8.8	23.2	16.8	16.5	14.8	14.8
100–149 percent	14.0	14.7	17.0	17.7	17.3	42.2	33.9	32.6	30.5	26.0
150–199 percent	18.1	22.5	24.5	27.5	26.2	54.3	44.6	43.0	41.1	38.4
200 percent or more	23.1	31.3	34.1	38.4	37.1	67.8	57.6	54.9	50.6	50.0
Geographic region[4]										
Northeast	20.6	27.0	31.0	32.3	37.7	60.7	48.0	44.2	42.5	36.2
Midwest	20.8	21.2	23.9	28.2	25.6	60.9	56.7	53.8	50.4	51.5
South	11.9	18.5	21.2	23.7	23.6	59.5	47.0	45.7	42.4	43.2
West	26.0	31.9	33.6	36.5	34.9	45.8	34.5	34.3	30.8	29.8
Location of residence[4]										
Within MSA[7]	21.7	27.4	29.7	32.9	32.1	54.8	43.7	42.6	39.5	38.6
Outside MSA[7]	8.4	11.2	13.7	15.8	17.0	65.5	57.6	54.5	50.5	51.5

[1]Persons reporting private health insurance coverage are considered to have health maintenance organization (HMO) coverage if they responded positively to the question "Is this plan an HMO or IPA (individual practice association)?" Does not include Medicaid or Medicare HMO plans.
[2]Preliminary data. The questionnaire changed compared with previous years. See Appendix II, Health insurance coverage.
[3]Includes all other races not shown separately and unknown poverty level.
[4]Age adjusted. See Appendix II for age-adjustment procedure.
[5]The race groups white, black, and Asian or Pacific Islander include persons of Hispanic and non-Hispanic origin; persons of Hispanic origin may be of any race.
[6]Poverty level is based on family income and family size using Bureau of the Census poverty thresholds. See Appendix II.
[7]Metropolitan statistical area.

SOURCES: Centers for Disease Control and Prevention, National Center for Health Statistics. Data computed by the Division of Health and Utilization Analysis from the National Health Interview Survey.

Table 132. Health maintenance organizations (HMO's) and enrollment, according to model type, geographic region, and Federal program: United States, selected years 1976–98

[Data are based on a census of health maintenance organizations]

Plans and enrollment	1976	1980	1985[1]	1990	1992	1993	1994[2]	1995[2]	1996[2]	1997[2]	1998[2]
Plans						Number					
All plans	174	235	478	572	555	551	543	562	630	652	651
Model type:[3]											
Individual practice association[4]	41	97	244	360	340	332	321	332	367	284	317
Group[5]	122	138	234	212	166	150	118	108	122	98	116
Mixed	- - -	- - -	- - -	- - -	49	69	104	122	141	258	212
Geographic region:											
Northeast	29	55	81	115	111	102	101	100	111	110	107
Midwest	52	72	157	160	165	169	159	157	182	184	185
South	23	45	141	176	161	167	173	196	218	236	237
West	70	63	99	121	118	113	110	109	119	121	122
Enrollment						Number of persons in millions					
Total	6.0	9.1	21.0	33.0	36.1	38.4	45.1	50.9	59.1	66.8	76.6
Model type:[3]											
Individual practice association[4]	0.4	1.7	6.4	13.7	14.7	15.3	17.8	20.1	26.0	26.7	32.6
Group[5]	5.6	7.4	14.6	19.3	16.5	15.4	13.9	13.3	14.1	11.0	13.8
Mixed	- - -	- - -	- - -	- - -	4.9	7.7	13.4	17.6	19.0	29.0	30.1
Federal program:[6]											
Medicaid[7]	- - -	0.3	0.6	1.2	1.7	1.7	2.6	3.5	4.7	5.6	7.8
Medicare	- - -	0.4	1.1	1.8	2.2	2.2	2.5	2.9	3.7	4.8	5.7
						Percent of HMO enrollees					
Model type:[3]											
Individual practice association[4]	6.6	18.7	30.4	41.6	40.7	39.8	39.4	39.4	44.1	39.9	42.6
Group[5]	93.4	81.3	69.6	58.4	45.9	40.1	30.7	26.0	23.7	16.5	18.0
Mixed	- - -	- - -	- - -	- - -	13.5	20.1	29.9	34.5	32.2	43.4	39.2
Federal program:[6]											
Medicaid[7]	- - -	2.9	2.7	3.5	4.8	4.4	5.8	6.9	8.0	8.2	10.2
Medicare	- - -	4.3	5.1	5.4	6.0	5.7	5.5	5.7	6.3	7.2	7.4
						Percent of population enrolled in HMO's					
Total	2.8	4.0	8.9	13.4	14.3	15.1	17.3	19.4	22.3	25.2	28.6
Geographic region:											
Northeast	2.0	3.1	7.9	14.6	16.1	18.0	20.8	24.4	25.9	32.4	37.8
Midwest	1.5	2.8	9.7	12.6	12.8	13.2	15.2	16.4	18.8	19.5	22.7
South	0.4	0.8	3.8	7.1	7.8	8.4	10.2	12.4	15.2	17.9	21.0
West	9.7	12.2	17.3	23.2	24.7	25.1	27.4	28.6	33.2	36.4	39.1

- - - Data not available.

[1] Increases partly due to changes in reporting methods. See Appendix I, InterStudy.
[2] Open-ended enrollment in HMO plans, amounting to 11.6 million on Jan. 1, 1998, is included from 1994 onwards. See Appendix II, Health maintenance organization.
[3] In 1976, 11 HMO's with 35,000 enrollment did not report model type. In 1997, 11 HMO's with 153,000 enrollment did not report model type. In 1998, 6 HMO's with 109,000 enrollment did not report model type.
[4] An HMO operating under an individual practice association model contracts with an association of physicians from various settings (a mixture of solo and group practices) to provide health services.
[5] Group includes staff, group, and network model types.
[6] Federal program enrollment in HMO's refers to enrollment by Medicaid or Medicare beneficiaries, where the Medicaid or Medicare program contracts directly with the HMO to pay the appropriate annual premium.
[7] Data for 1990 and later include enrollment in managed care health insuring organizations.

NOTES: Data as of June 30 in 1976–80, December 31 in 1985, and January 1 in 1990–98. Medicaid enrollment in 1990 is as of June 30. HMO's in Guam are included starting in 1994; HMO's in Puerto Rico, starting in 1998. In 1998 HMO enrollment in Guam was 84,000 and in Puerto Rico, 390,000. Some numbers for 1997 have been revised and differ from the previous edition of *Health, United States*. Data for additional years are available (see Appendix III).

SOURCES: Office of Health Maintenance Organizations: Summary of the National HMO census of prepaid plans—June 1976 and National HMO Census 1980. Public Health Service. Washington. U.S. Government Printing Office. DHHS Pub. No. (PHS) 80–50159; InterStudy: National HMO Census: Annual Report on the Growth of HMO's in the U.S., 1984–1985 Editions; The InterStudy Edge, 1990, vol. 2; Competitive Edge, vols. 1–8, 1991–1998; 1986 December Update of Medicare Enrollment in HMO's. 1988 January Update of Medicare Enrollment in HMO's. Excelsior, Minnesota (Copyrights 1983–98: Used with the permission of InterStudy); U.S. Bureau of the Census. Current Population Reports. Series P–25, Nos. 998 and 1058. Washington: U.S. Government Printing Office, Dec. 1986 and Mar. 1990. U.S. Dept. of Commerce. Press release CB 91–100. Mar. 11, 1991; Health Care Financing Administration: Unpublished data; Centers for Disease Control and Prevention, National Center for Health Statistics: Data computed by the Division of Health and Utilization Analysis.

[Data are based on a survey of employers]

Size of establishment and type of benefit	All			Professional, technical, and related			Clerical and sales			Blue-collar and service		
	1990	1994	1996	1990	1994	1996	1990	1994	1996	1990	1994	1996
Small private establishments[1]	Percent of all employees											
Participation in medical care benefit:												
Full-time employees	69	66	64	82	80	76	75	70	69	60	57	56
Part-time employees	6	7	6	6	11	14	7	9	9	6	5	3
Type of medical care benefit among participating full-time employees	Percent of participating full-time employees											
Fee arrangement	100	100	100	100	100	100	100	100	100	100	100	100
Traditional fee-for-service	74	55	36	69	53	31	77	55	34	73	57	41
Preferred provider organization (PPO)	13	24	35	16	27	41	13	24	36	11	23	32
Health maintenance organization (HMO)	14	19	27	15	20	27	10	19	28	15	20	25
Other	0	1	2	0	0	1	0	2	2	0	0	2
Individual coverage:												
Employee contributions not required	58	47	48	56	49	49	53	44	46	62	48	48
Employee contributions required	42	53	52	44	51	51	47	56	54	38	52	51
Family coverage:												
Employee contributions not required	32	19	24	28	17	21	29	15	20	37	23	29
Employee contributions required	68	81	75	72	83	78	71	85	80	63	77	70
	Average monthly contribution											
Individual coverage:												
Average monthly employee contribution:												
Total	$ 25	$ 41	$ 43	$ 24	$ 47	$ 41	$ 24	$ 41	$ 42	$ 27	$ 38	$ 44
Non-HMO	25	39	43	24	46	40	24	38	43	28	36	45
HMO	25	49	41	24	48	42	27	50	42	25	47	41
Family coverage:												
Average monthly employee contribution:												
Total	109	160	182	112	181	190	106	160	181	111	149	177
Non-HMO	104	151	181	110	173	192	102	155	181	101	137	175
HMO	135	190	182	118	204	183	134	178	183	145	191	182

See footnotes at end of table.

Table 133 (page 2 of 2). Medical care benefits for employees of private establishments by size of establishment and occupation: United States, selected years 1990–96

[Data are based on a survey of employers]

Size of establishment and type of benefit	All 1991	All 1993	All 1995	Professional, technical, and related 1991	Professional, technical, and related 1993	Professional, technical, and related 1995	Clerical and sales 1991	Clerical and sales 1993	Clerical and sales 1995	Blue-collar and service 1991	Blue-collar and service 1993	Blue-collar and service 1995
Medium and large private establishments[2]				Percent of all employees								
Participation in medical care benefit:												
Full-time employees	83	82	77	85	84	80	81	79	76	84	82	75
Part-time employees	28	24	19	42	33	31	26	22	20	26	24	15
Type of medical care benefit among participating full-time employees				Percent of participating full-time employees								
Fee arrangement	100	100	100	100	100	100	100	100	100	100	100	100
Traditional fee-for-service	67	50	37	62	41	29	59	42	30	73	59	45
Preferred provider organization (PPO)	16	26	34	19	29	36	21	30	36	12	22	33
Health maintenance organization (HMO)	17	23	27	18	28	33	19	27	32	14	18	21
Other	0	1	1	1	2	1	0	1	2	0	1	1
Individual coverage:												
Employee contributions not required	49	38	33	45	32	21	43	33	24	55	44	44
Employee contributions required	51	62	67	55	68	79	57	67	76	45	56	56
Family coverage:												
Employee contributions not required	31	22	22	25	15	11	27	18	15	37	29	33
Employee contributions required	69	78	78	75	85	89	73	82	85	63	71	67
				Average monthly contribution								
Individual coverage:												
Average monthly employee contribution:												
Total	$ 27	$ 32	$ 34	$ 26	$ 32	$ 35	$ 28	$ 34	$ 36	$ 26	$ 30	$ 32
Non-HMO	26	31	33	26	32	33	27	34	34	25	30	32
HMO	29	32	36	29	32	38	32	34	39	28	30	32
Family coverage:												
Average monthly employee contribution:												
Total	97	107	118	96	114	120	108	115	127	91	99	112
Non-HMO	92	102	112	93	113	116	104	112	120	84	92	106
HMO	118	122	133	110	117	128	121	125	141	122	124	130

[1]Less than 100 employees in all private nonfarm industries.
[2]100 or more employees in all private nonfarm industries.

NOTE: In 1992–93, 88 percent of full-time employees in private establishments were offered health care plans by their employers (96 percent in medium and large private establishments and 80 percent in small private establishments).

SOURCES: U.S. Department of Labor, Bureau of Labor Statistics, Employee benefits in small private establishments, 1990 Bulletin 2388, September 1991, 1994 Bulletin 2475, April 1996, and news release USDL 98–240, June 15, 1998. Employee benefits in medium and large private establishments, 1991 Bulletin 2422, May 1993, 1993 Bulletin 2456, Nov. 1994, and news release USDL 97–246. July 25, 1997. Blostin AP and Pfuntner JN. Employee medical care contributions on the rise. Compensation and Working Conditions, Spring 1998.

Table 134. Medicare enrollees and expenditures and percent distribution, according to type of service: United States and other areas, selected years 1967–97

[Data are compiled by the Health Care Financing Administration]

Type of service	1967	1970	1975	1980	1985	1990	1995	1996	1997[1]
Enrollees					Number in millions				
Total[2]	19.5	20.5	25.0	28.5	31.1	34.2	37.5	38.1	38.4
Hospital insurance	19.5	20.4	24.6	28.1	30.6	33.7	37.1	37.7	38.1
Supplementary medical insurance	17.9	19.6	23.9	27.4	30.0	32.6	35.7	36.1	36.5
Expenditures[3]					Amount in millions				
Total	$4,737	$7,493	$16,316	$36,822	$72,294	$110,984	$184,204	$200,338	$214,304
Total hospital insurance[4]	3,430	5,281	11,581	25,577	48,414	66,997	117,604	129,929	140,180
Inpatient hospital	3,034	4,827	10,877	24,116	44,940	59,451	89,127	97,802	103,642
Skilled nursing facility	282	246	278	395	548	2,575	9,595	11,129	12,681
Home health agency	29	51	160	540	1,913	3,666	15,571	17,527	20,163
Hospice	...	...	...	...	43	358	1,883	1,999	2,120
Administrative expenses[5]	77	157	266	526	970	947	1,428	1,472	1,574
Total supplementary medical insurance	1,307	2,212	4,735	11,245	23,880	43,987	66,600	70,409	74,124
Physician	1,128	1,790	3,416	8,187	17,312	29,609	40,475	41,238	42,399
Outpatient hospital	33	114	643	1,897	4,319	8,482	15,625	16,456	17,423
Home health agency	10	34	95	234	38	74	200	219	220
Group practice prepayment	19	26	80	203	720	2,827	6,608	8,847	10,980
Independent laboratory	7	11	39	114	558	1,476	2,065	1,839	1,734
Administrative expenses[5]	110	237	462	610	933	1,519	1,627	1,810	1,368
					Percent distribution of expenditures				
Total hospital insurance[4]	100.0	100.0	100.0	100.0	100.0	100.0	100.0	100.0	100.0
Inpatient hospital	88.5	91.4	93.9	94.3	92.8	88.7	75.8	75.3	73.9
Skilled nursing facility	8.2	4.7	2.4	1.5	1.1	3.8	8.2	8.6	9.0
Home health agency	0.8	1.0	1.4	2.1	4.0	5.5	13.2	13.5	14.4
Hospice	...	...	...	...	0.1	0.5	1.6	1.5	1.5
Administrative expenses[5]	2.2	3.0	2.3	2.1	2.0	1.4	1.2	1.1	1.1
Total supplementary medical insurance	100.0	100.0	100.0	100.0	100.0	100.0	100.0	100.0	100.0
Physician	86.3	80.9	72.1	72.8	72.5	67.3	60.8	58.6	57.2
Outpatient hospital	2.5	5.2	13.6	16.9	18.1	19.3	23.5	23.4	23.5
Home health agency	0.8	1.5	2.0	2.1	0.2	0.2	0.3	0.3	0.3
Group practice prepayment	1.5	1.2	1.7	1.8	3.0	6.4	9.9	12.6	14.8
Independent laboratory	0.5	0.5	0.8	1.0	2.3	3.4	3.1	2.6	2.3
Administrative expenses[5]	8.4	10.7	9.8	5.4	3.9	3.5	2.4	2.6	1.8

... Category not applicable.
[1]Preliminary figures.
[2]Number enrolled in the hospital insurance and/or supplementary medical insurance programs on July 1.
[3]Managed care expenditures are excluded.
[4]In 1967 includes coverage for outpatient hospital diagnostic services.
[5]Includes research, costs of experiments and demonstration projects, and peer review activity.

NOTES: Table includes data for Medicare enrollees residing in Puerto Rico, Virgin Islands, Guam, other outlying areas, foreign countries, and unknown residence. Some numbers in this table have been revised and differ from previous editions of *Health, United States*. Data for additional years are available (see Appendix III).

SOURCE: Health Care Financing Administration. Office of Medicare Cost Estimates, Office of the Actuary and Bureau of Data Management and Strategy. Washington.

Table 135. Medicare enrollment, persons served, and payments for Medicare enrollees 65 years of age and over, according to selected characteristics: United States and other areas, selected years 1977–96

[Data are compiled by the Health Care Financing Administration]

Characteristic	Enrollment in millions[1]				Persons served per 1,000 enrollees[2]				Payments per person served[3]				Payments per enrollee[3]			
	1977	1987	1995	1996	1977	1987	1995	1996	1977	1987	1995	1996	1977	1987	1995	1996
Total	23.8	29.4	33.1	33.4	570	754	826	816	$1,332	$3,025	$5,074	$5,330	$ 759	$2,281	$4,193	$4,348
Age																
65–66 years	3.3	4.0	3.8	3.8	533	700	809	792	1,075	2,214	3,146	3,250	573	1,550	2,546	2,574
67–68 years	3.2	3.7	3.8	3.8	511	667	746	727	1,173	2,536	3,936	4,118	599	1,691	2,937	2,994
69–70 years	2.9	3.4	3.7	3.7	531	705	773	760	1,211	2,700	4,205	4,340	643	1,902	3,249	3,296
71–72 years	2.6	3.1	3.6	3.6	555	740	790	781	1,228	2,904	4,538	4,748	681	2,150	3,586	3,709
73–74 years	2.3	2.9	3.3	3.3	576	762	817	805	1,319	3,048	4,911	5,119	759	2,322	4,010	4,120
75–79 years	4.5	5.7	6.6	6.7	597	787	845	833	1,430	3,312	5,464	5,751	853	2,608	4,616	4,788
80–84 years	3.0	3.7	4.5	4.6	623	828	890	882	1,549	3,496	6,299	6,600	965	2,894	5,603	5,818
85 years and over	2.1	3.0	3.8	3.9	652	841	911	912	1,636	3,708	6,980	7,311	1,068	3,119	6,356	6,666
Sex and age																
Male	9.6	11.8	13.4	13.6	546	712	784	769	1,505	3,432	5,450	5,756	821	2,443	4,275	4,428
65–66 years	- - -	1.8	1.8	1.8	- - -	640	755	736	- - -	2,560	3,516	3,620	- - -	1,639	2,655	2,663
67–68 years	- - -	1.6	1.7	1.7	- - -	623	707	686	- - -	2,955	4,401	4,816	- - -	1,841	3,110	3,166
69–70 years	- - -	1.5	1.7	1.7	- - -	667	737	721	- - -	3,116	4,740	4,827	- - -	2,078	3,491	3,482
71–72 years	- - -	1.3	1.5	1.6	- - -	711	757	745	- - -	3,399	5,032	5,322	- - -	2,416	3,810	3,965
73–74 years	- - -	1.2	1.4	1.4	- - -	735	782	770	- - -	3,587	5,420	5,697	- - -	2,635	4,241	4,387
75–79 years	- - -	2.2	2.6	2.7	- - -	764	816	798	- - -	3,775	6,026	6,387	- - -	2,883	4,915	5,099
80–84 years	- - -	1.3	1.6	1.6	- - -	806	869	854	- - -	3,997	6,895	7,289	- - -	3,222	5,994	6,222
85 years and over	- - -	0.8	1.1	1.1	- - -	808	874	863	- - -	4,227	7,636	8,173	- - -	3,417	6,671	7,055
Female.	14.2	17.6	19.7	19.8	586	782	855	847	1,223	2,778	4,840	5,066	717	2,173	4,136	4,293
65–66 years	- - -	2.2	2.0	2.0	- - -	750	856	841	- - -	1,970	2,865	3,740	- - -	1,477	2,453	2,498
67–68 years	- - -	2.0	2.1	2.0	- - -	702	779	762	- - -	2,236	3,584	3,980	- - -	1,569	2,793	2,849
69–70 years	- - -	1.9	2.1	2.0	- - -	734	801	791	- - -	2,404	3,812	4,339	- - -	1,765	3,055	3,146
71–72 years	- - -	1.8	2.0	2.0	- - -	762	816	809	- - -	2,557	4,183	4,719	- - -	1,950	3,412	3,511
73–74 years	- - -	1.7	2.0	1.9	- - -	781	842	831	- - -	2,687	4,560	3,451	- - -	2,099	3,839	3,922
75–79 years	- - -	3.5	4.0	4.0	- - -	802	864	856	- - -	3,032	5,106	5,348	- - -	2,433	4,414	4,577
80–84 years	- - -	2.4	2.9	2.9	- - -	839	901	897	- - -	3,244	5,980	6,232	- - -	2,722	5,387	5,592
85 years and over	- - -	2.2	2.8	2.8	- - -	854	925	931	- - -	3,518	6,743	7,004	- - -	3,004	6,235	6,517
Geographic region[4]																
Northeast	5.7	6.6	7.1	7.1	613	793	865	840	1,426	3,171	5,503	5,810	874	2,513	4,757	4,879
Midwest	6.3	7.4	8.0	8.0	541	756	892	897	1,401	2,969	4,555	4,740	757	2,246	4,062	4,250
South.	7.5	9.6	11.2	11.3	556	768	869	866	1,198	2,893	5,263	5,564	666	2,221	4,576	4,816
West	3.8	5.2	6.2	6.3	632	726	663	637	1,341	3,222	5,036	5,282	848	2,339	3,340	3,364

- - - Data not available.
[1] Includes fee-for-service and managed care enrollees and is as of July 1 each year.
[2] Excludes managed care enrollees.
[3] Excludes amounts for managed care services.
[4] Includes residents of the United States. Excludes unknown residence.

NOTES: Table includes data for Medicare enrollees residing in Puerto Rico, Virgin Islands, Guam, other outlying areas, foreign countries, and unknown residence. Data for additional years are available (see Appendix III).

SOURCE: Health Care Financing Administration. Bureau of Data Management and Strategy. Unpublished data.

Table 136. Medicaid recipients and medical vendor payments, according to basis of eligibility: United States, selected fiscal years 1972–97

[Data are compiled by the Health Care Financing Administration]

Basis of eligibility	1972	1975	1980	1985	1990	1994	1995	1996	1997
Recipients					Number in millions				
All recipients	17.6	22.0	21.6	21.8	25.3	35.1	36.3	36.1	33.6
					Percent of recipients[1]				
Aged (65 years and over)	18.8	16.4	15.9	14.0	12.7	11.5	11.4	11.9	11.8
Blind and disabled	9.8	11.2	13.5	13.8	14.7	15.6	16.1	17.2	18.3
Adults in families with dependent children[2]	17.8	20.6	22.6	25.3	23.8	21.6	21.0	19.7	20.2
Children under age 21[3]	44.5	43.6	43.2	44.7	44.4	49.0	47.3	46.3	45.5
Other Title XIX[4]	9.0	8.2	6.9	5.6	3.9	1.7	1.7	1.8	4.3
Vendor payments[5]					Amount in billions				
All payments	$ 6.3	$ 12.2	$ 23.3	$ 37.5	$ 64.9	$107.9	$120.1	$121.7	$123.6
					Percent distribution				
Total	100.0	100.0	100.0	100.0	100.0	100.0	100.0	100.0	100.0
Aged (65 years and over)	30.6	35.6	37.5	37.6	33.2	30.9	30.4	30.4	30.5
Blind and disabled	22.2	25.7	32.7	35.9	37.6	39.1	41.1	42.8	43.8
Adults in families with dependent children[2]	15.3	16.8	13.9	12.7	13.2	12.6	11.2	10.1	10.0
Children under age 21[3]	18.1	17.9	13.4	11.8	14.0	16.0	15.0	14.4	12.7
Other Title XIX[4]	13.9	4.0	2.6	2.1	1.6	1.2	1.2	1.2	3.0
Vendor payments per recipient[5]					Amount				
All recipients	$ 358	$ 556	$1,079	$1,719	$2,568	$3,080	$3,311	$3,369	$3,679
Aged (65 years and over)	580	1,206	2,540	4,605	6,717	8,264	8,868	8,622	9,539
Blind and disabled	807	1,276	2,618	4,459	6,564	7,735	8,435	8,369	8,832
Adults in families with dependent children[2]	307	455	662	860	1,429	1,791	1,777	1,722	1,810
Children under age 21[3]	145	228	335	452	811	1,007	1,047	1,048	1,027
Other Title XIX[4]	555	273	398	657	1,062	2,165	2,380	2,152	2,599

[1]Recipients included in more than one category for 1980 and 1985. From 1990 to 1996 between 0.2 and 2.5 percent of recipients have unknown basis of eligibility. In 1997 unknowns are included in Other Title XIX.
[2]Includes adults in the Aid to Families with Dependent Children (AFDC) program.
[3]Includes children in the AFDC program.
[4]Includes some participants in the Supplemental Security Income program and other people deemed medically needy in participating States.
[5]Payments exclude disproportionate share hospital payments ($16 billion in 1997) and payments to health maintenance organizations ($18 billion in 1997).

NOTES: 1972 and 1975 data are for fiscal year ending June 30. All other years are for fiscal year ending September 30. Data for additional years are available (see Appendix III). 1997 data for Hawaii not reported.

SOURCE: Health Care Financing Administration. Office of Information Services, Enterprise Databases Group, Division of Information Distribution. Unpublished data.

Table 137. Medicaid recipients and medical vendor payments, according to type of service: United States, selected fiscal years 1972–97

[Data are compiled by the Health Care Financing Administration]

Type of service	1972	1975	1980	1985	1990	1994	1995	1996	1997
Recipients	Number in millions								
All recipients	17.6	22.0	21.6	21.8	25.3	35.1	36.3	36.1	33.6
	Percent of recipients								
Inpatient general hospitals	16.1	15.6	17.0	15.7	18.2	16.7	15.3	14.8	14.1
Inpatient mental hospitals	0.2	0.3	0.3	0.3	0.4	0.2	0.2	0.3	0.3
Mentally retarded intermediate care facilities	---	0.3	0.6	0.7	0.6	0.5	0.4	0.4	0.4
Nursing facilities	---	---	---	---	---	4.7	4.6	4.4	4.8
Skilled	3.1	2.9	2.8	2.5	2.4	---	---	---	---
Intermediate care	---	3.1	3.7	3.8	3.4	---	---	---	---
Physician	69.8	69.1	63.7	66.0	67.6	69.2	65.6	63.3	63.0
Dental	13.6	17.9	21.5	21.4	18.0	18.1	17.6	17.2	17.7
Other practitioner	9.1	12.1	15.0	15.4	15.3	15.4	15.2	14.8	15.3
Outpatient hospital	29.6	33.8	44.9	46.2	49.0	47.2	46.1	44.0	40.6
Clinic	2.8	4.9	7.1	9.7	11.1	15.0	14.7	14.0	14.0
Laboratory and radiological	20.0	21.5	14.9	29.1	35.5	38.3	36.0	34.9	33.0
Home health	0.6	1.6	1.8	2.5	2.8	3.9	4.5	4.8	5.5
Prescribed drugs	63.3	64.3	63.4	63.8	68.5	69.8	65.4	62.5	62.4
Family planning	...	5.5	5.2	7.5	6.9	7.3	6.9	6.6	6.2
Early and periodic screening	...	...	...	8.7	11.7	18.4	18.2	18.2	19.2
Rural health clinic	...	...	...	0.4	0.9	2.7	3.4	3.9	4.3
Other care	14.4	13.2	11.9	15.5	20.3	28.4	31.5	36.3	36.9
Vendor payments[1]	Amount in billions								
All payments	$ 6.3	$ 12.2	$ 23.3	$ 37.5	$ 64.9	$ 107.9	$ 120.1	$ 121.7	$ 123.6
	Percent distribution								
Total	100.0	100.0	100.0	100.0	100.0	100.0	100.0	100.0	100.0
Inpatient general hospitals	40.6	27.6	27.5	25.2	25.7	24.2	21.9	20.7	18.7
Inpatient mental hospitals	1.8	3.3	3.3	3.2	2.6	1.9	2.1	1.7	1.6
Mentally retarded intermediate care facilities	---	3.1	8.5	12.6	11.3	7.7	8.6	7.9	7.9
Nursing facilities	---	---	---	---	---	24.9	24.2	24.3	24.7
Skilled	23.3	19.9	15.8	13.5	12.4	---	---	---	---
Intermediate care	---	15.4	18.0	17.4	14.9	---	---	---	---
Physician	12.6	10.0	8.0	6.3	6.2	6.7	6.1	5.9	5.7
Dental	2.7	2.8	2.0	1.2	0.9	0.9	0.8	0.8	0.8
Other practitioner	0.9	1.0	0.8	0.7	0.6	1.0	0.8	0.9	0.8
Outpatient hospital	5.8	3.0	4.7	4.8	5.1	5.9	5.5	5.3	5.0
Clinic	0.7	3.2	1.4	1.9	2.6	3.5	3.6	3.5	3.4
Laboratory and radiological	1.3	1.0	0.5	0.9	1.1	1.1	1.0	1.0	0.8
Home health	0.4	0.6	1.4	3.0	5.2	6.5	7.8	8.9	9.9
Prescribed drugs	8.1	6.7	5.7	6.2	6.8	8.2	8.1	8.8	9.7
Family planning	...	0.5	0.3	0.5	0.4	0.5	0.4	0.4	0.3
Early and periodic screening	...	...	...	0.2	0.3	0.9	1.0	1.1	1.3
Rural health clinic	...	...	...	0.0	0.1	0.2	0.2	0.2	0.2
Other care	1.8	1.9	1.9	2.5	3.7	6.0	7.7	8.4	8.9
Vendor payments per recipient[1]	Amount								
Total payment per recipient	$ 358	$ 556	$ 1,079	$ 1,719	$ 2,568	$ 3,080	$ 3,311	$ 3,369	$ 3,679
Inpatient general hospitals	903	983	1,742	2,753	3,630	4,462	4,735	4,696	4,878
Inpatient mental hospitals	2,825	6,045	11,742	19,867	18,548	24,024	29,847	21,873	23,026
Mentally retarded intermediate care facilities	---	5,507	16,438	32,102	50,048	52,269	68,613	68,232	72,033
Nursing facilities	---	---	---	---	---	16,424	17,424	18,589	19,029
Skilled	2,665	3,864	6,081	9,274	13,356	---	---	---	---
Intermediate care	---	2,764	5,326	7,882	11,236	---	---	---	---
Physician	65	81	136	163	235	296	309	317	333
Dental	71	86	99	98	130	153	160	166	175
Other practitioner	37	48	61	75	96	192	178	205	190
Outpatient hospital	70	50	113	178	269	383	397	409	453
Clinic	82	358	209	337	602	714	804	833	902
Laboratory and radiological	23		38	53	80	88	90	96	93
Home health	229		847	2,094	4,733	5,124	5,740	6,293	6,575
Prescribed drugs	46	58	96	166	256	363	413	474	571
Family planning	...	55	72	119	151	201	206	200	200
Early and periodic screening	...	...	...	45	67	152	177	212	251
Rural health clinic	...	...	...	81	154	199	174	215	213
Other care	44	80	172	274	465	656	807	782	891

--- Data not available.

... Category not applicable.

[1]Excludes disproportionate share hospital payments ($16 billion in 1997) and payments to health maintenance organizations ($18 billion in 1997).

NOTES: 1972 and 1975 data are for fiscal year ending June 30. All other years are for fiscal year ending September 30. Data for additional years are available (see Appendix III). 1997 data for Hawaii not reported.

SOURCE: Health Care Financing Administration. Office of Information Services, Enterprise Databases Group, Division of Information Distribution. Unpublished data.

Table 138. Department of Veterans Affairs health care expenditures and use, and persons treated according to selected characteristics: United States, selected fiscal years 1970–97

[Data are compiled by Department of Veterans Affairs]

	1970	1980	1990	1992	1993	1994	1995	1996	1997
Health care expenditures				Amount in millions					
All expenditures[1]	$1,689	$5,981	$11,500	$13,682	$14,612	$15,401	$16,126	$16,373	$17,149
				Percent distribution					
All services	100.0	100.0	100.0	100.0	100.0	100.0	100.0	100.0	100.0
Inpatient hospital	71.3	64.3	57.5	55.8	54.8	53.8	49.0	46.3	43.1
Outpatient care	14.0	19.1	25.3	27.1	28.0	28.4	30.2	33.6	37.1
Nursing home care	5.5	7.1	9.5	10.0	10.4	10.5	10.0	10.1	10.2
All other[2]	9.1	9.6	7.7	7.1	6.8	7.3	10.8	10.0	9.6
Health care use				Number in thousands					
Inpatient hospital stays[3]	787	1,248	1,029	935	920	907	879	807	671
Outpatient visits	7,312	17,971	22,602	23,902	24,236	25,158	27,527	29,295	31,919
Nursing home stays[4]	47	57	75	75	78	78	79	79	87
Inpatients[5]									
Total	- - -	- - -	598	564	556	547	527	491	417
				Percent distribution					
Total	- - -	- - -	100.0	100.0	100.0	100.0	100.0	100.0	100.0
Veterans with service-connected disability	- - -	- - -	38.9	39.0	39.4	39.1	39.3	39.5	39.2
Veterans without service-connected disability	- - -	- - -	60.3	60.1	59.6	60.0	59.9	59.6	59.7
Low income	- - -	- - -	54.8	55.7	55.2	56.6	56.2	55.7	55.5
Exempt[6]	- - -	- - -	2.5	2.7	2.4	0.9	0.8	0.8	0.9
Other[7]	- - -	- - -	2.8	1.6	1.9	2.4	2.8	3.0	3.2
Unknown	- - -	- - -	0.2	0.1	0.1	0.1	0.1	0.1	0.1
Nonveterans	- - -	- - -	0.8	0.9	1.0	0.9	0.8	0.8	1.0
Outpatients[5]				Number in thousands					
Total	- - -	- - -	2,564	2,639	2,684	2,714	2,790	2,846	2,958
				Percent distribution					
Total	- - -	- - -	100.0	100.0	100.0	100.0	100.0	100.0	100.0
Veterans with service-connected disability	- - -	- - -	38.3	37.8	37.4	37.4	37.5	37.8	37.9
Veterans without service-connected disability	- - -	- - -	49.8	50.9	50.6	50.5	50.5	50.2	51.5
Low income	- - -	- - -	41.1	42.4	41.5	42.6	42.2	41.9	41.9
Exempt[6]	- - -	- - -	2.9	2.8	2.6	1.0	0.9	0.9	0.7
Other[7]	- - -	- - -	3.6	2.6	2.9	3.6	4.2	4.7	5.9
Unknown	- - -	- - -	2.2	3.1	3.6	3.3	3.2	2.8	3.0
Nonveterans	- - -	- - -	11.8	11.3	12.0	12.1	12.0	12.1	10.6

- - - Data not available.

[1]Health care expenditures exclude construction, medical administration, and miscellaneous operating expenses.
[2]Includes miscellaneous benefits and services, contract hospitals, education and training, subsidies to State veterans hospitals, nursing homes, and domiciliaries, and the Civilian Health and Medical Program of the Department of Veterans Affairs.
[3]One-day dialysis patients were included in fiscal year 1980. Interfacility transfers were included beginning in fiscal year 1990.
[4]Includes Department of Veterans Affairs nursing home and domiciliary stays, and community nursing home stays.
[5]Individuals.
[6]Prisoner of war, exposed to Agent Orange, and so forth. Prior to fiscal year 1994, veterans who reported exposure to Agent Orange were classified as Exempt. Beginning in fiscal year 1994 those veterans reporting Agent Orange exposure but not treated for it were means tested and placed in the low income or other group depending on income.
[7]Financial means-tested veterans who receive medical care subject to copayments according to income level.

NOTES: Figures may not add to totals due to rounding. In 1970 and 1980, the fiscal year ended June 30; for all other years the fiscal year ends September 30. The veteran population was estimated at 25.6 million in 1997 with 36 percent age 65 or over, compared with 11 percent in 1980. Twenty-six percent had served during World War II, 17 percent during the Korean conflict, 32 percent during the Vietnam era, 7 percent during the Persian Gulf War, and 23 percent during peacetime. Beginning in fiscal year 1995 categories for health care expenditures and health care use were revised. Data for additional years are available (see Appendix III).

SOURCE: Department of Veterans Affairs, Office of Policy and Planning, National Center for Veteran Analysis and Statistics. Unpublished data.

Table 139. Hospital care expenditures by geographic division and State and average annual percent change: United States, selected years 1980–93

[Data are compiled by the Health Care Financing Administration]

Geographic division and State[1]	Amount in millions						Average annual percent change	
	1980	1985	1990	1991	1992	1993	1980–90	1990–93
United States[2]	$101,510	$166,545	$254,239	$279,820	$303,461	$323,919	9.6	8.4
New England	6,467	10,332	15,540	16,773	17,855	19,056	9.2	7.0
Maine	460	735	1,119	1,207	1,280	1,376	9.3	7.1
New Hampshire	313	590	1,056	1,102	1,233	1,388	12.9	9.5
Vermont	174	290	447	494	532	562	9.9	7.9
Massachusetts	3,646	5,628	8,159	8,826	9,380	10,034	8.4	7.1
Rhode Island	481	760	1,095	1,177	1,237	1,314	8.6	6.3
Connecticut	1,396	2,328	3,664	3,967	4,193	4,380	10.1	6.1
Middle Atlantic	18,361	29,462	45,472	49,673	53,779	57,854	9.5	8.4
New York	9,582	14,585	22,739	24,784	26,387	28,001	9.0	7.2
New Jersey	2,763	4,751	7,857	8,586	9,406	10,312	11.0	9.5
Pennsylvania	6,017	10,126	14,876	16,303	17,987	19,540	9.5	9.5
East North Central	19,590	30,093	42,984	47,026	50,835	54,172	8.2	8.0
Ohio	4,808	8,026	11,419	12,359	13,394	14,305	9.0	7.8
Indiana	2,125	3,399	5,288	5,918	6,473	6,998	9.5	9.8
Illinois	6,217	8,998	12,400	13,560	14,744	15,621	7.1	8.0
Michigan	4,482	6,882	9,500	10,309	11,008	11,711	7.8	7.2
Wisconsin	1,959	2,788	4,377	4,880	5,216	5,537	8.4	8.2
West North Central	7,810	12,261	18,012	19,664	21,116	22,252	8.7	7.3
Minnesota	1,740	2,716	4,094	4,473	4,674	4,796	8.9	5.4
Iowa	1,179	1,733	2,634	2,856	2,996	3,111	8.4	5.7
Missouri	2,532	4,172	5,986	6,527	7,077	7,652	9.0	8.5
North Dakota	313	524	717	786	853	903	8.6	8.0
South Dakota	275	450	694	786	863	920	9.7	9.9
Nebraska	681	1,060	1,587	1,749	1,881	2,003	8.8	8.1
Kansas	1,090	1,607	2,300	2,487	2,771	2,868	7.8	7.6
South Atlantic	15,588	26,925	44,077	48,917	52,971	56,711	11.0	8.8
Delaware	259	434	709	777	854	937	10.6	9.7
Maryland	2,034	2,980	4,655	5,097	5,516	5,926	8.6	8.4
District of Columbia	913	1,469	2,133	2,291	2,437	2,612	8.9	7.0
Virginia	2,077	3,530	5,661	6,240	6,618	7,031	10.5	7.5
West Virginia	831	1,219	1,763	1,977	2,190	2,346	7.8	10.0
North Carolina	1,963	3,250	5,901	6,658	7,311	7,801	11.6	9.8
South Carolina	978	1,753	3,108	3,588	3,962	4,221	12.3	10.7
Georgia	2,148	3,885	6,685	7,398	8,092	8,704	12.0	9.2
Florida	4,385	8,404	13,462	14,890	15,992	17,131	11.9	8.4
East South Central	5,713	9,673	15,149	16,955	18,715	19,921	10.2	9.6
Kentucky	1,230	2,157	3,437	3,900	4,268	4,515	10.8	9.5
Tennessee	2,027	3,483	5,511	6,146	6,761	7,208	10.5	9.4
Alabama	1,590	2,606	4,015	4,511	5,028	5,301	9.7	9.7
Mississippi	867	1,427	2,187	2,398	2,658	2,897	9.7	9.8
West South Central	9,210	16,230	25,344	28,335	31,236	33,601	10.7	9.9
Arkansas	746	1,313	2,109	2,336	2,546	2,723	11.0	8.9
Louisiana	1,744	3,155	4,627	5,164	5,575	5,956	10.2	8.8
Oklahoma	1,177	1,896	2,674	2,938	3,182	3,329	8.6	7.6
Texas	5,543	9,866	15,935	17,897	19,932	21,592	11.1	10.7
Mountain	4,255	7,652	11,748	13,092	14,223	15,095	10.7	8.7
Montana	264	438	679	764	841	894	9.9	9.6
Idaho	243	419	665	752	844	900	10.6	10.6
Wyoming	146	248	353	381	396	417	9.2	5.7
Colorado	1,218	2,087	3,101	3,480	3,776	3,932	9.8	8.2
New Mexico	451	873	1,364	1,538	1,703	1,848	11.7	10.7
Arizona	1,093	2,103	3,218	3,532	3,765	3,999	11.4	7.5
Utah	453	816	1,325	1,483	1,631	1,743	11.3	9.6
Nevada	387	667	1,043	1,162	1,267	1,362	10.4	9.3
Pacific	14,515	23,918	35,912	39,384	42,731	45,259	9.5	8.0
Washington	1,396	2,516	3,961	4,546	5,090	5,305	11.0	10.2
Oregon	928	1,486	2,297	2,403	2,714	2,966	9.5	8.9
California	11,632	18,883	27,949	30,554	32,880	34,827	9.2	7.6
Alaska	199	385	557	631	690	701	10.8	8.0
Hawaii	360	648	1,148	1,250	1,358	1,460	12.3	8.3

[1]States where services were provided.
[2]These estimates differ from National Health Expenditures estimates presented elsewhere in *Health, United States*. See Appendix I, Health Care Financing Administration.

NOTE: Figures may not sum to totals due to rounding.

SOURCE: Health Care Financing Administration, Office of the Actuary. Estimates prepared by the Office of National Health Statistics.

Table 140. Physician service expenditures by geographic division and State and average annual percent change: United States, selected years 1980–93

[Data are compiled by the Health Care Financing Administration]

Geographic division and State[1]	Amount in millions						Average annual percent change	
	1980	1985	1990	1991	1992	1993	1980–90	1990–93
United States[2]	$45,245	$83,636	$140,499	$150,318	$161,783	$171,226	12.0	6.8
New England	2,072	4,010	7,656	8,088	8,678	9,250	14.0	6.5
Maine	142	275	480	520	570	601	13.0	7.8
New Hampshire	130	281	491	583	719	780	14.2	16.7
Vermont	68	131	221	229	248	265	12.5	6.2
Massachusetts	978	1,890	3,766	3,892	4,130	4,442	14.4	5.7
Rhode Island	166	304	514	527	543	575	12.0	3.8
Connecticut	589	1,127	2,185	2,336	2,468	2,587	14.0	5.8
Middle Atlantic	6,636	12,255	20,470	22,035	24,044	25,238	11.9	7.2
New York	3,332	5,822	9,697	10,238	11,287	12,003	11.3	7.4
New Jersey	1,353	2,533	4,519	4,771	5,526	5,776	12.8	8.5
Pennsylvania	1,950	3,901	6,254	7,026	7,230	7,460	12.4	6.1
East North Central	8,078	13,646	21,823	23,280	24,837	26,275	10.4	6.4
Ohio	2,130	3,692	6,048	6,486	6,786	7,118	11.0	5.6
Indiana	891	1,607	2,680	2,821	3,061	3,263	11.6	6.8
Illinois	2,118	3,672	5,864	6,191	6,707	6,970	10.7	5.9
Michigan	2,002	3,080	4,668	5,017	5,224	5,562	8.8	6.0
Wisconsin	938	1,595	2,564	2,765	3,059	3,362	10.6	9.5
West North Central	3,286	5,739	9,125	9,594	10,395	10,987	10.8	6.4
Minnesota	944	1,765	2,957	3,202	3,322	3,617	12.1	6.9
Iowa	488	769	1,142	1,178	1,294	1,376	8.9	6.4
Missouri	877	1,537	2,485	2,581	2,879	2,958	11.0	6.0
North Dakota	139	288	368	371	433	445	10.2	6.5
South Dakota	102	173	274	280	319	342	10.4	7.7
Nebraska	276	433	688	700	785	825	9.6	6.2
Kansas	461	774	1,211	1,280	1,362	1,425	10.1	5.6
South Atlantic	7,141	14,169	25,449	26,853	28,588	30,041	13.6	5.7
Delaware	120	214	377	405	439	466	12.1	7.3
Maryland	835	1,702	2,968	3,249	3,498	3,704	13.5	7.7
District of Columbia	237	362	657	662	651	672	10.7	0.8
Virginia	886	1,772	3,172	3,462	3,565	3,769	13.6	5.9
West Virginia	330	642	856	882	973	988	10.0	4.9
North Carolina	866	1,543	3,005	3,213	3,458	3,717	13.2	7.3
South Carolina	399	734	1,325	1,423	1,552	1,685	12.8	8.3
Georgia	987	1,930	3,645	3,957	4,321	4,543	14.0	7.6
Florida	2,482	5,272	9,444	9,600	10,131	10,498	14.3	3.6
East South Central	2,361	4,188	7,379	8,051	8,418	8,913	12.1	6.5
Kentucky	562	955	1,639	1,762	1,950	2,038	11.3	7.5
Tennessee	841	1,499	2,569	2,822	2,988	3,137	11.8	6.9
Alabama	632	1,167	2,247	2,477	2,466	2,631	13.5	5.4
Mississippi	327	568	925	990	1,015	1,107	11.0	6.2
West South Central	4,649	8,666	13,566	14,280	15,334	15,947	11.3	5.5
Arkansas	374	680	1,134	1,228	1,217	1,244	11.7	3.1
Louisiana	743	1,424	2,129	2,282	2,450	2,537	11.1	6.0
Oklahoma	536	972	1,382	1,431	1,558	1,640	9.9	5.9
Texas	2,996	5,590	8,920	9,340	10,108	10,526	11.5	5.7
Mountain	2,211	4,336	7,347	7,731	8,357	8,897	12.8	6.6
Montana	138	205	311	325	350	392	8.5	8.0
Idaho	140	235	374	410	453	486	10.3	9.1
Wyoming	64	118	146	142	152	160	8.6	3.1
Colorado	600	1,230	1,891	2,032	2,242	2,452	12.2	9.0
New Mexico	182	368	574	590	665	716	12.2	7.6
Arizona	635	1,287	2,500	2,559	2,676	2,799	14.7	3.8
Utah	244	472	739	794	832	864	11.7	5.3
Nevada	207	421	812	879	988	1,029	14.6	8.2
Pacific	8,811	16,627	27,682	30,406	33,132	35,677	12.1	8.8
Washington	909	1,667	2,834	3,155	3,413	3,720	12.0	9.5
Oregon	596	990	1,597	1,626	1,798	1,904	10.4	6.0
California	6,959	13,311	22,365	24,654	26,903	28,981	12.4	9.0
Alaska	97	214	258	265	276	301	10.3	5.3
Hawaii	249	444	629	706	742	771	9.7	7.0

[1]States where services were provided.
[2]These estimates differ from National Health Expenditures estimates presented elsewhere in *Health, United States*. See Appendix I, Health Care Financing Administration.

NOTE: Figures may not sum to totals due to rounding.

SOURCE: Health Care Financing Administration, Office of the Actuary. Estimates prepared by the Office of National Health Statistics.

Table 141. Expenditures for purchases of prescription drugs by geographic division and State and average annual percent change: United States, selected years 1980–93

[Data are compiled by the Health Care Financing Administration]

Geographic division and State[1]	Amount in millions						Average annual percent change	
	1980	1985	1990	1991	1992	1993	1980–90	1990–93
United States	$12,049	$21,405	$38,198	$42,755	$45,730	$48,840	12.2	8.5
New England	625	1,217	2,250	2,463	2,578	2,710	13.7	6.4
Maine	51	93	174	192	202	213	13.1	7.0
New Hampshire	39	77	160	174	185	197	15.2	7.2
Vermont	22	43	86	95	101	108	14.6	7.9
Massachusetts	290	596	1,113	1,214	1,270	1,337	14.4	6.3
Rhode Island	48	96	174	190	198	206	13.7	5.8
Connecticut	174	312	544	597	622	650	12.1	6.1
Middle Atlantic	1,817	3,334	5,911	6,513	6,859	7,219	12.5	6.9
New York	820	1,506	2,665	2,929	3,077	3,232	12.5	6.6
New Jersey	381	723	1,298	1,432	1,515	1,601	13.0	7.2
Pennsylvania	616	1,105	1,948	2,152	2,267	2,386	12.2	7.0
East North Central	2,219	3,850	6,691	7,437	7,895	8,360	11.7	7.7
Ohio	607	1,010	1,684	1,869	1,982	2,095	10.7	7.6
Indiana	305	508	874	974	1,038	1,106	11.1	8.2
Illinois	561	1,006	1,771	1,964	2,084	2,206	12.2	7.6
Michigan	527	939	1,654	1,837	1,947	2,054	12.1	7.5
Wisconsin	218	387	708	791	844	899	12.5	8.3
West North Central	887	1,495	2,557	2,835	3,012	3,195	11.2	7.7
Minnesota	191	324	580	648	691	739	11.7	8.4
Iowa	156	255	419	463	490	516	10.4	7.2
Missouri	274	461	783	868	919	975	11.1	7.6
North Dakota	28	51	86	93	98	103	11.9	6.2
South Dakota	30	50	82	91	97	104	10.6	8.2
Nebraska	80	136	235	261	277	293	11.4	7.6
Kansas	128	218	373	412	439	465	11.3	7.6
South Atlantic	1,997	3,694	7,181	8,120	8,746	9,412	13.7	9.4
Delaware	25	49	98	111	120	129	14.6	9.6
Maryland	226	443	888	998	1,069	1,140	14.7	8.7
District of Columbia	32	57	93	99	101	103	11.3	3.5
Virginia	275	522	1,026	1,154	1,248	1,343	14.1	9.4
West Virginia	116	204	333	369	389	412	11.1	7.4
North Carolina	340	569	1,061	1,199	1,287	1,392	12.1	9.5
South Carolina	154	268	511	580	622	665	12.7	9.2
Georgia	294	540	1,035	1,176	1,283	1,397	13.4	10.5
Florida	536	1,041	2,135	2,435	2,627	2,832	14.8	9.9
East South Central	890	1,537	2,659	2,969	3,175	3,402	11.6	8.6
Kentucky	225	392	667	741	791	846	11.5	8.2
Tennessee	288	500	886	996	1,072	1,153	11.9	9.2
Alabama	235	404	707	790	845	904	11.6	8.5
Mississippi	142	241	399	442	468	499	10.9	7.7
West South Central	1,431	2,440	3,846	4,331	4,671	5,039	10.4	9.4
Arkansas	153	235	382	425	452	484	9.6	8.2
Louisiana	254	440	668	740	788	832	10.2	7.6
Oklahoma	175	299	450	500	535	569	9.9	8.1
Texas	848	1,467	2,346	2,666	2,896	3,153	10.7	10.4
Mountain	489	916	1,738	1,998	2,201	2,436	13.5	11.9
Montana	31	54	90	101	110	120	11.2	10.1
Idaho	44	74	129	149	164	182	11.4	12.2
Wyoming	23	37	49	55	59	64	7.9	9.3
Colorado	127	223	379	434	481	534	11.6	12.1
New Mexico	52	101	190	216	237	259	13.8	10.9
Arizona	123	250	526	600	659	728	15.6	11.4
Utah	54	110	218	249	274	302	15.0	11.5
Nevada	36	67	158	193	218	246	15.9	15.9
Pacific	1,694	2,921	5,365	6,089	6,593	7,067	12.2	9.6
Washington	212	340	618	711	781	853	11.3	11.3
Oregon	125	187	318	364	396	431	9.8	10.7
California	1,296	2,274	4,222	4,776	5,155	5,501	12.5	9.2
Alaska	16	34	58	69	77	85	13.7	13.6
Hawaii	44	87	148	169	184	197	12.9	10.0

[1]State where prescriptions were provided.

NOTES: Prescription drug expenditures are limited to spending for products purchased in retail outlets. The value of drugs and other products provided by hospitals, nursing homes, or other health professionals is included in estimates of spending for these providers' services. Figures may not sum to totals due to rounding.

SOURCE: Health Care Financing Administration, Office of the Actuary. Estimates prepared by the Office of National Health Statistics.

Table 142. State mental health agency per capita expenditures for mental health services and average annual percent change by geographic division and State: United States, selected fiscal years 1981–93

[Data are based on reporting by State mental health agencies]

Geographic division and State	1981	1983	1985	1987	1990[1]	1993[1,2]	Average annual percent change 1981–93
			Amount per capita				
United States.	$ 27	$31	$35	$ 38	$ 48	$ 54	6.0
New England:							
Maine	25	32	36	42	67	70	8.9
New Hampshire	35	39	42	36	63	78	7.0
Vermont.	32	40	44	44	54	74	7.2
Massachusetts	32	36	46	62	84	83	8.3
Rhode Island	36	32	35	41	50	61	4.5
Connecticut	32	39	44	56	73	82	8.2
Middle Atlantic:							
New York	67	74	90	99	118	131	5.8
New Jersey	26	31	36	43	57	68	8.2
Pennsylvania	41	47	52	50	57	68	4.4
East North Central:							
Ohio	25	29	30	34	41	47	5.5
Indiana	19	23	27	31	47	39	6.3
Illinois	18	21	24	25	34	36	6.0
Michigan	33	39	49	61	74	75	7.2
Wisconsin	22	27	28	31	37	35	3.8
West North Central:							
Minnesota[3]	17	30	32	42	54	69	8.7
Iowa	8	10	11	12	17	13	4.2
Missouri.	24	25	28	32	35	41	4.7
North Dakota	39	42	36	42	40	43	0.9
South Dakota	17	21	22	27	25	47	8.8
Nebraska	17	19	21	21	29	34	6.2
Kansas	18	22	27	28	35	48	8.8
South Atlantic:							
Delaware	44	51	46	41	55	56	2.0
Maryland	33	37	40	49	61	64	5.7
District of Columbia[4]	- - -	23	28	130	268	315	- - -
Virginia	23	29	32	35	45	40	4.8
West Virginia	20	20	22	23	24	22	1.0
North Carolina	24	29	38	41	46	50	6.4
South Carolina	31	33	33	45	51	56	5.1
Georgia	25	26	23	32	51	49	5.7
Florida	20	23	26	25	37	31	3.8
East South Central:							
Kentucky	15	17	19	23	23	25	4.5
Tennessee	18	20	23	24	29	37	6.3
Alabama	20	24	28	29	38	43	6.6
Mississippi	14	16	24	22	34	41	9.6
West South Central:							
Arkansas	17	20	24	24	26	30	5.0
Louisiana	19	23	26	25	28	39	6.2
Oklahoma	22	33	31	30	36	38	4.6
Texas	13	16	17	19	23	31	7.4
Mountain:							
Montana	25	28	29	28	28	34	2.8
Idaho.	13	15	15	17	20	26	5.7
Wyoming	23	28	31	30	35	42	5.1
Colorado	24	25	28	30	34	41	4.6
New Mexico	24	25	25	24	23	24	0.1
Arizona	10	10	12	16	27	60	16.1
Utah	13	16	17	19	21	25	5.4
Nevada	22	25	26	28	33	32	3.3
Pacific:							
Washington	18	24	30	37	43	66	11.5
Oregon	21	21	25	28	41	60	9.4
California	28	29	34	30	42	50	4.8
Alaska	38	41	45	50	72	86	7.1
Hawaii	19	22	23	26	38	71	11.7

- - - Data not available.

[1] Puerto Rico is included in U.S. total.

[2] Guam is included in U.S. total.

[3] Data for 1981 not comparable with 1983–93 data for Minnesota. Average annual percent change is for 1983–93.

[4] Transfer of St. Elizabeths Hospital from the National Institute of Mental Health to the District of Columbia Office of Mental Health took place over the years 1985–93.

NOTE: Expenditures for mental illness, excluding mental retardation and substance abuse.

SOURCES: National Association of State Mental Health Program Directors and the National Association of State Mental Health Program Directors Research Institute, Inc.: Final Report: Funding sources and expenditures of State mental health agencies: Revenue/expenditure study results, fiscal year 1990. Nov. 1992; Funding sources and expenditures of State mental health agencies: Supplemental report fiscal year 1993. Mar. 1996.

Table 143. Medicare enrollees, enrollees in managed care, payments per enrollee, and short-stay hospital utilization by geographic division and State: United States, 1990 and 1996

[Data are compiled by the Health Care Financing Administration]

Geographic division and State	Enrollment in thousands 1996	Percent of enrollees in managed care 1990	Percent of enrollees in managed care 1996	Payments per enrollee 1990	Payments per enrollee 1996[1]	Short-stay hospital utilization — Discharges per 1,000 enrollees 1990	Short-stay hospital utilization — Discharges per 1,000 enrollees 1996[1]	Short-stay hospital utilization — Average length of stay in days 1990	Short-stay hospital utilization — Average length of stay in days 1996
United States	37,300	5.7	11.8	$3,012	$5,048	316	359	8.8	6.5
New England	2,070	3.4	8.5	3,083	5,418	299	329	10.4	6.5
Maine	206	0.1	0.1	2,410	3,949	301	321	9.3	6.1
New Hampshire	158	0.3	1.0	2,558	4,021	292	282	9.2	6.5
Vermont	85	0.0	1.3	2,297	3,962	281	289	9.7	6.5
Massachusetts	946	5.6	14.4	3,443	6,266	326	365	10.0	6.4
Rhode Island	168	3.7	9.1	2,833	5,230	299	336	10.0	7.0
Connecticut	507	2.1	4.1	3,043	5,385	252	295	10.4	6.9
Middle Atlantic	5,899	4.1	11.0	3,413	5,430	327	373	11.4	8.4
New York	2,638	5.9	10.8	3,525	5,541	299	357	13.1	9.6
New Jersey	1,182	3.2	7.0	3,008	5,353	330	360	11.7	8.7
Pennsylvania	2,080	2.2	13.6	3,496	5,333	361	402	9.5	6.9
East North Central	6,254	2.8	4.0	3,068	4,675	330	353	8.6	6.3
Ohio	1,683	2.2	4.1	3,268	4,614	351	360	8.6	6.2
Indiana	823	2.7	2.8	2,819	4,357	337	342	8.3	6.0
Illinois	1,626	4.8	7.5	3,080	4,940	336	379	8.9	6.4
Michigan	1,359	1.5	1.1	3,290	5,118	307	347	8.9	6.7
Wisconsin	763	2.2	2.4	2,489	3,809	306	311	7.7	5.9
West North Central	2,802	7.0	7.3	2,560	4,069	323	344	7.8	5.9
Minnesota	636	21.9	17.7	2,186	3,856	283	339	6.7	5.3
Iowa	474	3.0	3.2	2,375	3,643	320	336	8.1	5.8
Missouri	837	3.1	6.6	2,966	4,591	346	359	8.6	6.4
North Dakota	102	0.8	0.6	2,534	3,568	338	326	7.2	5.8
South Dakota	117	0.0	0.1	2,264	3,525	344	351	7.2	5.6
Nebraska	251	1.8	2.4	2,319	3,512	300	299	7.6	5.6
Kansas	385	3.4	3.8	2,782	4,476	346	360	7.7	5.9
South Atlantic	7,097	4.7	9.1	2,935	5,045	303	351	8.8	6.5
Delaware	106	0.2	4.3	3,024	4,514	315	311	9.3	7.3
Maryland	615	1.2	5.6	3,665	5,320	345	373	9.4	6.5
District of Columbia	78	2.9	8.7	4,024	6,631	321	388	11.6	8.1
Virginia	840	1.4	2.9	2,726	4,182	343	348	8.9	6.6
West Virginia	332	9.8	7.7	2,648	4,593	370	420	8.2	6.3
North Carolina	1,049	0.4	0.7	2,479	4,217	303	339	9.6	6.8
South Carolina	523	0.1	0.4	2,287	4,316	276	336	9.4	6.9
Georgia	860	0.3	0.7	3,046	5,081	373	377	7.9	6.2
Florida	2,693	10.0	19.8	3,090	5,901	256	338	8.6	6.2
East South Central	2,439	1.1	1.9	2,940	5,031	385	408	8.2	6.3
Kentucky	598	2.9	2.9	2,884	4,492	381	397	8.3	6.2
Tennessee	784	0.4	0.4	2,982	5,227	363	384	8.3	6.4
Alabama	654	0.9	3.5	3,106	5,113	400	419	8.1	6.1
Mississippi	404	0.0	0.5	2,681	5,299	407	452	7.8	6.8
West South Central	3,624	0.9	7.6	3,120	5,709	350	370	8.1	6.3
Arkansas	427	0.3	1.0	2,764	4,303	376	370	8.1	6.4
Louisiana	586	0.0	7.5	3,722	6,553	399	430	7.9	6.3
Oklahoma	492	0.6	4.7	2,812	5,201	361	362	8.0	6.2
Texas	2,119	1.3	9.6	3,099	5,905	328	356	8.2	6.3
Mountain	2,018	8.3	20.9	2,644	4,299	274	307	7.0	5.3
Montana	131	0.3	0.4	2,517	3,532	342	313	6.6	5.3
Idaho	155	0.5	2.8	2,216	3,683	260	283	6.2	4.8
Wyoming	61	0.9	2.9	2,626	4,034	342	309	6.7	5.1
Colorado	435	13.3	24.7	2,524	4,767	264	313	7.3	5.3
New Mexico	217	7.8	16.1	2,512	3,906	298	297	6.8	5.6
Arizona	617	11.7	32.0	2,934	4,537	274	339	7.0	5.2
Utah	193	1.5	10.1	2,370	4,197	236	244	6.3	4.9
Nevada	209	8.2	26.7	2,922	4,593	248	315	8.1	6.0
Pacific	5,097	17.6	33.6	2,873	5,379	258	368	7.2	5.5
Washington	702	10.4	19.8	2,515	4,005	262	288	6.7	4.9
Oregon	481	18.1	35.3	2,047	3,999	244	339	6.2	4.7
California	3,724	18.7	36.6	3,079	5,986	262	397	7.3	5.6
Alaska	36	0.6	0.6	3,223	4,538	260	273	7.7	6.4
Hawaii	154	26.3	31.2	2,044	3,565	208	303	10.1	8.2

[1] These data are not comparable with 1990 data because they do not include Medicare managed care enrollees.

NOTES: Figures may not sum to totals due to rounding. Data for additional years are available (see Appendix III).

SOURCES: Health Care Financing Administration, Bureau of Data Management and Strategy. Data for the Medicare Decision Support System; Data development by the Office of Research and Demonstrations.

Table 144. Medicaid recipients, recipients in managed care, payments per recipient, and recipients per 100 persons below the poverty level by geographic division and State: United States, selected fiscal years 1989–97

[Data are compiled by the Health Care Financing Administration]

Geographic division and State	Recipients in thousands 1996	Recipients in thousands 1997	Percent of recipients in managed care 1996	Percent of recipients in managed care 1997	Payments per recipient 1990	Payments per recipient 1996	Payments per recipient 1997	Recipients per 100 persons below the poverty level 1989–90	Recipients per 100 persons below the poverty level 1996–97
United States	36,118	33,579	40	48	$ 2,568	$3,369	$3,679	75	97
New England:									
Maine	167	167	1	8	3,248	4,321	4,662	88	129
New Hampshire	100	95	16	13	5,423	5,496	5,818	53	107
Vermont	102	109	–	24	2,530	2,954	2,824	108	165
Massachusetts[1]	715	723	70	64	4,622	5,285	5,329	103	106
Rhode Island	130	117	63	62	[2]3,778	5,280	6,320	[2]163	110
Connecticut	329	202	61	64	4,829	6,179	9,927	167	79
Middle Atlantic:									
New York	3,281	3,152	23	29	5,099	6,811	6,771	95	107
New Jersey	714	538	43	56	4,054	5,217	6,635	83	86
Pennsylvania	1,168	1,025	53	55	2,449	3,993	4,575	88	81
East North Central:									
Ohio	1,478	1,396	32	32	2,566	3,729	4,190	98	108
Indiana	594	515	31	54	3,859	4,130	4,628	45	118
Illinois	1,454	1,400	13	14	2,271	3,689	4,131	69	103
Michigan	1,172	1,133	73	78	2,094	2,867	3,170	85	111
Wisconsin	434	392	32	49	3,179	4,384	4,790	95	94
West North Central:									
Minnesota	455	371	33	42	3,709	5,342	6,350	70	90
Iowa	308	294	41	41	2,589	3,534	3,691	80	110
Missouri	636	540	35	43	2,002	3,171	3,880	63	104
North Dakota	61	61	55	54	3,955	4,889	5,373	58	78
South Dakota	77	75	65	69	3,368	4,114	4,221	51	76
Nebraska	191	203	27	65	2,595	3,548	3,424	61	119
Kansas	251	233	32	51	2,524	3,425	3,947	71	90
South Atlantic:									
Delaware	82	84	78	81	3,004	3,773	3,273	68	123
Maryland	399	402	64	75	3,300	5,138	5,474	74	85
District of Columbia	143	128	55	65	2,629	4,955	5,439	86	112
Virginia	623	595	68	59	2,596	2,849	3,121	53	74
West Virginia	395	359	30	40	1,443	2,855	3,500	80	124
North Carolina	1,130	1,113	37	43	2,531	3,255	3,404	66	130
South Carolina	503	520	1	4	2,343	3,026	3,092	52	104
Georgia	1,185	1,208	32	64	3,190	2,604	2,557	64	108
Florida	1,638	1,597	64	64	2,273	2,851	3,058	55	79
East South Central:									
Kentucky	641	664	53	51	2,089	3,014	3,415	81	102
Tennessee	1,409	1,416	100	100	1,896	2,049	2,074	67	169
Alabama	546	546	11	82	1,731	2,675	2,877	43	87
Mississippi	510	504	7	15	1,354	2,633	2,826	67	98
West South Central:									
Arkansas	363	370	39	60	2,267	3,375	3,514	55	76
Louisiana	778	746	6	6	2,247	3,154	3,129	58	97
Oklahoma	358	316	19	51	2,516	2,852	3,287	56	67
Texas	2,572	2,539	4	13	1,928	2,672	2,893	47	79
Mountain:									
Montana	101	96	59	88	2,793	3,478	3,325	47	67
Idaho	119	115	37	40	2,973	3,402	3,757	36	72
Wyoming	51	49	1	–	2,036	3,571	3,771	[2]59	81
Colorado	271	251	80	81	2,705	3,815	4,470	45	71
New Mexico	318	320	45	57	2,120	2,757	2,568	39	74
Arizona[3]	528	541	86	81	- - -	- - -	- - -	- - -	- - -
Utah	152	145	82	79	2,279	2,775	2,927	72	88
Nevada	109	106	41	30	3,161	3,361	3,531	37	67
Pacific:									
Washington	621	630	100	100	2,128	2,242	2,210	98	105
Oregon	450	531	91	83	2,283	2,915	2,776	74	128
California	5,107	4,855	23	39	1,795	2,178	2,355	88	91
Alaska	69	73	–	–	3,562	4,027	4,392	70	129
Hawaii[4]	41	- - -	80	81	2,252	6,574	- - -	73	- - -

– Quantity zero.
- - - Data not available.
[1]Data for categorically eligible blind Medicaid recipients in 1990 are estimated by the Bureau of Data Management and Strategy, HCFA.
[2]Data are estimated by the Bureau of Data Management and Strategy, Health Care Financing Administration (HCFA).
[3]Arizona has a limited Medicaid program, with care financed largely on a capitated basis.
[4]1997 data for Hawaii not reported.
NOTE: Payments exclude disproportionate share hospital payments ($16 billion in 1997) and payments to health maintenance organizations ($18 billion in 1997).
SOURCES: Health Care Financing Administration, Bureau of Data Management and Strategy, Office of Systems Management, Division of Program Systems and the Office of Managed Care; Department of Commerce, Bureau of the Census, Housing and Household Economic Statistics Division. Data computed by the Centers for Disease Control and Prevention, National Center for Health Statistics, Division of Health and Utilization Analysis.

Table 145. Persons enrolled in health maintenance organizations (HMO's) by geographic division and State: United States, selected years 1980–98

[Data are based on a census of health maintenance organizations]

Geographic division and State	Number in thousands 1998	Percent of population							
		1980	1985	1990	1994	1995	1996	1997	1998
United States[1]	76,634	4.0	7.9	13.5	17.3	19.4	22.3	25.2	28.6
New England:									
Maine	237	0.4	0.3	2.6	5.1	7.0	9.5	15.9	19.1
New Hampshire	396	1.2	5.6	9.6	14.2	18.5	21.9	23.9	33.8
Vermont	–	–	–	6.4	11.2	12.5	13.4	–	–
Massachusetts	3,314	2.9	13.7	26.5	34.5	39.0	39.0	44.6	54.2
Rhode Island	294	3.7	9.1	20.6	26.6	19.6	23.7	11.8	29.8
Connecticut	1,404	2.4	7.1	19.9	21.2	21.2	29.8	34.7	42.9
Middle Atlantic:									
New York	6,860	5.5	8.0	15.1	23.4	26.6	29.2	35.7	37.8
New Jersey	2,522	2.0	5.6	12.3	11.4	14.7	23.0	27.5	31.3
Pennsylvania	4,457	1.2	5.0	12.5	18.3	21.5	27.4	29.9	37.1
East North Central:									
Ohio	2,620	2.2	6.7	13.3	15.2	16.3	18.5	17.6	23.4
Indiana	821	0.5	3.6	6.1	7.4	8.3	9.9	11.9	14.0
Illinois	2,474	1.9	7.1	12.6	16.2	17.2	20.0	17.1	20.8
Michigan	2,470	2.4	9.9	15.2	18.3	20.5	22.2	23.5	25.3
Wisconsin	1,590	8.5	17.8	21.7	22.4	24.0	27.6	24.9	30.8
West North Central:									
Minnesota	1,520	9.9	22.2	16.4	25.4	26.5	28.6	32.7	32.4
Iowa	139	0.2	4.8	10.1	4.6	4.5	4.9	4.6	4.9
Missouri	1,823	2.3	6.0	8.2	15.0	18.5	24.0	30.2	33.7
North Dakota	14	0.4	2.5	1.7	0.7	1.2	1.2	1.7	2.2
South Dakota	37	–	–	3.3	2.9	2.8	2.8	3.5	5.1
Nebraska	280	1.1	1.8	5.1	6.9	8.6	10.8	15.4	16.9
Kansas	374		3.3	7.9	5.2	4.7	6.3	11.5	14.4
South Atlantic:									
Delaware	352	–	3.9	17.5	16.6	18.4	29.3	38.8	48.1
Maryland	2,220	2.0	4.8	14.2	24.5	29.5	30.9	38.0	43.6
District of Columbia[2]	172	- - -	- - -	- - -	- - -	- - -	- - -	34.1	33.0
Virginia	1,137	–	1.1	6.1	7.2	7.7	8.7	15.7	16.9
West Virginia	194	0.7	1.7	3.9	4.1	5.8	7.0	9.4	10.7
North Carolina	1,269	0.6	1.6	4.8	6.7	8.3	11.1	14.6	17.1
South Carolina	372	0.2	1.0	1.9	3.6	5.5	9.0	8.4	9.9
Georgia	1,161	0.1	2.9	4.8	6.7	7.6	9.4	12.7	15.5
Florida	4,615	1.5	5.6	10.6	15.7	18.8	23.0	29.0	31.5
East South Central:									
Kentucky	1,087	0.9	1.6	5.7	10.6	16.1	15.3	27.4	35.1
Tennessee	1,293	–	1.8	3.7	11.0	12.2	13.9	15.3	24.1
Alabama	469	0.3	0.9	5.3	6.2	7.3	7.9	9.8	10.8
Mississippi	99	–	–	–	0.1	0.7	1.2	2.4	3.6
West South Central:									
Arkansas	271	–	0.1	2.2	5.4	3.8	15.2	8.7	10.7
Louisiana	723	0.6	0.9	5.4	7.5	7.2	11.0	14.7	16.6
Oklahoma	458	–	2.1	5.5	7.1	7.6	10.3	12.4	13.8
Texas	3,461	0.6	3.4	6.9	9.1	12.0	12.3	15.3	17.8
Mountain:									
Montana	34	–	–	1.0	1.6	2.4	2.9	3.1	3.9
Idaho	69	1.2	–	1.8	1.1	1.4	3.7	4.3	5.7
Wyoming	4	–	–	–	–	–	–	0.4	0.7
Colorado	1,419	6.9	10.8	20.0	22.2	23.3	25.8	31.1	36.4
New Mexico	558	1.4	2.0	12.7	12.7	15.1	15.5	21.0	32.3
Arizona	1,378	6.0	10.3	16.2	22.5	25.8	29.0	28.8	30.3
Utah	732	0.6	8.8	13.9	23.4	25.1	30.1	40.7	35.6
Nevada	450	–	5.8	8.5	11.9	15.9	18.7	20.8	26.8
Pacific:									
Washington	1,474	9.4	8.7	14.6	21.0	18.7	23.2	25.1	26.3
Oregon	1,469	12.0	14.0	24.7	29.6	40.0	44.8	47.2	45.3
California	15,184	16.8	22.5	30.7	33.7	36.0	40.3	43.8	47.1
Alaska	–	–	–	–	–	–	–	–	–
Hawaii	389	15.3	18.1	21.6	21.1	21.0	21.6	25.0	32.8

– Quantity zero.

- - - Data not available.

[1]HMO's in Guam are included starting in 1994; HMO's in Puerto Rico, starting in 1998. In 1998 HMO enrollment in Guam was 84,000 and in Puerto Rico, 390,000.
[2]Data for the District of Columbia (DC) were not included for 1980–96 because the data were not adjusted for the high proportion of enrollees of DC-based HMO's living in Maryland and Virginia.

NOTES: Data for 1980–90 are for pure HMO enrollment at midyear. Data for 1994–98 are for pure and open-ended enrollment as of January 1. In 1990 open-ended enrollment accounted for 3 percent of HMO enrollment compared with 15 percent in 1998. See Appendix II, Health maintenance organization.

SOURCE: The InterStudy Edge, Managed care: A decade in review 1980–1990. The InterStudy Competitive Edge, vols 4–8, 1994–1998. St. Paul, Minnesota (Copyrights 1991, 1994–1998: Used with the permission of InterStudy).

Table 146. Persons without health care coverage by geographic division and State: United States, selected years 1987–97

[Data are based on household interviews of the civilian noninstitutionalized population]

Geographic division and State	Number in thousands 1997	Percent of population								
		1987	1990	1991	1992	1993	1994	1995	1996	1997
United States.	43,448	12.9	13.9	14.1	15.0	15.3	15.2	15.4	15.6	16.1
New England:										
Maine	182	8.4	11.2	11.1	11.1	11.1	13.1	13.5	12.1	14.9
New Hampshire	141	10.1	9.9	10.1	12.6	12.5	11.9	10.1	9.6	11.8
Vermont.	55	9.8	9.5	12.7	9.5	11.9	8.6	13.0	11.0	9.5
Massachusetts	755	6.3	9.1	10.9	10.6	11.7	12.5	11.1	12.4	12.6
Rhode Island	96	6.8	11.1	10.1	9.5	10.3	11.5	12.9	9.9	10.2
Connecticut	395	6.4	6.9	7.5	8.2	10.0	10.4	8.8	11.0	12.0
Middle Atlantic:										
New York.	3,174	11.6	12.1	12.3	13.9	13.9	16.0	15.2	17.0	17.5
New Jersey	1,320	7.9	10.0	10.8	13.3	13.7	13.0	14.2	16.8	16.5
Pennsylvania	1,209	7.2	10.1	7.8	8.7	10.8	10.6	10.0	9.5	10.1
East North Central:										
Ohio	1,297	9.2	10.3	10.3	11.0	11.1	11.0	11.9	11.5	11.5
Indiana	669	13.4	10.7	13.0	11.0	11.9	10.5	12.6	10.6	11.4
Illinois	1,506	9.7	10.9	11.5	13.2	12.6	11.4	11.0	11.3	12.4
Michigan	1,133	8.4	9.4	9.0	10.0	11.2	10.8	9.7	8.9	11.6
Wisconsin	409	6.5	6.7	8.0	9.1	8.7	8.9	7.3	8.4	8.0
West North Central:										
Minnesota	438	6.6	8.9	9.3	8.1	10.1	9.5	8.0	10.2	9.2
Iowa	340	7.3	8.1	8.8	10.3	9.2	9.7	11.3	11.6	12.0
Missouri	669	10.5	12.7	12.2	14.4	12.2	12.2	14.6	13.2	12.6
North Dakota	97	7.7	6.3	7.6	8.2	13.4	8.4	8.2	9.8	15.2
South Dakota	84	13.7	11.6	9.9	15.1	13.0	10.0	9.4	9.5	11.8
Nebraska	180	9.6	8.5	8.2	9.4	11.9	10.7	9.0	11.4	10.8
Kansas	304	10.3	10.8	11.4	10.9	12.7	12.9	12.4	11.4	11.7
South Atlantic:										
Delaware	98	10.5	13.9	13.2	11.2	13.4	13.5	15.8	13.3	13.1
Maryland	677	9.8	12.7	13.1	11.3	13.5	12.6	15.3	11.4	13.4
District of Columbia.	84	15.6	19.2	25.7	21.8	20.7	16.4	17.3	14.8	16.2
Virginia	854	10.4	15.7	16.3	14.6	13.0	12.0	13.5	12.5	12.6
West Virginia	300	13.5	13.8	15.7	15.4	18.3	16.2	15.3	14.9	17.2
North Carolina	1,141	13.3	13.8	14.9	13.9	14.0	13.3	14.3	16.0	15.5
South Carolina	640	11.1	16.2	13.1	17.2	16.9	14.2	14.6	17.1	16.8
Georgia	1,344	13.0	15.3	14.1	19.1	18.4	16.2	17.9	17.8	17.6
Florida.	2,817	17.4	18.0	18.6	19.8	19.6	17.2	18.3	18.9	19.6
East South Central:										
Kentucky	587	15.2	13.2	13.1	14.6	12.5	15.2	14.6	15.4	15.0
Tennessee	756	14.5	13.7	13.4	13.6	13.2	10.2	14.8	15.2	13.6
Alabama	659	15.8	17.4	17.9	16.8	17.2	19.2	13.5	12.8	15.5
Mississippi	550	17.1	19.9	18.9	19.4	17.9	17.8	19.7	18.5	20.1
West South Central:										
Arkansas	639	20.7	17.4	15.7	19.9	19.7	17.4	18.0	21.7	24.4
Louisiana	827	17.1	19.7	20.7	22.3	23.9	19.2	20.5	20.8	14.9
Oklahoma	593	18.1	18.6	18.2	22.0	23.6	17.8	19.2	17.0	17.8
Texas	4,836	21.1	21.1	22.1	23.1	21.8	24.2	24.5	24.3	24.5
Mountain:										
Montana	174	15.5	14.0	12.7	9.4	15.3	13.6	12.7	13.6	19.5
Idaho.	223	15.3	15.2	17.8	16.5	14.8	14.0	14.0	16.5	17.7
Wyoming	76	11.4	12.5	11.3	11.7	15.0	15.4	15.9	13.4	15.5
Colorado	592	13.8	14.7	10.1	12.7	12.6	12.4	14.8	16.6	15.1
New Mexico	413	22.7	22.2	21.5	19.8	22.0	23.1	25.6	22.3	22.6
Arizona	1,141	18.4	15.5	16.9	15.5	20.2	20.2	20.4	24.1	24.5
Utah	280	12.4	9.0	13.8	11.8	11.3	11.5	11.8	12.0	13.4
Nevada	301	15.9	16.5	18.7	23.0	18.1	15.7	18.7	15.6	17.5
Pacific:										
Washington	655	13.0	11.4	10.4	10.4	12.6	12.7	12.4	13.5	11.4
Oregon	440	15.0	12.4	14.2	13.6	14.7	13.1	12.5	15.3	13.3
California	7,095	16.8	19.1	18.7	20.0	19.7	21.1	20.6	20.1	21.5
Alaska	116	16.2	15.4	13.2	16.8	13.3	13.3	12.5	13.4	18.1
Hawaii	89	7.5	7.3	7.0	6.1	11.1	9.2	8.9	8.6	7.5

NOTES: New health insurance questions were introduced for a quarter sample for 1993 data and the full sample for 1994 data. Starting with 1993 data, the collection method changed from paper and pencil to computer-assisted interviewing. 1990 census population controls were implemented starting with 1992 data. Estimates of the percent of persons lacking health care coverage based on the National Health Interview Survey (NHIS) (table 129) are slightly higher than those based on the March Current Population Survey (CPS). See Appendix II, health insurance coverage.

SOURCES: U.S. Bureau of the Census: Household Economic Studies. Current population reports, series P–60, no 190. Washington: U.S. Government Printing Office. Nov. 1995; press release CB98–172, Sept. 28, 1998; and unpublished data from the Current Population Survey provided by the Income Statistics Branch.

Appendix Contents ....

Appendix Contents

Appendix I

Sources of Data

Introduction

This report consolidates the most current data on the health of the population of the United States, the availability and use of health resources, and health care expenditures. The information was obtained from the data files and/or published reports of many governmental and nongovernmental agencies and organizations. In each case, the sponsoring agency or organization collected data using its own methods and procedures. Therefore, the data in this report vary considerably with respect to source, method of collection, definitions, and reference period.

Much of the data presented in the detailed tables are from the ongoing data collection systems of the National Center for Health Statistics. For an overview of these systems, see: Kovar MG. Data systems of the National Center for Health Statistics. National Center for Health Statistics. Vital Health Stat 1(23). 1989. However, health care personnel data come primarily from the Bureau of Health Professions, Health Resources and Services Administration, and the American Medical Association. National health expenditures data were compiled by the office of the Actuary, Health Care Financing Administration.

Although a detailed description and comprehensive evaluation of each data source is beyond the scope of this appendix, users should be aware of the general strengths and weaknesses of the different data collection systems. For example, population-based surveys obtain socioeconomic data, data on family characteristics, and information on the impact of an illness, such as days lost from work or limitation of activity. They are limited by the amount of information a respondent remembers or is willing to report. Detailed medical information, such as precise diagnoses or the types of operations performed, may not be known and so will not be reported. Health care providers, such as physicians and hospitals, usually have good diagnostic information but little or no information about the socioeconomic characteristics of individuals or the impact of illnesses on individuals.

The populations covered by different data collection systems may not be the same and understanding the differences is critical to interpreting the data. Data on vital statistics and national expenditures cover the entire population. Most data on morbidity and utilization of health resources cover only the civilian noninstitutionalized population. Thus, statistics are not included for military personnel who are usually young; for institutionalized people who may be any age; or for nursing home residents who are usually old.

All data collection systems are subject to error, and records may be incomplete or contain inaccurate information. People may not remember essential information, a question may not mean the same thing to different respondents, and some institutions or individuals may not respond at all. It is not always possible to measure the magnitude of these errors or their impact on the data. Where possible, the tables have notes describing the universe and the method of data collection to enable the user to place his or her own evaluation on the data. In many instances data do not add to totals because of rounding.

Some information is collected in more than one survey and estimates of the same statistic may vary among surveys. For example, cigarette use is measured by the Health Interview Survey, the National Household Survey of Drug Abuse, and the Monitoring the Future Survey. Estimates of cigarette use may differ among surveys because of different survey methodologies, sampling frames, questionnaires, definitions, and tabulation categories.

Overall estimates generally have relatively small sampling errors, but estimates for certain population subgroups may be based on small numbers and have relatively large sampling errors. Numbers of births and deaths from the vital statistics system represent complete counts (except for births in those States where data are based on a 50-percent sample for certain years). Therefore, they are not subject to sampling error. However, when the figures are used for analytical purposes, such as the comparison of rates over a period, the number of events that actually occurred may be considered as one of a large series of possible results that could have arisen under the same

326

circumstances. When the number of events is small and the probability of such an event is small, considerable caution must be observed in interpreting the conditions described by the figures. Estimates that are unreliable because of large sampling errors or small numbers of events have been noted with asterisks in selected tables. The criteria used to designate unreliable estimates are indicated as notes to the applicable tables.

The descriptive summaries that follow provide a general overview of study design, methods of data collection, and reliability and validity of the data. More complete and detailed discussions are found in the publications referenced at the end of each summary. The data set or source is listed under the agency or organization that sponsored the data collection.

Department of Health and Human Services

Centers for Disease Control and Prevention

National Center for Health Statistics

National Vital Statistics System

Through the National Vital Statistics System, the National Center for Health Statistics (NCHS) collects and publishes data on births, deaths, marriages, and divorces in the United States. Fetal deaths are classified and tabulated separately from other deaths. The Division of Vital Statistics obtains information on births and deaths from the registration offices of all States, New York City, the District of Columbia, Puerto Rico, the U.S. Virgin Islands, and Guam. Geographic coverage for births and deaths has been complete since 1933. U.S. data shown in detailed tables in this book are for the 50 States and the District of Columbia, unless otherwise specified.

Until 1972 microfilm copies of all death certificates and a 50-percent sample of birth certificates were received from all registration areas and processed by NCHS. In 1972 some States began sending their data to NCHS through the Cooperative Health Statistics System (CHSS). States that participated in the CHSS program processed 100 percent of their death and birth records and sent the entire data file to NCHS on computer tapes. Currently, the data are sent to NCHS through the Vital Statistics Cooperative Program (VSCP), following the same procedures as the CHSS. The number of participating States grew from 6 in 1972 to 46 in 1984. Starting in 1985 all 50 States and the District of Columbia participated in VSCP.

In most areas practically all births and deaths are registered. The most recent test of the completeness of birth registration, conducted on a sample of births from 1964 to 1968, showed that 99.3 percent of all births in the United States during that period were registered. No comparable information is available for deaths, but it is generally believed that death registration in the United States is at least as complete as birth registration.

Demographic information on the birth certificate such as race and ethnicity is provided by the mother at the time of birth. Medical and health information is based on hospital records. Demographic information on the death certificate is provided by the funeral director based on information supplied by an informant. Medical certification of cause of death is provided by a physician, medical examiner, or coroner.

U.S. Standard Certificates—U.S. Standard Live Birth and Death Certificates and Fetal Death Reports are revised periodically, allowing careful evaluation of each item and addition, modification, and deletion of items. Beginning with 1989, revised standard certificates replaced the 1978 versions. The 1989 revision of the birth certificate includes items to identify the Hispanic parentage of newborns and to expand information about maternal and infant health characteristics. The 1989 revision of the death certificate includes items on educational attainment and Hispanic origin of decedents as well as changes to improve the medical certification of cause of death. Standard certificates recommended by NCHS are modified in each registration area to serve the area's needs. However, most certificates conform closely in content and arrangement to the standard certificate, and all certificates contain a minimum data set specified by NCHS. For selected items, reporting areas expanded during the years spanned by this report. For items on the birth certificate, the number of reporting States increased for mother's education, prenatal care, marital status, Hispanic parentage, and tobacco use; and on the death certificate, for educational attainment and Hispanic origin of the decedent.

Maternal age—Mother's age was reported on the birth certificate by all States. Data are presented for mothers age 10–49 years through 1996 and 10–54 years starting in 1997, based on mother's date of birth or age as reported on the birth certificate. The age of mother is edited for upper and lower limits. When the age of the mother is computed to be under 10 years or 55 years or over (50 years or over in 1964–96), it is considered not stated and imputed according to the age of the mother from the previous birth record of the same race and total birth order (total of fetal deaths and live births). Before 1963 not stated ages were distributed in proportion to the known ages for each racial group. Beginning in 1997, the birth rate for the maternal age group 45–49 years includes data for mothers age 50–54 years in the numerator and is based on the population of women 45–49 years in the denominator.

Maternal education—Mother's education was reported on the birth certificate by 38 States in 1970. Data were not available from Alabama, Arkansas, California, Connecticut, Delaware, District of Columbia, Georgia, Idaho, Maryland, New Mexico, Pennsylvania, Texas, and Washington. In 1975 these data were available from 4 additional States, Connecticut, Delaware, Georgia, Maryland, and the District of Columbia, increasing the number of States reporting mother's education to 42 and the District of Columbia. Between 1980 and 1988 only three States, California, Texas, and Washington did not report mother's education. In 1988 mother's education was also missing from New York State outside of New York City. In 1989–91 mother's education was missing only from Washington and New York State outside of New York City. Starting in 1992 mother's education

was reported by all 50 States and the District of Columbia.

Prenatal care—Prenatal care was reported on the birth certificate by 39 States and the District of Columbia in 1970. Data were not available from Alabama, Alaska, Arkansas, Connecticut, Delaware, Georgia, Idaho, Massachusetts, New Mexico, Pennsylvania, and Virginia. In 1975 these data were available from 3 additional States, Connecticut, Delaware, and Georgia, increasing the number of States reporting prenatal care to 42 and the District of Columbia. Starting in 1980 prenatal care information was available for the entire United States.

Marital status—Mother's marital status was reported on the birth certificate by 39 States and the District of Columbia in 1970, and by 38 states and the District of Columbia in 1975. The incidence of births to unmarried women in States with no direct question on marital status was assumed to be the same as the incidence in reporting States in the same geographic division. Starting in 1980 for States without a direct question, marital status was inferred by comparing the parents' and child's surnames and other information concerning the father. In 1980 through 1996 marital status was reported on the birth certificates of 41–45 states. Beginning in 1997, all but four States (Connecticut, Michigan, Nevada, and New York) included a direct question on their birth certificates.

Hispanic births—In 1980 and 1981 information on births of Hispanic parentage was reported on the birth certificate by the following 22 States: Arizona, Arkansas, California, Colorado, Florida, Georgia, Hawaii, Illinois, Indiana, Kansas, Maine, Mississippi, Nebraska, Nevada, New Jersey, New Mexico, New York, North Dakota, Ohio, Texas, Utah, and Wyoming. In 1982 Tennessee, and in 1983 the District of Columbia began reporting this information. Between 1983 and 1987 information on births of Hispanic parentage was available for 23 States and the District of Columbia. In 1988 this information became available for Alabama, Connecticut, Kentucky, Massachusetts, Montana, North Carolina, and Washington, increasing the number of States reporting information on births of Hispanic parentage to 30 States and the District of Columbia. In 1989 this information became available from an additional 17 States, increasing the number of Hispanic-reporting States to 47 and the District of Columbia. In 1989 only Louisiana, New Hampshire, and Oklahoma did not report Hispanic parentage on the birth certificate. In 1990 Louisiana began reporting Hispanic parentage. Hispanic origin of the mother was reported on the birth certificates of 49 States and the District of Columbia in 1991 and 1992; only New Hampshire did not provide this information. Starting in 1993 Hispanic origin of mother was reported by all 50 States and the District of Columbia. In 1990, 99 percent of birth records included information on mother's origin.

Tobacco use—Information on tobacco use during pregnancy became available for the first time in 1989 with the revision of the U.S. Standard Birth Certificate. In 1989 data on tobacco use were collected by 43 States and the District of Columbia. The following States did not require the reporting of tobacco use on the birth certificate: California, Indiana, Louisiana, Nebraska, New York, Oklahoma, and South Dakota. In 1990 information on tobacco use became available from Louisiana and Nebraska increasing the number of reporting States to 45 and the District of Columbia. In 1991–93 information on tobacco use was available for 46 States and the District of Columbia with the addition of Oklahoma to the reporting area; and in 1994–97, for 46 States, the District of Columbia, and New York City.

Education of decedent—Information on educational attainment of decedents became available for the first time in 1989 due to the revision of the U.S. Standard Certificate of Death. Mortality data by educational attainment for 1989 was based on data from 20 States and by 1994–96 increased to 45 States and the District of Columbia. In 1994–96 the following States either did not report educational attainment on the death certificate or the information was more than 20 percent incomplete: Georgia, Kentucky, Oklahoma, Rhode Island, and South Dakota. In 1997 information on decedent's education became available from

Oklahoma, increasing the reporting area to 46 States and the District of Columbia. Information on the death certificate about the decedent's educational attainment is reported by the funeral director based on information provided by an informant such as next of kin.

Calculation of unbiased death rates by educational attainment based on the National Vital Statistics System requires that the reporting of education on the death certificate be complete and consistent with the reporting of education on the Current Population Survey, the source of population estimates that form the denominators for death rates. Death records with education not stated have not been included in the calculation of rates. Therefore the levels of the rates shown in this report are underestimated by approximately the percent not stated, which ranged from 3 to 5 percent.

The validity of information about the decedent's education was evaluated by comparing self-reported education obtained in the Current Population Survey with education on the death certificate for decedents in the National Longitudinal Mortality Survey (NLMS). (Sorlie PD, Johnson NJ: Validity of education information on the death certificate, *Epidemiology* 7(4):437–439, 1996.) Another analysis compared self-reported education collected in the first National Health and Nutrition Examination Survey (NHANES I) with education on the death certificate for decedents in the NHANES I Epidemiologic Followup Study. (Makuc DM, Feldman JJ, Mussolino ME: Validity of education and age as reported on death certificates, American Statistical Association 1996 Proceedings of the Social Statistics Section, 102–6, 1997.) Results of both studies indicated that there is a tendency for some people who did not graduate from high school to be reported as high school graduates on the death certificate. This tendency results in overstating the death rate for high school graduates and understating the death rate for the group with less than 12 years of education. The bias was greater among older than younger decedents and somewhat greater among black than white decedents.

In addition, educational gradients in death rates based on the National Vital Statistics System were compared with those based on the NLMS, a prospective study of persons in the Current Population Survey. Results of these comparisons indicate that educational gradients in death rates based on the National Vital Statistics System were reasonably similar to those based on the NLMS for white persons 25–64 years of age and black persons 25–44 years of age. The number of deaths for persons of Hispanic origin in the NLMS was too small to permit comparison for this ethnic group.

Hispanic deaths—In 1985 mortality data by Hispanic origin of decedent were based on deaths to residents of the following 17 States and the District of Columbia whose data on the death certificate were at least 90 percent complete on a place-of-occurrence basis and of comparable format: Arizona, Arkansas, California, Colorado, Georgia, Hawaii, Illinois, Indiana, Kansas, Mississippi, Nebraska, New York, North Dakota, Ohio, Texas, Utah, and Wyoming. In 1986 New Jersey began reporting Hispanic origin of decedent, increasing the number of reporting States to 18 and the District of Columbia in 1986 and 1987. In 1988 Alabama, Kentucky, Maine, Montana, North Carolina, Oregon, Rhode Island, and Washington were added to the reporting area, increasing the number of States to 26 and the District of Columbia. In 1989 an additional 18 States were added, increasing the Hispanic reporting area to 44 States and the District of Columbia. In 1989 only Connecticut, Louisiana, Maryland, New Hampshire, Oklahoma, and Virginia were not included in the reporting area. Starting with 1990 data in this book, the criterion was changed to include States whose data were at least 80 percent complete. In 1990 Maryland, Virginia, and Connecticut, in 1991 Louisiana, and in 1993 New Hampshire were added, increasing the reporting area for Hispanic origin of decedent to 47 States and the District of Columbia in 1990, 48 States and the District of Columbia in 1991 and 1992, and 49 States and the District of Columbia in 1993–96. Only Oklahoma did not provide this information in

1993–96. Starting in 1997 Hispanic origin of decedent was reported by all 50 States and the District of Columbia. Based on data from the U.S. Bureau of the Census, the 1990 reporting area encompassed 99.6 percent of the U.S. Hispanic population. In 1990 more than 96 percent of death records included information on origin of decedent.

Alaska data—For 1995 the number of deaths occurring in Alaska is in error for selected causes because NCHS did not receive changes resulting from amended records and because of errors in processing the cause of death data. Differences are concentrated among selected causes of death, principally Symptoms, signs, and ill-defined conditions (ICD-9 Nos. 780–799) and external causes.

For more information, see: National Center for Health Statistics, Technical Appendix, *Vital Statistics of the United States, 1992*, Vol. I, Natality, DHHS Pub. No. (PHS)96–1100 and Vol. II, Mortality, Part A, DHHS Pub. No. (PHS) 96–1101, Public Health Service. Washington. U.S. Government Printing Office, 1996.

National Linked File of Live Births and Infant Deaths

National linked files of live births and infant deaths are data sets for research on infant mortality. To create these data sets, death certificates are linked with corresponding birth certificates for infants who die in the United States before their first birthday. Linked data files include all of the variables on the national natality file, including the more accurate racial and ethnic information, as well as the variables on the national mortality file, including cause of death and age at death. The linkage makes available for the analysis of infant mortality extensive information from the birth certificate about the pregnancy, maternal risk factors, and infant characteristics and health items at birth. Each year, 97–98 percent of infant death records are linked to their corresponding birth records.

National linked files of live births and infant deaths were first produced for the 1983 birth cohort. Birth cohort linked file data are available for 1983–91 and period linked file data for 1995 and 1996. While birth cohort linked files have methodological advantages, their production incurs substantial delays in data availability, since it is necessary to wait until the close of a second data year to include all infant deaths to the birth cohort. Starting with data year 1995, more timely linked file data are produced in a period data format, preceding the release of the corresponding birth cohort format. Other changes to the data set starting with 1995 data include the addition of record weights to correct for the 2.2–2.5 percent of records that could not be linked and the addition of an imputation for not stated birthweight. For more information, see: Prager K. Infant mortality by birthweight and other characteristics: United States, 1985 birth cohort. National Center for Health Statistics. Vital Health Stat 20(24). 1994; MacDorman MF, Atkinson JO. Infant mortality statistics from the 1996 period linked birth/death data set. Monthly vital statistics report; vol 46 no 12, supp. Hyattsville, Maryland: National Center for Health Statistics. 1998.

Compressed Mortality File

The Compressed Mortality File (CMF) used to compute death rates by urbanization level is a county level national mortality and population database. The mortality data base of CMF is derived from the detailed mortality files of the National Vital Statistics System starting with 1968. The population data base of CMF is derived from intercensal and postcensal population estimates and census counts of the resident population of each U.S. county by age, race, and sex. Counties are categorized according to level of urbanization based on an NCHS-modified version of the 1993 rural-urban continuum codes for metropolitan and nonmetropolitan counties developed by the Economic Research Service, U.S. Department of Agriculture. See Appendix II, Urbanization. For more information about the CMF, contact: D. Ingram, Analytic Studies Branch, Division of Health and Utilization Analysis, National Center for Health Statistics, 6525 Belcrest Road, Hyattsville, MD 20782.

National Survey of Family Growth

Data from the National Survey of Family Growth (NSFG) are based on samples of women ages 15–44 years in the civilian noninstitutionalized population of the United States. The first and second cycles, conducted in 1973 and 1976, excluded most women who had never been married. The third, fourth, and fifth cycles, conducted in 1982, 1988, and 1995, included all women ages 15–44 years.

The purpose of the survey is to provide national data on factors affecting birth and pregnancy rates, adoption, and maternal and infant health. These factors include sexual activity, marriage, divorce and remarriage, unmarried cohabitation, contraception and sterilization, infertility, breastfeeding, pregnancy loss, low birthweight, and use of medical care for family planning and infertility.

Interviews are conducted in person by professional female interviewers using a standardized questionnaire. In 1973–88 the average interview length was about 1 hour. In 1995 the average interview lasted about 1 hour and 45 minutes. In all cycles black women were sampled at higher rates than white women, so that detailed statistics for black women could be produced.

Interviewing for Cycle 1 of NSFG was conducted from June 1973 to February 1974. Counties and independent cities of the United States were sampled to form a frame of primary sampling units (PSU's), and 101 PSU's were selected. From these 101 PSU's, 10,879 women 15–44 years of age were selected; 9,797 of these were interviewed. Most never-married women were excluded from the 1973 NSFG.

Interviewing for Cycle 2 of NSFG was conducted from January to September 1976. From 79 PSU's, 10,202 eligible women were identified; of these, 8,611 were interviewed. Again, most never-married women were excluded from the sample for the 1976 NSFG.

Interviewing for Cycle 3 of NSFG was conducted from August 1982 to February 1983. The sample design was similar to that in Cycle 2: 31,027 households were selected in 79 PSU'S. Household screener interviews were completed in 29,511 households (95.1 percent). Of the 9,964 eligible women identified, 7,969 were interviewed. For the first time in NSFG, Cycle 3 included women of all marital statuses.

Interviewing for Cycle 4 was conducted between January and August 1988. The sample was obtained from households that had been interviewed in the National Health Interview Survey in the 18 months between October 1, 1985, and March 31, 1987. For the first time, women living in Alaska and Hawaii were included so that the survey covered women from the noninstitutionalized population of the entire United States. The sample was drawn from 156 PSU's; 10,566 eligible women ages 15–44 years were sampled. Interviews were completed with 8,450 women.

Between July and November of 1990, 5,686 women were interviewed by telephone in the first NSFG telephone reinterview. The average length of interview in 1990 was 20 minutes. The response rate for the 1990 telephone reinterview was 68 percent of those responding to the 1988 survey and still eligible for the 1990 survey.

Interviewing for Cycle 5 of NSFG was conducted between January and October of 1995. The sample was obtained from households that had been interviewed in 198 PSU's in the National Health Interview Survey in 1993. Of the 13,795 eligible women in the sample, 10,847 were interviewed. For the first time, Hispanic as well as black women were sampled at a higher rate than other women.

In order to make national estimates from the sample for the millions of women ages 15–44 years in the United States, data for the interviewed sample women were (a) inflated by the reciprocal of the probability of selection at each stage of sampling (for example, if there was a 1 in 5,000 chance that a woman would be selected for the sample, her sampling weight was 5,000), (b) adjusted for nonresponse, and (c) forced to agree with benchmark population values based on data from the Current Population Survey of the U.S. Bureau of the Census (this la   is called "poststratification").

Quality control procedures for selecting and training interviewers, coding, editing, and processing the data, were built into NSFG to minimize nonsampling error.

More information on the methodology of NSFG is available in the following reports: French DK. National Survey of Family Growth, Cycle I: Sample design, estimation procedures, and variance estimation. National Center for Health Statistics. Vital Health Stat 2(76). 1978; Grady WR. National Survey of Family Growth, Cycle II: Sample design, estimation procedures, and variance estimation. National Center for Health Statistics. Vital Health Stat 2(87). 1981; Bachrach CA, Horn MC, Mosher WD, Shimizu I. National Survey of Family Growth, Cycle III: Sample design, weighting, and variance estimation. National Center for Health Statistics. Vital Health Stat 2(98). 1985; Judkins DR, Mosher WD, Botman SL. National Survey of Family Growth: Design, estimation, and inference. National Center for Health Statistics. Vital Health Stat 2(109). 1991; Goksel H, Judkins DR, Mosher WD. Nonresponse adjustments for a telephone followup to a National In-Person Survey. Journal of Official Statistics 8(4):417–32. 1992; Kelly JE, Mosher WD, Duffer AP, Kinsey SH. Plan and operation of the 1995 National Survey of Family Growth. Vital Health Stat 1(36). 1997; Potter FJ, Iannacchione VG, Mosher WD, Mason RE, Kavee JD. Sampling weights, imputation, and variance estimation in the 1995 National Survey of Family Growth. Vital Health Stat 2(124). 1998.

National Health Interview Survey

The National Health Interview Survey (NHIS) is a continuing nationwide sample survey in which data are collected through personal household interviews. Information is obtained on personal and demographic characteristics including race and ethnicity by self-reporting or as reported by an informant. Information is also obtained on illnesses, injuries, impairments, chronic conditions, utilization of health resources, and other health topics. The household questionnaire is reviewed each year with special health topics being added or deleted. For most health topics data are collected over an entire calendar year.

The sample design plan of NHIS follows a multistage probability design that permits a continuous sampling of the civilian noninstitutionalized population residing in the United States. The survey is designed in such a way that the sample scheduled for each week is representative of the target population and the weekly samples are additive over time. The response rate for the ongoing portion of the survey (core) has been between 94 and 98 percent over the years. Response rates for special health topics (supplements) have generally been lower. For example the response rate was 80 percent for the 1994 Year 2000 Supplement, which included questions about cigarette smoking and use of such preventive services as mammography.

In 1985 NHIS adopted several new sample design features although, conceptually, the sampling plan remained the same as the previous design. Two major changes included reducing the number of primary sampling locations from 376 to 198 for sampling efficiency and oversampling the black population to improve the precision of the statistics. The sample was designed so that a typical NHIS sample for the data collection years 1985–94 consisted of approximately 7,500 segments containing about 59,000 assigned households. Of these households, an expected 10,000 were vacant, demolished, or occupied by persons not in the target population of the survey. The expected sample of 49,000 occupied households yielded a probability sample of about 127,000 persons. In 1994 there was a sample of 116,179 persons.

In 1995 the NHIS sample was redesigned again. Major design changes included increasing the number of primary sampling units from 198 to 358 and oversampling the black and Hispanic populations to improve the precision of the statistics. The sample was designed so that a typical NHIS sample for the data collection years 1995–2004 will consist of approximately 7,000 segments. The expected sample of 44,000 occupied respondent households will yield a probability sample of about 106,000 persons. In 1995 there was a sample of 102,467 persons. In 1996 there was a smaller sample of 63,402 persons because part

of the sample was reserved for use in testing the new questionnaire instrument (1997).

In 1997 the questionnaire was redesigned and data were collected using a computer assisted personal interview (CAPI). The CAPI instrument was administered using a laptop computer with interviewers entering responses directly in the computer during the interview. In 1997 the interviewed sample consisted of 39,832 households yielding 40,623 families or 103,477 persons. Because of the extensive redesign of the questionnaire and the introduction of the CAPI method of data collection, 1997 data may differ from earlier years.

A description of the survey design, the methods used in estimation, and the general qualifications of the data obtained from the survey are presented in: Massey JT, Moore TF, Parsons VL, Tadros W. Design and estimation for the National Health Interview Survey, 1985–94. National Center for Health Statistics. Vital Health Stat 2(110). 1989; Kovar MG, Poe GS. The National Health Interview Survey design, 1973–84, and procedures, 1975–83. National Center for Health Statistics. Vital Health Stat 1(18). 1985; Hendershot G, Adams P, Marano M, Benaissa S. Current estimates from the National Health Interview Survey, 1996. National Center for Health Statistics. Vital Health Stat 10(200). 1999.

National Immunization Survey

The National Immunization Survey (NIS) is a continuing nationwide telephone sample survey togather data on children 19–35 months of age. Estimates of vaccine-specific coverage are available for national, State, and 28 urban areas considered to be high risk for undervaccination.

NIS uses a two-phase sample design. First, a random-digit-dialing (RDD) sample of telephone numbers is drawn. When households with age-eligible children are contacted, the interviewer collects information on the vaccinations received by all age-eligible children. In 1997 the overall response rate was 69 percent, yielding data for 32,742 children aged 19–35 months. The interviewer also collects information on the vaccination providers. In the second phase, all vaccination providers are contacted by mail. Vaccination information from providers was obtained for 68 percent of all children who were eligible for provider followup in 1997. Providers' responses are combined with information obtained from the households to provide a more accurate estimate of vaccination coverage levels. Final estimates are adjusted for noncoverage of nontelephone households.

A description of the survey design and the methods used in estimation are presented in: Massey JT. Estimating the response rate in a two stage telephone survey. Proceedings of the Section on Survey Research Methods. Alexandria, Virginia: American Statistical Association. 1995.

National Health and Nutrition Examination Survey

For the first program or cycle of the National Health Examination Survey (NHES I), 1960–62, data were collected on the total prevalence of certain chronic diseases as well as the distributions of various physical and physiological measures, including blood pressure and serum cholesterol levels. For that program, a highly stratified, multistage probability sample of 7,710 adults, of whom 86.5 percent were examined, was selected to represent the 111 million civilian noninstitutionalized adults 18–79 years of age in the United States at that time. The sample areas consisted of 42 primary sampling units (PSU's) from the 1,900 geographic units.

NHES II (1963–65) and NHES III (1966–70) examined probability samples of the nation's noninstitutionalized children between the ages of 6 and 11 years (NHES II) and 12 and 17 years (NHES III) focusing on factors related to growth and development. Both cycles were multistage, stratified probability samples of clusters of households in land-based segments and used the same 40 PSU's. NHES II sampled 7,417 children with a response rate of 96 percent. NHES III sampled 7,514 youth with a response rate of 90 percent.

For more information on NHES I, see: Gordon T, Miller HW. Cycle I of the Health Examination Survey:

Sample and response, United States, 1960–62. National Center for Health Statistics. Vital Health Stat 11(1). 1974. For more information on NHES II, see: Plan, operation, and response results of a program of children's examinations. National Center for Health Statistics. Vital Health Stat 1(5). 1967. For more information on NHES III, see: Schaible, WL. Quality control in a National Health Examination Survey. National Center for Health Statistics. Vital Health Stat 2(44). 1972.

In 1971 a nutrition surveillance component was added and the survey name was changed to the National Health and Nutrition Examination Survey (NHANES). In NHANES I, conducted from 1971 to 1974, a major purpose was to measure and monitor indicators of the nutrition and health status of the American people through dietary intake data, biochemical tests, physical measurements, and clinical assessments for evidence of nutritional deficiency. Detailed examinations were given by dentists, ophthalmologists, and dermatologists with an assessment of need for treatment. In addition, data were obtained for a subsample of adults on overall health care needs and behavior, and more detailed examination data were collected on cardiovascular, respiratory, arthritic, and hearing conditions.

The NHANES I target population was the civilian noninstitutionalized population 1–74 years of age residing in the coterminous United States, except for people residing on any of the reservation lands set aside for the use of American Indians. The sample design was a multistage, stratified probability sample of clusters of persons in land-based segments. The sample areas consisted of 65 PSU's selected from the 1,900 PSU's in the coterminous United States. A subsample of persons 25–74 years of age was selected to receive the more detailed health examination. Groups at high risk of malnutrition were oversampled at known rates throughout the process. Household interviews were completed for more than 96 percent of the 28,043 persons selected for the NHANES I sample, and about 75 percent (20,749) were examined.

For NHANES II, conducted from 1976 to 1980, the nutrition component was expanded from the one fielded for NHANES I. In the medical area primary emphasis was placed on diabetes, kidney and liver functions, allergy, and speech pathology. The NHANES II target population was the civilian noninstitutionalized population 6 months–74 years of age residing in the United States, including Alaska and Hawaii.

NHANES II utilized a multistage probability design that involved selection of PSU's, segments (clusters of households) within PSU's, households, eligible persons, and finally, sample persons. The sample design provided for oversampling among those persons 6 months–5 years of age, those 60–74 years of age, and those living in poverty areas. A sample of 27,801 persons was selected for NHANES II. Of this sample 20,322 (73.1 percent) were examined. Race information for NHANES I and NHANES II was determined primarily by interviewer observation.

The estimation procedure used to produce national statistics for NHANES I and NHANES II involved inflation by the reciprocal of the probability of selection, adjustment for nonresponse, and poststratified ratio adjustment to population totals. Sampling errors also were estimated to measure the reliability of the statistics.

For more information on NHANES I, see: Miller HW. Plan and operation of the Health and Nutrition Examination Survey, United States, 1971–73. National Center for Health Statistics. Vital Health Stat 1(10a) and 1(10b). 1977 and 1978; and Engel A, Murphy RS, Maurer K, Collins E. Plan and operation of the NHANES I Augmentation Survey of Adults 25–74 years, United States 1974–75. National Center for Health Statistics. Vital Health Stat 1(14). 1978.

For more information on NHANES II, see: McDowell A, Engel A, Massey JT, Maurer K. Plan and operation of the second National Health and Nutrition Examination Survey, 1976–80. National Center for Health Statistics. Vital Health Stat 1(15). 1981. For information on nutritional applications of these surveys, see: Yetley E, Johnson C. 1987.

Nutritional applications of the Health and Nutrition Examination Surveys (HANES). Ann Rev Nutr 7:441–63.

The Hispanic Health and Nutrition Examination Survey (HHANES), conducted during 1982–84, was similar in content and design to the previous National Health and Nutrition Examination Surveys. The major difference between HHANES and the previous national surveys is that HHANES employed a probability sample of three special subgroups of the population living in selected areas of the United States rather than a national probability sample. The three HHANES universes included approximately 84, 57, and 59 percent of the respective 1980 Mexican-, Cuban-, and Puerto Rican-origin populations in the continental United States. The Hispanic ethnicity of these populations was determined by self-report.

In the HHANES three geographically and ethnically distinct populations were studied: Mexican Americans living in Texas, New Mexico, Arizona, Colorado, and California; Cuban Americans living in Dade County, Florida; and Puerto Ricans living in parts of New York, New Jersey, and Connecticut. In the Southwest 9,894 persons were selected (75 percent or 7,462 were examined), in Dade County 2,244 persons were selected (60 percent or 1,357 were examined), and in the Northeast 3,786 persons were selected (75 percent or 2,834 were examined).

For more information on HHANES, see: Maurer KR. Plan and operation of the Hispanic Health and Nutrition Examination Survey, 1982–84. National Center for Health Statistics. Vital Health Stat 1(19). 1985.

The third National Health and Nutrition Examination Survey (NHANES III) is a 6-year survey covering the years 1988–94. Over the 6-year period, 39,695 persons were selected for the survey of which 30,818 (77.6 percent) were examined in the mobile examination center.

The NHANES III target population is the civilian noninstitutionalized population 2 months of age and over. The sample design provides for oversampling among children 2–35 months of age, persons 70 years of age and over, black Americans, and Mexican Americans. Race is reported for the household by the respondent.

Although some of the specific health areas have changed from earlier NHANES surveys, the following goals of the NHANES III are similar to those of earlier NHANES surveys:

- to estimate the national prevalence of selected diseases and risk factors
- to estimate national population reference distributions of selected health parameters
- to document and investigate reasons for secular trends in selected diseases and risk factors

Two new additional goals for the NHANES III survey are:

- to contribute to an understanding of disease etiology
- to investigate the natural history of selected diseases

For more information on NHANES III, see: Ezzati TM, Massey JT, Waksberg J, et al. Sample design: Third National Health and Nutrition Examination Survey. National Center for Health Statistics. Vital Health Stat 2(113). 1992; Plan and operation of the Third National Health and Nutrition Examination Survey, 1988–94. National Center for Health Statistics. Vital Health Stat 1(32). 1994.

National Health Provider Inventory (National Master Facility Inventory)

The National Master Facility Inventories (NMFI's) were a series of surveys of inpatient health facilities in the United States. They included hospitals, nursing and related care homes, and other custodial care facilities. The last NMFI was conducted in 1982. In 1986 a different inventory was conducted, the Inventory of Long-Term Care Places (ILTCP). This was a survey of nursing and related care homes and facilities for the mentally retarded. In 1991 the National Health Provider Inventory (NHPI), which was a survey of nursing homes, board and care homes, home health

agencies, and hospices, was conducted. The NMFI, ILTCP, and NHPI were used as a basis for sampling frames for other surveys conducted by the National Center for Health Statistics (National Nursing Home Survey and National Home and Hospice Care Survey).

National Home and Hospice Care Survey

The National Home and Hospice Care Survey (NHHCS) is a sample survey of health agencies and hospices. Initiated in 1992, it was also conducted in 1993, 1994, and 1996. The original sampling frame consisted of all home health care agencies and hospices identified in the 1991 National Health Provider Inventory (NHPI). The 1992 sample contained 1,500 agencies. These agencies were revisited during the 1993 survey (excluding agencies that had been found to be out of scope for the survey). In 1994 in-scope agencies identified in the 1993 survey were revisited, with 100 newly identified agencies added to the sample. For 1996 the universe was again updated and a new sample of 1,200 agencies was drawn.

The sample design for the 1992–94 NHHCS was a stratified three-stage probability design. Primary sampling units were selected at the first stage, agencies were selected at the second stage, and current patients and discharges were selected at the third stage. The sample design for the 1996 NHHCS has a two-stage probability design in which agencies were selected at the first stage and current patients and discharges were selected at the second stage. Current patients were on the rolls of the agency as of midnight on the day before the survey. Discharges were selected to estimate the number of discharges from the agency during the year before the survey.

After the samples were selected, a patient questionnaire was completed for each current patient and discharge by interviewing the staff member most familiar with the care provided to the patients. The respondent was requested to refer to the medical records for each patient. For additional information see: Haupt BJ. Development of the National Home and

Hospice Care Survey. National Center for Health Statistics. Vital Health Stat 1(33). 1994.

National Hospital Discharge Survey

The National Hospital Discharge Survey (NHDS) is a continuing nationwide sample survey of short-stay hospitals in the United States. The scope of NHDS encompasses patients discharged from noninstitutional hospitals, exclusive of military and Department of Veterans Affairs hospitals, located in the 50 States and the District of Columbia. Only hospitals having six or more beds for patient use are included in the survey and before 1988 those in which the average length of stay for all patients was less than 30 days. In 1988 the scope was altered slightly to include all general and children's general hospitals regardless of the length of stay. Although all discharges of patients from these hospitals are within the scope of the survey, discharges of newborn infants from all hospitals are excluded from this report.

The original sample was selected in 1964 from a frame of short-stay hospitals listed in the National Master Facility Inventory. A two-stage stratified sample design was used, and hospitals were stratified according to bed size and geographic region. Sample hospitals were selected with probabilities ranging from certainty for the largest hospitals to 1 in 40 for the smallest hospitals. Within each sample hospital, a systematic random sample of discharges was selected from the daily listing sheet. Initially, the within-hospital sampling rates for selecting discharges varied inversely with the probability of hospital selection so that the overall probability of selecting a discharge was approximately the same across the sample. Those rates were adjusted for individual hospitals in subsequent years to control the reporting burden of those hospitals.

In 1985, for the first time, two data collection procedures were used for the survey. The first was the traditional manual system of sample selection and data abstraction. In the manual system, sample selection and transcription of information from the hospital records to abstract forms were performed by either the hospital staff or representatives of NCHS or both. The second was an automated method, used in approximately 17 percent of the sample hospitals in 1985, involving the purchase of data tapes from commercial abstracting services. These tapes were then subjected to NCHS sampling, editing, and weighting procedures.

In 1988 NHDS was redesigned. The hospitals with the most beds and/or discharges annually were selected with certainty, but the remaining sample was selected using a three-stage stratified design. The first stage is a sample of PSU's used by the National Health Interview Survey. Within PSU's, hospitals were stratified or arrayed by abstracting status (whether subscribing to a commercial abstracting service) and within abstracting status arrayed by type of service and bed size. Within these strata and arrays, a systematic sampling scheme with probability proportional to the annual number of discharges was used to select hospitals. The rates for systematic sampling of discharges within hospitals vary inversely with probability of hospital selection within PSU. Discharge records from hospitals submitting data via commercial abstracting services and selected State data systems (approximately 38 percent of sample hospitals in 1996) were arrayed by primary diagnoses, patient sex and age group, and date of discharge before sampling. Otherwise, the procedures for sampling discharges within hospitals are the same as those used in the prior design.

In 1994 the hospital sample was updated by continuing the sampling process among hospitals that were NHDS-eligible for the sampling frame in 1994 but not in 1991. The additional hospitals were added at the end of the list for the strata where they belonged, and the systematic sampling was continued as if the additional hospitals had been present during the initial sample selection. Hospitals that were no longer NHDS-eligible were deleted. A similar updating process occurred in 1991.

The basic unit of estimation for NHDS is the sample patient abstract. The estimation procedure involves inflation by the reciprocal of the probability

Sources of Data

of selection, adjustment for nonresponding hospitals and missing abstracts, and ratio adjustments to fixed totals. In 1996, 525 hospitals were selected, 507 were within scope, 480 participated, and 282,000 medical records were abstracted.

For more detailed information on the design of NHDS and the magnitude of sampling errors associated with the NHDS estimates, see: Graves EJ, Owings MF. 1996 Summary: National Hospital Discharge Survey. Advance data from vital and health statistics; no 301. Hyattsville, Maryland: National Center for Health Statistics. 1998; and Haupt BJ, Kozak LJ. Estimates from two survey designs: National Hospital Discharge Survey. National Center for Health Statistics. Vital Health Stat 13(111). 1992.

National Survey of Ambulatory Surgery

The National Survey of Ambulatory Surgery (NSAS) is a nationwide sample survey of ambulatory surgery patient discharges from short-stay non-Federal hospitals and freestanding surgery centers. NSAS was conducted annually between 1994 and 1996. The sample consisted of eligible hospitals listed in the 1993 SMG Hospital Market Database and the 1993 SMG Freestanding Outpatient Surgery Center Database or Medicare Provider-of-Service files. Facilities specializing in dentistry, podiatry, abortion, family planning, or birthing were excluded.

A three-state stratified cluster design was used, and facilities were stratified according to primary sampling unit (PSU). The second stage consisted of the selection of facilities from sample PSU's, and the third stage consisted of a systematic random sample of cases from all locations within a facility where ambulatory surgery was performed. Locations within hospitals dedicated exclusively to dentistry, podiatry, pain block, abortion, or small procedures (sometimes referred to as "lump and bump" rooms) were not included. In 1996 of the 751 hospitals and freestanding ambulatory surgery centers selected for the survey, 601 were in-scope, and 488 responded for an overall response rate of 81 percent. These facilities provided information for approximately 125,000 ambulatory

surgery discharges. Up to six procedures were coded to the *International Classification of Diseases, 9th Revision, Clinical Modification*. Estimates were derived using a multistage estimation procedure: inflation by reciprocals of the probabilities of selection; adjustment for nonresponse; and population weighting ratio adjustments.

For more detailed information on the design of NSAS, see: McLemore T, Lawrence L. Plan and Operation of the National Survey of Ambulatory Surgery. National Center for Health Statistics. Vital Health Stat 1(37). 1997.

National Nursing Home Survey

NCHS has conducted five National Nursing Home Surveys. The first survey was conducted from August 1973 to April 1974; the second survey from May 1977 to December 1977; the third from August 1985 to January 1986; the fourth from July 1995 to December 1995; and the fifth from July 1997 to December 1997.

Much of the background information and experience used to develop the first National Nursing Home Survey was obtained from a series of three ad hoc sample surveys of nursing and personal care homes called the Resident Places Surveys (RPS-1, -2, -3). The three surveys were conducted by the National Center for Health Statistics during April–June 1963, May–June 1964, and June–August 1969. During the first survey, RPS-1, data were collected on nursing homes, chronic disease and geriatric hospitals, nursing home units, and chronic disease wards of general and mental hospitals. RPS-2 concentrated mainly on nursing homes and geriatric hospitals. During the third survey, RPS-3, nursing and personal care homes in the coterminous United States were sampled.

For the initial National Nursing Home Survey (NNHS) conducted in 1973–74, the universe included only those nursing homes that provided some level of nursing care. Homes providing only personal or domiciliary care were excluded. The sample of 2,118 homes was selected from the 17,685 homes that provided some level of nursing care and were listed in the 1971 National Master Facility Inventory (NMFI) or those that opened for business in 1972. Data were obtained from about 20,600 staff and 19,000 residents. Response rates were 97 percent for facilities, 88 percent for expenditures, 98 percent for residents, and 82 percent for staff.

The scope of the 1977 NNHS encompassed all types of nursing homes, including personal care and domiciliary care homes. The sample of about 1,700 facilities was selected from 23,105 nursing homes in the sampling frame, which consisted of all homes listed in the 1973 NMFI and those opening for business between 1973 and December 1976. Data were obtained from about 13,600 staff, 7,000 residents, and 5,100 discharged residents. Response rates were 95 percent for facilities, 85 percent for expenses, 81 percent for staff, 99 percent for residents, and 97 percent for discharges.

The scope of the 1985 NNHS was similar to the 1973–74 survey in that it excluded personal or domiciliary care homes. The sample of 1,220 homes was selected from a sampling frame of 20,479 nursing and related care homes. The frame consisted of all homes in the 1982 NMFI; homes identified in the 1982 Complement Survey of NMFI as "missing" from the 1982 NMFI; facilities that opened for business between 1982 and June 1984; and hospital-based nursing homes obtained from the Health Care Financing Administration. Information on the facility was collected through a personal interview with the administrator. Accountants were asked to complete a questionnaire on expenditures or provide a financial statement. Resident data were provided by a nurse familiar with the care provided to the resident. The nurse relied on the medical record and personal knowledge of the resident. In addition to employee data that were collected during the interview with the administrator, a sample of registered nurses completed a self-administered questionnaire. Discharge data were based on information recorded in the medical record. Additional data about the current and discharged residents were obtained in telephone interviews with next of kin. Data were obtained from 1,079 facilities, 2,763 registered nurses, 5,243 current residents, and 6,023 discharges. Response rates were 93 percent for

facilities, 68 percent for expenses, 80 percent for registered nurses, 97 percent for residents, 95 percent for discharges, and 90 percent for next of kin.

The scope of the 1995 and 1997 NNHS was similar to the 1985 and the 1973–74 NNHS in that they included only nursing homes that provided some level of nursing care. Homes providing only personal or domiciliary care were excluded. The 1995 sample of 1,500 homes was selected from a sampling frame of 17,500 nursing homes. The frame consisted of an updated version of the 1991 National Health Provider Inventory (NHPI). Data were obtained from about 1,400 nursing homes and 8,000 current residents. Data on current residents were provided by a staff member familiar with the care received by residents and from information contained in resident's medical records.

The 1997 sample of 1,488 nursing homes was the same basic sample used in 1995. Excluded were out-of-scope and out-of-business places identified in the 1995 survey and included were a small number of additions to the sample from a supplemental frame of places not in the 1995 frame. The 1997 NNHS included the discharge component not available in the 1995 survey.

Statistics for all five surveys were derived by a ratio-estimation procedure. Statistics were adjusted for failure of a home to respond, failure to fill out one of the questionnaires, and failure to complete an item on a questionnaire.

For more information on the 1973–74 NNHS, see: Meiners MR. Selected operating and financial characteristics of nursing homes, United States, 1973–74 National Nursing Home Survey. National Center for Health Statistics. Vital Health Stat 13(22). 1975. For more information on the 1977 NNHS, see: Van Nostrand JF, Zappolo A, Hing E, et al. The National Nursing Home Survey, 1977 summary for the United States. National Center for Health Statistics. Vital Health Stat 13(43). 1979. For more information on the 1985 NNHS, see: Hing E, Sekscenski E, Strahan G. The National Nursing Home Survey: 1985 summary for the United States. National Center for Health Statistics. Vital Health Stat 13(97). 1985. For more information on the 1995 NNHS, see: Strahan G. An overview of nursing homes and their current residents: Data from the 1995 National Nursing Home Survey. Advance data from vital and health statistics; no 280. Hyattsville, Maryland: National Center for Health Statistics. 1997. For more information on the 1997 NNHS, see the Advance Data report available in the summer of 1999.

National Ambulatory Medical Care Survey

The National Ambulatory Medical Care Survey (NAMCS) is a continuing national probability sample of ambulatory medical encounters. The scope of the survey covers physician-patient encounters in the offices of non-Federally employed physicians classified by the American Medical Association or American Osteopathic Association as "office-based, patient care" physicians. Patient encounters with physicians engaged in prepaid practices (health maintenance organizations (HMO's), independent practice organizations (IPA's), and other prepaid practices) are included in NAMCS. Excluded are visits to hospital-based physicians, visits to specialists in anesthesiology, pathology, and radiology, and visits to physicians who are principally engaged in teaching, research, or administration. Telephone contacts and nonoffice visits are excluded, also.

A multistage probability design is employed. The first-stage sample consists of 84 primary sampling units (PSU's) in 1985 and 112 PSU's in 1992 selected from about 1,900 such units into which the United States has been divided. In each sample PSU, a sample of practicing non-Federal office-based physicians is selected from master files maintained by the American Medical Association and the American Osteopathic Association. The final stage involves systematic random samples of office visits during randomly assigned 7-day reporting periods. In 1985 the survey excluded Alaska and Hawaii. Starting in 1989 the survey included all 50 States.

For the 1997 survey a sample of 2,498 physicians was selected. The physician response rate for 1997 was 69 percent, providing data on 24,715 records.

The estimation procedure used in NAMCS basically has three components: inflation by the reciprocal of the probability of selection, adjustment for nonresponse, and ratio adjustment to fixed totals.

For more detailed information on NAMCS, see: Woodwell, DA. National Ambulatory Medical Care Survey: 1997 summary. Advance data from vital and health statistics; no 305. Hyattsville, Maryland: National Center for Health Statistics. 1999.

National Hospital Ambulatory Medical Care Survey

The National Hospital Ambulatory Medical Care Survey (NHAMCS), initiated in 1992, is a continuing annual national probability sample of visits by patients to emergency departments (ED's) and outpatient departments (OPD's) of non-Federal, short-stay, or general hospitals. Telephone contacts are excluded.

A four-stage probability sample design is used in NHAMCS, involving samples of primary sampling units (PSU's), hospitals with ED's and/or OPD's within PSU's, ED's within hospitals and/or clinics within OPD's, and patient visits within ED's and/or clinics. In 1997 the hospital response rate for NHAMCS was 95 percent. Hospital staff were asked to complete Patient Record forms for a systematic random sample of patient visits occurring during a randomly assigned 4-week reporting period. In 1997 the number of Patient Record forms completed for ED's was 22,209 and for OPD's was 30,107.

For more detailed information on NHAMCS, see: McCaig LF, McLemore T. Plan and operation of the National Hospital Ambulatory Medical Care Survey. National Center for Health Statistics. Vital Health Stat 1(34). 1994.

National Center for HIV, STD, and TB Prevention

AIDS Surveillance

Acquired immunodeficiency syndrome (AIDS) surveillance is conducted by health departments in each State, territory, and the District of Columbia. Although surveillance activities range from passive to active, most areas employ multifaceted active surveillance programs, which include four major reporting sources of AIDS information: hospitals and hospital-based physicians, physicians in nonhospital practice, public and private clinics, and medical record systems (death certificates, tumor registries, hospital discharge abstracts, and communicable disease reports). Using a standard confidential case report form, the health departments collect information without personal identifiers, which is coded and computerized either at the Centers for Disease Control and Prevention (CDC) or at health departments from which it is then transmitted electronically to CDC.

AIDS surveillance data are used to detect epidemiologic trends, to identify unusual cases requiring followup, and for semiannual publication in the *HIV/AIDS Surveillance Report*. Studies to determine the completeness of reporting of AIDS cases meeting the national surveillance definition suggest reporting at greater than or equal to 90 percent.

For more information on AIDS surveillance, see: Centers for Disease Control and Prevention. *HIV/AIDS Surveillance Report*, published semiannually; or contact: Chief, Surveillance Branch, Division of HIV/AIDS, National Center for HIV, STD, and TB Prevention (NCHSTP), Centers for Disease Control and Prevention, Atlanta, GA 30333; or visit the NCHSTP home page at http://www.cdc.gov/nchstp/od/nchstp.html.

Epidemiology Program Office

National Notifiable Diseases Surveillance System

The Epidemiology Program Office (EPO) of CDC, in partnership with the Council of State and Territorial Epidemiologists (CSTE), operates the National Notifiable Diseases Surveillance System. The purpose of this system is primarily to provide weekly provisional information on the occurrence of diseases defined as notifiable by CSTE. In addition, the system also provides summary data on an annual basis. State epidemiologists report cases of notifiable diseases to EPO, and EPO tabulates and publishes these data in the *Morbidity and Mortality Weekly Report* (MMWR)

and the. *Summary of Notifiable Diseases, United States* (entitled *Annual Summary* before 1985). Notifiable disease surveillance is conducted by public health practitioners at local, State, and national levels to support disease prevention and control activities.

Notifiable disease reports are received from 52 areas in the United States and 5 territories. To calculate U.S. rates, data reported by 50 States, New York City, and the District of Columbia, are used. (New York State is reported as Upstate New York, which excludes New York City.)

CSTE and CDC annually review the status of national infectious disease surveillance and recommend additions or deletions to the list of nationally notifiable diseases based on the need to respond to emerging priorities. For example, genital chlamydial infections became nationally notifiable in 1995. However, reporting nationally notifiable diseases to CDC by States is voluntary. Reporting is currently mandated by law or regulation only at the State level. Therefore, the list of diseases that are considered notifiable varies slightly by State. For example, reporting of mumps to CDC is not done by some States in which this disease is not notifiable to local or State authorities.

Completeness of reporting varies because not all cases receive medical care and not all treated conditions are reported. Estimates of underreporting of some diseases have been made. For example, it is estimated that only 22 percent of cases of congenital rubella syndrome are reported. Only 10–15 percent of all measles cases were reported before the institution of the Measles Elimination Program in 1978. Recent investigations suggest that fewer than 50 percent of measles cases were reported following an outbreak in an inner city and that 40 percent of hospitalized measles cases are currently reported. Data from a study of pertussis suggest that only one-third of severe cases causing hospitalization or death are reported. Data from a study of tetanus deaths suggest that only 40 percent of tetanus cases are reported to CDC.

For more information, see: Centers for Disease Control and Prevention, Summary of Notifiable Diseases, United States, 1997. *Morbidity and Mortality*

Appendix I ....

Sources of Data

Weekly Report, 46(53), Public Health Service, DHHS, Atlanta, GA, 1998; or write: Chief, Surveillance Systems Branch, Division of Public Health Surveillance and Informatics. Epidemiology Program Office, Centers for Disease Control and Prevention, 1600 Clifton Road, MS C08, Atlanta, GA 30333; or visit the EPO home page at http://www.cdc.gov/epo.

National Center for Chronic Disease Prevention and Health Promotion

Abortion Surveillance

In 1969 CDC began abortion surveillance to document the number and characteristics of women obtaining legal induced abortions, monitor unintended pregnancy, and assist efforts to identify and reduce preventable causes of morbidity and mortality associated with abortions. For each year since 1969 abortion data have been available from 52 reporting areas: 50 States, the District of Columbia, and New York City. The total number of legal induced abortions is available from all reporting areas; however, not all areas collect information regarding the characteristics of women who obtain abortions. Furthermore the number of States reporting each characteristic and the number of States with complete data for each characteristic vary from year to year. State data with more than 15 percent unknown for a given characteristic are excluded from the analysis of that characteristic.

For 47 reporting areas, data concerning the number and characteristics of women who obtain legal induced abortions are provided by central health agencies such as State health departments and the health departments of New York City and the District of Columbia. For the other five areas, data concerning the number of abortions are provided by hospitals and other medical facilities. In general the procedures are reported by the State in which the procedure is performed. However, two reporting areas (the District of Columbia and Wisconsin) report abortions by State of residence; occurrence data are unavailable for these areas.

The total number of abortions reported to CDC is about 10 percent less than the total estimated independently by the Alan Guttmacher Institute, a not-for-profit organization for reproductive health research, policy analysis, and public education.

For more information, see: Centers for Disease Control and Prevention, CDC Surveillance Summaries, July 3, 1998. *Morbidity and Mortality Weekly Report* 1998;47 (NoSS-2), Abortion Surveillance - United States, 1995; or contact: Director, Division of Reproductive Health, National Center for Chronic Disease Prevention and Health Promotion (NCCDPHP), Centers for Disease Control and Prevention Atlanta, GA 30333; or visit the NCCDPHP home page at http://www.cdc.gov.nccdphp.

National Institute for Occupational Safety and Health

National Traumatic Occupational Fatalities Surveillance System

The National Traumatic Occupational Fatalities (NTOF) surveillance system is compiled by the National Institute for Occupational Safety and Health (NIOSH) based on information taken from death certificates. Certificates are collected from 52 vital statistics reporting units (the 50 States, New York City, and the District of Columbia) based on the following criteria: age 16 years or over, an external cause of death (ICD-9, E800-E999), and a positive response to the "Injury at work?" item.

For the period of this analysis there were no standardized guidelines regarding the completion of the "Injury at work?" item on the death certificate, thus, numbers and rates of occupational injury deaths from NTOF should be regarded as the lower bound for the true number of these events. Operational guidelines for the completion of the "Injury at work?" item have been developed by NIOSH in conjunction with the National Center for Health Statistics, the National Association for Public Health Statistics and Information Systems, and the National Center for Environmental Health and were disseminated in 1992 for implementation in 1993. This should improve death certificate-based surveillance of work-related injuries.

The denominator data for the calculation of rates by industry division were obtained from the U.S. Bureau of Labor Statistics' annual average employment data. All of the rates presented are for the U.S. civilian labor force.

For further information on NTOF, see DHHS (NIOSH). Publication No. 93–108, *Fatal Injuries to Workers in the United States, 1980–1989: A Decade of Surveillance*; or contact: Director, Division of Safety Research, National Institute for Occupational Safety and Health, 1095 Willowdale Road, Mailstop P-1172, Morgantown, WV 26505; or visit the NIOSH home page at http://www.cdc.gov/niosh.

Health Resources and Services Administration

Bureau of Health Professions

Physician Supply Projections

Physician supply projections in this report are based on a model developed by the Bureau of Health Professions to forecast the supply of physicians by specialty, activity, and State of practice. The 1995 supply of active physicians (M.D.'s) was used as the starting point for the most recent projections of active physicians. The major source of data used to obtain 1995 figures was the American Medical Association (AMA) Physician Masterfile.

In the first stage of the projections, graduates from U.S. schools of allopathic (M.D.) and osteopathic (D.O.) medicine and internationally trained additions were estimated on a year-by-year basis. Estimates of first-year enrollments, student attrition, other medical school-related trends, and a model of net internationally trained medical graduate immigration were used in deriving these annual additions. These year-by-year additions were then combined with the already existing active supply in a given year to produce a preliminary estimate of the active work force in each succeeding year. These estimates were then reduced to account for mortality and retirement.

Gender-specific mortality and retirement losses were computed by 5-year age cohorts on an annual basis, using age distributions and mortality and retirement rates based on the AMA data.

For more information, see: Bureau of Health Professions, *Health Personnel in the United States Ninth Report to Congress, 1993*, DHHS Pub. No. HRS-P-OD-94–1, Health Resources and Services Administration, Rockville, MD.

Nurse Supply Estimates

Nursing estimates in this report are based on a model developed by the Bureau of Health Professions to meet the requirements of Section 951, P.L. 94–63. The model estimates the following for each State: (a) population of nurses currently licensed to practice; (b) supply of full- and part-time practicing nurses (or available to practice); and (c) full-time equivalent supply of nurses practicing full time plus one-half of those practicing part time (or available on that basis).

The three estimates are divided into three levels of highest educational preparation: associate degree or diploma, baccalaureate, and master's and doctorate.

Among the factors considered are new graduates, changes in educational status, nursing employment rates, age, migration patterns, death rates, and licensure phenomena. The base data for the model are derived from the National Sample Surveys of Registered Nurses, conducted by the Division of Nursing, Bureau of Health Professions, HRSA. Other data sources include National League for Nursing for data on nursing education and National Council of State Boards of Nursing for data on licensure.

Substance Abuse and Mental Health Services Administration

Office of Applied Studies

National Household Surveys on Drug Abuse

Data on trends in use of marijuana, cigarettes, alcohol, and cocaine among persons 12 years of age

Sources of Data

and over are from the National Household Survey on Drug Abuse (NHSDA). The 1997 survey is the 17th in a series that began in 1971 under the auspices of the National Commission on Marijuana and Drug Abuse. From 1974 to September 1992, the survey was sponsored by the National Institute on Drug Abuse. Since October 1992, the survey has been sponsored by the Substance Abuse and Mental Health Services Administration (SAMHSA).

Since 1991 the National Household Survey on Drug Abuse has covered the civilian noninstitutionalized population 12 years of age and over in the United States. This includes civilians living on military bases and persons living in noninstitutionalized group quarters, such as college dormitories, rooming houses, and shelters. Hawaii and Alaska were included for the first time in 1991.

In 1994 the survey underwent major changes that affect the reporting of substance abuse prevalence rates. New questionnaire and data editing procedures were implemented to improve the measurement of trends in prevalence and to enhance the timeliness and quality of the data. Because it was anticipated that the new methodology would affect the estimates of prevalence, the 1994 NHSDA was designed to generate two sets of estimates. The first set, called the 1994-A estimates, was based on the same questionnaire and editing method that were used in 1993. The second set, called the 1994-B estimates, was based on the new questionnaire and editing methodology. A description of this new methodology can be found in Advance Report 10, available from SAMHSA. Because of the 1994 changes, many of the estimates from the 1994-A and earlier NHSDA's are not comparable with estimates from the 1994-B and later NHSDA's. To be able to describe long-term trends in drug use accurately, an adjustment procedure was developed and applied to the pre-1994 estimates. This adjustment uses the 1994 split sample design to estimate the magnitude of the impact of the new methodology for each drug category. The adjusted estimates are presented in this volume of *Health, United States*. A description of the adjustment method can be found in Advance Report Number 18, Appendix A, available from SAMHSA.

The 1997 survey employed a multistage probability sample design. Young people (age 12–34 years), black Americans, and Hispanics were oversampled. The sample included 24,505 respondents. The screening and interview response rates were 92.7 percent and 78.3 percent, respectively.

For more information on the National Household Survey on Drug Abuse (NHSDA), see: NHSDA Series: H-5 National Household Survey on Drug Abuse Main Findings 1996, H-6 Preliminary Results from the 1997 National Household Survey on Drug Abuse, H-7 National Household Survey on Drug Abuse: Population Estimates 1997; or write: Office of Applied Studies, Substance Abuse and Mental Health Services Administration, Room 16C-06, 5600 Fishers Lane, Rockville, MD 20857; or visit the SAMHSA home page at http://www.samhsa.gov.

Drug Abuse Warning Network

The Drug Abuse Warning Network (DAWN) is a large-scale, ongoing drug abuse data collection system based on information from emergency room and medical examiner facilities. DAWN collects information about those drug abuse occurrences that have resulted in a medical crisis or death. The major objectives of the DAWN data system include the monitoring of drug abuse patterns and trends, the identification of substances associated with drug abuse episodes, and the assessment of drug-related consequences and other health hazards.

Hospitals eligible for DAWN are non-Federal, short-stay general hospitals that have a 24-hour emergency room. Since 1988 the DAWN emergency room data have been collected from a representative sample of these hospitals located throughout the coterminous United States, including 21 oversampled metropolitan areas. Within each facility, a designated DAWN reporter is responsible for identifying drug abuse episodes by reviewing official records and transcribing and submitting data on each case. The data from this sample are used to generate estimates of the total number of emergency room drug abuse episodes and drug mentions in all such hospitals. A response rate of 74 percent was obtained in the 1996 survey.

A methodology for generating comparable estimates for years before 1988 was developed, taking advantage of historical data on the characteristics of the universe of eligible hospitals and the extensive data files compiled over the years by DAWN. After the new probability sample for DAWN was implemented in 1988, old and new DAWN sample data were collected for a period of 1 year. This overlap period was used to evaluate various procedures for weighting the old sample data (from 1978 to 1987). The procedure that consistently produced reliable estimates for a particular metropolitan area was selected as the weighting scheme for that area and used to generate all estimates for that area for years before 1988. These historical estimates are available in Advance Report 16, available from SAMHSA.

For further information, see: Series I, Number 14-A The Drug Abuse Warning Network (DAWN) Annual Data, 1994; Advance Report 14: Historical Estimates from the Drug Abuse Warning Network; DAWN Series: D-5 Mid-Year 1997 Preliminary Emergency Department Data from the Drug Abuse Warning Network and D-6 Drug Abuse Warning Network - Annual Medical Examiner Data 1996 or write: Office of Applied Studies, Substance Abuse and Mental Health Services Administration, Room 16C-06, 5600 Fishers Lane, Rockville, MD 20857; or visit the SAMHSA home page at http://www.samhsa.gov.

Uniform Facility Data Set

The Uniform Facility Data Set (UFDS), is part of the Drug and Alcohol Services Information System (DASIS) maintained by the Substance Abuse and Mental Health Services Administration. UFDS is a census of all substance abuse treatment and prevention facilities that are licensed, certified, or otherwise recognized by the individual State substance abuse agencies, and an additional group of substance abuse treatment facilities identified from other sources. It seeks information from all specialized facilities that

treat substance abuse. These include facilities that only treat substance abuse, as well as specialty substance abuse units operating within larger mental health (for example, community mental health centers), general health (for example, hospitals), social service (for example, family assistance centers), and criminal justice (for example, probation departments) agencies. UFDS solicits data concerning facility and client characteristics for a specific reference day (on or about October 1) including number of individuals in treatment, substance of abuse (alcohol, drugs, or both), types of services, and source of revenue. Public and private facilities are included.

Treatment facilities contacted through UFDS are identified from the National Master Facility Inventory (NMFI), which lists all State-sanctioned substance abuse treatment and prevention facilities and additional treatment facilities identified through business directories and other sources. In 1996, only State-sanctioned facilities were included in the published tables. The 1997 data include, for the first time, the facilities identified through business directories and other sources. Response rates to the survey were 86 and 88 percent in 1996 and 1997 respectively.

For further information on UFDS, contact: Office of Applied Studies, Substance Abuse and Mental Health Services Administration, Room 16–105, 5600 Fishers Lane, Rockville, MD 20857; or visit the OAS statistical information section of the SAMHSA home page: http://www.samhsa.gov.

Center for Mental Health Services

Surveys of Mental Health Organizations

The Survey and Analysis Branch of the Division of State and Community Systems Development conducts a biennial inventory of mental health organizations (IMHO) and general hospital mental health services (GHMHS). One version is designed for specialty mental health organizations and another for non-Federal general hospitals with separate psychiatric services. The response rate to most of the items on these inventories is relatively high (90 percent or better) as is the rate for data presented in this report. However, for some inventory items, the response rate may be somewhat lower.

IMHO and GHMHS are the primary sources for Center for Mental Health Services data included in this report. This data system is based on questionnaires mailed every other year to mental health organizations in the United States, including psychiatric hospitals, non-Federal general hospitals with psychiatric services, Department of Veterans Affairs psychiatric services, residential treatment centers for emotionally disturbed children, freestanding outpatient psychiatric clinics, partial care organizations, freestanding day-night organizations, and multiservice mental health organizations, not elsewhere classified.

Federally funded community mental health centers (CMHC's) were included separately through 1980. In 1981, with the advent of block grants, the changes in definition of CMHC's and the discontinuation of CMHC monitoring by the Center for Mental Health Services, organizations formerly classified as CMHC's have been reclassified as other organization types, primarily "multiservice mental health organizations, not elsewhere classified," and "freestanding psychiatric outpatient clinics."

Beginning in 1983 any organization that provides services in any combination of two or more services (for example, outpatient plus partial care, residential treatment plus outpatient plus partial care) and is neither a hospital nor a residential treatment center for emotionally disturbed children is classified as a multiservice mental health organization.

Other surveys conducted by the Survey and Analysis Branch encompass samples of patients admitted to State and county mental hospitals, private mental hospitals, multiservice mental health organizations, the psychiatric services of non-Federal general hospitals and Department of Veterans Affairs medical centers, residential treatment centers for emotionally disturbed children, and freestanding outpatient and partial care programs. The purpose of these surveys is to determine the sociodemographic, clinical, and treatment characteristics of patients served by these facilities.

For more information, write: Survey and Analysis Branch, Division of State and Community Systems Development, Center for Mental Health Services, Room 15C-O4, 5600 Fishers Lane, Rockville, MD 20857. For further information on mental health, see: Center for Mental Health Services, *Mental Health, United States, 1998.* Manderscheid R, Henderson MJ, eds. DHHS Pub. No. (SMA) 99–3285. Washington: Superintendent of Documents, U.S. Government Printing Office. 1998; or visit the Center for Mental Health Services home page at http://www.samhsa.gov/cmhs/cmhs.htm.

National Institutes of Health

National Cancer Institute

Surveillance, Epidemiology, and End Results Program

In the Surveillance, Epidemiology, and End Results (SEER) Program the National Cancer Institute (NCI) contracts with 11 population-based registries throughout the United States to provide data on all residents diagnosed with cancer during the year and to provide current followup information on all previously diagnosed patients.

This report covers residents of one of the following geographic areas at the time of their initial diagnosis of cancer: Atlanta, Georgia; Detroit, Michigan; Seattle-Puget Sound, Washington; San Francisco-Oakland, California; Connecticut; Iowa; New Mexico; Utah; and Hawaii.

Population estimates used to calculate incidence rates are obtained from the U.S. Bureau of the Census. NCI uses estimation procedures as needed to obtain estimates for years and races not included in the data provided by the U.S. Bureau of the Census. Rates presented in this report may differ somewhat from previous reports due to revised population estimates and the addition and deletion of small numbers of incidence cases.

Life tables used to determine normal life expectancy when calculating relative survival rates were obtained from NCHS and in-house calculations. Separate life tables are used for each race-sex-specific group included in the SEER Program.

For further information, see: National Cancer Institute, *Cancer Statistics Review, 1973–95* by L.A.G. Ries, et al. Public Health Service. Bethesda, MD, 1998; or visit the SEER home page: http://www-seer.ims.nci.nih.gov.

National Institute on Drug Abuse

Monitoring the Future Study (High School Senior Survey)

Monitoring the Future Study (MTF) is a large-scale epidemiological survey of drug use and related attitudes. It was initiated by the National Institute on Drug Abuse (NIDA) in 1975 and is conducted annually through a NIDA grant awarded to the University of Michigan's Institute for Social Research. MTF is composed of three substudies: (a) annual survey of high school seniors initiated in 1975; (b) ongoing panel studies of representative samples from each graduating class that have been conducted by mail since 1976; and (c) annual surveys of 8th and 10th graders initiated in 1991.

The survey design is a multistage random sample with stage one being the selection of particular geographic areas, stage two the selection of one or more schools in each area, and stage three the selection of students within each school. Data are collected using self-administered questionnaires administered in the classroom by representatives of the Institute for Social Research. Dropouts and students who are absent on the day of the survey are excluded. Recognizing that the dropout population is at higher risk for drug use, this survey was expanded to include similar nationally representative samples of 8th and 10th graders in 1991. Statistics that are published in the Dropout Rates in the United States: 1996 (published by the National Center for Educational Statistics, Pub. No. 98–250) stated that among persons 15–16 years of age, 3.5 percent have dropped out of school. Among persons 17 years of age, 3.4 percent have dropped out of school, while the dropout percent increases to 5.9 percent of persons 18 years of age, and to 8.9 percent for persons 19 years of age. Therefore, surveying eighth graders (where drop out rates are much lower than for high school seniors) should be effective for picking up students at higher risk for drug use.

Approximately 50,000 8th, 10th, and 12th graders are surveyed annually. In 1998 the annual senior samples are comprised of 15,780 seniors in 144 public and private high schools nationwide, selected to be representative of all seniors in the continental United States. The 10th grade samples involve about 15,419 students in 129 schools in 1998, and the 1998 eighth grade samples have 18,667 students in 149 schools.

For further information on Monitoring the Future Study, see: National Institute on Drug Abuse, National Survey Results on Drug Use from Monitoring the Future Study, 1975–1997, vol I, secondary school students. NIH Pub. No. 98–4345. Washington: Public Health Service. 1998; or visit the NIDA home page at http://www.nida.nih.gov or University of Michigan's website, http://www.isr.umich.edu/src/mtf/.

Health Care Financing Administration

Office of the Actuary

Estimates of National Health Expenditures

Estimates of expenditures for health (National Health Accounts) are compiled annually by type of expenditure and source of funds.

Estimates of expenditures for health services come from an array of sources. The American Hospital Association (AHA) data on hospital finances are the primary source for estimates relating to hospital care. The salaries of physicians and dentists on the staffs of hospitals, hospital outpatient clinics, hospital-based home health agencies, and nursing home care provided in the hospital setting are considered to be components of hospital care. Expenditures for home health care and for services of health professionals (for example, doctors, chiropractors, private duty nurses, therapists,

Sources of Data

and podiatrists) are estimated primarily using a combination of data from the U.S. Bureau of the Census' Service Annual Survey and the quinquennial Census of Service Industries.

The estimates of retail spending for prescription drugs are based on results of a HCFA-sponsored study conducted by the Actuarial Research Corporation and on industry data on prescription drug transactions. Expenditures for other medical nondurables and vision products and other medical durables purchased in retail outlets are based on estimates of personal consumption expenditures prepared by the U.S. Department of Commerce's Bureau of Economic Analysis, U.S. Bureau of Labor Statistics/Consumer Expenditure Survey, and the 1987 National Medical Expenditure Survey conducted by the Agency for Health Care Policy and Research. Those durable and nondurable products provided to inpatients in hospitals or nursing homes, and those provided by licensed professionals or through home health agencies are excluded here, but are included with the expenditure estimates of the provider service category.

Nursing home expenditures cover care rendered in establishments providing inpatient nursing and health-related personal care through active treatment programs for medical and health-related conditions. These establishments cover skilled nursing and intermediate care facilities, including those for the mentally retarded. Spending estimates are based upon data from the U.S. Bureau of the Census Services Annual Survey, and the quinequennial Census of Service Industries.

Expenditures for construction include those spent on the erection or renovation of hospitals, nursing homes, medical clinics, and medical research facilities, but not for private office buildings providing office space for private practitioners. Expenditures for noncommercial research (the cost of commercial research by drug companies is assumed to be imbedded in the price charged for the product; to include this item again would result in double counting) are developed from information gathered by the National Institutes of Health.

Source of funding estimates likewise come from a multiplicity of sources. Data on the Federal health programs are taken from administrative records maintained by the servicing agencies. Among the sources used to estimate State and local government spending for health are the U.S. Bureau of the Census' *Government Finances* and Social Security Administration reports on State-operated Workers' Compensation programs. Federal and State-local expenditures for education and training of medical personnel are excluded from these measures where they are separable. For the private financing of health care, data on the financial experience of health insurance organizations come from special Health Care Financing Administration analyses of private health insurers, and from the Bureau of Labor Statistics' survey on the cost of employer-sponsored health insurance and on consumer expenditures. Information on out-of-pocket spending from the U.S. Bureau of the Census' Services Annual Survey, U.S. Bureau of Labor Statistics' Consumer Expenditure Survey, the 1987 National Medical Expenditure Survey conducted by the Agency for Health Care Policy and Research, and from private surveys conducted by the American Hospital Association, American Medical Association, and the American Dental Association are used to develop estimates of direct spending by customers.

For more specific information on definitions, sources and methods used in the National Health Accounts, see: National Health Accounts: Lessons from the U.S. Experience, by Lazenby HC, Levit KR, Waldo DR, et al. Health Care Financing Review, vol 14 no 4. Health Care Financing Administration. Washington: Public Health Service. 1992 and National Health Expenditures, 1994, Levit KR, Lazenby HC, Sivarajan L, et al. Health Care Financing Review, vol 17 no 3. Health Care Financing Administration. Washington: Public Health Service. 1996.

Estimates of State Health Expenditures

Estimates of spending by State are created using the same definitions of health care sectors used in producing the National Health Expenditures (NHE).

The same data sources used in creating NHE are also used to create State estimates whenever possible. Frequently, however, surveys that are used to create valid national estimates lack sufficient size to create valid State level estimates. In these cases, alternative data sources that best represent the State-by-State distribution of spending are substituted and the U.S. aggregate expenditures for the specific type of service or source of funds are used to control the level of State-by-State distributions. This procedure implicitly assumes that national spending estimates can be created more accurately than State specific expenditures.

Despite definitional correspondence, NHE differ from the sum of State estimates. NHE include expenditures for persons living in U.S. territories and for military and Federal civilian employees and their families stationed overseas. The sum of the State level expenditures exclude health spending for those groups. For hospital care, exclusion of purchases of services in non-U.S. areas accounts for a 0.9 percent reduction in hospital expenditures from those measured as part of NHE.

For more information, contact: Office of the Actuary, Health Care Financing Administration, 7500 Security Blvd., Baltimore, MD 21244–1850.

Medicare National Claims History Files

The Medicare Common Working File (CWF) is a Medicare Part A and Part B benefit coordination and claims validation system. There are two National Claims History (NCH) files, the NCH 100 percent-Nearline File, and the NCH Beneficiary Program Liability (BPL) File. The NCH files contain claims records and Medicare beneficiary information. The NCH 100 percent Nearline File contains all institutional and physician/supplier claims from the CWF. It provides records of every claim submitted, including all adjustment claims. The NCH BPL file contains Medicare Part A and Part B beneficiary liability information (such as deductible and coinsurance amounts remaining). The records include all Part A and Part B utilization and entitlement data.

Records for 1997 were maintained on more than 38 million enrollees and 48,826 institutional providers including 6,246 hospitals, 14,619 skilled nursing facilities, 10,487 home health agencies, 2,239 hospices, 2,689 outpatient physical therapy, 472 comprehensive outpatient rehabilitation facilities, 3,274 end state renal dialysis facilities, 3,447 rural health clinics, 1,175 community mental health centers, 2,406 ambulatory surgical centers, and 1,772 federally qualified health centers. About 708 million claims were processed in fiscal year 1996.

Data from the NCH files provide information about enrollee use of benefits for a point in time or over an extended period. Statistical reports are produced on enrollment, characteristics of participating providers, reimbursement, and services used.

For further information on the NCH files see: Health Care Financing Administration, Office of Information Services, Enterprise Data Base Group, Division of Information Distribution, Data Users Reference Guide or call the Medicare Hotline at 410–786–3689.

For further information on Medicare visit the HCFA home page at http://www.hcfa.gov.

Medicaid Data System

The majority of Medicaid data are compiled from forms submitted annually by State Medicaid agencies to the Health Care Financing Administration (HCFA) for Federal fiscal years ending September 30 on the Form HCFA-2082, *Statistical Report on Medical Care: Eligibles, Recipients, Payments, and Services*.

When using the data keep the following caveats in mind:

■ Counts of recipients and eligibles categorized by basis of eligibility generally count each person only once based on the person's basis of eligibility as of first appearance on the Medicaid rolls during the Federal fiscal year covered by the report. Note, however, that some States report duplicated counts of recipients; that is, they report an individual in as many categories as the individual had different eligibility statuses during the year. In such cases, the sum of all basis-of-eligibility cells will be greater than the "total recipients" number.

■ Expenditure data include payments for all claims adjudicated or paid during the fiscal year covered by the report. Note that this is not the same as summing payments for services that were rendered during the reporting period.

■ Some States fail to submit the HCFA-2082 for a particular year. When this happens, HCFA estimates the current year's HCFA-2082 data for missing States based upon prior year's submissions and information the State entered on Form HCFA-64 (the form States use to claim reimbursement for Federal matching funds for Medicaid).

■ HCFA-2082's submitted by States frequently contain obvious errors in one or more cells in the form. For cells obviously in error, HCFA estimates values that appear to be more reasonable.

The Medicaid data presented in *Health, United States* are from the Medicaid statistical system (using form HCFA-2082) and may differ from data presented elsewhere using the quarterly financial reports (form HCFA-64) submitted by States for reimbursement. Vendor payments from the Medicaid statistical system exclude disproportionate share hospital payments ($17 billion in 1993) and payments to health maintenance organizations and Medicare ($6 billion in 1993).

For further information on Medicaid data, see: *Health Care Financing Review: Medicare and Medicaid Statistical Supplement, 1995*, HCFA Pub. No. 0374, Health Care Financing Administration, Baltimore, MD. U.S. Government Printing Office, Sept. 1995; or visit the HCFA home page at http://www.hcfa.gov.

Online Survey Certification and Reporting Database

The Online Survey Certification and Reporting (OSCAR) database has been maintained by the Health Care Financing Administration (HCFA) since 1992. OSCAR is an updated version of the Medicare and Medicaid Automated Certification System that has been in existence since 1972. OSCAR is an administrative database containing detailed information on all Medicare and Medicaid health care providers in addition to all currently certified Medicare and Medicaid nursing home facilities in the United States and Territories. (Data for the territories are not shown in this report.) The purpose of the nursing home facility survey certification process is to ensure that nursing facilities meet the current HCFA long-term care requirements and thus can participate in serving Medicare and Medicaid beneficiaries. Included in the OSCAR database are all certified nursing facilities, certified hospital-based nursing homes, and certified units for other types of nursing home facilities (for example, life care communities or board and care homes). Facilities not included in OSCAR are all noncertified facilities (that is, facilities that are only licensed by the State and are limited to private payment sources), and nursing homes that are part of the Department of Veterans Affairs. Also excluded are nursing homes that are intermediate care facilities for the mentally retarded.

Information on the number of beds, residents, and resident characteristics are collected during an inspection of all certified facilities. All certified nursing homes are inspected by representatives of the State survey agency (generally the Department of Health) at least once every 15 months. The information present on OSCAR is based on each facility's own administrative record system in addition to interviews with key administrative staff members.

For more information, see: HCFA: OSCAR data users reference guide, 1995, available from HCFA, Health Standards and Quality Bureau, HCFA/HSQB S2–11–07, 7500 Security Boulevard, Baltimore, MD 21244; or visit the HCFA home page at http://www.hcfa.gov.

Department of Commerce

Bureau of the Census

Census of Population

The census of population has been taken in the United States every 10 years since 1790. In the 1990 census, data were collected on sex, race, age, and marital status from 100 percent of the enumerated population. More detailed information such as income, education, housing, occupation, and industry were collected from a representative sample of the population. For most of the country, one out of six households (about 17 percent) received the more detailed questionnaire. In places of residence estimated to have less than 2,500 population, 50 percent of households received the long form.

For more information on the 1990 census, see: U.S. Bureau of the Census, *1990 Census of Population, General Population Characteristics*, Series 1990, CP-1; or visit the Census Bureau home page at http://www.census.gov.

Current Population Survey

The Current Population Survey (CPS) is a household sample survey of the civilian noninstitutionalized population conducted monthly by the U.S. Bureau of the Census. CPS provides estimates of employment, unemployment, and other characteristics of the general labor force, the population as a whole, and various other subgroups of the population.

The 1998 CPS sample is located in 754 sample areas, with coverage in every State and the District of Columbia. In an average month during 1998, the number of housing units or living quarters eligible for interview was about 50,000; of these about 7 percent were, for various reasons, unavailable for interview. In 1994 major changes were introduced, which included a complete redesign of the questionnaire and the introduction of computer-assisted interviewing for the entire survey. In addition, there were revisions to some of the labor force concepts and definitions.

The estimation procedure used involves inflation by the reciprocal of the probability of selection, adjustment for nonresponse, and ratio adjustment. Beginning in 1994 new population controls based on the 1990 census adjusted for the estimated population undercount were utilized.

For more information, see: U.S. Bureau of the Census, *The Current Population Survey, Design and Methodology*, Technical Paper 40, Washington, U.S. Government Printing Office, Jan. 1978; U.S. Department of Labor, Bureau of Labor Statistics, Employment and Earnings, Feb. 1994, vol 41 no 2 and Feb. 1995, vol 42 no 2, Washington: U.S. Government Printing Office, Feb. 1994 and Feb. 1995; or visit the CPS home page at http://www.bls.census.gov.

Population Estimates

National population estimates are derived by using decennial census data as benchmarks and data available from various agencies as follows: births and deaths (National Center for Health Statistics); immigrants (Immigration and Naturalization Service); Armed Forces (Department of Defense); net movement between Puerto Rico and the U.S. mainland (Puerto Rico Planning Board); and Federal employees abroad (Office of Personnel Management and Department of Defense). State estimates are based on similar data and also on a variety of data series, including school statistics from State departments of education and parochial school systems. Current estimates are consistent with official decennial census figures and do not reflect estimated decennial census underenumeration.

After decennial population censuses, intercensal population estimates for the preceding decade are prepared to replace postcensal estimates. Intercensal population estimates are more accurate than postcensal estimates because they take into account the census of population at the beginning and end of the decade. Intercensal estimates have been prepared for the 1960's, 1970's, and 1980's to correct the "error of closure" or difference between the estimated population at the end of the decade and the census count for that date. The error of closure at the national level was quite small during the 1960's (379,000). However, for the 1970's it amounted to almost 5 million and for the 1980's, 1.5 million.

For more information, see: U.S. Bureau of the Census, U.S. population estimated by age, sex, race, and Hispanic origin: 1990–96, release PPL-57, March 1997; or visit the Census Bureau home page: http://www.census.gov.

Department of Labor

Bureau of Labor Statistics

Annual Survey of Occupational Injuries and Illnesses

Since 1971 the Bureau of Labor Statistics (BLS) has conducted an annual survey of establishments in the private sector to collect statistics on occupational injuries and illnesses. The Survey of Occupational Injuries and Illnesses is based on records that employers maintain under the Occupational Safety and Health Act. Excluded from the survey are self-employed individuals; farmers with fewer than 11 employees; employers regulated by other Federal safety and health laws; and Federal, State, and local government agencies.

Data are obtained from a sample of approximately 250,000 establishments, that is, single physical locations where business is conducted or where services of industrial operations are performed. An independent sample is selected for each State and the District of Columbia that represents industries in that jurisdiction. BLS includes all the State samples in the national sample.

Establishments included in the survey are instructed in a mailed questionnaire to provide summary totals of all entries for the previous calendar year to its Log and Summary of Occupational Injuries and Illnesses (OSHA No. 200 form). Additionally, from the selected establishments, approximately 550,000 injuries and illnesses with days away from work are sampled in order to obtain demographic and detailed case characteristic information. An

occupational injury is any injury, such as a cut, fracture, sprain, or amputation, that results from a work-related event or from a single instantaneous exposure in the work environment. An occupational illness is any abnormal condition or disorder, other than one resulting from an occupational injury, caused by exposure to factors associated with employment. It includes acute and chronic illnesses or disease that may be caused by inhalation, absorption, ingestion, or direct contact. Lost workday cases are cases that involve days away from work, or days of restricted work activity, or both. The response rate is about 92 percent.

For more information, see: Bureau of Labor Statistics, Occupational Injuries and Illnesses: Counts, Rates, and Characteristics, 1993. BLS Bulletin 2478, U.S. Department of Labor, Washington, D.C., August 1996; or visit the BLS home page at http://www.bls.gov.

Consumer Price Index

The Consumer Price Index (CPI) is a monthly measure of the average change in the prices paid by urban consumers for a fixed market basket of goods and services. The all-urban index (CPI-U) introduced in 1978 covers residents of metropolitan areas as well as residents of urban parts of non-metropolitan areas (about 87 percent of the United States population in 1990).

In calculating the index, price changes for the various items in each location were averaged together with weights that represent their importance in the spending of all urban consumers. Local data were then combined to obtain a U.S. city average.

The index measures price changes from a designated reference date, 1982–84, which equals 100. An increase of 22 percent, for example, is shown as 122. This change can also be expressed in dollars as follows: the price of a base period "market basket" of goods and services bought by all urban consumers has risen from $10 in 1982–84 to $16.30 in 1998.

The current revision of CPI, projected to be completed in 2000, reflects spending patterns based on the Survey of Consumer Expenditures from 1993 to 1995, the 1990 Census of Population, and the ongoing Point-of-Purchase Survey. Using an improved sample design, prices for the goods and services required to calculate the index are collected in urban areas throughout the country and from retail and service establishments. Data on rents are collected from tenants of rented housing and residents of owner-occupied housing units. Food, fuels, and other goods and services are priced monthly in urban locations. Price information is obtained through visits or calls by trained BLS field representatives using computer-assisted telephone interviews.

The earlier 1987 revision changed the treatment of health insurance in the cost-weight definitions for medical care items. This change has no effect on the final index result but provides a clearer picture of the role of health insurance in the CPI. As part of the revision, three new indexes have been created by separating previously combined items, for example, eye care from other professional services and inpatient and outpatient treatment from other hospital and medical care services.

Effective January 1997 the hospital index was restructured by combining the three categories room, inpatient services and outpatient services into one category, hospital services. Differentiation between inpatient and outpatient and among service types are under this broad category. In addition new procedures for hospital data collection identify a payor, diagnosis, and the payor's reimbursement arrangement from selected hospital bills.

A new geographic sample and item structure were introduced in January 1998 and expenditure weights were updated to 1993 to 1995. Pricing of a new housing sample using computer-assisted data collection was started in June 1998. In January 1999 the index will be rebased from the 1982–84 time period to 1993–95.

For more information, see: Bureau of Labor Statistics, *Handbook of Methods*, BLS Bulletin 2490, U.S. Department of Labor, Washington, Apr. 1997; IK Ford and P Sturm. CPI revision provides more

accuracy in the medical care services component, *Monthly Labor Review*, U.S. Department of Labor, Bureau of Labor Statistics, Washington, Apr. 1988; or visit the BLS home page at http://www.bls.gov.

Employment and Earnings

The Division of Monthly Industry Employment Statistics and the Division of Employment and Unemployment Analysis of the Bureau of Labor Statistics publish data on employment and earnings. The data are collected by the U.S. Bureau of the Census, State Employment Security Agencies, and State Departments of Labor in cooperation with BLS.

The major data source is the Current Population Survey (CPS), a household interview survey conducted monthly by the U.S. Bureau of the Census to collect labor force data for BLS. CPS is described separately in this appendix. Data based on establishment records are also compiled each month from mail questionnaires by BLS, in cooperation with State agencies.

For more information, see: U.S. Department of Labor, Bureau of Labor Statistics, *Employment and Earnings*, Jan. 1999, vol 46 no 1, Washington: U.S. Government Printing Office. Jan. 1999.

Employer Costs for Employee Compensation

Employer costs for employee compensation cover all occupations in private industry, excluding farms and households and State and local governments. These cost levels are published once a year with the payroll period including March 12th as the reference period.

The cost levels are based on compensation cost data collected for the Bureau of Labor Statistics Employment Cost Index (ECI), released quarterly. Employee Benefits Survey (EBS) data are jointly collected with ECI data. Cost data were collected from the ECI's March 1993 sample that consisted of about 23,000 occupations within 4,500 sample establishments in private industry and 7,000 occupations within 1,000 establishments in State and local governments. The sample establishments are classified industry categories based on the 1987 Standard Industrial Classification (SIC) system, as defined by the U.S. Office of

Management and Budget. Within an establishment, specific job categories are selected to represent broader major occupational groups such as professional specialty and technical occupations. The cost levels are calculated with current employment weights each year.

For more information, see: U.S. Department of Labor, Bureau of Labor Statistics, *Employment Cost Indexes and Levels, 1975–95*, Bulletin 2466, Oct. 1995.

Department of Veterans Affairs

Data are obtained from the Department of Veterans Affairs (VA) administrative data systems. These include budget, patient treatment, patient census, and patient outpatient clinic information. Data from the three patient files are collected locally at each VA medical center and are transmitted to the national databank at the VA Austin Automated Center where they are stored and used to provide nationwide statistics, reports, and comparisons.

The Patient Treatment File

The patient treatment file (PTF) collects data, at the time of the patient's discharge, on each episode of inpatient care provided to patients at VA hospitals, VA nursing homes, VA domiciliaries, community nursing homes, and other non-VA facilities. The PTF record contains the scrambled social security number, dates of inpatient treatment, date of birth, State and county of residence, type of disposition, place of disposition after discharge, as well as the ICD–9–CM diagnostic and procedure or operative codes for each episode of care.

The Patient Census File

The patient census file collects data on each patient remaining in a VA medical facility at midnight on a selected date of each year, normally September 30. This file includes patients admitted to VA hospitals, VA nursing homes, and VA domiciliaries. The census record includes information similar to that reported in the patient treatment file record.

The Outpatient Clinic File

The outpatient clinic file (OPC) collects data on each instance of medical treatment provided to a veteran in an outpatient setting. The OPC record includes the age, scrambled social security number, State and county of residence, VA eligibility code, clinic(s) visited, purpose of visit, and the date of visit for each episode of care.

For more information, write: Department of Veterans Affairs, National Center for Veteran Analysis and Statistics, Biometrics Division 008C12, 810 Vermont Ave., NW, Washington, DC 20420; or visit the VA home page at http://www.va.gov.

Environmental Protection Agency

Aerometric Information Retrieval System (AIRS)

The Environmental Protection Agency's Aerometric Information Retrieval System (AIRS) compiles data on ambient air levels of particulate matter smaller than 10 microns (PM-10), lead, carbon monoxide, sulphur dioxide, nitrogen dioxide, and tropospheric ozone. These pollutants were identified in the Clean Air Act of 1970 and in its 1977 and 1990 amendments because they pose significant threats to public health. The National Ambient Air Quality Standards (NAAQS) define for each pollutant the maximum concentration level (micrograms per cubic meter) that cannot be exceeded during specific time intervals. Data shown in this publication reflect attainment of NAAQS during a 12-month period based on analysis using county level air monitoring data from AIRS and population data from the Bureau of the Census.

Data are collected at State and local air pollution monitoring sites. Each site provides data for one or more of the six pollutants. The number of sites has varied, but generally increased over the years. In 1993 there were 4,469 sites, 4,668 sites in 1994, and 4,800 sites in 1995. The monitoring sites are located primarily in heavily populated urban areas. Air quality

Sources of Data

for less populated areas is assessed through a combination of data from supplemental monitors and air pollution models.

For more information, see: Environmental Protection Agency, *National Air Quality and Emissions Trend Report, 1994*, EPA-454/R-95–014, Research Triangle Park, NC, Oct. 1995, or write: Office of Air Quality Planning and Standards, Environmental Protection Agency, Research Triangle Park, NC 27711. For additional information on this measure and similar measures used to track the Healthy People 2000 Objectives and Health Status Indicators, see: National Center for Health Statistics, *Monitoring Air Quality in Healthy People 2000*, Statistical Notes, No. 9. Hyattsville, Maryland: 1995; or visit the EPA AIRS home page at http://www.epa.gov/airs/airs.html.

United Nations

Demographic Yearbook

The Statistical Office of the United Nations prepares the *Demographic Yearbook*, a comprehensive collection of international demographic statistics.

Questionnaires are sent annually and monthly to more than 220 national statistical services and other appropriate government offices. Data forwarded on these questionnaires are supplemented, to the extent possible, by data taken from official national publications and by correspondence with the national statistical services. To ensure comparability, rates, ratios, and percents have been calculated in the statistical office of the United Nations.

Lack of international comparability between estimates arises from differences in concepts, definitions, and time of data collection. The comparability of population data is affected by several factors, including (a) the definitions of the total population, (b) the definitions used to classify the population into its urban and rural components, (c) the difficulties relating to age reporting, (d) the extent of over- or underenumeration, and (e) the quality of population estimates. The completeness and accuracy of vital statistics data also vary from one country to

another. Differences in statistical definitions of vital events may also influence comparability.

For more information, see: United Nations, *Demographic Yearbook 1996*, United Nations, New York, NY. 1998; or visit the United Nations home page at http://www.un.org or their website locator at http://www.unsystem.org.

World Health Statistics Annual

The World Health Organization (WHO) prepares the *World Health Statistics Annual*, an annual volume of information on vital statistics and causes of death designed for use by the medical and public health professions. Each volume is the result of a joint effort by the national health and statistical administrations of many countries, the United Nations, and WHO. United Nations estimates of vital rates and population size and composition, where available, are reprinted directly in the *Statistics Annual*. For those countries for which the United Nations does not prepare demographic estimates, primarily smaller populations, the latest available data reported to the United Nations and based on reasonably complete coverage of events are used.

Information published on late fetal and infant mortality is based entirely on official national data either reported directly or made available to WHO.

Selected life table functions are calculated from the application of a uniform methodology to national mortality data provided to WHO, in order to enhance their value for international comparisons. The life table procedure used by WHO may often lead to discrepancies with national figures published by countries, due to differences in methodology or degree of age detail maintained in calculations.

The international comparability of estimates published in the *World Health Statistics Annual* is affected by the same problems discussed above for the *Demographic Yearbook*. Cross-national differences in statistical definitions of vital events, in the completeness and accuracy of vital statistics data, and in the comparability of population data are the primary factors affecting comparability.

For more information, see: World Health Organization, *World Health Statistics Annual 1996*, World Health Organization, Geneva, Switzerland, 1998; or visit the WHO home page at http://www.who.org.

Alan Guttmacher Institute

Abortion Survey

The Alan Guttmacher Institute (AGI) conducts an annual survey of abortion providers. Data are collected from hospitals, nonhospital clinics, and physicians identified as providers of abortion services. A universal survey of 3,092 hospitals, nonhospital clinics, and individual physicians was compiled. To assess the completeness of the provider and abortion counts, supplemental surveys were conducted of a sample of obstetrician-gynecologists and a sample of hospitals (not in original universe) that were identified as providing abortion services through the American Hospital Association Survey.

The number of abortions estimated by AGI through the mid to late 1980's was about 20 percent more than the number reported to the Centers for Disease Control and Prevention (CDC). Since 1989 the AGI estimates have been about 12 percent higher than those reported by CDC.

For more information, write: The Alan Guttmacher Institute, 120 Wall Street, New York, NY 10005; or visit AGI's home page at http://www.agi-usa.org.

American Association of Colleges of Osteopathic Medicine

The American Association of Colleges of Osteopathic Medicine (AACOM) compiles data on various aspects of osteopathic medical education for distribution to the profession, the government, and the public. Questionnaires are sent annually to all schools of osteopathic medicine requesting information on characteristics of applicants and students, curricula, faculty, grants, contracts, revenues, and expenditures. The response rate is 100 percent.

For more information, see: *Annual Statistical Report, 1997*, American Association of Colleges of Osteopathic Medicine: Rockville, Maryland. 1997; or visit the AACOM home page at http://www.aacom.org.

American Association of Colleges of Pharmacy

The American Association of Colleges of Pharmacy (AACP) compiles data on the Colleges of Pharmacy, including information on student enrollment and types of degrees conferred. Data are collected through an annual survey; the response rate is 100 percent.

For further information, see: Profile of Pharmacy Students. The American Association of Colleges of Pharmacy, 1426 Prince Street, Alexandria, VA 22314; or visit the AACP home page at http://www.aacp.org.

American Association of Colleges of Podiatric Medicine

The American Association of Colleges of Podiatric Medicine (AACPM) compiles data on the Colleges of Podiatric Medicine, including information on the schools and enrollment. Data are collected annually through written questionnaires. The response rate is 100 percent.

For further information, write: The American Association of Colleges of Podiatric Medicine, 1350 Piccard Drive, Suite 322, Rockville, MD 20850–4307; or visit the AACPM home page at http://www.aacpm.org.

American Dent. l Association

The Division of Educational Measurement of the American Dental Association (ADA) conducts annual surveys of predoctoral dental educational institutions. The questionnaire, mailed to all dental schools, collects information on student characteristics, financial management, and curricula.

For more information, see: American Dental Association, *1996/97 Survey of predoctoral dental educational institutions*. Chicago, Illinois, 1997; or visit the ADA home page at http://www.ada.org.

American Hospital Association

Annual Survey of Hospitals

Data from the American Hospital Association (AHA) annual survey are based on questionnaires sent to all hospitals, AHA-registered and nonregistered, in the United States and its associated areas. U.S. government hospitals located outside the United States were excluded. Questionnaires were mailed to all hospitals on AHA files. For nonreporting hospitals and for the survey questionnaires of reporting hospitals on which some information was missing, estimates were made for all data except those on beds, bassinets, and facilities. Data for beds and bassinets of nonreporting hospitals were based on the most recent information available from those hospitals. Facilities and services and inpatient service area data include only reporting hospitals and, therefore, do not include estimates.

Estimates of other types of missing data were based on data reported the previous year, if available. When unavailable, the estimates were based on data furnished by reporting hospitals similar in size, control, major service provided, length of stay, and geographic and demographic characteristics.

For more information on the AHA Annual Survey of Hospitals, see: American Hospital Association, (Health Forum), *Hospital Statistics, 1999 ed.* Chicago. 1999; or visit an AHA page at http://www.aha.org.

American Medical Association

Physician Masterfile

A masterfile of physicians has been maintained by the American Medical Association (AMA) since 1906. The Physician Masterfile contains data on almost every physician in the United States, members and nonmembers of AMA, and on those graduates of American medical schools temporarily practicing overseas. The file also includes graduates of

international medical schools who are in the United States and meet education standards for primary recognition as physicians.

A file is initiated on each individual upon entry into medical school or, in the case of international graduates, upon entry into the United States. Between 1969–85 a mail questionnaire survey was conducted every 4 years to update the file information on professional activities, self-designated area of specialization, and present employment status. Since 1985 approximately one-third of all physicians are surveyed each year.

For more information on the AMA Physician Masterfile, see: Division of Survey and Data Resources, American Medical Association, *Physician Characteristics and Distribution in the U.S.*, 1999 ed. Chicago. 1999; or visit the AMA home page at http://www.ama-assn.org.

Annual Census of Hospitals

From 1920 to 1953 the Council on Medical Education and Hospitals of the AMA conducted annual censuses of all hospitals registered by AMA.

In each annual census, questionnaires were sent to hospitals asking for the number of beds, bassinets, births, patients admitted, average census of patients, lists of staff doctors and interns, and other information of importance at the particular time. Response rates were always nearly 100 percent.

The community hospital data from 1940 and 1950 presented in this report were calculated using published figures from the AMA Annual Census of Hospitals. Although the hospital classification scheme used by AMA in published reports is not strictly comparable with the definition of community hospitals, methods were employed to achieve the greatest comparability possible.

For more information on the AMA Annual Census of Hospitals, see: American Medical Association, Hospital service in the United States, *Journal of the American Medical Association,* 16(11):1055–1144. 1941; or visit the AMA home page at http://www.ama-assn.org.

Sources of Data

Association of American Medical Colleges

The Association of American Medical Colleges (AAMC) collects information on student enrollment in medical schools through the annual Liaison Committee on Medical Education questionnaire, the fall enrollment questionnaire, and the American Medical College Application Service (AMCAS) data system. Other data sources are the institutional profile system, the premedical students questionnaire, the minority student opportunities in medicine questionnaire, the faculty roster system, data from the Medical College Admission Test, and one-time surveys developed for special projects.

For more information, see: Association of American Medical Colleges: *Statistical Information Related to Medical Education.* Washington. 1997; or visit the AAMC home page at http://www.aamc.org.

Association of Schools and Colleges of Optometry

The Association of Schools and Colleges of Optometry (ASCO) compiles data on the various aspects of optometric education including data on schools and enrollment. Questionnaires are sent annually to all the schools and colleges of optometry. The response rate is 100 percent.

For further information, write: Annual Survey of Optometric Educational Institutions, Association of Schools and Colleges of Optometry, 6110 Executive Blvd., Suite 690, Rockville, MD 20852; or visit the ASCO home page at http://www.opted.org.

Association of Schools of Public Health

The Association of Schools of Public Health (ASPH) compiles data on the 28 schools of public health in the United States and Puerto Rico. Questionnaires are sent annually to all member schools, and the response rate is 100 percent.

Unlike health professional schools that emphasize specific clinical occupations, schools of public health offer study in specialty areas such as biostatistics, epidemiology, environmental and occupational health, health administration, health planning, nutrition, maternal and child health, social and behavioral sciences, and other population-based sciences.

For further information, write: Association of Schools of Public Health, 1660 L Street, NW, Suite 204, Washington, D.C. 20036–5603; or visit the ASPH home page at http://www.asph.org.

InterStudy

National Health Maintenance Organization Census

From 1976 to 1980 the Office of Health Maintenance Organizations conducted a census of health maintenance organizations (HMO's). Since 1981 InterStudy has conducted the census. A questionnaire is sent to all HMO's in the United States asking for updated enrollment, profit status, and Federal qualification status. New HMO's are also asked to provide information on model type. When necessary, information is obtained, supplemented, or clarified by telephone. For nonresponding HMO's State-supplied information or the most current available data are used.

In 1985 a large increase in the number of HMO's and enrollment was partly attributable to a change in the categories of HMO's included in the census: Medicaid-only and Medicare-only HMO's have been added. Also component HMO's, which have their own discrete management, can be listed separately; whereas, previously the oldest HMO reported for all of its component or expansion sites, even when the components had different operational dates or were different model types.

For further information, see: *The InterStudy Competitive Edge,* 1995. InterStudy Publications, St. Paul, MN 55104; or visit the InterStudy home page at http://www.hmodata.com.

National League for Nursing

The division of research of the National League for Nursing (NLN) conducts The Annual Survey of Schools of Nursing in October of each year. Questionnaires are sent to all graduate nursing

Sources of Data

programs (master's and doctoral), baccalaureate programs designed exclusively for registered nurses, basic registered nursing programs (baccalaureate, associate degree, and diploma), and licensed practical nursing programs. Data on enrollments, first-time admissions, and graduates are completed for all nursing education programs. Response rates of approximately 80 percent are achieved for other areas of inquiry.

For more information, see: National League for Nursing, *Nursing Data Review*, 1997, New York, NY; or visit the NLN home page at http://www.nln.org.

The glossary is an alphabetical listing of terms used in *Health, United States*. It includes cross references to related terms and synonyms. It also contains the standard populations used for age adjustment and *International Classification of Diseases* (ICD) codes for cause of death and diagnostic and procedure categories.

Abortion—The Centers for Disease Control and Prevention's (CDC) surveillance system counts legal induced abortions only. For surveillance purposes, legal abortion is defined as a procedure performed by a licensed physician or someone acting under the supervision of a licensed physician to induce the termination of a pregnancy.

Acquired immunodeficiency syndrome (AIDS)—All 50 States and the District of Columbia report AIDS cases to CDC using a uniform case definition and case report form. The case reporting definitions were expanded in 1985 *(MMWR* 1985; 34:373–5); 1987 *(MMWR* 1987; 36 (supp. no. 1S): 1S–15S); and 1993 *(MMWR* 1992; 41 (no. RR-17): 1–19). These data are published semiannually by CDC in HIV/AIDS Surveillance Report. See related *Human immunodeficiency virus (HIV) infection*.

Active physician—See *Physician*.

Addition—An addition to a psychiatric organization is defined by the Center for Mental Health Services as a new admission, a readmission, a return from long-term leave, or a transfer from another service of the same organization or another organization. See related *Mental health disorder; Mental health organization; Mental health service type*.

Admission—The American Hospital Association defines admissions as patients, excluding newborns, accepted for inpatient services during the survey reporting period. See related *Days of care; Discharge; Patient*.

Age—Age is reported as age at last birthday, that is, age in completed years, often calculated by subtracting date of birth from the reference date, with the reference date being the date of the examination, interview, or other contact with an individual.

Age adjustment—Age adjustment, using the direct method, is the application of age-specific rates in a population of interest to a standardized age distribution in order to eliminate differences in observed rates that result from age differences in population composition. This adjustment is usually done when comparing two or more populations at one point in time or one population at two or more points in time.

Age-adjusted death rates are calculated by the direct method as follows:

$$\sum_{i=1}^{n} r_i \times (p_i/P)$$

where r_i = age-specific death rates for the population of interest

p_i = standard population in age group i

$P = \sum_{i=1}^{n} p_i$ for the age groups that comprise the age range of the rate being age adjusted

n = total number of age groups over the age range of the age-adjusted rate

Mortality data—Death rates are age adjusted to the U.S. standard million population (relative age distribution of 1940 enumerated population of the United States totaling 1,000,000) (table I).

Table I. Standard million age distribution used to adjust death rates to the U.S. population in 1940

Age	Standard million
All ages	1,000,000
Under 1 year	15,343
1–4 years	64,718
5–14 years	170,355
15–24 years	181,677
25–34 years	162,066
35–44 years	139,237
45–54 years	117,811
55–64 years	80,294
65–74 years	48,426
75–84 years	17,303
85 years and over	2,770

Age-adjusted death rates are calculated using age-specific death rates per 100,000 population rounded to 1 decimal place. Adjustment is based on 11 age groups with 2 exceptions. First, age-adjusted death rates for black males and black females in 1950 are based on nine age groups, with under 1 year and 1–4 years of age combined as one group and 75–84 years and 85 years of age and over combined as one group. Second, age-adjusted death rates by educational attainment for the age group 25–64 years are based on four 10-year age groups (25–34 years, 35–44 years, 45–54 years, and 55–64 years).

The rate for years of potential life lost (YPLL) before age 75 years is age adjusted to the U.S. standard million population (table I) and is based on eight age groups (under 1 year, 1–14 years, 15–24 years, and 10-year age groups through 65–74 years).

Maternal mortality rates for Complications of pregnancy, childbirth, and the puerperium are calculated as the number of deaths per 100,000 live births. These rates are age adjusted to the 1970 distribution of live births by mother's age in the United States as shown in table II. See related *Rate: Death and related rates; Years of potential life lost.*

National Health Interview Survey—Data from the National Health Interview Survey (NHIS) are age adjusted to the 1970 civilian noninstitutionalized population shown in table III. The 1970 civilian noninstitutionalized population is derived as follows: Civilian noninstitutionalized population = civilian population on July 1, 1970 – institutionalized

population. Institutionalized population = (1 – proportion of total population not institutionalized on April 1, 1970) × total population on July 1, 1970.

Most of the data from NHIS (except as noted below and in table III) are age adjusted using four age groups: under 15 years, 15–44 years, 45–64 years, and 65 years and over. The NHIS data on health status and

Table III. Populations and age groups used to age adjust NCHS survey data

Population, survey, and age	Number in thousands
U.S. civilian noninstitutionalized population in 1970 NHIS, NHDS, NSAS, NAMCS, and NHAMCS	
All ages.	199,584
Under 15 years	57,745
15–44 years	81,189
45–64 years	41,537
65 years and over	19,113
65–74 years.	12,224
75 years and over	6,889
NHIS smoking data	
18 years and over	130,158
25 years and over	107,694
18–24 years	22,464
25–34 years	24,430
35–44 years	22,614
45–64 years	41,537
65 years and over	19,113
NHIS health status and health care coverage data	
All ages.	199,584
Under 18 years	69,426
18–44 years	69,508
45–64 years	41,537
65–74 years	12,224
75 years and over	6,889
U.S. resident population in 1980 NHES and NHANES	
6–11 years	20,834
6–8 years	9,777
9–11 years	11,057
12–17 years	23,410
12–14 years.	10,945
15–17 years.	12,465
20–74 years.	144,120
20–34 years.	58,401
35–44 years.	25,635
45–54 years.	22,800
55–64 years.	21,703
65–74 years.	15,581

SOURCE: Calculated from U.S. Bureau of Census: Estimates of the Population of the United States by Age, Sex, and Race: 1970 to 1977. Population Estimates and Projections. *Current Population Reports.* Series P–25, No. 721, Washington. U.S. Government Printing Office, April 1978.

Table II. Numbers of live births and mother's age groups used to adjust maternal mortality rates to live births in the United States in 1970

Mother's age	Number
All ages.	3,731,386
Under 20 years	656,460
20–24 years	1,418,874
25–29 years	994,904
30–34 years	427,806
35 years and over	233,342

SOURCE: U.S. Bureau of the Census: Population estimates and projections. *Current Population Reports.* Series P-25, No. 499. Washington. U.S. Government Printing Office, May 1973.

health care coverage are age adjusted for the population under 65 years of age using three age groups: under 18 years, 18–44 years, and 45–64 years; and for the population 65 years and over using two age groups: 65–74 years and 75 years and over. The NHIS data on smoking in the population 18 years and over are age adjusted using five age groups: 18–24 years, 25–34 years, 35–44 years, 45–64 years, and 65 years and over. The NHIS data on smoking in the population 25 years and over are age adjusted using four age groups: 25–34 years, 35–44 years, 45–64 years, and 65 years and over. The NHIS data on no usual source of health care among adults are age adjusted using three groups: 18–24 years, 25–44 years, and 45–64 years.

Health Care Surveys—Data from the four health care surveys, National Hospital Discharge Survey (NHDS), National Survey of Ambulatory Surgery (NSAS), National Ambulatory Medical Care Survey (NAMCS), and National Hospital Ambulatory Medical Care Survey (NHAMCS) are age adjusted to the 1970 civilian noninstitutionalized population using five age groups: under 15 years, 15–44 years, 45–64 years, 65–74 years, and 75 years and over (table III).

National Health and Nutrition Examination Survey— Data from the National Health Examination Survey (NHES) and the National Health and Nutrition Examination Survey (NHANES) are age adjusted to the 1980 U.S. resident population using five age groups for adults: 20–34 years, 35–44 years, 45–54 years, 55–64 years, and 65–74 years (table III). Data for children aged 6–11 years and 12–17 years are age adjusted within each group using two subgroups: 6–8 years and 9–11 years; and 12–14 years and 15–17 years (table III).

AIDS—See *Acquired immunodeficiency syndrome.*

Air quality standards—See *National ambient air quality standards.*

Air pollution—See *Pollutant.*

Alcohol abuse treatment clients—See *Substance abuse treatment clients.*

Ambulatory care—Health care provided to persons without their admission to a health facility.

Ambulatory surgery—According to the National Survey of Ambulatory Surgery (NSAS), ambulatory surgery refers to previously scheduled surgical and nonsurgical procedures performed on an outpatient basis in a hospital or freestanding ambulatory surgery center's general or main operating rooms, satellite operating rooms, cystoscopy rooms, endoscopy rooms, cardiac catheterization labs, and laser procedure rooms. Procedures performed in locations dedicated exclusively to dentistry, podiatry, abortion, pain block, or small procedures were not included.

In NSAS, data on up to six surgical and non-surgical procedures are collected and coded. See related *Outpatient surgery.*

Average annual rate of change (percent change)—In this report average annual rates of change or growth rates are calculated as follows:

$$[(P_n / P_o)^{1/N} - 1] \times 100$$

where P_n = later time period
 P_o = earlier time period
 N = number of years in interval.

This geometric rate of change assumes that a variable increases or decreases at the same rate during each year between the two time periods.

Average length of stay—In the National Health Interview Survey, the average length of stay per discharged patient is computed by dividing the total number of hospital days for a specified group by the total number of discharges for that group. Similarly, in the National Hospital Discharge Survey, the average length of stay is computed by dividing the total number of days of care, counting the date of admission but not the date of discharge, by the number of patients discharged. The American Hospital Association computes the average length of stay by dividing the number of inpatient days by the number of admissions. See related *Days of care; Discharge; Patient.*

Bed—Any bed that is set up and staffed for use by inpatients is counted as a bed in a facility. For the American Hospital Association the count is the average number of beds, cribs, and pediatric bassinets during the entire reporting period. In the Health Care Financing Administration's Online Survey Certification and Reporting database, all beds in certified facilities are counted on the day of certification inspection. The World Health Organization defines a hospital bed as one regularly maintained and staffed for the accommodation and full-time care of a succession of inpatients and situated in a part of the hospital where continuous medical care for inpatients is provided. The Center for Mental Health Services counts the number of beds set up and staffed for use in inpatient and residential treatment services on the last day of the survey reporting period. See related *Hospital; Mental health organization; Mental health service type; Occupancy rate.*

Birth cohort—A birth cohort consists of all persons born within a given period of time, such as a calendar year.

Birth rate—See *Rate: Birth and related rates.*

Birthweight—The first weight of the newborn obtained after birth. Low birthweight is defined as less than 2,500 grams or 5 pounds 8 ounces. Very low birthweight is defined as less than 1,500 grams or 3 pounds 4 ounces. Before 1979 low birthweight was defined as 2,500 grams or less and very low birthweight as 1,500 grams or less.

Body mass index (BMI)— BMI is a measure that adjusts body weight for height. It is calculated as weight in kilograms divided by height in meters squared. Sex- and age-specific cut points of BMI are used in this book in the definition of overweight for children and adolescents. Healthy weight for adults is defined as a BMI of 19 to less than 25; overweight, as greater than or equal to a BMI of 25; and obesity, as greater than or equal to a BMI of 30. BMI cut points are defined in the Report of the Dietary Guidelines Advisory Committee on the Dietary Guidelines for Americans, 1995. U.S. Department of Agriculture, Agricultural Research Service, Dietary Guidelines

Table IV. Revision of the *International Classification of Diseases*, according to year of conference by which adopted and years in use in the United States

Revision of the International Classification of Diseases	Year of conference by which adopted	Years in use in United States
First.	1900	1900–1909
Second.	1909	1910–1920
Third	1920	1921–1929
Fourth	1929	1930–1938
Fifth.	1938	1939–1948
Sixth	1948	1949–1957
Seventh	1955	1958–1967
Eighth	1965	1968–1978
Ninth	1975	1979–present

Advisory Committee. 1995. pp.23–4; Clinical Guidelines on the Identification, Evaluation, and Treatment of Overweight and Obesity in Adults: The Evidence Report. National Institutes of Health. National Heart, Lung, and Blood Institute. in press; and in the Healthy People 2010 Objectives: Draft for Public Comment. September 15, 1998. Objectives 2.1, 2.2, and 2.3.

Cause of death—For the purpose of national mortality statistics, every death is attributed to one underlying condition, based on information reported on the death certificate and utilizing the international rules for selecting the underlying cause of death from the reported conditions. Beginning with 1979 the *International Classification of Diseases, Ninth Revision* (ICD-9) has been used for coding cause of death. Data from earlier time periods were coded using the appropriate revision of the ICD for that time period. (See tables IV and V.) Changes in classification of causes of death in successive revisions of the ICD may introduce discontinuities in cause-of-death statistics over time. For further discussion, see Technical Appendix in National Center for Health Statistics: *Vital Statistics of the United States, 1990, Volume II, Mortality, Part A.* DHHS Pub. No. (PHS) 95–1101, Public Health Service, Washington, U.S. Government Printing Office, 1994. See related *Human immunodeficiency virus infection; International Classification of Diseases, Ninth Revision.*

Cause-of-death ranking—Cause-of-death ranking for infants is based on the List of 61 Selected Causes of Infant Death and HIV infection (ICD-9 Nos.

Appendix II ....

Table V. Cause-of-death codes, according to applicable revision of *International Classification of Diseases*

Cause of death	Code numbers			
	Sixth Revision	Seventh Revision	Eighth Revision	Ninth Revision
Communicable diseases	. . .	. . .	. . .	001–139, 460–466, 480–487
Chronic and other non-communicable diseases	. . .	. . .	. . .	140–459, 467–479, 488–799
Injury and adverse effects	. . .	. . .	. . .	E800–E999
Meningococcal infection	. . .	. . .	. . .	036
Septicemia	. . .	. . .	. . .	038
Human immunodeficiency virus infection[1] . . .	. . .	. . .	. . .	*042–*044
Malignant neoplasms	140–205	140–205	140–209	140–208
Colorectal	153–154	153–154	153–154	153, 154
Malignant neoplasm of peritoneum and pleura		. . .	158, 163.0	158, 163
Respiratory system	160–164	160–164	160–163	160–165
Malignant neoplasm of trachea, bronchus and lung				162
Breast	170	170	174	174–175
Prostate	177	177	185	185
Benign neoplasms				210–239
Diabetes mellitus	260	260	250	250
Anemias	. . .	. . .	. . .	280–285
Meningitis	. . .	. . .	. . .	320–322
Alzheimer's disease				331.0
Diseases of heart	410–443	400–402, 410–443	390–398, 402, 404, 410–429	390–398, 402, 404–429
Ischemic heart disease	. . .	. . .	. . .	410–414
Cerebrovascular diseases	330–334	330–334	430–438	430–438
Atherosclerosis			. . .	440
Pneumonia and influenza	480–483, 490–493	480–483, 490–493	470–474, 480–486	480–487
Chronic obstructive pulmonary diseases	241, 501, 502, 527.1	241, 501, 502, 527.1	490–493, 519.3	490–496
Coalworkers' pneumoconiosis	. . .	. . .	515.1	500
Asbestosis			515.2	501
Silicosis			515.0	502
Chronic liver disease and cirrhosis	581	581	571	571
Nephritis, nephrotic syndrome, and nephrosis	. . .	. . .	. . .	580–589
Complications of pregnancy, childbirth, and the puerperium	640–689	640–689	630–678	630–676
Congenital anomalies	. . .	. . .	. . .	740–759
Certain conditions originating in the perinatal period	. . .	. . .	. . .	760–779
Newborn affected by maternal complications of pregnancy	. . .	. . .	. . .	761
Newborn affected by complications of placenta, cord, and membranes	. . .	. . .	. . .	762
Disorders relating to short gestation and unspecified low birthweight	. . .	. . .	. . .	765
Birth trauma	. . .	. . .	. . .	767
Intrauterine hypoxia and birth asphyxia . . .	. . .	. . .	. . .	768
Respiratory distress syndrome	. . .	. . .	. . .	769
Infections specific to the perinatal period . .	. . .	. . .	. . .	771
Sudden infant death syndrome				798.0
Unintentional injuries[2]	E800–E962	E800–E962	E800–E949	E800–E949
Motor vehicle-related injuries[2]	E810–E835	E810–E835	E810–E823	E810–E825
Suicide	E963, E970–E979	E963, E970–E979	E950–E959	E950–E959
Homicide and legal intervention	E964, E980–E985	E964, E980–E985	E960–E978	E960–E978
Firearm-related injuries	. . .	. . .	E922, E955, E965, E970, E985	E922, E955.0–E955.4, E965.0–E965.4, E970, E985.0–E985.4

. . .   Category not applicable.

[1]Categories for coding human immunodeficiency virus infection were introduced in 1987. The * indicates codes are not part of the Ninth Revision.

[2]In the public health community, the term "unintentional injuries" is preferred to "accidents and adverse effects" and "motor vehicle-related injuries" to "motor vehicle accidents."

*042–*044). Cause-of-death ranking for other ages is based on the List of 72 Selected Causes of Death, HIV infection, and Alzheimer's disease. The List of 72 Selected Causes of Death was adapted from one of the special lists for mortality tabulations recommended by the World Health Organization for use with the *Ninth Revision of the International Classification of Diseases*. Two group titles—Certain conditions originating in the perinatal period and Symptoms, signs, and ill-defined conditions—are not ranked from the List of 61 Selected Causes of Infant Death; and two group titles—Major cardiovascular diseases and Symptoms, signs, and ill-defined conditions—are not ranked from the List of 72 Selected Causes. In addition, category titles that begin with the words "Other" and "All other" are not ranked. The remaining category titles are ranked according to number of deaths to determine the leading causes of death. When one of the titles that represent a subtotal is ranked (for example, unintentional injuries), its component parts are not ranked (in this case, motor vehicle crashes and all other unintentional injuries). See related *International Classification of Diseases, Ninth Revision*.

Civilian noninstitutionalized population; Civilian population—See *Population*.

Cocaine-related emergency room episodes—The Drug Abuse Warning Network monitors selected adverse medical consequences of cocaine and other drug abuse episodes by measuring contacts with hospital emergency rooms. Contacts may be for drug overdose, unexpected drug reactions, chronic abuse, detoxification, or other reasons in which drug use is known to have occurred.

Cohort fertility—Cohort fertility refers to the fertility of the same women at successive ages. Women born during a 12-month period comprise a birth cohort. Cohort fertility for birth cohorts of women is measured by central birth rates, which represent the number of births occurring to women of an exact age divided by the number of women of that exact age. Cumulative birth rates by a given exact age represent the total childbearing experience of women in a cohort up to

that age. Cumulative birth rates are sums of central birth rates for specified cohorts and show the number of children ever born up to the indicated age. For example, the cumulative birth rate for women exactly 30 years of age as of January 1, 1960, is the sum of the central birth rates for the 1930 birth cohort for the years 1944 (when its members were age 14) through 1959 (when they were age 29). Cumulative birth rates are also calculated for specific birth orders at each exact age of woman. The percent of women who have not had at least one live birth by a certain age is found by subtracting the cumulative first birth rate for women of that age from 1,000 and dividing by 10. For method of calculation, see Heuser RL. *Fertility tables for birth cohorts by color: United States, 1917–73*. Rockville, Maryland. NCHS. 1976. See related *Rate: Birth and related rates*.

Community hospitals—See *Hospital*.

Compensation—See *Employer costs for employee compensation*.

Completed fertility rate—See *Rate: Birth and related rates*.

Condition—A health condition is a departure from a state of physical or mental well-being. An impairment is a health condition that includes chronic or permanent health defects resulting from disease, injury, or congenital malformations. All health conditions, except impairments, are coded according to the *International Classification of Diseases, Ninth Revision, Clinical Modification (ICD–9–CM)*.

Based on duration, there are two categories of conditions, acute and chronic. In the National Health Interview Survey, an *acute condition* is a condition that has lasted less than 3 months and has involved either a physician visit (medical attention) or restricted activity. A *chronic condition* refers to any condition lasting 3 months or more or is a condition classified as chronic regardless of its time of onset (for example, diabetes, heart conditions, emphysema, and arthritis). The National Nursing Home Survey uses a specific list of chronic conditions, also disregarding time of onset. See related *International Classification of Diseases, Ninth Revision, Clinical Modification.*

Consumer Price Index (CPI)—CPI is prepared by the U.S. Bureau of Labor Statistics. It is a monthly measure of the average change in the prices paid by urban consumers for a fixed market basket of goods and services. The medical care component of CPI shows trends in medical care prices based on specific indicators of hospital, medical, dental, and drug prices. A revision of the definition of CPI has been in use since January 1988. See related *Gross domestic product; Health expenditures, national.*

Crude birth rate; Crude death rate—See *Rate: Birth and related rates; Rate: Death and related rates.*

Current smoker—In 1992 the definition of current smoker in the National Health Interview Survey (NHIS) was modified to specifically include persons who smoked on "some days." Before 1992 a current smoker was defined by the following questions from the NHIS survey "Have you ever smoked 100 cigarettes in your lifetime?" and "Do you smoke now?" (traditional definition). In 1992 data were collected for half the respondents using the traditional smoking questions and for the other half of respondents using a revised smoking question ("Do you smoke every day, some days, or not at all?"). An unpublished analysis of the 1992 traditional smoking measure revealed that the crude percent of current smokers 18 years of age and over remained the same as 1991. The statistics for 1992 combine data collected using the traditional and the revised questions. For further information on survey methodology and sample sizes pertaining to the NHIS cigarette data for data years 1965–92 and other sources of cigarette smoking data available from the National Center for Health Statistics, see: National Center for Health Statistics, *Biographies and Data Sources, Smoking Data Guide,* No. 1, DHHS Pub. No. (PHS) 91–1308-1, Public Health Service. Washington. U.S. Government Printing Office. 1991.

Starting with 1993 data estimates of cigarette smoking prevalence are based on the revised definition

that is considered a more complete estimate of smoking prevalence. In 1993–95 estimates of cigarette smoking prevalence were based on a half-sample. Smoking data were not collected in 1996.

Days of care—According to the American Hospital Association, days, hospital days, or inpatient days are the number of adult and pediatric days of care rendered during the entire reporting period. Days of care for newborns are excluded.

In the National Health Interview Survey, hospital days during the year refer to the total number of hospital days occurring in the 12-month period before the interview week. A hospital day is a night spent in the hospital for persons admitted as inpatients.

In the National Hospital Discharge Survey, days of care refers to the total number of patient days accumulated by patients at the time of discharge from non-Federal short-stay hospitals during a reporting period. All days from and including the date of admission but not including the date of discharge are counted. See related *Admission; Average length of stay; Discharge; Hospital; Patient.*

Death rate—See *Rate: Death and related rates.*

Dental visit—The National Health Interview Survey considers dental visits to be visits to a dentist's office for treatment or advice, including services by a technician or hygienist acting under the dentist's supervision. Services provided to hospital inpatients are not included. Dental visits are based on a 12-month recall period.

Diagnosis—See *First-listed diagnosis.*

Diagnostic and other nonsurgical procedures—See *Procedure.*

Discharge—The National Health Interview Survey defines a hospital discharge as the completion of any continuous period of stay of one night or more in a hospital as an inpatient, not including the period of stay of a well newborn infant. According to the National Hospital Discharge Survey and the American Hospital Association, discharge is the formal release of an inpatient by a hospital (excluding newborn infants), that is, the termination of a period of hospitalization (including stays of 0 nights) by death or by disposition to a place of residence, nursing home, or another hospital. See related *Admission; Average length of stay; Days of care; Patient.*

Domiciliary care homes—See *Nursing home.*

Drug abuse treatment clients—See *Substance abuse treatment clients.*

Emergency department—According to the National Hospital Ambulatory Medical Care Survey (NHAMCS), an emergency department is a hospital facility for the provision of unscheduled outpatient services to patients whose conditions require immediate care and is staffed 24 hours a day. Off-site emergency departments open less than 24 hours are included if staffed by the hospital's emergency department. An emergency department visit is a direct personal exchange between a patient and a physician or other health care providers working under the physician's supervision, for the purpose of seeking care and receiving personal health services. See related *Hospital; Outpatient department.*

Employer costs for employee compensation—A measure of the average cost per employee hour worked to employers for wages and salaries and benefits. Wages and salaries are defined as the hourly straight-time wage rate, or for workers not paid on an hourly basis, straight-time earnings divided by the corresponding hours. Straight-time wage and salary rates are total earnings before payroll deductions, excluding premium pay for overtime and for work on weekends and holidays, shift differentials, nonproduction bonuses, and lump-sum payments provided in lieu of wage increases. Production bonuses, incentive earnings, commission payments, and cost-of-living adjustments are included in straight-time wage and salary rates. Benefits covered are paid leave—paid vacations, holidays, sick leave, and other leave; supplemental pay—premium pay for overtime and work on weekends and holidays, shift differentials, nonproduction bonuses, and lump-sum payments

provided in lieu of wage increases; insurance benefits—life, health, and sickness and accident insurance; retirement and savings benefits—pension and other retirement plans and savings and thrift plans; legally required benefits—social security, railroad retirement and supplemental retirement, railroad unemployment insurance, Federal and State unemployment insurance, workers' compensation, and other benefits required by law, such as State temporary disability insurance; and other benefits—severance pay and supplemental unemployment plans.

Expenditures—See *Health expenditures, national.*

Family income—For purposes of the National Health Interview Survey and National Health and Nutrition Examination Survey, all people within a household related to each other by blood, marriage, or adoption constitute a family. Each member of a family is classified according to the total income of the family. Unrelated individuals are classified according to their own income. Family income is the total income received by the members of a family (or by an unrelated individual) in the 12 months before the interview. Family income includes wages, salaries, rents from property, interest, dividends, profits and fees from their own businesses, pensions, and help from relatives. Family income has generally been categorized into approximate quintiles in the tables.

Federal hospitals—See *Hospital.*

Federal physicians—See *Physician.*

Fee-for-service health insurance—This is private (commercial) health insurance that reimburses health care providers on the basis of a fee for each health service provided to the insured person. Also known as indemnity health insurance. See related *Health insurance coverage.*

Fertility rate—See *Rate: Birth and related rates.*

Fetal death—In the World Health Organization's definition, also adopted by the United Nations and the National Center for Health Statistics, a fetal death is death before the complete expulsion or extraction from its mother of a product of conception, irrespective of the duration of pregnancy; the death is indicated by the fact that after such separation, the fetus does not breathe or show any other evidence of life, such as beating of the heart, pulsation of the umbilical cord, or definite movement of voluntary muscles. For statistical purposes, fetal deaths are classified according to gestational age. In this report tabulations are shown for fetal deaths with stated or presumed gestation of 20 weeks or more and of 28 weeks or more, the latter gestational age group also known as late fetal deaths. See related *Gestation; Live birth; Rate: Death and related rates.*

First-listed diagnosis—In the National Hospital Discharge Survey this is the first recorded final diagnosis on the medical record face sheet (summary sheet).

General hospitals—See *Hospital.*

General hospitals providing separate psychiatric services—See *Mental health organization.*

Geographic region and division—The 50 States and the District of Columbia are grouped for statistical purposes by the U.S. Bureau of the Census into 4 geographic regions and 9 divisions. The groupings are as follows:

■ Northeast
New England
Maine, New Hampshire, Vermont, Massachusetts, Rhode Island, Connecticut
Middle Atlantic
New York, New Jersey, Pennsylvania

■ Midwest
East North Central
Ohio, Indiana, Illinois, Michigan, Wisconsin
West North Central
Minnesota, Iowa, Missouri, North Dakota, South Dakota, Nebraska, Kansas

■ South
South Atlantic
Delaware, Maryland, District of Columbia, Virginia, West Virginia, North Carolina, South Carolina, Georgia, Florida
East South Central
Kentucky, Tennessee, Alabama, Mississippi
West South Central
Arkansas, Louisiana, Oklahoma, Texas

■ West
Mountain
Montana, Idaho, Wyoming, Colorado, New Mexico, Arizona, Utah, Nevada
Pacific
Washington, Oregon, California, Alaska, Hawaii

Gestation—For the National Vital Statistics System and the Centers for Disease Control and Prevention's Abortion Surveillance, the period of gestation is defined as beginning with the first day of the last normal menstrual period and ending with the day of birth or day of termination of pregnancy. See related *Abortion; Fetal death; Live birth.*

Gross domestic product (GDP)—GDP is the market value of the goods and services produced by labor and property located in the United States. As long as the labor and property are located in the United States, the suppliers (that is, the workers and, for property, the owners) may be either U.S. residents or residents of the rest of the world. See related *Consumer Price Index; Health expenditures, national.*

Health expenditures, national—See related *Consumer Price Index; Gross domestic product.*

Health services and supplies expenditures—These are outlays for goods and services relating directly to patient care plus expenses for administering health insurance programs and government public health activities. This category is equivalent to total national health expenditures minus expenditures for research and construction.

National health expenditures—This measure estimates the amount spent for all health services and supplies and health-related research and construction activities consumed in the United States during the calendar year. Detailed estimates are available by source of expenditures (for example, out-of-pocket payments, private health insurance, and government programs), type of expenditures (for example, hospital care, physician services, and drugs), and are in current dollars for the year of report. Data are compiled from a variety of sources.

Nursing home expenditures—These cover care rendered in skilled nursing and intermediate care facilities, including those for the mentally retarded. The costs of long-term care provided by hospitals are excluded.

Personal health care expenditures—These are outlays for goods and services relating directly to patient care. The expenditures in this category are total national health expenditures minus expenditures for research and construction, expenses for administering health insurance programs, and government public health activities.

Private expenditures—These are outlays for services provided or paid for by nongovernmental sources—consumers, insurance companies, private industry, philanthropic, and other nonpatient care sources.

Public expenditures—These are outlays for services provided or paid for by Federal, State, and local government agencies or expenditures required by governmental mandate (such as, workmen's compensation insurance payments).

Health insurance coverage—National Health Interview Survey (NHIS) respondents were asked about their health insurance coverage at the time of the interview in 1984, 1989, and 1997 and in the previous month in 1993–96. Questions on health insurance coverage were expanded starting in 1993 compared with previous years. In 1997 the entire questionnaire

was redesigned and data were collected using a computer assisted personal interview (CAPI).

Respondents are covered by private health insurance if they indicate private health insurance or if they are covered by a single service hospital plan, except in 1997 when no information on single service plans was obtained. Private health insurance includes managed care such as health maintenance organizations (HMO's).

Until 1996 persons were defined as having Medicaid or other public assistance coverage if they indicated that they had either Medicaid or other public assistance, or if they reported receiving Aid to Families with Dependent Children (AFDC) or Supplementary Security Income (SSI). After welfare reform in late 1996, Medicaid was delinked from AFDC and SSI. In 1997 persons were considered to be covered by Medicaid if they reported Medicaid or a State-sponsored health program.

Medicare or military health plan coverage is also determined in the interview, and in 1997 other government-sponsored program was determined.

If respondents do not report coverage under one of the above types of plans and they have unknown coverage on either private health insurance or Medicaid then they are considered to have unknown coverage.

The remaining respondents are considered uninsured. The uninsured are persons who do not have coverage under private health insurance, Medicare, Medicaid, public assistance, a State-sponsored health plan, other government-sponsored programs, or a military health plan. Persons with only Indian Health Service coverage are considered uninsured. Estimates of the percent of persons who are uninsured based on the NHIS (table 129) are slightly higher than those based on the March Current Population Survey (CPS) (table 146). The NHIS asks about coverage at the time of the survey (or in some survey years, coverage during the previous month), whereas the CPS asks about coverage over the previous calendar year. This may result in higher estimates of Medicaid and other health insurance coverage and correspondingly lower estimates of persons without health care coverage in the CPS compared with the NHIS. In addition, the CPS estimate is for persons of all ages whereas the NHIS estimate is for persons under age 65. See related *Fee-for-service health insurance; Health maintenance organization; Managed care; Medicaid; Medicare.*

Health maintenance organization (HMO)—An HMO is a prepaid health plan delivering comprehensive care to members through designated providers, having a fixed monthly payment for health care services, and requiring members to be in a plan for a specified period of time (usually 1 year). Pure HMO enrollees use only the prepaid capitated health services of the HMO's panel of medical care providers. Open-ended HMO enrollees use the prepaid HMO health services but in addition may receive medical care from providers who are not part of the HMO's panel. There is usually a substantial deductible, copayment, or coinsurance associated with the use of nonpanel providers. These open-ended products are governed by State HMO regulations. HMO model types are:

Group—An HMO that delivers health services through a physician group that is controlled by the HMO unit or an HMO that contracts with one or more independent group practices to provide health services.

Individual practice association (IPA)—An HMO that contracts directly with physicians in independent practice, and/or contracts with one or more associations of physicians in independent practice, and/or contracts with one or more multispecialty group practices. The plan is predominantly organized around solo-single-specialty practices.

Mixed—An HMO that combines features of group and IPA. This category was introduced in mid-1990 because HMO's are continually changing and many now combine features of group and IPA plans in a single plan.

See related *Managed care.*

Health services and supplies expenditures—See *Health expenditures, national.*

Health status, respondent-assessed—Health status was measured in the National Health Interview Survey by asking the respondent, "Would you say _____'s health is excellent, very good, good, fair, or poor?"

Hispanic origin—Hispanic origin includes persons of Mexican, Puerto Rican, Cuban, Central and South American, and other or unknown Latin American or Spanish origins. Persons of Hispanic origin may be of any race. See related *Race.*

HIV—See *Human immunodeficiency virus infection.*

Home health care—Home health care as defined by the National Home and Hospice Care Survey is care provided to individuals and families in their place of residence for promoting, maintaining, or restoring health; or for minimizing the effects of disability and illness including terminal illness.

Hospice care—Hospice care as defined by the National Home and Hospice Care Survey is a program of palliative and supportive care services providing physical, psychological, social, and spiritual care for dying persons, their families, and other loved ones. Hospice services are available in home and inpatient settings.

Hospital—According to the American Hospital Association, hospitals are licensed institutions with at least six beds whose primary function is to provide diagnostic and therapeutic patient services for medical conditions by an organized physician staff, and have continuous nursing services under the supervision of registered nurses. The World Health Organization considers an establishment to be a hospital if it is permanently staffed by at least one physician, can offer inpatient accommodation, and can provide active medical and nursing care. Hospitals may be classified by type of service, ownership, size in terms of number of beds, and length of stay. In the National Hospital Ambulatory Medical Care Survey (NHAMCS) hospitals include all those with an average length of stay for all patients of less than 30 days (short-stay) or hospitals whose specialty is general (medical or surgical) or children's general. Federal hospitals and hospital units of institutions and hospitals with fewer than six beds staffed for patient use are excluded. See related *Average length of stay; Bed; Days of care; Emergency department; Outpatient department; Patient.*

Community hospitals traditionally included all non-Federal short-stay hospitals except facilities for the mentally retarded. In the revised definition the following additional sites are excluded: hospital units of institutions, and alcoholism and chemical dependency facilities.

Federal hospitals are operated by the Federal Government.

For profit hospitals are operated for profit by individuals, partnerships, or corporations.

General hospitals provide diagnostic, treatment, and surgical services for patients with a variety of medical conditions. According to the World Health Organization, these hospitals provide medical and nursing care for more than one category of medical discipline (for example, general medicine, specialized medicine, general surgery, specialized surgery, and obstetrics). Excluded are hospitals, usually in rural areas, that provide a more limited range of care.

Nonprofit hospitals are operated by a church or other nonprofit organization.

Psychiatric hospitals are ones whose major type of service is psychiatric care. See *Mental health organization.*

Registered hospitals are hospitals registered with the American Hospital Association. About 98 percent of hospitals are registered.

Short-stay hospitals in the National Hospital Discharge Survey are those in which the average length of stay is less than 30 days. The National Health Interview Survey defines short-stay hospitals as any hospital or hospital department in which the type of service provided is general; maternity; eye, ear, nose, and throat; children's; or osteopathic.

Specialty hospitals, such as psychiatric, tuberculosis, chronic disease, rehabilitation, maternity, and alcoholic or narcotic, provide a particular type of service to the majority of their patients.

Hospital-based physician—See *Physician.*

Hospital days—See *Days of care.*

Human immunodeficiency virus (HIV) infection—Mortality coding: Beginning with data for 1987, NCHS introduced category numbers *042–*044 for classifying and coding HIV infection as a cause of death. HIV infection was formerly referred to as human T-cell lymphotropic virus-III/lymphadenopathy-associated virus (HTLV-III/LAV) infection. The asterisk before the category numbers indicates that these codes are not part of the *Ninth Revision of the International Classification of Diseases* (ICD-9). Before 1987 deaths involving HIV infection were classified to Deficiency of cell-mediated immunity (ICD-9 279.1) contained in the title All other diseases; to Pneumocystosis (ICD-9 136.3) contained in the title All other infectious and parasitic diseases; to Malignant neoplasms, including neoplasms of lymphatic and hematopoietic tissues; and to a number of other causes. Therefore, before 1987, death statistics for HIV infection are not strictly comparable with data for 1987 and later years, and are not shown in this report.

Morbidity coding: The National Hospital Discharge Survey codes diagnosis data using the *International Classification of Diseases, Ninth Revision, Clinical Modification* (ICD-9-CM). Discharges with diagnosis of HIV as shown in *Health, United States*, have at least one HIV diagnosis listed on the face sheet of the medical record and are not limited to the first-listed diagnosis. During 1984 and

Table VI. Codes for industries, according to the *Standard Industrial Classification (SIC) Manual*

Industry	Code numbers
Agriculture, forestry, and fishing	01–09
Mining	10–14
Construction	15–17
Manufacturing	20–39
Transportation, communication, and public utilities	40–49
Wholesale trade	50–51
Retail trade	52–59
Finance, insurance, and real estate	60–67
Services	70–89
Public administration	91–97

1985 only data for AIDS (ICD–9–CM 279.19) were included. In 1986–94, discharges with the following diagnoses were included: acquired immunodeficiency syndrome (AIDS), human immunodeficiency virus (HIV) infection and associated conditions, and positive serological or viral culture findings for HIV (ICD–9–CM 042–044, 279.19, and 795.8). Beginning in 1995 discharges with the following diagnoses were included: human immunodeficiency virus (HIV) disease and asymptomatic human immunodeficiency virus (HIV) infection status (ICD–9–CM 042 and V08). See related *Acquired immunodeficiency syndrome; Cause of death; International Classification of Diseases, Ninth Revision; International Classification of Diseases, Ninth Revision, Clinical Modification.*

ICD; ICD codes—See *Cause of death; International Classification of Diseases, Ninth Revision.*

Incidence—Incidence is the number of cases of disease having their onset during a prescribed period of time. It is often expressed as a rate (for example, the incidence of measles per 1,000 children 5–15 years of age during a specified year). Incidence is a measure of morbidity or other events that occur within a specified period of time. See related *Prevalence.*

Individual practice association (IPA)—See *Health maintenance organization (HMO).*

Industry of employment—Industries are classified according to the *Standard Industrial Classification (SIC) Manual* of the Office of

Management and Budget. Three editions of the SIC are used for coding industry data in *Health, United States*: the 1972 edition; the 1977 supplement to the 1972 edition; and the 1987 edition.

The changes between versions include a few detailed titles created to correct or clarify industries or to recognize changes within the industry. Codes for major industrial divisions (table VI) were not changed between versions.

The category "Private sector" includes all industrial divisions except public administration and military. The category "Civilian sector" includes "Private sector" and the public administration division. The category "Not classified" is comprised of the following entries from the death certificate: housewife, student, or self-employed; information inadequate to code industry; establishments not elsewhere classified.

Infant death—An infant death is the death of a live-born child before his or her first birthday. Deaths in the first year of life may be further classified according to age as neonatal and postneonatal. Neonatal deaths are those that occur before the 28th day of life; postneonatal deaths are those that occur between 28 and 365 days of age. See *Live birth; Rate: Death and related rates.*

Inpatient care—See *Mental health service type.*

Inpatient days—See *Days of care.*

Insured—See *Health insurance coverage.*

Intermediate care facilities—See *Nursing home.*

International Classification of Diseases, Ninth Revision (ICD-9)—The *International Classification of Diseases* (ICD) classifies mortality information for statistical purposes. The ICD was first used in 1900 and has been revised about every 10 years since then. The ICD-9, published in 1977, is used to code U.S. mortality data beginning with data year 1979. (See tables IV and V.) See related *Cause of death; International Classification of Diseases, Ninth Revision, Clinical Modification.*

Table VII. Codes for diagnostic categories from the *International Classification of Diseases, Ninth Revision, Clinical Modification*

Diagnostic category	Code numbers
Females with delivery	V27
Human immunodeficiency virus (HIV) (1984–85)	279.19
(1986–94)	042–044, 279.19, 795.8
(Beginning in 1995)	042, V08
Malignant neoplasms	140–208
Large intestine and rectum	153–154, 197.5
Trachea, bronchus, and lung	162, 197.0, 197.3
Breast	174–175, 198.81
Prostate	185
Diabetes	250
Psychoses	293–299
Diseases of the nervous system and sense organs	320–389
Diseases of the circulatory system	390–459
Diseases of heart	391–392.0, 393–398, 402, 404, 410–416, 420–429
Ischemic heart disease	410–414
Acute myocardial infarction	410
Congestive heart failure	428.0
Cerebrovascular diseases	430–438
Diseases of the respiratory system	460–519
Bronchitis	466.0, 490–491
Pneumonia	466.1, 480–487.0
Asthma	493
Hyperplasia of prostate	600
Decubitus ulcers	707.0
Diseases of the musculoskeletal system and connective tissue	710–739
Osteoarthritis	715
Intervertebral disc disorders	722
Injuries and poisoning	800–999
Fracture, all sites	800–829
Fracture of neck of femur (hip)	820

International Classification of Diseases, Ninth Revision, Clinical Modification (ICD–9–CM)—The ICD–9–CM is based on and is completely compatible with the *International Classification of Diseases, Ninth Revision*. The ICD–9–CM is used to code morbidity data and the ICD-9 is used to code mortality data. Diagnostic groupings and code number inclusions for ICD–9–CM are shown in table VII; surgical and nonsurgical operations, diagnostic procedures, and therapeutic procedures and code number inclusions are shown in table VIII.

ICD-9 and ICD–9–CM are arranged in 17 main chapters. Most of the diseases are arranged according to their principal anatomical site, with special chapters for infective and parasitic diseases; neoplasms; endocrine, metabolic, and nutritional diseases; mental diseases; complications of pregnancy and childbirth; certain diseases peculiar to the perinatal period; and ill-defined conditions. In addition, two supplemental classifications are provided: the classification of factors influencing health status and contact with health service and the classification of external causes of injury and poisoning. See related *Condition; International Classification of Diseases, Ninth Revision; Mental health disorder*.

Late fetal death rate—See *Rate: Death and related rates*.

Leading causes of death—See *Cause-of-death ranking*.

Length of stay—See *Average length of stay*.

Life expectancy—Life expectancy is the average number of years of life remaining to a person at a particular age and is based on a given set of age-specific death rates, generally the mortality conditions existing in the period mentioned. Life expectancy may be determined by race, sex, or other characteristics using age-specific death rates for the population with that characteristic. See related *Rate: Death and related rates*.

Table VIII. Codes for procedure categories from the *International Classification of Diseases, Ninth Revision, Clinical Modification*

Procedure category	Code numbers
Extraction of lens	13.1–13.6
Insertion of prosthetic lens (pseudophakos)	13.7
Myringotomy with insertion of tube	20.01
Tonsillectomy, with or without adenoidectomy	28.2–28.3
Coronary angioplasty (Prior to 1997)	36.0
(Beginning in 1997)	36.01–36.05, 36.09
Coronary artery bypass graft	36.1
Cardiac catheterization	37.21–37.23
Pacemaker insertion or replacement	37.7–37.8
Carotid endarterectomy	38.12
Endoscopy of large or small intestine with or without biopsy	45.11–45.14, 45.16, 45.21–45.25
Cholecystectomy	51.2
Prostatectomy	60.2–60.6
Bilateral destruction or occlusion of fallopian tubes	66.2–66.3
Hysterectomy	68.3–68.7, 68.9
Cesarean section	74.0–74.2, 74.4, 74.99
Repair of current obstetrical laceration	75.5–75.6
Reduction of fracture	76.7, 79.0–79.3
Arthroscopy of knee	80.26
Excision or destruction of intervertebral disc	80.5
Total hip replacement	81.51
Lumpectomy	85.21
Mastectomy	85.4
Angiocardiography with contrast material	88.5

Limitation of activity—In the National Health Interview Survey limitation of activity refers to a long-term reduction in a person's capacity to perform the usual kind or amount of activities associated with his or her age group. Each person is classified according to the extent to which his or her activities are limited, as follows:

■ Persons unable to carry on major activity;
■ Persons limited in the amount or kind of major activity performed;
■ Persons not limited in major activity but otherwise limited; and
■ Persons not limited in activity.

See related *Condition; Major activity*.

Live birth—In the World Health Organization's definition, also adopted by the United Nations and the National Center for Health Statistics, a live birth is the complete expulsion or extraction from its mother of a product of conception, irrespective of the duration of the pregnancy, which, after such separation, breathes or shows any other evidence of life such as heartbeat, umbilical cord pulsation, or definite movement of voluntary muscles, whether the umbilical cord has

been cut or the placenta is attached. Each product of such a birth is considered live born. See related *Gestation; Rate: Birth and related rates*.

Live-birth order—In the National Vital Statistics System this item from the birth certificate refers to the total number of live births the mother has had, including the present birth as recorded on the birth certificate. Fetal deaths are excluded. See related *Live birth*.

Low birthweight—See *Birthweight*.

Major activity (or usual activity)—This is the principal activity of a person or of his or her age-sex group. For children 1–5 years of age, the major activity refers to ordinary play with other children; for children 5–17 years of age, the major activity refers to school attendance; for adults 18–69 years of age, the major activity usually refers to a job, housework, or school attendance; for persons 70 years of age and over, the major activity refers to the capacity for independent living (bathe, shop, dress, or eat without needing the help of another person). See related *Limitation of activity*.

Managed care—Managed care is a health care plan that integrates the financing and delivery of health care services by using arrangements with selected health care providers to provide services for covered individuals. Plans are generally financed using capitation fees. There are signifcant financial incentives for members of the plan to use the health care providers associated with the plan. The plan includes formal programs for quality assurance and utilization review. Health maintenance organizations (HMO's), preferred provider organizations (PPO's), and point of service (POS) plans are examples of managed care. See related *Health maintenance organization; Preferred provider organization.*

Marital status—Marital status is classified through self-reporting into the categories married and unmarried. The term married encompasses all married people including those separated from their spouses. Unmarried includes those who are single (never married), divorced, or widowed. The Abortion Surveillance Reports of the Centers for Disease Control and Prevention classified separated people as unmarried before 1978.

Maternal mortality rate—See *Rate: Death and related rates.*

Medicaid—This program is State operated and administered but has Federal financial participation. Within certain broad federally determined guidelines, States decide who is eligible; the amount, duration, and scope of services covered; rates of payment for providers; and methods of administering the program. Medicaid provides health care services for certain low-income persons. Medicaid does not provide health services to all poor people in every State. It categorically covers participants in the Aid to Families with Dependent Children program and in the Supplemental Security Income program. In most States it also covers certain other people deemed to be medically needy. The program was authorized in 1965 by Title XIX of the Social Security Act. See related *Health expenditures, national; Health maintenance organization; Medicare.*

Medical specialties—See *Physician specialty.*

Medical vendor payments—Under the Medicaid program, medical vendor payments are payments (expenditures) to medical vendors from the State through a fiscal agent or to a health insurance plan. Adjustments are made for Indian Health Service payments to Medicaid, cost settlements, third party recoupments, refunds, voided checks, and other financial settlements that cannot be related to specific provided claims. Excluded are payments made for medical care under the emergency assistance provisions, payments made from State medical assistance funds that are not federally matchable, disproportionate share hospital payments, cost sharing or enrollment fees collected from recipients or a third party, and administration and training costs.

Medicare—This is a nationwide health insurance program providing health insurance protection to people 65 years of age and over, people entitled to social security disability payments for 2 years or more, and people with end-stage renal disease, regardless of income. The program was enacted July 30, 1965, as Title XVIII, *Health Insurance for the Aged of the Social Security Act*, and became effective on July 1, 1966. It consists of two separate but coordinated programs, hospital insurance (Part A) and supplementary medical insurance (Part B). See related *Health expenditures, national; Health maintenance organization; Medicaid.*

Mental health disorder—The Center for Mental Health Services defines a mental health disorder as any of several disorders listed in the *International Classification of Diseases, Ninth Revision, Clinical Modification* (ICD–9–CM) or *Diagnostic and Statistical Manual of Mental Disorders, Third Edition* (DSM-IIIR). Table IX shows diagnostic categories and code numbers for ICD–9–CM/DSM-IIIR and corresponding codes for the *International Classification of Diseases, Adapted for Use in the United States, Eighth Revision* (ICDA-8) and *Diagnostic and Statistical Manual of Mental*

Disorders, Second Edition (DSM-II). See related *International Classification of Diseases, Clinical Modification.*

Mental health organization—The Center for Mental Health Services defines a mental health organization as an administratively distinct public or private agency or institution whose primary concern is the provision of direct mental health services to the mentally ill or emotionally disturbed. Excluded are private office-based practices of psychiatrists, psychologists, and other mental health providers; psychiatric services of all types of hospitals or outpatient clinics operated by Federal agencies other than the Department of Veterans Affairs (for example, Public Health Service, Indian Health Service, Department of Defense, and Bureau of Prisons); general hospitals that have no separate psychiatric services, but admit psychiatric patients to nonpsychiatric units; and psychiatric services of schools, colleges, halfway houses, community residential organizations, local and county jails, State prisons, and other human service providers. The major types of mental health organizations are described below.

Freestanding psychiatric outpatient clinics provide only outpatient services on either a regular or emergency basis. The medical responsibility for services is generally assumed by a psychiatrist.

General hospitals providing separate psychiatric services are non-Federal general hospitals that provide psychiatric services in either a separate psychiatric inpatient, outpatient, or partial hospitalization service with assigned staff and space.

Multiservice mental health organizations directly provide two or more of the program elements defined under Mental health service type and are not classifiable as a psychiatric hospital, general hospital, or a residential treatment center for emotionally disturbed children. (The classification of a psychiatric or general hospital or a residential treatment center for emotionally disturbed children takes precedence over a multiservice classification, even if two or more services are offered.)

Partial care organizations provide a program of ambulatory mental health services.

Private mental hospitals are operated by a sole proprietor, partnership, limited partnership, corporation, or nonprofit organization, primarily for the care of persons with mental disorders.

Psychiatric hospitals are hospitals primarily concerned with providing inpatient care and treatment for the mentally ill. Psychiatric inpatient units of Department of Veterans Affairs general hospitals and Department of Veterans Affairs neuropsychiatric hospitals are combined into the category Department of Veterans Affairs psychiatric hospitals because of their similarity in size, operation, and length of stay.

Residential treatment centers for emotionally disturbed children must meet all of the following criteria: (a) Not licensed as a psychiatric hospital and primary purpose is to provide individually planned mental health treatment services in conjunction with residential care; (b) Include a clinical program that is directed by a psychiatrist, psychologist, social worker, or psychiatric nurse with a graduate degree; (c) Serve children and

Table IX. Mental health codes, according to applicable revision of the *Diagnostic and Statistical Manual of Mental Disorders* and *International Classification of Diseases*

Diagnostic category	DSM-II/ICDA-8	DSM-IIIR/ICD-9-CM
Alcohol related	291, 303, 309.13	291, 303, 305.0
Drug related	294.3, 304, 309.14	292, 304, 305.1–305.9, 327, 328
Organic disorders (other than alcoholism and drug)	290, 292, 293, 294 (except 294.3), 309.0, 309.2–309.9	290, 293, 294, 310
Affective disorders	296, 298.0, 300.4	296, 298.0, 300.4, 301.11, 301.13
Schizophrenia	295	295

youth primarily under the age of 18; and (d) Primary diagnosis for the majority of admissions is mental illness, classified as other than mental retardation, developmental disability, and substance-related disorders, according to DSM-II/ICDA-8 or DSM-IIIR/ICD–9–CM codes. See related *Table IX. Mental health codes.*

State and county mental hospitals are under the auspices of a State or county government or operated jointly by a State and county government.

See related *Addition; Mental health service type.*

Mental health service type—refers to the following kinds of mental health services:

Inpatient care is the provision of 24-hour mental health care in a mental health hospital setting.

Outpatient care is the provision of ambulatory mental health services for less than 3 hours at a single visit on an individual, group, or family basis, usually in a clinic or similar organization. Emergency care on a walk-in basis, as well as care provided by mobile teams who visit patients outside these organizations are included. "Hotline" services are excluded.

Partial care treatment is a planned program of mental health treatment services generally provided in visits of 3 or more hours to groups of patients. Included are treatment programs that emphasize intensive short-term therapy and rehabilitation; programs that focus on recreation, and/or occupational program activities, including sheltered workshops; and education and training programs, including special education classes, therapeutic nursery schools, and vocational training.

Residential treatment care is the provision of overnight mental health care in conjunction with an intensive treatment program in a setting other than a hospital. Facilities may offer care to

emotionally disturbed children or mentally ill adults.

See related *Addition; Mental health organization.*

Metropolitan statistical area (MSA)—The definitions and titles of MSA's are established by the U.S. Office of Management and Budget with the advice of the Federal Committee on Metropolitan Statistical Areas. Generally speaking, an MSA consists of a county or group of counties containing at least one city (or twin cities) having a population of 50,000 or more plus adjacent counties that are metropolitan in character and are economically and socially integrated with the central city. In New England, towns and cities rather than counties are the units used in defining MSA's. There is no limit to the number of adjacent counties included in the MSA as long as they are integrated with the central city. Nor is an MSA limited to a single State; boundaries may cross State lines. Metropolitan population, as used in this report in connection with data from the National Health Interview Survey, is based on MSA's as defined in the 1980 census and does not include any subsequent additions or changes.

Multiservice mental health organizations—See *Mental health organization.*

National ambient air quality standards—The Federal Clean Air Act of 1970, amended in 1977 and 1990, required the Environmental Protection Agency (EPA) to establish National Ambient Air Quality Standards. EPA has set specific standards for each of six major pollutants: carbon monoxide, lead, nitrogen dioxide, ozone, sulfur dioxide, and particulate matter whose aerodynamic size is equal to or less than 10 microns (PM-10). Each pollutant standard represents a maximum concentration level (micrograms per cubic meter) that cannot be exceeded during a specified time interval. A county meets the national ambient air quality standards if none of the six pollutants exceed the standard during a 12-month period. See *related Particulate matter; Pollutant.*

Neonatal mortality rate—See *Rate: Death and related rates*.

Non-Federal physicians—See *Physician*.

Nonpatient revenue—Nonpatient revenues are those revenues received for which no direct patient care services are rendered. The most widely recognized source of nonpatient revenues is philanthropy. Philanthropic support may be direct from individuals or may be obtained through philanthropic fund raising organizations such as the United Way. Support may also be obtained from foundations or corporations. Philanthropic revenues may be designated for direct patient care use or may be contained in an endowment fund where only the current income may be tapped.

Nonprofit hospitals—See *Hospital*.

Notifiable disease—A notifiable disease is one that, when diagnosed, health providers are required, usually by law, to report to State or local public health officials. Notifiable diseases are those of public interest by reason of their contagiousness, severity, or frequency.

Nursing care—The following definition of nursing care applies to data collected in National Nursing Home Surveys through 1977. Nursing care is the provision of any of the following services: application of dressings or bandages; bowel and bladder retraining; catheterization; enema; full bed bath; hypodermic, intramuscular, or intravenous injection; irrigation; nasal feeding; oxygen therapy; and temperature-pulse-respiration or blood pressure measurement. See related *Nursing home*.

Nursing care homes—See *Nursing home*.

Nursing home—In the Online Certification and Reporting database, a nursing home is a facility that is certified and meets the Health Care Financing Administration's long-term care requirements for Medicare and Medicaid eligibility. In the National Master Facility Inventory and the National Nursing Home Survey a nursing home is an establishment with three or more beds that provides nursing or personal care services to the aged, infirm, or chronically ill. The following definitions of nursing home types apply to data collected in National Nursing Home Surveys through 1977.

Nursing care homes must employ one or more full-time registered or licensed practical nurses and must provide nursing care to at least one-half the residents.

Personal care homes with nursing have some but fewer than one-half the residents receiving nursing care. In addition, such homes must employ one or more registered or licensed practical nurses or must provide administration of medications and treatments in accordance with physicians' orders, supervision of self-administered medications, or three or more personal services.

Personal care homes without nursing have no residents who are receiving nursing care. These homes provide administration of medications and treatments in accordance with physicians' orders, supervision of self-administered medications, or three or more personal services.

Domiciliary care homes primarily provide supervisory care but also provide one or two personal services.

Nursing homes are certified by the Medicare and/or Medicaid program. The following definitions of certification levels apply to data collected in National Nursing Home Surveys of 1973–74, 1977, and 1985.

Skilled nursing facilities provide the most intensive nursing care available outside of a hospital. Facilities certified by Medicare provide posthospital care to eligible Medicare enrollees. Facilities certified by Medicaid as skilled nursing facilities provide skilled nursing services on a daily basis to individuals eligible for Medicaid benefits.

Intermediate care facilities are certified by the Medicaid program to provide health-related services on a regular basis to Medicaid eligibles who do not require hospital or skilled nursing facility care but do require institutional care above the level of room and board.

Not certified facilities are not certified as providers of care by Medicare or Medicaid.

See related *Nursing care; Resident.*

Nursing home expenditures—See *Health expenditures, national.*

Occupancy rate—The American Hospital Association defines hospital occupancy rate as the average daily census divided by the average number of hospital beds during a reporting period. Average daily census is defined by the American Hospital Association as the average number of inpatients, excluding newborns, receiving care each day during a reporting period. The occupancy rate for facilities other than hospitals is calculated as the number of residents reported at the time of the interview divided by the number of beds reported. In the Online Survey Certification and Reporting database, occupancy is the total number of residents on the day of certification inspection divided by the total number of beds on the day of certification.

Office—In the National Health Interview Survey, an office refers to the office of any physician in private practice not located in a hospital. In the National Ambulatory Medical Care Survey, an office is any location for a physician's ambulatory practice other than hospitals, nursing homes, other extended care facilities, patients' homes, industrial clinics, college clinics, and family planning clinics. However, private offices in hospitals are included. See related *Office visit; Outpatient visit; Physician; Physician contact.*

Office-based physician—See *Physician.*

Office visit—In the National Ambulatory Medical Care Survey, an office visit is any direct personal exchange between an ambulatory patient and a physician or members of his or her staff for the purposes of seeking care and rendering health services. See related *Outpatient visit; Physician contact.*

Operations—See *Procedure.*

Outpatient department—According to the National Hospital Ambulatory Medical Care Survey (NHAMCS), an outpatient department (OPD) is a hospital facility where nonurgent ambulatory medical care is provided. The following are examples of the types of OPD's excluded from the NHAMCS: ambulatory surgical centers, chemotherapy, employee health services, renal dialysis, methadone maintenance, and radiology. An outpatient department visit is a direct personal exchange between a patient and a physician or other health care provider working under the physician's supervision for the purpose of seeking care and receiving personal health services. See related *Emergency department; Hospital.*

Outpatient surgery—According to the American Hospital Association, outpatient surgery is performed on patients who do not remain in the hospital overnight and occurs in inpatient operating suites, outpatient surgery suites, or procedure rooms within an outpatient care facility. Outpatient surgery is a surgical operation, whether major or minor, performed in operating or procedure rooms. A surgical operation involving more than one surgical procedure is considered one surgical operation. See related *Ambulatory surgery.*

Outpatient visit—The American Hospital Association defines outpatient visits as visits for receipt of medical, dental, or other services by patients who are not lodged in the hospital. Each appearance by an outpatient to each unit of the hospital is counted individually as an outpatient visit. See related *Office visit; Physician contact.*

Partial care organization—See *Mental health organization.*

Partial care treatment—See *Mental health service type.*

Particulate matter—Particulate matter is defined as particles of solid or liquid matter in the air, including nontoxic materials (soot, dust, and dirt) and toxic materials (for example, lead, asbestos, suspended sulfates, and nitrates). See related *National ambient air quality standards; Pollutant.*

Patient—A patient is a person who is formally admitted to the inpatient service of a hospital for observation, care, diagnosis, or treatment. See related *Admission; Average length of stay; Days of care; Discharge; Hospital.*

Percent change—See *Average annual rate of change.*

Perinatal mortality rate, ratio—See *Rate: Death and related rates.*

Personal care homes with or without nursing—See *Nursing home.*

Personal health care expenditures—See *Health expenditures, national.*

Physician—Physicians, through self-reporting, are classified by the American Medical Association and others as licensed doctors of medicine or osteopathy, as follows:

Active (or professionally active) physicians are currently practicing medicine for a minimum of 20 hours per week. Excluded are physicians who are inactive practicing medicine less than 20 hours per week, have unknown addresses, or specialties not classified (when specialty information is presented).

Federal physicians are employed by the Federal Government; non-Federal or civilian physicians are not.

Hospital-based physicians spend the plurality of their time as salaried physicians in hospitals.

Office-based physicians spend the plurality of their time working in practices based in private offices.

Data for physicians are presented by type of education (doctor of medicine and doctor of osteopathy), place of education (U.S. medical graduates and international medical graduates); activity status (professionally active and inactive); employment setting (Federal and non-Federal); area of specialty; and geographic area. See related *Office; Physician specialty.*

Physician contact—In the National Health Interview Survey, a physician contact is defined as a consultation with a physician in person or by telephone, for examination, diagnosis, treatment, or advice. The service may be provided by the physician or by another person working under the physician's supervision. Contacts involving services provided on a mass basis (for example, blood pressure screenings) and contacts for hospital inpatients are not included.

Place of contact includes office, hospital outpatient clinics, emergency room, telephone (advice given by a physician in a telephone call), home (any place in which a person was staying at the time a physician was called there), clinics, HMO's, and other places located outside a hospital.

In the National Health Interview Survey, analyses of the annual number of physician contacts and place of contact are based upon data collected using a 2-week recall period and are adjusted to produce annual estimates. Analyses of children without a physician contact during the past 12-month period are based upon a different question that uses a 12-month recall period. Analyses of the interval since last physician contact are based upon the length of time before the week of interview in which the physician was last consulted. See related *Office; Office visit.*

Physician specialty—A physician specialty is any specific branch of medicine in which a physician may concentrate. Data are based on physician self-reports of their primary area of speciality. Physician data are broadly categorized into two general areas of practice: generalists and specialists.

Generalist physicians are synonymous with primary care generalists and only include physicians practicing in the general fields of family and general practice, general internal medicine, and general pediatrics. They specifically exclude primary care specialists.

Primary care specialists practice in the subspecialties of general and family practice, internal medicine, and pediatrics. The primary care subspecialties for family practice include geriatric medicine and sports medicine. Primary care subspecialties for internal medicine include diabetes, endocrinology and metabolism, hematology, hepatology, cardiac electrophysiology, infectious diseases, diagnostic laboratory immunology, geriatric medicine, sports medicine, nephrology, nutrition, medical oncology, and rheumatology. Primary care subspecialties for pediatrics include adolescent medicine, critical care pediatrics, neonatal-perinatal medicine, pediatric allergy, pediatric cardiology, pediatric endocrinology, pediatric pulmonology, pediatric emergency medicine, pediatric gastroenterology, pediatric hematology/oncology, diagnostic laboratory immunology, pediatric nephrology, pediatric rheumatology, and sports medicine.

Specialist physicians practice in the primary care specialties, in addition to all other specialist fields not included in the generalist definition. Specialist fields include allergy and immunology, aerospace medicine, anesthesiology, cardiovascular diseases, child and adolescent psychiatry, colon and rectal surgery, dermatology, diagnostic radiology, forensic pathology, gastroenterology, general surgery, medical genetics, neurology, nuclear medicine, neurological surgery, obstetrics and gynecology, occupational medicine, ophthalmology, orthopedic surgery, otolaryngology, psychiatry, public health and general preventive medicine, physical medicine and rehabilitation, plastic surgery, anatomic and clinical pathology, pulmonary diseases, radiation oncology, thoracic surgery, urology, addiction medicine, critical care medicine, legal medicine, and clinical pharmacology.

See related *Physician.*

Pollutant—A pollutant is any substance that renders the atmosphere or water foul or noxious to health. See related *National ambient air quality standards; Particulate matter.*

Population—The U.S. Bureau of the Census collects and publishes data on populations in the United States according to several different definitions. Various statistical systems then use the appropriate population for calculating rates.

Total population is the population of the United States, including all members of the Armed Forces living in foreign countries, Puerto Rico, Guam, and the U.S. Virgin Islands. Other Americans abroad (for example, civilian Federal employees and dependents of members of the Armed Forces or other Federal employees) are not included.

Resident population includes persons whose usual place of residence (that is, the place where one usually lives and sleeps) is in one of the 50 States or the District of Columbia. It includes members of the Armed Forces stationed in the United States and their families. It excludes international military, naval, and diplomatic personnel and their families located here and residing in embassies or similar quarters. Also excluded are international workers and international students in this country and Americans living abroad. The resident population is usually the denominator when calculating birth and death rates and incidence of disease. The resident population is also the denominator for selected population-based rates that use numerator data from the National Nursing Home Survey.

Civilian population is the resident population excluding members of the Armed Forces. However, families of members of the Armed Forces are included. This population is the denominator in rates calculated for the NCHS National Hospital Discharge Survey.

Civilian noninstitutionalized population is the civilian population not residing in institutions. Institutions include correctional institutions, detention homes, and training schools for juvenile delinquents; homes for the aged and dependent (for example, nursing homes and convalescent homes); homes for dependent and neglected children; homes and schools for the mentally or physically handicapped; homes for unwed mothers; psychiatric, tuberculosis, and chronic disease hospitals; and residential treatment centers. This population is the denominator in rates calculated for the NCHS National Health Interview Survey; National Health and Nutrition Examination Survey; National Ambulatory Medical Care Survey; and the National Hospital Ambulatory Medical Care Survey.

Postneonatal mortality rate—See *Rate: Death and related rates*.

Poverty level—Poverty statistics are based on definitions originally developed by the Social Security Administration. These include a set of money income thresholds that vary by family size and composition. Families or individuals with income below their appropriate thresholds are classified as below the poverty level. These thresholds are updated annually by the U.S. Bureau of the Census to reflect changes in the Consumer Price Index for all urban consumers (CPI-U). For example, the average poverty threshold for a family of four was $16,036 in 1996 and $13,359 in 1990. For more information, see U.S. Bureau of the Census: *Money Income of Households, Families, and Persons in the United States, 1996*. Series P-60. Washington. U.S. Government Printing office. See related *Consumer Price Index*.

Preferred provider organization (PPO)—Health plan generally consisting of hospital and physician providers. The PPO provides health care services to plan members usually at discounted rates in return for expedited claims payment. Plan members can use PPO or non-PPO health care providers, however, financial incentives are built into the benefit structure to encourage utilization of PPO providers. See related *Managed care*.

Prevalence—Prevalence is the number of cases of a disease, infected persons, or persons with some other attribute present during a particular interval of time. It is often expressed as a rate (for example, the prevalence of diabetes per 1,000 persons during a year). See related *Incidence*.

Primary admission diagnosis—In the National Home and Hospice Care Survey the primary admission diagnosis is the first-listed diagnosis at admission on the patient's medical record as provided by the agency staff member most familiar with the care provided to the patient.

Primary care specialties—See *Physician specialty*.

Private expenditures—See *Health expenditures, national*.

Procedure—The National Hospital Discharge Survey (NHDS) and the National Survey of Ambulatory Surgery (NSAS) define a procedure as a surgical or nonsurgical operation, diagnostic procedure, or therapeutic procedure (such as respiratory therapy) recorded on the medical record of discharged patients. A maximum of four procedures per discharge in NHDS and up to six procedures per discharge in NSAS were recorded and coded to the *International Classification of Diseases, Ninth Revision, Clinical Modification*. Previous editions of *Health, United States* classified procedures into surgical and diagnostic and other nonsurgical procedures. The distinction between surgical and diagnostic and nonsurgical procedures has become less meaningful due to the development of minimally invasive and noninvasive procedures thus the practice of classifying procedures has been discontinued. See related *Ambulatory surgery; Outpatient surgery*.

Proprietary hospitals—See *Hospital*.

Psychiatric hospitals—See *Hospital; Mental health organization*.

Public expenditures—See *Health expenditures, national*.

Public health activities—Public health activities may include any of the following essential services of public health—surveillance, investigations, education, community mobilization, workforce training, research, and personal care services delivered or funded by governmental agencies.

Race—Beginning in 1976 the Federal Government's data systems classified individuals into the following racial groups: American Indian or Alaska Native, Asian or Pacific Islander, black, and white. Depending on the data source, the classification by race may be based on self-classification or on observation by an interviewer or other persons filling out the questionnaire. Starting in 1989, data from the National Vital Statistics System for newborn infants and fetal deaths are tabulated according to race of mother, and trend data by race shown in this report have been retabulated by race of mother for all years, beginning with 1980. Before 1980 data were tabulated by race of newborn and fetus according to race of both parents. If the parents were of different races and one parent was white, the child was classified according to the race of the other parent. When neither parent was white, the child was classified according to father's race, with one exception: if either parent was Hawaiian, the child was classified Hawaiian. Before 1964 the National Vital Statistics System classified all births for which race was unknown as white. Beginning in 1964 these births were classified according to information on the previous record.

In *Health, United States*, trends of birth rates, birth characteristics, and infant and maternal mortality rates are calculated according to race of mother unless specified otherwise. Vital event rates for the American Indian or Alaska Native population shown in this book are based on the total U.S. resident population of American Indians and Alaska Natives as enumerated by the U.S. Bureau of Census. In contrast the Indian Health Service calculates vital event rates for this population based on U.S. Bureau of Census county data for American Indians and Alaska Natives who reside on or near reservations. See related *Hispanic origin*.

Rate—A rate is a measure of some event, disease, or condition in relation to a unit of population, along with some specification of time. See related *Age adjustment; Population*.

■ *Birth and related rates*

Birth rate is calculated by dividing the number of live births in a population in a year by the midyear resident population. For census years, rates are based on unrounded census counts of the resident population, as of April 1. For the noncensus years of 1981–89 and 1991, rates are based on national estimates of the resident population, as of July 1, rounded to 1,000's. Population estimates for 5-year age groups are generated by summing unrounded population estimates before rounding to 1,000's. Starting in 1992 rates are based on unrounded national population estimates. Birth rates are expressed as the number of live births per 1,000 population. The rate may be restricted to births to women of specific age, race, marital status, or geographic location (specific rate), or it may be related to the entire population (crude rate). See related *Cohort fertility; Live birth*.

Fertility rate is the total number of live births, regardless of age of mother, per 1,000 women of reproductive age, 15–44 years.

■ *Death and related rates*

Death rate is calculated by dividing the number of deaths in a population in a year by the midyear resident population. For census years, rates are based on unrounded census counts of the resident population, as of April 1. For the noncensus years of 1981–89 and 1991, rates are based on national estimates of the resident population, as of July 1, rounded to 1,000's. Population estimates for 10-year age groups are generated by summing unrounded population estimates before rounding to 1,000's. Starting in 1992 rates are based on unrounded national population estimates. Rates for the Hispanic and non-Hispanic white populations in each year are based on unrounded State population estimates for States in the Hispanic reporting area. Death rates are expressed as the number of deaths per 100,000 population. The rate may be restricted to deaths in specific age, race, sex, or geographic groups or from specific causes of death (specific rate) or it may be related to the entire population (crude rate).

Fetal death rate is the number of fetal deaths with stated or presumed gestation of 20 weeks or more divided by the sum of live births plus fetal deaths, stated per 1,000 live births plus fetal deaths. *Late fetal death rate* is the number of fetal deaths with stated or presumed gestation of 28 weeks or more divided by the sum of live births plus late fetal deaths, stated per 1,000 live births plus late fetal deaths. See related *Fetal death; Gestation.*

Infant mortality rate based on period files is calculated by dividing the number of infant deaths during a calendar year by the number of live births reported in the same year. It is expressed as the number of infant deaths per 1,000 live births. *Neonatal mortality rate* is the number of deaths of children under 28 days of age, per 1,000 live births. *Postneonatal mortality rate* is the number of deaths of children that occur between 28 days and 365 days after birth, per 1,000 live births. See related *Infant death.*

Birth cohort infant mortality rates are based on linked birth and infant death files. In contrast to period rates in which the births and infant deaths occur in the same period or calendar year, infant deaths comprising the numerator of a birth cohort rate may have occurred in the same year as, or in the year following the year of birth. The birth cohort infant mortality rate is expressed as the number of infant deaths per 1,000 live births. See related *Birth cohort.*

Perinatal relates to the period surrounding the birth event. Rates and ratios are based on events reported in a calendar year. *Perinatal mortality rate* is the sum of late fetal deaths plus infant deaths within 7 days of birth divided by the sum

of live births plus late fetal deaths, stated per 1,000 live births plus late fetal deaths. *Perinatal mortality ratio* is the sum of late fetal deaths plus infant deaths within 7 days of birth divided by the number of live births, stated per 1,000 live births.

Feto-infant mortality rate is the sum of late fetal deaths plus all infant deaths divided by the sum of live births plus late fetal deaths, stated per 1,000 live births plus late fetal deaths. See related *Fetal death; Gestation; Infant death; Live birth.*

Maternal death is one for which the certifying physician has designated a maternal condition as the underlying cause of death. Maternal conditions are those assigned to Complications of pregnancy, childbirth, and the puerperium, ICD–9 codes 630–676. (See related table V.) *Maternal mortality rate* is defined as the number of maternal deaths per 100,000 live births. The maternal mortality rate is a measure of the likelihood that a pregnant woman will die from maternal causes. The number of live births used in the denominator is a proxy for the population of pregnant women who are at risk of a maternal death.

Region—See *Geographic region and division.*

Registered hospitals—See *Hospital.*

Registered nursing education—Registered nursing data are shown by level of educational preparation. Baccalaureate education requires at least 4 years of college or university; associate degree programs are based in community colleges and are usually 2 years in length; and diploma programs are based in hospitals and are usually 3 years in length.

Registration area—The United States has separate registration areas for birth, death, marriage, and divorce statistics. In general, registration areas correspond to States and include two separate registration areas for the District of Columbia and New York City. All States have adopted laws that require the registration of births and deaths and the reporting of fetal deaths. It is believed that more than 99 percent of the births and deaths occurring in this country are registered.

The *death registration area* was established in 1900 with 10 States and the District of Columbia, and the *birth registration area* was established in 1915, also with 10 States and the District of Columbia. Both areas have covered the entire United States since 1933. Currently, Puerto Rico, U.S. Virgin Islands, and Guam comprise separate registration areas, although their data are not included in statistical tabulations of U.S. resident data. See related *Reporting area.*

Relative survival rate—The relative survival rate is the ratio of the observed survival rate for the patient group to the expected survival rate for persons in the general population similar to the patient group with respect to age, sex, race, and calendar year of observation. The 5-year relative survival rate is used to estimate the proportion of cancer patients potentially curable. Because over one-half of all cancers occur in persons 65 years of age and over, many of these individuals die of other causes with no evidence of recurrence of their cancer. Thus, because it is obtained by adjusting observed survival for the normal life expectancy of the general population of the same age, the relative survival rate is an estimate of the chance of surviving the effects of cancer.

Reporting area—In the National Vital Statistics System, the reporting area for such basic items on the birth and death certificates as age, race, and sex, is based on data from residents of all 50 States in the United States and the District of Columbia. The reporting area for selected items such as Hispanic origin, educational attainment, and marital status, is based on data from those States that require the item to be reported, whose data meet a minimum level of completeness (such as, 80 or 90 percent), and are considered to be sufficiently comparable to be used for analysis. In 1993–96 the reporting area for Hispanic origin of decedent on the death certificate included 49 States and the District of Columbia. See related

Registration area; National Vital Statistics System in Appendix I.

Resident—In the Online Certification and Reporting database, all residents in certified facilities are counted on the day of certification inspection. In the National Nursing Home Survey, a resident is a person on the roster of the nursing home as of the night before the survey. Included are all residents for whom beds are maintained even though they may be on overnight leave or in a hospital. See related *Nursing home.*

Resident population—See *Population.*

Residential treatment care—See *Mental health service type.*

Residential treatment centers for emotionally disturbed children—See *Mental health organization.*

Self-assessment of health—See *Health status, respondent-assessed.*

Short-stay hospitals—See *Hospital.*

Skilled nursing facilities—See *Nursing home.*

Smoker—See *Current smoker.*

Specialty hospitals—See *Hospital.*

State health agency—The agency or department within State government headed by the State or territorial health official. Generally, the State health agency is responsible for setting statewide public health priorities, carrying out national and State mandates, responding to public health hazards, and assuring access to health care for underserved State residents.

Substance abuse treatment clients—In the Substance Abuse and Mental Health Services Administration's Uniform Facilities Data Set substance abuse treatment clients have been admitted to treatment and have been seen on a scheduled appointment basis at least once in the month before the survey reference date or were inpatients on the survey reference date. Types of treatment include 24-hour detoxification, 24-hour rehabilitation or residential care, and outpatient care.

Surgical operations—See *Procedure.*

Surgical specialties—See *Physician specialty.*

Uninsured—See *Health insurance coverage.*

Urbanization—In this report death rates are presented according to level of urbanization of the decedent's county of residence. Metropolitan and nonmetropolitan counties are categorized into urbanization levels based on an NCHS-modification of the 1993 rural-urban continuum codes. The 1993 rural-urban continuum codes were developed by the Economic Research Service, U.S. Department of Agriculture using the 1993 U.S. Office of Management and Budget definition of metropolitan statistical areas (MSA's). The codes classify metropolitan counties by population size and level of urbanization and nonmetropolitan counties by level of urbanization and proximity to metropolitan areas. NCHS modified the 1993 rural-urban continuum codes to make the definition of core and fringe metropolitan counties comparable to the definitions used for the 1983 codes. For this report, the 10 categories of counties have been collapsed into 5 categories (a) core metropolitan counties contain the primary central city of an MSA with a 1990 population of 1 million or more; (b) fringe metropolitan counties are the noncore counties of an MSA with 1990 population of 1 million or more; (c) medium or small metropolitan counties are in MSA's with 1990 population under 1 million; (d) urban nonmetropolitan counties are not in MSA's and have 2,500 or more urban residents in 1990; and (e) rural counties are not in MSA's and have fewer than 2,500 urban residents in 1990. See related *Metropolitan statistical area (MSA).*

Usual source of care—Usual source of care was measured in the National Health Interview Survey (NHIS) in 1991 by asking the respondent, "Is there a particular clinic, health center, doctor's office, or other place that you usually go to if you are sick or need advice about your health?" In 1993 and 1994 the respondent was asked, "Is there a particular person or place that __ usually goes to when ___ is sick or needs advice about __ health?" In the 1995 and 1996 NHIS, the respondent was asked "Is there one doctor, person, or place that __ usually goes to when __ is sick or needs advice about ___ health?" Persons who reported multiple sources of care are defined as having a usual source of care. Additionally, persons who reported the emergency room as their usual source of care are defined as having no usual source of care for the purposes of this report.

Wages and salaries—See *Employer costs for employee compensation.*

Years of potential life lost—Years of potential life lost (YPLL) is a measure of premature mortality. Starting with *Health, United States, 1996–97*, YPLL is presented for persons under 75 years of age because the average life expectancy in the United States is over 75 years. YPLL-75 is calculated using the following eight age groups: under 1 year, 1–14 years, 15–24 years, 25–34 years, 35–44 years, 45–54 years, 55–64 years, 65–74 years. The number of deaths for each age group is multiplied by the years of life lost, calculated as the difference between age 75 years and the midpoint of the age group. For the eight age groups the midpoints are 0.5, 7.5, 19.5, 29.5, 39.5, 49.5, 59.5, and 69.5. For example, the death of a person 15–24 years of age counts as 55.5 years of life lost. Years of potential life lost is derived by summing years of life lost over all age groups. In *Health, United States, 1995* and earlier editions, YPLL was presented for persons under 65 years of age. For more information, see Centers for Disease Control. *MMWR*. Vol 35 no 25S, suppl. 1986.

Detailed Tables With Additional Years of Data Available in Electronic Spreadsheet Files

Many of the detailed tables in this report present data for extended time periods. Because of space limitations on the printed page, only selected years of data are shown to highlight major trends. For the tables listed below, additional years of data are available in electronic spreadsheet files that may be accessed through the internet and on CD-ROM.

To access the files on the internet, go to the FTP server on the NCHS homepage at www.cdc.gov/nchswww and select "Data Warehouse" and *Health, United States*.

Spreadsheet files are also available on a CD-ROM entitled "Publications from the National Center for Health Statistics," featuring *Health, United States, 1999*, vol 1 no 5, 1999. The CD-ROM may be purchased from the Government Printing Office or the National Technical Information Service.

Table number	Table topic	Additional data years available
1	Resident population	1981–89, 1991–95
2	Poverty	1986–89
3	Fertility rates and birth rates	1981–84, 1986–89
5	Live births	1971–74, 1976–79, 1981–84, 1986–89, 1991–93
6	Prenatal care	1981–84, 1986–89
7	Teenage childbearing	1981–84, 1986–89
8	Nonmarital childbearing	1981–84, 1986–89
9	Maternal education	1981–84, 1986–89
11	Low birthweight	1981–84, 1986–89
15	Abortions	1981–84, 1986–88
16	Abortions	1981–84, 1986–88
17	Contraception	1990
19	Infant mortality rates	1984, 1985–86, 1988–89
20	Infant mortality rates	1984, 1985–86, 1988–89
21	Infant mortality rates	1984
22	Infant mortality rates	1981–84, 1986–88
28	Life expectancy	1975, 1981–84
29	Age-adjusted death rates by State	1992–94, 1993–95, 1994–96
30	Age-adjusted death rates for selected causes	1991–93
31	Years of potential life lost	1985, 1991–96
36	Death rates for all causes	1981–84, 1986–89, 1991–94
37	Diseases of heart	1981–84, 1986–89, 1991–93
38	Cerebrovascular diseases	1981–84, 1986–89, 1991–93
39	Malignant neoplasms	1981–84, 1986–89, 1991–93
40	Malignant neoplasms of respiratory system	1981–84, 1986–89, 1991–93
41	Malignant neoplasm of breast	1981–84, 1986–89, 1991–93
42	Chronic obstructive pulmonary diseases	1981–84, 1986–89
43	Human immunodeficiency virus (HIV) infection	1988
44	Maternal mortality	1981–84, 1986–89, 1991–93
45	Motor vehicle-related injuries	1981–84, 1986–89, 1991–93
46	Homicide	1981–84, 1986–89, 1991–93
47	Suicide	1981–84, 1986–89, 1991–93
48	Firearm-related injuries	1981–84, 1986–87 1989, 1991–92
49	Occupational diseases	1979, 1981–84, 1986–88
50	Occupational injury deaths	1981–84, 1986–88
53	Notifiable diseases	1985, 1988–89, 1991–93
61	Cigarette smoking	1987–88

Table number	Table topic	Additional data years available
62	Cigarette smoking	1987–88
64	Use of selected substances	1982, 1988
65	Use of selected substances	1981–84, 1986, 1987–88
66	Cocaine-related emergency room episodes	1986–89
74	Occupational injuries	1931–84, 1986–88
75	Physician contacts	1985–86
77	Physician contacts	1990–92, 1993–95
83	Ambulatory care visits	1993–94
87	Additions to mental health organizations	1986, 1988
90	Discharges	1988–89
91	Discharges	1989, 1994
96	Hospital admissions	1991–93
101	Persons employed	1983–84, 1986–89, 1991
103	Physicians	1970, 1987, 1989, 1992–94
106	Staff in mental health organizations	1986, 1988
110	Hospitals	1991–93
112	Community hospital beds	1985, 1988–89, 1995–96
113	Occupancy rates	1985, 1988–89, 1995–96
117	Consumer Price Index	1965, 1975
122	Employers' costs and health insurance	1992–93, 1995–96
123	Hospital expenses	1991–92, 1994
127	Funding for health research	1984, 1986–89, 1991–92
132	Health maintenance organizations	1984, 1986–87, 1989, 1991
134	Medicare	1988–89, 1991–94
135	Medicare	1967, 1991–94
136	Medicaid	1986–89, 1991–93
137	Medicaid	1986–89, 1991–93
138	Department of Veterans Affairs	1985, 1988–89, 1991
143	Medicare	1994–95

(Numbers refer to table numbers)

Index to Detailed Tables ....

Index to Detailed Tables ....

Index to Detailed Tables ....

Index to Detailed Tables ....

Index to Detailed Tables ....